MEDIEVAL MEDICINE

READINGS IN MEDIEVAL CIVILIZATIONS AND CULTURES: XV

series editor: Paul Edward Dutton

MEDIEVAL MEDICINE

A READER

edited by

FAITH WALLIS

University of Toronto Press

LIBRARY AND ARCHIVES CANADA CATALOGUING IN PUBLICATION

Medieval medicine : a reader / edited by Faith Wallis.

Includes bibliographical references and index.
ISBN 978-1-4426-0169-7 (bound). – ISBN 978-1-4426-0103-1 (pbk.)

1. Medicine, Medieval.   2. Medicine, Medieval – Sources.   I. Wallis, Faith

R141.M43 2010   610.902   C2010-900973-8

We welcome comments and suggestions regarding any aspect of our publications – please feel free to contact us at news@utphighereducation.com or visit our internet site at www.utphighereducation.com.

North America
5201 Dufferin Street
Toronto, Ontario, Canada, M3H 5T8

2250 Military Road
Tonawanda, New York, USA, 14150

UK, Ireland, and continental Europe
NBN International
Estover Road, Plymouth, PL6 7PY, UK

TEL: 44 (0) 1752 202301
FAX ORDER LINE: 44 (0) 1752 202333
enquiries@nbninternational.com

ORDERS PHONE: 1-800-565-9523
ORDERS FAX: 1-800-221-9985
ORDERS EMAIL: utpbooks@utpress.utoronto.ca

The University of Toronto Press acknowledges the financial support for its publishing activities of the Government of Canada through the Book Publishing Industry Development Program (BPIDP).

Book design and composition by George Kirkpatrick.

For my aunt, Faith Townesend

Revelation 22:1–2

CONTENTS

ACKNOWLEDGMENTS

This book was beta-tested by my students at McGill University, especially those in HIST 356 "Medicine in the Medieval West," who responded with great forbearance, intelligence, and good humor. Comments, communications, and corrections were generously provided by Klaus-Dietrich Fischer, Michael R. McVaugh, Luke Demaitre, Geneviève Dumas, Dorothy Bray, and Eliza Glaze. I owe a special debt of gratitude to the series editor, Paul Edward Dutton, for his meticulous reading of the manuscript and his warm encouragement, and to Martin Boyne for his painstaking and thoughtful copy-editing. My dear husband Kendall, a brilliant reference librarian, solved innumerable problems (bibliographic and otherwise) and gallantly proofread the whole text. He has also signed on for a fifth decade of sharing bed and board with me; a girl can't get much luckier than that. This book is dedicated to my aunt and namesake Faith Townesend, through whom I first glimpsed the world of medicine.

INTRODUCTION

Healing, both as a constellation of ideas and as a repertory of practices, is surely one of the most ancient and persistent elements of human culture. Material remains from prehistoric sites are eloquent: our distant ancestors thought that disease had a cause and that someone could use that knowledge to help the sick person. Human remains indicate that these people could repair broken bones and even drill a hole into the skull of a living person. The "Ice Man" who perished on the high alpine pass of the Tisenjoch between Italy and Austria around 2700 BCE had already recovered from several broken ribs long before he set out on his last and fateful journey; he also carried in his travel gear dried birch fungus to treat diseases and wounds. Medicine, if not as old as the hills, is at least as old as the human ambition to climb over hills.

Until fairly recently, medical historians have seen their role as that of archaeologists, excavating the origins of modern medicine. The first to specialize in this field in the nineteenth and early twentieth centuries were doctors themselves, and they read the story of medicine as a continuous epic of progress. In the English-speaking world, the best-known spokesman for this model was the Canadian physician and educator Sir William Osler (1849–1919). During Osler's lifetime, medicine was shedding its past as a gentlemanly learned profession in favor of a new identity grounded in experimental methods and laboratory science. Osler's textbook *The Principles and Practice of Medicine*, published in 1892, was a spectacular best-seller precisely because it captured this emerging scientific identity. But Osler also enjoyed buying and reading rare and historic books on medicine; his collection is now the core of the Osler Library of the History of Medicine at McGill University. He wrote essays on historical figures and events and promoted the cult of great doctors of the past by sponsoring monuments and societies in their honor. The message that this charismatic physician relayed to his colleagues and to the public was that the new scientific medicine was the latest chapter in a chronicle that went back to Hippocrates, and even beyond. The hero of the story was medicine itself, and the narrative was Darwinian. Osler's overview of medical history is tellingly entitled *The Evolution of Modern Medicine*. Modern scientific medicine is the product of an impersonal historic process that is inevitable and progressive. As in natural selection, the critical event is the random variation that proves to be adaptive. In epic medical history, this is the "breakthrough" – the exceptional concept, discovery or innovation that is "ahead of its time." Its scientific truth guarantees that it will survive to reproduce itself in the modern paradigm. False ideas and useless practices are bred out.

In *The Evolution of Modern Medicine*, Osler opens his chapter on medieval medicine as follows:

> There are waste places of the earth which fill one with terror − not simply because they are waste; one has not such feelings in the desert nor in the vast solitude of the ocean. Very different is it where the desolation has overtaken a brilliant and flourishing product of man's head and hand. To know that
>
>> ... the Lion and the Lizard keep
>> the Courts where Jamshyd gloried and drank deep
>
> sends a chill to the heart, and one trembles with a sense of human instability. With this feeling we enter the Middle Ages.[1]

He closes the chapter in this vein: "[I]n medicine the Middle Ages represent a restatement from century to century of the facts and theories of the Greeks modified here and there by Arabian practice. There was, in Francis Bacon's phrase, much iteration, small addition. The schools bowed in humble, slavish submission to Galen and Hippocrates, taking everything from them but their spirit...."[2] Even today, Osler's negative caricature of medieval medicine persists not only in popular culture, but even in textbooks destined for university classrooms. Alongside laments over intellectual stagnation, these accounts display sensational images of appalling hygienic conditions: the Middle Ages were a thousand years without a bath. If there is anything interesting about medieval medicine, it is its helplessness in the face of leprosy and plague. Even though the first disease has a history stretching back millennia before the medieval period, and the second was far more prevalent in the Renaissance and early modern periods, leprosy and plague have become "medieval" diseases. Medieval society, if it did not actually invent these ailments, at least encouraged them, and probably deserved them, by being so stupid and dirty.

Since World War II, another style of medical history has grown up alongside the evolutionary model. Though it incorporates a variety of theoretical approaches, it is broadly referred to as the social history of medicine. For the most part, it is practiced by professional historians who are not physicians, and is taught in history departments rather than medical faculties, though

---

1 William Osler, *The Evolution of Modern Medicine: A Series of Lectures Delivered at Yale University on the Silliman Foundation in April, 1913* (New Haven: Yale University Press, 1921), p. 84. The embedded quotation is from Edward Fitzgerald, *The Rubaiyat of Omar Khayyam*, quatrain 18.

2 Osler, p. 125.

Europe was, as everyone knows, permeated by Christianity: its religious world-view and system of values, its theology, its worship, its piety, and of course its institutions. The "evolution" narrative of medical history, emerging in the midst of the nineteenth-century struggle between religion and science for cultural authority in the West, assumed that the religious dimension of medieval civilization was inherently hostile to medicine, or at least to secular medical learning and practice. The medieval hospital was a problem, because it seemed to have no doctors. Was it, then, really a hospital? No solution seemed possible until medical historians started to be recruited from the ranks of people whose initial training lay in medieval church history or the history of medieval spirituality. They merged with another stream of historians of social and political institutions and together began rewriting the history of the medieval hospital. What is especially refreshing about this new hospital history is that it sets aside the sterile debate over whether medieval hospitals were "real" hospitals that provided "real" medical care. In the older paradigm, medical care was distinguished from the provision of shelter and nursing; a "real" hospital would prominently, and preferably exclusively, provide something beyond mere care. What the new hospital history brings to the debate is an understanding that whether a doctor was present or not, and however they framed their mandate, medieval hospital staff cared for sick people in accordance with mainstream learned traditions of medicine. They embedded this care, however, in a comprehensive religious context. This had two aspects. First, tending to the needs of the sick was one of an array of works of charity offered to the poor. Charity was the vocation of the hospital, and medicine was not separated from clothing the naked, feeding the hungry, or burying the dead. Second, the hospital was a religious community dedicated to the worship of God. This worship, centered on the sacraments, the singing of the office, and the reading of Scripture, was inseparable from charity, including medical care. Beds were arranged so that the sick could see the altar where the mass was celebrated, the consecrated host was carried around the wards in procession, painted altarpieces depicted themes of redemptive suffering, and all these were held to exert healing power in the fullest and most concrete sense. This spiritual therapeutics was not distinct from, let alone opposed to, the healing power of herbs, plasters, or bloodletting. In the Bible, Jesus Christ healed the sick by making ointments as well as by exorcism; Christ the heavenly Physician was also eclectic in his methods.

This volume aims to tell the story of medieval medicine through textual records that trace historical change over time and reveal a distinctively medieval social and cultural context. It is divided into three parts. The first two parts are narrative in their focus, because, to put it bluntly, Osler was wrong. Medicine did not stand still but was transformed significantly over the medieval centuries, the major watershed being the two centuries from 1050 to 1250. This watershed divides the history of medieval medicine into two periods, which I call the "age of *medicina*" and the "age of *physica*." *Medicina* and *physica* lend their names to the first two sections of this book: "*Medicina*: Healers and Healing in Early Medieval Europe (500–1100)," and "*Physica*: The Advent and Impact of Academic Medicine (1100–1500)."

It will come as no surprise that the Latin word *medicina* means "medicine"; it is perhaps less obvious that the Latinized Greek word *physica* (literally "natural philosophy") can also mean "medicine," or rather, it came to mean medicine in the watershed centuries. That it did so is one of the major reasons why this watershed is such a significant one. *Medicina* in the pre-watershed age, from late antiquity to the threshold of the twelfth century, connoted several things, similar to the many meanings of "medicine" in Modern English: a body of knowledge (as in "my sister is studying medicine"), a practice or art carried out by more or less recognized specialists ("he is practicing medicine in Toronto"), or a synonym for medication ("are you taking medicine for that cold?"). These multiple and ambiguous meanings are typical of early medieval experience. Hagiographers or theologians could condemn the implicit rationalism of *medicina* as a branch of secular learning (knowledge), or make invidious comparisons between the *medicina* of doctors and the healing power of saints (practice), and then in a perfectly matter-of-fact way send *medicina* (medication) to their clerical and monastic colleagues, complete with a recipe and advice on dosage. For the most part, *medicina* in the Early Middle Ages connoted something concrete and practical; this facilitated dialogue between Greco-Roman practical medicine on the one hand and the Christian commitment to charitable care of the sick on the other. The Church Fathers authorized a fairly generous and inclusive attitude to ancient secular learning, and so some medical "theory" (anatomy, physiology, pathology, etc.) could be admitted to encyclopedias such as the *Etymologies* of Isidore of Seville. What was missing in the West in the early medieval centuries was a visible and articulate class of students and professional practitioners of medicine. Institutional support for teaching and regulating medicine had never been very strong in the Roman Empire, and with the devolution of the western empire into the new sub-Roman "barbarian" kingdoms, secular medicine became to an even greater extent an informally transmitted art. In consequence, it was an art that could be practiced by people without professional aspirations, such as clergy or monks. In the case of Anglo-Saxon England, for example, we have no clear idea whether Bald, who commissioned *Bald's Leechbook*, was a lay practitioner, a cleric, or simply an interested amateur. This rich but unconsolidated medical scene of the "age of *medicina*" is reflected in the texts on medical learning and practice that have come down to us.

The story of medieval medicine took a decisive turn in the eleventh century, when *medicina* acquired a new synonym: *physica*. Ushering in these changes – but also, of course, driven by them – was an influx of new medical information in textual form. Much of this was, indeed, old medical information: ancient medical treatises now made available in Latin through translations from Greek and Arabic. In a twelfth-century biography of one translator, Constantine the African, we see the emerging distinction between *medicina* and *physica*. In Rome, the merchant Constantine meets a famous *medicus* and through him learns to diagnose diseases from urine. Constantine then asks the *medicus* whether there are many books in Latin about *physica*.

[The *medicus*] answered that he had none, but that he had learned through much diligence and drill. So Constantine, returning to Africa, devoted himself to the study of *physica* for three continuous years; then came back, bringing with him many books. (doc. 32)

The distinction is implicit, but clear. *Medicina* is a practical art acquired through craft training and experience. *Physica* resides in books – but not in the kind of books available to early medieval western readers. *Physica* was a type of book-learning about medicine that was imported from the Arab world, though its roots were in ancient Greece.

The term *physica* denotes the branch of philosophy concerned with the natural world. Until the age of the Enlightenment, *physica* or "natural philosophy" encompassed all reflection on the qualities and operations of the material universe; it was only in the nineteenth century that the term was supplanted by "science." To call medicine *physica* was to make certain claims about the character of medical knowledge. It was knowledge about the essential nature of things, the materials they are made of, and their inherent qualities. Medicine was also about physical processes such as growth, decay, and change; it was interested in fundamental questions about what causes things to be as they are and to become other than what they are. Medicine was philosophy, then, not just because it was encyclopedic in scope, but because its basic concepts and intellectual methods were those of natural philosophy.

The translation movement coincided with a new approach to studying medicine through the formal, systematic reading and analysis of texts, including analysis of their problematic and dubious points. This kind of study was not carried out in solitude or through a sort of apprenticeship, whether in a secular milieu or in a monastery. Instead, it took place in a group – a *schola* or "school" – under the leadership of a teacher, a *magister* or *doctor*. In the rapidly changing intellectual world of the twelfth century, schools of this new type were emerging all over western Europe, teaching old subjects such as grammar, logic, and law, and new ones, notably theology. Perhaps the most important contribution of the Middle Ages to the overall historical development of medicine in the western world was the fact that medicine participated in this academic turn. Eventually medicine was established as a discipline within the nascent university, and it continues to be taught there today. It was not, however, inevitable that medicine would become a school subject. Medicine could be based on book learning, but it was also an art or practice. Many other kinds of art had an ancient textual heritage but did not qualify for the schools (one thinks, for example, of architecture). Medicine succeeded in establishing itself in the schools because it successfully argued that it was a branch of philosophy; philosophy was the goal of the study of the liberal arts, and the arts were legitimate subjects for the schools. But how could medicine argue that it was actually philosophy? Here is where the word *physica* came to the rescue.

Natural philosophy or *physica* examines the natural world and its processes. The human body was understood to be part of this natural world, and its changes from health to sickness and back to health were subject to the laws of nature; indeed, the birth of Greek *physica* with the pre-Socratic philosophers is closely linked to the emergence of a reflective type of medical discourse associated with the name of Hippocrates. Centuries before the emergence of the new schools of the twelfth century, Carolingian thinkers speculated on the divisions of philosophy that they found in manuals like Isidore of Seville's *Etymologies*, and classified medicine under *physica*. Twelfth-century teachers of medicine traded on that connection to introduce their subject into the schools. As *physica*, medical knowledge was unambiguously *scientia*, that is, organized knowledge based on first principles. As such, it could be conveyed through rationalized instruction – what medieval people called *doctrina*. The academic turn of the twelfth century is the reason English speakers today call medical practitioners "physicians," and why physicians are addressed with the title "doctor" – that is, "teacher." Needless to say, the textual record of medical knowledge in the "age of *physica*" looks very different from that in the "age of *medicina*."

Medicine's academic turn coincided with both the emergence of a secularized profession within a more urban and commercial economy, and an expanding court society. It also erected a boundary between licit and illicit medicine, and it appealed to rulers to police that boundary. On the one side stood a kind of medicine defined by a distinctive cognitive style – rationalized, literate, theoretically informed – and exercised by men who could claim academic credentials. On the other stood those who did not possess these credentials, but who not infrequently absorbed and imitated the academic approach. Concurrently, the Church's ongoing processes of reform in theology and pastoral care stimulated new approaches to the relationship of religion and healing. Part III of this book, "Medicine and Society, 1100–1500," draws on a rich lode of documentation that gives us a detailed and multidimensional picture of medicine in action. This action was, of course, largely a matter of interaction: the encounters of doctors with patients, of learned masters with informally trained empirics, of professionals with the state. Threading through these encounters are shared representations of disease causation and expectations about responsible behavior (on the part of both healer and patient). There was, in short, a coherent culture of health and healing in late medieval Europe. One index of this coherence is the fact that medicine was satirized and criticized in the popular arena.

So abundant is the information about health and healers in the later medieval period that this entire anthology might have been devoted to that theme. I have therefore been obliged, with a somewhat heavy heart, to set certain topics aside completely, rather than attempt to include a token document on everything. With a few exceptions, I have omitted the rich legal literature on doctors and their practices as well as records of medieval medical guilds. The expanding realm of public health is another topic that I have, with great regret, passed over. In order to tie Part III to the narrative story of medical knowledge and learning laid out in Parts I and II, I have emphasized the social role of practices and practitioners that medieval records call "medical"; documents about informal healers, midwives, barbers, and apothecaries will have to wait for another book. Many anthologies of translated primary sources about the Black Death are readily available, and so the role of the plague in this volume is confined to illustrating some aspects of medieval ideas about medical intervention. I have also concentrated exclusively on western Europe, and have only dealt with such Byzantine and Arabic sources as were available to western readers.

To compensate in some measure for these limitations and omissions, I have striven to make available texts that convey something of the beauty, coherence, and intricacy of the medieval picture of the human body – a picture composed of homey analogies like cooking, and elusive forces like spirits and faculties. I have also sought out texts that convey the distinctive contours of the medieval conception of disease and that give voice to medical teachers, students, doctors, patients, and by-standers. These people were persuaded that knowledge of disease was, at the very least, possible, and that action grounded in knowledge might make a difference; their hopes and struggles deserve our sympathy and respectful attention. Finally, I have thought it important to include texts that speak to the bonds, at once intimate and tense, that united medicine and religion throughout the medieval millennium.

old-fashioned medical English, "consumption." Many medieval descriptions of "consumption" strongly suggest that the condition in question is pulmonary tuberculosis. It would, however, be a mistake to translate *phthisis* as "pulmonary tuberculosis." Not only can one waste away from diseases other than tuberculosis, but the term "pulmonary tuberculosis," coined by early nineteenth-century pathological anatomy, frames the disease as a particular diagnostic lesion (the tubercule) sited on a specific organ (the lung). The lesion is visible only on post-mortem examination and is produced by the action of an invading microorganism that can be identified only under a microscope. "Tuberculosis" is, therefore, something only the doctor sees, and he sees it only apart from the living patient. It does not represent what the patient experiences – or the doctor either, while the patient is alive – namely, the patient's severe emaciation, his "consumption." In modern medicine, consumption is only a symptom, the by-product of the pathological changes wrought by the bacillus, but in pre-modern medicine the symptom *was* the disease. For this reason, I have always translated *phthisis* as "consumption."

Even when it comes to relatively familiar terms, crucial distinctions are needed. "Fever" in the Middle Ages is "the same thing" as it is today, namely an elevated body temperature, but it did not *mean* the same thing, because we regard fever as a symptom, while pre-modern physicians saw it as a disease in its own right. The clinical picture of epilepsy was well established in antiquity and the Middle Ages and, while our ancestors ascribed a different cause to this condition, there is little doubt that medieval *epilepsia* and modern epilepsy are "the same thing." But with conditions such as "leprosy," "cancer," and "plague," equivalences are less secure. Modern scholars agree that by the Central Middle Ages at least, texts both medical and non-medical were painting a clinical picture of leprosy that matches what we now call Hansen's disease (see doc. 69). But this does not mean that everyone designated in a medieval text as a leper had Hansen's disease, or vice versa, nor would such an equation do justice to the cultural difference between medieval leprosy and modern Hansen's disease. Descriptions of the symptoms and course of the Black Death of 1347–50 are often precise and consistent, but this has by no means settled the question of whether the pestilence was bubonic plague as presently defined, namely the disease caused by *Yersinia pestis*. Even in modern usage "cancer" is a catch-all term; it was in the Middle Ages as well, but what the term caught then was both more and less than what it catches today. Medieval medical texts describe cancers that can be detected on the surface of the body; brain tumors, cancers of the internal organs, and leukemia lay outside their ken. On the other hand, medieval "cancer" also included an array of swellings, indurations, and skin conditions, which may or may not align with any modern species of cancer. The texts defined cancer both etiologically and clinically with considerable precision (see docs. 70–71), but it is important for us to exercise our imagination in order to see the disease with medieval eyes.

It can sometimes be useful for the purposes of historical analysis to try to determine what modern disease category might match a medieval description; indeed, it can actually enhance our understanding of what the medieval writer is attempting to convey. But, if not handled sensitively, retrospective diagnosis can become an unedifying guessing game that relegates the medieval medical world-view to the margins. So retrospective diagnosis must be undertaken with caution; what human beings – medieval or modern – see in the human body, or in the patterns of disease, is shaped not only by the possibilities and limitations of their experience, but by the structures and meanings that their culture bestows on this experience.

In rendering the names of medieval persons, I have adopted a policy of consistent inconsistency. The names of persons living before roughly 1200 are those commonly used in textbooks and reference works in English. In most cases, these are anglicized versions of Latin names: Isidore of Seville, Gregory of Tours, Constantine the African, and so forth. This is also the case for later medieval individuals whose names have well-established English forms, such as Petrarch and John of Burgundy. Other figures are identified by their name in the vernacular of their home country, followed by their distinguishing place of origin in English, e.g., Arnau of Vilanova, Henri of Mondeville, Aldobrandino of Siena, John of Gaddesden. Family names, however, are retained in the original vernacular, e.g., Mondino de'Liuzzi. Arabic writers are normally identified by their medieval Latin names, e.g., Avicenna. Titles of ancient and medieval works have been turned into English, save for texts that are always identified in the scholarly literature by their original title (e.g., *Isagoge, Colliget, Circa Instans*).

Finally, two brief remarks about the presentation of the texts. First, square brackets enclosing text in Roman type signal material supplied by the translator or by myself as editor in order to complete the meaning of a sentence: for example, "*Oxea* is [the name applied to] an acute disease ..." (doc. 1). Square brackets enclosing text in Italic type indicate material added by myself as editor to identify or clarify what is in the text: for example, "It is called the comitial disease because if, among the pagans, this seized anyone on a meeting day set for the Comitia [*the Roman political assembly*], this assembly was dismissed" (doc. 1). Second, in transcribing texts from previously published translations, I have modified punctuation and standardized orthography where necessary.

PART I.

MEDICINA: HEALERS AND HEALING IN EARLY MEDIEVAL EUROPE (500–1100)

Early medieval medicine in western Europe has been closely studied for a long time, yet its distinctive features are still not in sharp focus. For the pioneering medical historians of the nineteenth and early twentieth centuries, the age of medicina was all about the survival of a rather attenuated legacy of classical medical learning. As they sifted through these texts, however, they slowly came to appreciate the energy and creativity with which late antiquity and the early medieval period handled this medical inheritance. At a time when learning and literature were fading in the West, medical writing was, comparatively speaking, in a flourishing state. Much of it, to be sure, consisted of translated and repackaged Hippocratic, Galenic, and Methodist materials, but appropriation of this kind is evidence of the vitality of medicine. Chapter 1 presents texts that illustrate the essentially practical orientation of this enterprise of adaptation. Medical scientific theory was repackaged as well, though in more conventional formats.

Medicine was also digested into the new religious world-view of Christianity; indeed, the new religion's commitment to care of the sick as an ethical obligation contributed to the lively interest in practical medicine. Nonetheless, the Christian Gospel proclaims its own ideology of healing, as well as a special understanding of the spiritual meaning and destiny of the body. The saints, alive or dead, were also channels of God's therapy for medieval believers. In chapter 2, we will examine how early medieval people brought secular medicine into the embrace of religious healing. The process was not always conscious or willing, nor was the influence only in one direction.

It can be argued that the West crossed the threshold from antiquity to the medieval world around 600. By that time, all credible attempts to reunite the western provinces to the Roman Empire, now centered on the new capital of Constantinople, were at an end. The western provinces became independent kingdoms. Their rulers were "barbarians," but the Ostrogoths in sixth-century Italy, the Visigoths in Spain, and the Franks in what is now France, the Low Countries, and western Germany all imagined that they were continuing and even surpassing the Roman achievement. The threshold was also marked by economic decline, dwindling urban life, and the profound re-organization of the countryside. Though rarely mentioned in medical texts, plague was also a fact of life: the "Justinianic pandemic" that first appeared in 541 recurred at intervals until at least 750.

The new Europe of the sub-Roman and, later, the Carolingian age was also in the hands of a new elite: kings, their aristocratic followers, and men of the Church – priests, bishops, missionaries, and monks. Chapter 3 looks for traces of medical learning and medical activity in this shifting social landscape. The secular medical professional is not easy to spot, but we can catch a glimpse of him at royal courts. On the other hand, a distinctive style of clerical medicine was taking shape in the cloisters of monasteries and in the network of contacts maintained by bishops and missionaries. Finally, the rich vernacular literature of Anglo-Saxon England (chapter 4) furnishes a vivid demonstration of the inventive ways in which a particular early medieval culture adopted and adapted the medical heritage of antiquity.

CHAPTER ONE

THE FRAGMENTED HERITAGE OF ANCIENT MEDICINE

The transmission of the rich heritage of ancient medicine to the medieval world was fragmented in more ways than one. First, the ancient scientific theories of medicine, and the accumulated experience of medical practice, flowed through different channels – theory through the efforts made in the sixth century to translate some of the texts used in the medical school of Alexandria into Latin, and practice through a more diffuse process of repackaging information from the various therapeutic traditions. Second, the medical theory available in Latin was only the torso of an enormous body of Greek medical thought; practical medical literature in Latin, by contrast, was expanding and diversifying into fresh, often informal genres. The documents presented in this chapter illustrate these divergent fortunes.

In the medical school of Alexandria in late antiquity, students studied medicine as they would have studied philosophy. They read a canon of texts by Hippocrates and Galen, arranged in topical order, and each course took two or three years. Through later Arabic sources, we know about the Galenic course in some detail. It comprised works of an introductory character, followed by texts on anatomy, physiology, diseases and their causes, diagnosis, fevers, preventive medicine, and therapeutics. The surviving commentaries on these texts are a professor's or student's notes from one of these courses.

All teaching in Alexandria was conducted in Greek, but in sixth- and seventh-century Ravenna – the administrative capital of Late Roman, Ostrogothic, and Byzantine Italy – teachers tried to re-create the Alexandrian curriculum for a Latin-speaking audience. They translated the basic texts and (in some cases) composed commentaries in the Alexandrian style. Three texts illustrate the process by which this curriculum was, at least in part, transplanted to the milieu of post-Roman Europe. Isidore of Seville's Etymologies *(doc. 1), a vast storehouse of ancient erudition, presents an overview of medicine derived from introductory lectures at Alexandria. The foundational text of the Hippocratic canon, the* Aphorisms, *was translated and furnished with a full commentary (doc. 2), as was the first text in the Galen canon,* On Sects for Beginners *(doc. 3). The stream of ancient school medicine that trickled into the early medieval West was rather meager, but it conveyed some important ideas about the intellectual scope and cultural dignity of the subject.*

The literature of medical practice is more difficult to characterize, because it is both extensive and eclectic. It includes large-scale encyclopedic manuals such as the Therapeutics *of Alexander of Tralles (doc. 5), as well as more modest summaries of Galenic and Methodist medical practice (docs. 6–7, 10). On the other hand, medical writing* modeled on traditional Latin works designed for gentlemen and estate-holders (docs. 8–9) proliferated exuberantly. Both veins of medical writing reveal a society concerned to preserve what it could, and amass what it needed, in order to meet its medical needs.

I. THE ALEXANDRIAN CURRICULUM IN LATIN DRESS

1. ISIDORE OF SEVILLE: THE CANON OF MEDICINE

Isidore, bishop of Seville (d. 636), was an important leader of the church in Spain and a prolific writer on theology and church discipline. He was also deeply interested in clerical education, and composed a number of textbooks. His most influential work, however, was the Etymologies *(also called* The Origins*), an encyclopedia drawn largely from older Latin compendia, and structured around words and their meanings. Isidore's* Etymologies *is often decried as a typical product of a degenerate age, an incoherent rag-bag of poorly digested remnants of a once-great intellectual culture. On the other hand, it did preserve and disseminate a considerable amount of secular learning in a form both convenient and suitable for Christian readers. Moreover, Isidore's etymological method can be appreciated as a form of "art of memory" by which the whole semantic resonance of a term could be condensed for ready retrieval. It rested on the conviction that the full meaning and essential reality of every entity lay within the* origo *— the root or genesis — of its name.*

The sections on medicine in the Etymologies *echo the structure of the standard Alexandrian medical curriculum of late antiquity based on Hippocrates's* Aphorisms, Prognosis, *and* Regimen in Acute Diseases, *and Galen's* On Sects, Art of Medicine, Pulses, *and* Therapeutics. *This determined Isidore's choice of topics: (a) the history of medicine, (b) the theory of the four ˟humors, (c) the classification of diseases. It is noteworthy that his discussion of anatomy occurs in a totally different part of the* Etymologies, *namely book 11.*

Source: Selections from Isidore, *Etymologiae*, book 4, trans. William D. Sharpe, *Isidore of Seville: The Medical Writings*, Transactions of the American Philosophical Society, new series 54, pt. 2 (Philadelphia: American Philosophical Society, 1964), pp. 55–64. Original text ed. W.M. Lindsay, 2 vols. (Oxford: Clarendon Press, 1911). Latin.

1. Medicine

1. Medicine is that which either protects or restores bodily health: its subject matter deals with diseases and wounds.

2. There pertain to medicine not only those things which display the skill of those to whom the name physician (*medicus*) is properly applied, but also food and drink, shelter and clothing. In short, it includes every defense and fortification by which our body is kept [safe] from external attacks and accidents.

2. Its Name

The name of medicine (*medicina*) is thought to have been given it from "moderation" (*modus*), that is, from a due proportion, which advises that things be done not to excess, but little by little. For nature is pained by surfeit but rejoices in moderation. Whence also those who take drugs and antidotes constantly, or to the point of saturation, are sorely vexed, for every immoderation brings not health but danger.

3. The Founders of Medicine

1. Among the Greeks, the discoverer and founder of the art of medicine is said to have been Apollo. His son, Asclepius, added to it by his fame and works.

2. However, after Asclepius died from a lightning bolt, it is said that the healing art was forbidden and that the art died along with its founder, and was hidden for nearly five hundred years, until the time of Artaxerxes, king of Persia. At that time, Hippocrates, born on the island of Cos and whose father was Asclepius, restored it to light.

4. The Three Sects of Physicians

1. These three men founded as many sects. The first or Methodist was founded by Apollo, whose remedies are also discussed in poems. The second or Empiric, that is, the most fully tested, was established by Asclepius and is based upon observed factual experience alone, and not on mere signs and indications. The third or Logical, that is, rational sect, was founded by Hippocrates.

2. For having discussed the qualities of the ages of life, regions, and illness, Hippocrates thoroughly and rationally investigated the management of the art; diseases were searched through to their causes in the light of reason and their cure was rationally studied. The Empirics follow only experience; the Logical join reason to experience; the Methodists study the relationships of neither elements, times, ages, nor causes, but only the properties of the diseases themselves.

5. The Four Humors of the Body

1. Health (*sanitas*) consists in an integrity of the body and a harmonious proportion in its nature as regarding the hot and moist qualities embodied in the blood, wherefore it is called "health" as though the state of the blood (*sanguis*).

2. The word "disease" (*morbus*) is a general term which includes all bodily afflictions; our elders called it "disease" to indicate by this name the power

of death (*mors*), which could arise therefrom. Healing consists in a middle course between health and disease for, unless congruent with the disease, it does not conduce to health.

3. All diseases arise from the four humors: that is, from blood and yellow *bile, from black bile and *phlegm. Healthy people are maintained by them and the ill suffer from them. When any of the humors increase beyond the limits set by nature, they cause illnesses. Just as there are four elements, so also there are four humors, and each humor imitates its own proper element: blood the air; yellow bile fire; black bile earth; and phlegm water. Thus, there are four humors as well as four elements which preserve our bodies.

4. Blood derives its name from a Greek etymology, because it grows and sustains and lives. The Greeks call yellow bile [such] because it is bounded by the space of one day, whence also it is called *choler, that is, *fellicula*, for this is an effusion of bile (*fellis effusio*). For the Greeks call bile *chole*.

5. Black bile (*melancholia*) is so named because it is a mixture of the dregs from black blood with an abundance of bile; the Greeks call "black" *melas* and "bile" *chole*.

6. Blood (*sanguis*) is named in Latin because it is pleasant to the taste (*suavis*); whence also men in whom the humor blood predominates are pleasant and agreeable.

7. Phlegm (*phlegma*) however, is named because it is cold, for the Greeks call coldness *phlegmone*. By these four humors healthy people are maintained and the ill suffer from them, for when they increase beyond the limits set by nature, they cause illnesses. The acute diseases, which the Greeks call *oxea*, arise from blood and yellow bile, but the longstanding disorders, which the Greeks call *chronia*, come from phlegm and black bile.

6. Acute Diseases

1. *Oxea* is [the name applied to] an acute disease which either passes away quickly or kills speedily, such as pleurisy [or] phrenitis. The word for "acute" in Greek is *oxus*, which means "rapid." *Chronia* is [the name applied to] a protracted disease of the body which tarries for long periods of time, such as gout [or] *phthisis. Among the Greeks, *chronos* is said for "time." Certain diseases, however, are named after their own proper causes....

8. Pleurisy is a sharp pain of the side accompanied by a *fever and a bloody sputum: in Greek, the side is called *pleura*, whence the pleuritic disease derives its name.

9. Pneumonia (*peripleumonia*) is a disease of the lung marked by sharp pain and a sighing respiration. The Greeks call the lung *pleumon*, whence also this disease is named.

10. *Apoplexy is a sudden effusion of blood by which those who die are suffocated. It is called apoplexy because it is caused by a sudden lethal blow. The Greeks call a blow *apoplexis*....

15. Hydrophobia, that is, fear of water, for the Greeks call water *hudor*, fear *phobos*, whence also considering this fear of water the Latins called this disease "madness" (*lymphaticus*). It arises [either] from the bite of a rabid dog, or from spume falling from the air to the ground. Should man or beast touch this, he straightway becomes demented or is also made rabid.

16. A *carbuncle is named because in the beginning it is red like fire and in the end black like a dead coal (*carbo extinctus*).

17. Plague is a contagion which, when it takes hold of one person, quickly spreads to many. It arises from corrupt air, and by penetrating into the viscera settles there. Even though this disease often springs up from air-borne potencies, nevertheless it can never come about without the will of Almighty God.

7. Chronic Diseases

1. *Chronia* is a protracted disease which tarries for long periods of time, such as gout [or] phthisis, for *chronos* is said in Greek for "time."...

5. Epilepsy is named because hanging over the mind, it equally also possesses the body. The Greeks term anything "weighing upon," *epilepsia*. It arises whenever the black bile happens to develop in excess and is turned in its course to the brain. This disease is also called the "falling sickness," because the sick man, falling down, suffers convulsions.

6. These the common people call "lunatics" since under the influence of the moon's cycle (*lunae cursus*), the snare of demons catches them up. This also accounts for the term "ghost-ridden" (*larvaticus*). It is the same thing as the comitial disease, that is, a greater and divine disease by which those who have fallen to the ground are held – it is powerful enough to make a strong man fall down and froth at the mouth.

7. It is called the comitial disease because if, among the pagans, this seized anyone on a meeting day set for the Comitia [*the Roman political assembly*], this assembly was dismissed....

9. *Melancholia* is named from black bile: the Greeks call black *melas* and bile *chole*. Epilepsy arises in the *phantasy; melancholia in the reason; mania in the memory....

15. Pneumonia (*peripleumonia*) gets its name from the lungs, since it is a swelling of the lung marked by an effusion of blood-stained sputum....

23. *Dropsy (*hydropis*) takes its name from a watery humor of the skin, for the Greeks call water *hudor*. It is a subcutaneous accumulation of fluid, marked by a turgid swelling and a fetid, labored breath....

32. Calculus is a stone which arises in the bladder, whence it is also named (*i.e.* stone): however [the stone] is composed of phlegmatic matter....

35. Diarrhea is a continuous flow from the bowel not accompanied by vomiting.

36. Dysentery is a breach in the continuity, that is, an ulceration of the intestine. It arises following a *flux, which the Greeks call *diarroia*.

8. Diseases Which Appear on the Body's Surface

1. Mange (*alopicia*) is a loss of the hair in patches circumscribed by reddish-brown hairs having the color of copper, called by this name from a resemblance to the animal, the fox, which the Greeks call *alopex*....

5. Herpes (*serpedo*) is a redness of the skin accompanied by prominent pustules, and takes its name from "creeping" (*serpere*), because it creeps gradually along the members....

12. The disease *elephantiacus* is named from its similarity to the elephant, the skin of which is naturally hard and rough, and the name has been given to the disease among human beings because the surface of the body becomes similar to the skin of elephants, or because the pain is immense, like the animal itself from which its name has been taken....

14. Cancer is named from its resemblance to a certain marine animal [*cancer in Latin means "crab"*]: physicians say that it is a wound which admits of cure by no medications, and for this reason they usually cut off the member in which cancer has arisen from the body, so that [the patient] may live a little longer. In truth, death will yet come from it, although a little later....

13. The Study of Medicine

1. Some ask why the art of medicine is not included among the other liberal disciplines. It is because whereas they embrace individual subjects, medicine embraces them all. The physician ought to know literature (*grammatica*) to be able to understand or to explain what he reads.

2. Likewise also rhetoric, that he may delineate in true arguments the things which he discusses; dialectic so that he may study the causes and cures of infirmities in light of reason. Similarly also arithmetic, in view of the temporal relationships involved in the paroxysms of diseases and in diurnal cycles.

3. It is no different with respect to geometry [*literally "earth-measurement"*] because of the properties of regions and the locations of places. He should teach what must be observed in them by everyone. Moreover, music ought not to be unknown by him, for many things are said to be accomplished for ill men

through the use of this art, as is said of David who cleansed Saul of an unclean spirit through the art of melody [1 Sam. 16:14–21]. The physician Asclepiades also restored a certain insane man to his pristine health through music.

4. Finally, also, he ought to know astronomy, by which he should study the motions of the stars and the changes of the seasons, for as a certain physician said [*possibly Hippocrates, Airs, Waters, and Places* 2], our bodies are also changed with their courses.

5. Hence it is that medicine is called a second philosophy, for each discipline claims the whole of man for itself. Just as by philosophy the soul, so also by medicine the body is cured.

2. THE OLD LATIN COMMENTARY ON THE *APHORISMS* OF HIPPOCRATES

The Aphorisms *of Hippocrates, a collection of medical proverbs, summary observations, and rules of thumb, was one of the core texts of the Alexandrian medical curriculum. The first Latin translation of the* Aphorisms *and the anonymous commentary that accompanied it in the early medieval period were probably made at the same time and in the same milieu, namely sixth- or early seventh-century Italy. This Old Latin Commentary circulated with two different prologues, both of which reflect the Alexandrian method of expounding a medical text, modeled on the teaching of philosophy. The first prologue resembles an Alexandrian scholarly* isagoge *(introduction); it defines medicine as a domain of knowledge and outlines its various parts. Like philosophy, medicine is divided into theory and practice; theory in turn is divided into physiology, etiology, and semeiotics, and each of these parts is further subdivided. The message is that medicine is in its own right a learned and logical discipline, a "science" in the ancient and medieval sense of this term. A late Carolingian manuscript of this prologue from the Beneventan region (Glasgow University Library, Hunter 404) contains some interesting interpolations, which are incorporated in the translation below.*

Alexandrian commentaries often began with a stereotyped preface or prolegomenon *outlining preliminary questions to be covered before beginning to read a book, e.g., who the author was, what his purpose in writing was, etc. In Latin, this is known as an* accessus *(approach), and it serves to structure the second prologue. Note that the author recommends reading the* Oath *of Hippocrates, as well as the Hippocratic text entitled* Law. *Though there are no surviving early medieval translations of either text into Latin, there were certainly a number of paraphrases of the Oath (see doc. 87).*

Source: Prologue 1, trans. Faith Wallis from the edition by Giuseppe Flammini, "Le strutture prefatorie del commento all'antica traduzione latine degli 'Aforismi,'" in *Prefazioni, prologhi, proemi di opere tecnico-scientifiche latine*, ed. C. Santini and N. Scivoletto (Rome: Herder, 1992),

v. 2, pp. 591–92. Additional material from Hunter 404 based on the transcription of Faith Wallis. Prologue 2, trans. Faith Wallis from Flammini, pp. 605–6. Latin.

Prologue 1

Here begins the prologue to the commentary on the *Aphorisms*. Medicine is divided, according to the lesser partition, into two parts, which are theory and practice. Theory is what falls under the doctor's intellect; practice is what is done with the hands. Theory is divided into three, namely physiology, *etiology, and *semiotics. Physiology is that by which we understand the *physis* [*i.e.,* material nature] of things. Physiology itself [is divided] into six [parts]: elements, *humors, natures, members, *powers, perfections. (*Hunter 404 adds:* Hence the doctor ought to know the many arts of medicine which precede it: philosophy, geometry, and arithmetic. Preparatory to medicine are grammar, rhetoric, music, mathematics. [The doctor] should also know about herbs, medications, metals and elements.) The elements are four: fire, water, air and earth. (*Hunter 404 adds:* Hence also the human body is diversified, because these [elements] are opposed in their powers, and they create a certain *temperament; for instance, fire is a power of all burning things – the heavens, the sun, the stars and other things, and the Godhead itself is seen in fire. But if there were only fire, everything would be distempered by dissolving. Therefore the waters above the heavens were created [Genesis 1:7] to counteract it, so that by counteracting it, it might be tempered. And fire was created first, because all living things are vivified by fire, and because from fire, water ascends and [becomes] cloud, and becomes, so to speak, air. And what remains behind from this air becomes dense [earth]. The humors are four: blood, *phlegm, red *bile, and the melancholic humor. The natures are nine: four are simple, four composite, and one is temperate. The four simple natures are hot, cold, dry and moist, and the four composite [natures] are hot and dry, hot and moist, cold and dry, and cold and moist. Some members are *homeomerous and others are organic. The homeomerous are those solid members of which the body is made, that is, veins, arteries, sinews, bones, and what is similar to these, and to speak simply, that in which the part is subsumed under the term for the whole. Members are called "organic" when they are composed of these [homeomerous members], such as the hand, the foot, the head, and the like, where the part is not subsumed under the term for the whole. In us, some of the *powers pertain to the soul, others to nature. And of those pertaining to the soul, some are principal [powers], some are divided among the senses, and others are involved in motion. And the principal [powers are divided into] *fantasy (that is [the power] to receive images of everything), intellect (that is, to discern between false and true) and memory (that is, to retain all which they see and hear). The senses are five: sight, hearing, smell, taste and touch. And the motor powers of the soul are those which flow through the *nerves to stretch, bend, or turn the body. The powers of nature are divided into two: one by which we are nourished and the other by which we live. And [the power] by which we are nourished is divided into four: one which attracts food, one which holds on to it, one which *digests it, and one which expels what is superfluous from the body. The vital power governs the pulse, which opens and draws in air, and then closes and expels smoke. The perfections follow on from the powers.

Etiology is divided [in the first instance] into what happens from without, which the Greeks call *procatarctic, namely rage, tribulation, indigestion, sun-stroke, and the like. The Greeks term those causes that do not happen from without, but that take their origin from within the body *proeguminal. They call those diseases *synectic that are complete in themselves.

The theoretical part of semiotics is divided into three parts: to understand the present, to foresee the future, and to remember the past.

The practical part of medicine is divided into regimen and treatment. Regimen is to nourish children, restrain the elderly, and restore people after sickness. Treatment is divided into medication and surgery. Medications are either taken internally or applied externally. Those that are taken internally are taken either through the mouth or through the passageway [that is, the rectum]. Surgery is to cut or to stretch out what is superfluous in the body.

These are the parts of medicine.

Prologue 2

Because it is always necessary in every book that the headings required for the work first be set out, let it be said that today Hippocrates, like a generous *paterfamilias* who hastens to join the banquet of his teaching and decks the tables of knowledge, offers abundant riches by means of my discourse, so that anyone may be filled with whatever his mind desires.

The aim of the present book is briefly to expound chapters on the whole art [of medicine], but it would be much more exact to say that it makes haste to present almost everything that has been written down about [medical] teaching in compendious and distinct statements, as if excerpting for beginners. For in this book [Hippocrates] announces his view on human life and the nature of things, the breadth of the art [of medicine], the fleeting nature of time, the fallibility of experience, diseases and their circumstances, the diversity of places, airs, and waters, the methods of treatment, the sequence of the seasons, the variety of qualities – in short, the scope of this book contains summaries of the whole art [of medicine]. Such is its undeniable aim; for we say that what it aims at is the perfection of its end.

Usefulness. We say that a book is useful that contains within itself a summary of the whole art [of medicine], if this is really what this book intimates.

Now in ancient times there were many men named Hippocrates, and so some people say that this book is not by Hippocrates; but credit is given to him, because according to the judgment of Rufus [of Ephesus] both Pelos and Licos and many others agree that this is a genuine book by Hippocrates. Therefore we say that no one could have written such a book save Hippocrates, whom the philosophers call "the friend of nature." Some tentatively suggest that Democritus could have written such things; but he did not accomplish what Hippocrates did.

Under what division of the art of medicine should the present book be placed, seeing that medicine is both speculative and active? Speculation is comprehended in a short space of time, action cannot be comprehended in a long space of time. That which is comprehended in a short space of time always masters the other and he who does not fail to hold fast to these teachings will be as confident as it is possible to be. Therefore the present book should be placed in both [divisions].

The order in which [the book] ought to be read. In the case of beginners, this should be the third book they read and in the case of the learned, the final one. Let us see why. Those who wish to read medicine, because they are easily wearied, ought first to read the Oath of the said Hippocrates, and after the Oath, the *Law* (also called the *Treatise*), and thirdly, this book, in which the theory of the whole art is contained. But the educated should read this book last, so that everything they read in other books may be brought to mind in this one.

The mode of teaching. We say that there are five modes: three have an order, two do not. The intuitive (*intellectualis*) and part-by-part [mode] do not have order; analysis (*resolutivus*), synthesis (*complexivus*), and definition have an order, in which this mode is also ranged.

Into how many parts is the present book divided? ... Soranus [says it is divided] into three; Rufus, into four; Galen, into seven.

What is an aphorism? A brief statement that puts into writing the whole meaning of the subject under discussion.

3. TEACHING THE ALEXANDRIAN CURRICULUM IN SIXTH-CENTURY ITALY: AGNELLUS OF RAVENNA'S COMMENTARY ON GALEN'S *ON SECTS*

*Agnellus of Ravenna produced Latin commentaries on at least three of the introductory works of the Galen canon used in the school of Alexandria. In the manuscripts, Agnellus is given the title of "professor of medicine" (*iatrosophista*) and "chief court physician" (*archiatrus*), but attempts to flesh out his identity or to date his work more precisely than to the sixth century have been unsuccessful.*

Like the anonymous author of the Old Latin Commentary on the Aphorisms, *Agnellus followed the Alexandrian method of exposition. The text was apportioned out over a number of lectures. Each lecture began with an overview (*theoria*) followed by explanations, segment by segment, of the passage under review. Each passage was introduced by the phrase of the text with which it opens. In the translation below, the passage from Galen's text on which Agnellus is commenting (the* lemma*) is printed in bold type.*

Galen's On Sects *– the first book on the Alexandrian syllabus – is an introduction to the principles underpinning clinical judgment, framed as an analysis of three schools of thought about medicine. The Dogmatic or Rationalist school, represented (in Galen's view) by Hippocrates, held that knowledge of the ultimate cause of a disease was the key to managing therapy; the Empiricist school discounted the importance of remote or invisible causes and based therapy on tried-and-true experience; while the Methodists posited a single cause – excessive tension or relaxation – and designed their therapeutics to rectify this condition. Galen claimed to rise above the fray and to defend the unity of a truly scientific medicine. Nonetheless, the schema of the three sects proved to be an irresistibly memorable way of laying out the basic issues of medical theory, and Galen's own preferences and prejudices deeply influenced the way in which learned medieval doctors understood medicine. The disagreeable connotations of the word "sect" suggested that Empiricists and Methodists were "heretical" and that "reason" stood apart from and above mere "experience" and "method."*

Source: ed. and trans. David O. Davies, L.G. Westerink, *et al.* Agnellus of Ravenna, *Lectures on Galen's 'De sectis,'* Arethusa Monographs 8 (Buffalo: Dept. of Classics, SUNY Buffalo, 1981), pp. 51–55, 57, 61–65. Latin.

Lecture 12. The Empirical School of Medicine

The empiricists said the art of medicine has come into existence in the following way. We learned above what Galen's intention and purpose are, in which he makes three introductory remarks: in the first remark he mentions good health and thus encourages the minds of his audience: in the second remark, he discusses the instruments of the art; in the third, he discusses the sects of medicine, their agreements and disagreements.

But since we have already discussed these things, now let us begin to explain the schools in order. Following Galen, let us begin with the empirical school. There are some, however, who raise an objection and ask why he begins with the empirical school and not with the dogmatic, since the dogmatic is worthier and makes better use of reason than the empirical sect. We answer that the empirical school is simpler and simplicity is pleasing to those who are starting to learn an art; but the dogmatic doctrine is composed from many reasonings and goes over the heads of those who are new to the art.

The empiricists considered four sources, from which they derived their system: nature, chance, revelation, and similarity. The natural method: because they lived in a certain age and were unaware of what they should do with their sick and waited to see what happened to them naturally. And if nature restored itself on the *critical day, either through the bowels or through sweating and the patient was made healthy, they would call this the natural method. By chance: for example, someone wanted to drink cold water and got up, but not having the strength to walk, he fell down somewhere, and he bled, and his *fever was alleviated: they would say this happened by chance and called it chance. Through revelation: when people were lying sick, physicians, not knowing what they were to do for them, used to go to holy places, that is, to temples or cross-roads, and would ask oracles what they ought to do for their patients, – since they too had holy places just as we (speaking with due respect) have our churches. And if it was revealed to them and the idea flashed through their minds, to cure *erysipelas with *strychnos juice, they would do this and when the patient had been cured, they called this a revelation. On the basis of similarity: because those who had been cured by using, for example, strychnos juice for erysipelas, when they saw other patients suffering with erisypelas, approached them and presented the same cure by which they had been healed; and they called this similarity. The empiricists adopted these four: nature, chance, revelation, and similarity and thus assembled their art. The survey ends with these words.

The empiricists said that the art of medicine is composed in the following way. We said in the survey that the empiricists study four sources: nature, chance, revelation, and similarity, and from these they make up the empiricist's art of medicine. Some things, however, depend on ourselves, some do not. For prayer and work are in our power, but it is God who gives gold [and] silver, or slaves, or clothes. And similarly, in medicine it is for us to provide ointments and hot-packs on the critical days but for God it is to give sweat and a propitious *crisis....

Again they return to experience, and this is what especially

makes up their art of medicine: not only twice or three times but many times they have imitated what had helped before. Because the empiricists used what they had seen many times, not just once or twice, their sect is named accordingly; for experience means routine.

And memory of what they have seen many times. Those men who taught by seeing called it reporting; those who taught not by seeing but by hearing called it revelation.

Lecture 15. The Dogmatist or Rationalist School

Above we learned about the character of the empirical school, that it comprises those four categories, the natural, the fortuitous, the observational, and the imitative, and that as an instrument they used transposition by analogy; in examining these topics above, we finished the first part of the book. Coming now to the second part of the book, we discuss the position of the dogmatists' school. Here, some take issue with Galen, because he began from the empiricists' point and not with the dogmatists'. He began with the empiricists because theirs is the simpler doctrine; dogmatic doctrine is composed from many reasonings and passes over the heads of the students. The dogmatic doctor wants to know the natures of men.

Since we have mentioned nature, at this point let us say in how many ways the word nature is used. According to Hippocrates, the word nature is used in four ways. The first usage which Hippocrates states is that men, some in winter and some in summer, are given to be well and ill. The second use of nature which Hippocrates states is that people who have a long neck and a narrow chest and protruding shoulder-blades are prone to *consumption. The third use of the word nature which Hippocrates states is that it is a power which controls the nature of man. The fourth instance is that according to Hippocrates there are some natures which *digest barley-gruel and [do not digest] meat while others may digest meat but not gruel.

Thus, the first instance of the word nature is that in which men, some in summer and some in winter, are given to be well and ill. Warm natures are well in winter because they are tempered by the cold, but in summer they are ill because heated and weakened; on the other hand, cold natures are well because they are *tempered by the heat, but in winter they are ill because their coldness is increased. The second instance of nature: the doctor must know that those who have a long neck, narrow chest, and protruding shoulder-blades are called consumptive. The dogmatic physician must know that such people are apt to fall ill, he must always have in readiness a diet and medications of the kind that cures such cases. The third instance of nature, that it is a power that rules the human body: the dogmatic doctor must know that those who are quickly infuriated are hot natures; those who are slow to do so are cold natures. The fourth instance of the word nature: those who [do not] digest meat and do ... digest barley gruel by nature have colder stomachs, while those who digest meat and do not digest barley gruel by nature have warmer stomachs. The dogmatic doctor must know the natures of the waters and [the natures] of the [geographical] areas.

Some raise the objection, saying that the discussion is always on this same topic, of natures and causes. We say that it is not about this same thing, for water differs from water of a different nature just as does wine from wine and likewise the situation of one area differs from the situation of another. The second answer to the question is that causes are local, while natures are universal. The third answer to the question is that causes are relative, while natures are self-contained. Here ends the survey.

The rational method, however, enjoins us to learn the nature, namely, of the body which it professes to cure. The dogmatic doctor must know the natures of men, the natures of waters, and the natures of areas and the faculties of everything [*literally "the powers of all the causes"*], and the dogmatic doctor must know in what way things are involved with each other, and in what way their causes and the powers of remedies; and the dogmatic doctor must know the cures for things and prepare himself accordingly.

4. AN EARLY MEDIEVAL SUMMARY OF MEDICAL THEORY: *THE WISDOM OF THE ART OF MEDICINE*

The composite work known as The Wisdom of the Art of Medicine *(Sapientia artis medicinae) is contained in several early medieval manuscripts, but only one preserves the text in the form presented here. All other manuscripts contain one or two of the three parts, but not all three. This informal approach to transmitting medical writings is typical of the early medieval period. In one sense, it marks a loss of authority for the text, but one can also consider it as a sign of lively interest and creative adaptation. The* Wisdom of the Art of Medicine *is also typical of the way in which medical theory was boiled down to spare, didactic summaries. The emphasis on number is intriguing, as if counting diseases or bones offered some structure to compensate for the rather modest conceptual content. The three components of the text were probably composed in the sixth century.*

Source: trans. Faith Wallis from the edition by Montschil Wlaschky, "*Sapientia artis medicinae. Ein frühmittelalterliches Kompendium der Medizin,*" *Kyklos* 1 (1928): 103–13. Latin.

[Part 1]

1. **[Cosmic quaternities]** There are four winds, four corners of heaven, four seasons – spring, summer, autumn, and winter – and four *humors in the human body – red *bile, black bile, blood, and *phlegm.

2. **[Red bile]** Red bile is located on the right hand side, under the liver. These things are hot and sharp and cause bodies to be depleted in summer time, but plump and phlegmatic in the winter. Their fumes rise up to the human brain and cause heat in the head, earache, and migraine. [Choleric people] have a round and robust face, bulging eyes, and rough throat. They suffer from bitterness in the gullet and dry tongue. They are hot-tempered and changeable. But others are taciturn and are said to be reserved. They sleep on their right side. But some suffer from insomnia and have illusions because of the heat of their body. These have their health restored by cold water.

3. **[Black bile]** Black bile is situated on the left side, beneath the spleen. These things are salty and moist; they cause constipation and pain in the kidneys and various places. Their fumes ascend to the human brain and are responsible for headache and dizziness in the head and cause dripping of the uvula in winter. [Those in whom black bile dominates] have a long face; their prominent eyebrows make their eyes dark and they are prone to be solemn and inclined to sleep. Their bodies are given to morbid discharges; they are *melancholic and suffer from lung ailments and many bodily diseases.

4. **[Phlegm]** Some phlegm is situated in the head, some under the bladder, some in the kidneys, but it will be tempered in the stomach.

5. **[Blood]** Blood also draws off disease conditions (*morbositatem*) through the veins in due season.

6. **[Sinews]** Sinews contain bones, and bones sinews. The soul preserves the sinews. Blood governs the soul and the soul governs life. But *spirit is from the air.

7. **[Seasonal regimen]** In the month of March, from the fifteenth kalends [of April (18 March)] onwards, all the humors surge forth, and so do diseases, and morbid discharges, and the roots of herbs. Human bodies are irritated, and swell. Unhealthy conditions ought to be drawn off through the veins by bloodletting; bodies are *purged by cathartics. The humors dominate up

until the month of July. After the third ides of July [*13 July*], desist, O doctor, from bloodletting and purging, because the dog-days have begun, and the dog-day heat (*cynocaumata*) lasts 73 days. After the third ides of September [*11 September*], red bile bursts forth, and a superfluity of phlegm, and heat of the body follows. Autumn will last 64 days. Refrain from lovemaking, for it vitiates. Before the third kalends of December [*29 November*], black bile bursts forth, salty and moist, and one should make love [*one manuscript adds:* for those to whom this is permitted]. In winter, dripping of the uvula, phlegm, and many morbid discharges break out; up until the kalends of March [*1 March*], one will be more prone to discharges.

8. **[The fourfold kingdom of the body]** We divide the body into four parts: head, stomach, belly, and bladder. The head is an empire, the stomach a kingdom, the belly a hovel, but the bladder is a hired hand. If the head hurts, the stomach hurts; if the stomach hurts, the whole body is vexed with sickness and becomes feverish.

9. **[Pulse]** The pulse of *choleric people is hot and dry. The pulse of melancholic people is violent and slightly moist, so to speak. The pulse of phlegmatic people is cold and humid. The pulse of *sanguine people is violent and hot and moist.

10. **[The urines]** The urine of the liver is scurfy (*cantabrica*). The urine of the spleen resembles ash. The urine of the stomach will be ruddy and undigested before a meal; but clear urine proclaims good health.

11. **[The ages of man and the humors]** A child, from the day he is born until he is 14 years old, is phlegmatic and *rheumy. When he is 15, the heat of the blood comes upon him and there surges up in him red bile; and now it behooves to let blood. Red bile will dominate in him until he is 25; then black bile will surge up in him and will dominate until he is 52. Below the age of 30, it behooves him to take cathartics; nonetheless, should necessity arise, do not probe into his age but act according to reason, as it is written. After the age of 56 the humors of the body decline and the heat diminishes; phlegm and bodily rheum dominate. Then, leave off bloodletting and come to [the patient's] aid with cathartics and supporting therapies which are hot. And if in childhood the head is purged, let it be purged again because of heaviness of the head and blurring of vision; nor should he engage in sexual activity.

12. **[The number of bones]** The human head is positioned at four angles, but it rests at a fifth. There are eight bones in the face, but we divide the

jaws. There are 228 bones in the human body, but in women, 226 and in hermaphrodites (*frigiscis*), 227. There are 32 teeth and in women, 20.

[Part 2]

1. **[Cataracts]** The human eye has seven tunics and there are seven *cataracts. All their names are written here: *platorides, argyriides, graides, molybdites, amaurosis, placodes, serotaxis*. You couch *platorides* in the seventh year, *argyriides* in the eighth year and in the third year, if the person is old. You couch *graides* in the fourth year, and *placodes* in the second year. And if you find *molybdites, amaurosin*, and *serotaxis*, these are incurable.

2. Cure cataracts in the month of May and all summer and autumn. But when winter comes, leave off curing the eye. Cure cataracts like this: first you give to the stomach a cathartic of *gera* and *picra* [*that is, *hierapigra*]. After the third day you bleed the patient from the cephalic vein. After the fourth day you tie his hands to his right knee. You couch his left eye with your right hand. Couch him carefully, lest you touch the sense of sight and take out the eye. Another person should hold his head firmly so that it does not move, lest danger befall. Administer clean salty brine to the eyes and again place egg yolk over the eyes with soft wool. Let him lie in a secluded place for nine days, so that he does not hear any noise. Two times a day, you will treat his stomach with a *clyster. For his food, let him have new eggs and also barley-water. Refrain from wine and let him drink hot water for nine days, and on the tenth, let him have a bath and he will be better.

[Part 3]

1. **[The number of cures]** The human head has 24 cures, the eye has 12 cures, the thorax has 25 cures. There are 24 cures of the spleen. There are 33 cures of the liver. There are 22 cures of the stomach. There are 28 cures of *dropsy. There are 25 dropsiacal cures. There are 19 cures for impotence (*inopis*). There are 21 cures for ascites. There are 22 cures for *itroceps* [*hydrocele?*]. There are 33 cures for the intestine. There are 22 cures for the kidneys. There are 14 cures for the bladder. There are 27 cures for fever. There are 40 cures for coughing. There are 20 cures for the heart. There are 24 cures for paralysis. There are 29 cures for pleurisy. There are 27 cures for pneumonia. There are 21 cures for jaundice. There are 27 cures for epilepsy. There are 29 cures for *quinsy. There are 29 cures for angina. There are 23 cures for phlegm. There are 24 cures for the hips. There are 13 cures for the neck. There are 4 cures for the uvula. There are 16 cures of semi-*tertian fever.

There are 365 cures for gout. There is no cure for gout. And the human bones have 52 cures.

2. **[Frenzy]** What humor causes frenzy? It is caused by too much wine and cold water. First they come down with a semi-tertian fever from the cold. Due to this disorder, the veins emit a morbid discharge, and the brain is cut off, and they suffer from insomnia and become insane.

3. **[Paralysis]** What humor causes paralysis? From too much wine. First they come down with a semi-tertian fever from the cold, and the *nerves are twisted, and the veins and arteries are contracted.

4. **[Consumption]** What humor causes *consumption? From a morbid distillation of the head and a distillation of the uvula; and their lungs are riddled with holes and then they become consumptives.

5. **[Pleurisy]** What humor causes pleurisy? From too much cold wine, from cold water, from melancholy humor, and from too much phlegm and phlegmatic foods.

6. **[Liver disorders]** From what humor does the liver become irritated? From melancholy humor and too much morbid discharge because of cold. It descends from the head into the stomach and thence into the capillaries of the liver, and from this comes coagulation and irritation of the liver. And the right part of the stomach will swell up and will suffer from indigestion, and pain will throb in the right side.

7. **[Splenetic conditions]** Whence do splenetic conditions arise? From excessive fever and morbid discharge and cold water and hot water. A tumor of the spleen happens and there are morbid discharges, and the stomach is upset and a pain throbs in the left side, and they suffer from indigestion.

8. **[Sciatic conditions]** Whence do sciatic conditions arise? From melancholic humor. It descends from the head to the stomach, and descends into the liver and causes coagulation of phlegm and produces pain.

9. **[Arthritic conditions]** Whence do arthritic conditions arise? From melancholic humor. It descends through the bones and causes coagulation of the blood and produces pain.

10. **[Strangury]** Whence is *strangury generated? Melancholic humor descends and comes into the passages of the bladder and causes coagulation of phlegm.

11. **[Dysuria]** Whence is dysuria generated? Melancholy humor descends into the kidneys and causes coagulation of phlegm and filters through the veins into the bladder and produces pain in the kidneys and results in agonizing pains of the bladder.

12. **[Bladder stones]** Whence comes the stone? Blood and phlegm descend into the kidneys and from the kidneys into the bladder and makes a coagulation, and a stone is produced, just as mud [produces] a cucumber.

13. **[Inflammation of the lungs]** Whence does inflammation of the lungs arise? From excessive fever, for it burns in the lungs and dries up the phlegm and they become quite dry.

14. **[Lethargy]** Whence do lethargic conditions happen? Because of excessive sleep people suffer from heaviness and all their limbs waste away.

15. **[Jaundice]** Whence do jaundiced conditions happen? Because of excessive melancholy humor their gall erupts and the smoke of the bile ascends to the brain and makes the eyes yellow and they are said to be jaundiced.

16. **[Stomach and heart conditions]** What causes stomach and heart conditions? From excess smoke of the biles. There are stomach people and heart people and when people sweat quite a lot, they are heart people.

17. **[Beard, hair and nails]** From what humor are beard, hair, and nails produced? They are produced from the heat of the body and the sweetness of the blood.

18. **[What humor impedes beard growth]** What humor does not produce a beard? Because of the constriction of the humor, melancholics do not put forth hairs and they are phlegmatic.

19. **[Semen]** From what humor is semen in men derived? From the heat of the head and from phlegm that inhabits the kidneys.

II. MEDICAL PRACTICES IN A
CHANGING WORLD

5. AN ENCYCLOPEDIA OF PRACTICAL
MEDICINE FROM THE AGE OF JUSTINIAN:
ALEXANDER OF TRALLES

The Greek physician Alexander of Tralles came from a talented family: his brother Anthemius of Tralles was the architect of the great church of Hagia Sophia in Constantinople. He composed his major work, the Therapeutics *(*Therapeutica*) in the first half of the sixth century, possibly in Rome, where he spent much of his life. It was translated into Latin soon thereafter and in the process was reduced by about one-fifth, re-ordered from twelve books to three, and supplemented with extracts from two Greek medical writers, Philumenus (first or second century CE) and Philagrius (fourth century). This pattern of abbreviation and supplementation is typical of the medical literature, both Greek and Latin, of late antiquity and the early Middle Ages. The editing process tended to eliminate theoretical material (physiology, pathology, nosology, etc.), while preserving and enhancing practical information, particularly diagnostic and prognostic procedures; but it also contributed to the "decanonization" of medical literature, as texts lost their ascriptions to named authors or acquired pseudonymous authors. A few large-scale therapeutic manuals by named authorities escaped this fate, including Alexander's* Therapeutics, *the Latin adaptation of Galen's* Therapeutics *to Glaucon, and the* Synopsis *of Oribasius. But even these works were significantly transformed in the process of being translated.*

The fact that Alexander includes amulets in his Therapeutics *has raised a few eyebrows. They seem to be a concession to the whims of rich patients (Jacques Despars said as much about astrology: see doc. 66), but Alexander states that he has personally tried some, and found them effective. Ancient authorities like Dioscorides, Soranus, and even Galen himself report the use of amulets for digestive disorders, so Alexander was standing in a well-established tradition.*

Source: trans. Faith Wallis from Alexander of Tralles, *Therapeutica*, book 2, c. 131, 133, from MS Angers 457, fols. 113v–116v, collated with the Lyons 1504 *Practica Alexandri*, fols. 72v–74r. Latin.

Chapter 131. Signs That the Colic Is Generated by *Choleric Humor

It is known that a bout of colic is generated from hot, choleric, and acrid *humors because [patients] suffer from griping and burning, or their inner organs seem to be perforated; they have a dry tongue and suffer from thirst or insomnia, so that oftentimes they are driven mad, and their urine becomes bitter and those things which pass out of the belly are choleric. If hot foods and drinks or remedies are administered, these [symptoms] are greatly exacerbated and never without fever. Such are the signs that the bouts of colic are generated from choleric or hot humor.

Treatment If a Bout of Colic Is Generated from Choler

If a bout of colic is generated from choleric humor, remedies are to be administered in a fashion opposite to those used on patients who suffer from colic due to phlegm. First, their diet should be regulated. They should be given a simple *ptisane infusion, with nothing of any kind added to it save perhaps a small amount of salt. For choleric heat will be *tempered by it and expelled in the urine and from the belly. Hence this infusion should be given frequently. Cold egg yolks are to be provided.

Vegetables

Vegetables, given raw or cooked, are highly beneficial. Large, sweet lettuces are to be given, particularly to those who suffer from insomnia: [lettuces] are cold by nature and are larger in the summertime. All fruit which has the property of cooling and moistening should be given and none of these is thought to do any harm. Only squash is forbidden, because it has an inherent power to resist health and to do harm in cases of colic, and this is attested in all the books on diet. I know not only young people but even older ones who have been swiftly cured by following such a diet for a few days. But I know that they drink cold water in which is strength, and [do this] without injury; the vital places being preserved unharmed, they are completely relieved of pain. And when the cause from which the pain arose is completely averted, [the patient] arrives at a state of full health, and [I know this to happen] frequently in accessions of pain. Again, if he abstains from food and wine that have a biting quality and uses cold foods, he will be freed from this ailment. If he is afraid to drink cold water because of certain inflammations of the intestines, or because of weakness of the vital force, give him a large quantity of cold rose-water to drink, and give him an enema of oil of roses, and it will do a lot of good. Mix duck fat with [the oil of roses]. I know there is acridness and the biting quality of choleric humor in this. If shreds come out with the stool, a *decoction of ptisane with camomile oil, given as an enema, will help [the patient]. Egg yolk mixed with oil of roses also help, if given as an enema.

Fish

Fish which have firm flesh give relief, such as gilt-head, "blue-fish," sea-scorpion, *coctica* [*unidentified species*], squid, *tenceda* [*unidentified species*]. Also those which the Greeks call "shellfish" (*ostracoderinas*), that is scallops, oysters, and sea-snails. The sea-urchin helps [these patients], for it has within it a tempering and cooling liquor and it also possesses a *virtue which is good for the stomach – that is, it acts well upon the stomach and makes the belly relax, and it is a diuretic superior to everything mentioned above.

Meat

It is particularly fitting to give them meat which is not easily cooked, such as cows' feet, stomachs, pork tripe, and hooves that have been well cooked and cooled....

Baths

Baths may be taken in fresh water by almost everyone, particularly those who are middle-aged and who are warm by nature. If the air is temperate and the tub likewise moderate, they can be anointed with oil and hot water. They may be anointed with camomile oil on the places which hurt; do not rub the sore places with *nitre or marjoram or soap or the like. *Fomentations are also forbidden; and salty or alkaline waters, and all naturally hot waters, are forbidden.

Exercise

Exercise and movement and walking about may be done to relieve the ailment, but not much or very vigorously. For [patients] will not be able to bear it, but will rapidly become distempered and the pains will be sharper if they exercise more, or more vigorously. Let them abstain from all over-excitement and anxiety as much as possible, and from all heavy work. For if they behave themselves with moderation they will easily be cured....

Chapter 133.
Concerning Medicinal Talismans and *Potions and Amulets for Colic

Because many people who suffer from colic, and particularly the wealthy, do not wish to drink any [medicine], nor will they permit one to give them an enema, it is therefore necessary for us to say something about medicinal talismans and amulets. If these are provided, they are wont to relieve and reduce pain soon afterwards, and therefore I will not omit to write down those that have been proven effective by the ancients, or after them by us. So first, take wolf droppings, preferably from [a wolf] who has eaten bones; enclose them in an earthenware vessel and bind it on the right arm or shoulder – that is, the neck – or suspend it from the hips when the pain is severe. But take care that it never touches the ground; nor should [the patient] take it into the bath. *Another one.* And this is tried and true. Burn coral and grind it up and give about two or three spoonfuls in a drink to the [patient], fasting, for three or four days. This is good for colic. *Another one.* If he takes this coral in his food he will get better.... *Another one.* Engrave the stone called *medicon* with the image of Hercules strangling the lion and mount it on a gold ring and give it [to the patient] to wear on his finger and he will get well.... *Another very good one.* Take a little piece cut from the umbilical cord of a newborn child and enclose it in silver or gold. Let [the patient] carry this with him; he will always be free of pain.

6. GALEN ENLARGED FOR PRACTICE: PSEUDO-GALEN, *LIBER TERTIUS* ON PNEUMONIA AND PLEURISY

In the middle of the fifth century, and probably in North Africa, Galen's Therapeutics to Glaucon *was translated, or more precisely adapted, into Latin. This Latin version was in two books: the first dealt with *fevers, the second with a rather miscellaneous collection of conditions, ranging from morbid swellings of various kinds to abscesses, cancer, and leprosy. In early medieval manuscripts,* Therapeutics to Glaucon *is frequently augmented by a pseudonymous "Book Three," the* Liber tertius. *This is really a self-contained treatise on diseases, or* passionarius. *It follows the standard format for such works, working through conditions from head to toe.*

Around the same time, Therapeutics to Glaucon *picked up two further traveling companions: the* Aurelius *and its sibling text, the* Esculapius *(see doc. 7). Together, these treatises formed a stable text corpus. In the eleventh century, this corpus was re-organized, edited, and amplified by a certain Gariopontus. As the* Passionarius *of Gariopontus (or Galen), the old anthology continued to nurture medical writing well into the Scholastic period and beyond.*

The excerpt translated here concerns the distinction between pneumonia and pleurisy. Whether anyone could have learned how to diagnose and treat these conditions from such a condensed account is perhaps doubtful, though an experienced practitioner might have used it as a reference work and an aid to memory. But a text like this also served a wider purpose in transmitting the sophisticated intellectual heritage of Greek medical thinking, notably its precise technical vocabulary, and some inkling of the crucial importance that ancient medicine gave to differential diagnosis and to prognosis.

Source: trans. Faith Wallis: excerpts from the *Liber tertius*, ed. Klaus-Dietrich Fischer, in *Galenismo e medicina tardoantica: fonti greche, latine e arabe*, ed. Ivan Garofalo and Amneris Roselli (Naples: Istituto universitario orientale, 2003), pp. 308–11. Latin.

On Pneumonia

Pneumonia is an acute disease which takes its name from the affected place, for *pleumon* means "lung." These are the signs. There is pain throughout the chest, particularly on the right side under the breast. It stabs sharply, rising up to the shoulder-blades on the same side. There is a high fever and continual shortness of breath. [Patients] seek out cold things and they have a slight cough. The pain pierces the chest in a pronounced fashion. The pulse is broad and sluggish. What comes up is somewhat red and foamy. The complexion is flushed, notably the cheeks. The face is shiny and attractive, that is, more good-looking because of the redness. The [patients] cannot lie down flat, but prefer to sit up, and they frequently toss and turn. These things indicate that there is *humor in the lungs. But it is hot and fiery. One should ask [the patient] when he first took ill. For in women and children this condition (*causa*) occurs frequently, because these conditions arise in a hot and moist body. For in women and young people the body is hot and moist. In young people, this condition appears up to the age of thirty-five, and it is a danger to them and they rarely escape. But women either do not get it after the age of twenty-five, or if they get it, it is neither grievous nor dangerous and they are readily cured. This condition is engendered by the season of the year, for when there is seasonal heat, the air is made moist. Pneumonia is also caused by *catarrh and recent pleurisy, that is, pain in the side. Should fourteen days pass and the [patient] not thereafter cough or bring up *sanies, he will be cured rapidly. If after fourteen days he coughs or brings up sanies, one can say that he will be cured by the twenty-first day. But if the twenty-first day passes and these signs persist, the case is desperate and there is no doubt that he will die.

This treatment is to be applied. You will steam [the patient] with a moist dressing of oil, hot wine, and soft wool pads, particularly the whole right side of the chest, the throat, and the ligaments. Do this for three days. Make a salve of wax and cypress oil and ground mustard and apply it on small compresses, and apply *cupping glasses to the chest or the painful place. This is very beneficial. Give them food of this kind: soft-boiled eggs; broth of *ptisane with fish-sauce and pepper, or without fish-sauce; and they should take mead every day on an empty stomach. If possible, they should take this whenever they want to drink. In this mead, rue should be boiled, and bitter almonds or hyssop or oregano or the herb polygony; or give only the juice of polygony, for it is excellent and helps a lot....

On Pleurisy

Pleurisy is pain in the chest, and its signs are similar to liver disease and pneumonia. But pleurisy can be recognized by these signs. [Patients] are disturbed by very high fevers and unbearable pains in the left or right side. In [patients] in whom this pain arises in the flexible ribs or above the ribs, it sometimes strikes the uppermost ribs from the back and the whole side hurts. The pain extends even to the collar-bone and strikes behind the shoulder-blades and shoulders; even the groin can be tormented with pain. They cough constantly, not vigorously, but slightly – constantly, nonetheless, but lightly. They bring up blood and they sometimes bring up a reddish fluid with this blood. They suffer from insomnia and cannot lie on their right side, and if they go on like this for a long time, there is no question that they are in danger and will not be cured. But so that you will understand who can be cured and who can not, these are the signs. You should ask the patient if he received a blow on that side [of his body], or if he had fallen on it or bruised it a few days earlier. And if that is the case, he can easily be cured. If he is suffering from a cold condition or a *rheumatic one, it is more difficult to cure. If he previously had pain in his liver or lungs and then came down with pleurisy, the danger is great. And if his spleen hurts and pain in the spleen coincides with pain in the left side, then he is in grave danger. And if he had a sore throat previously, you will know that the pain in the side is from a rheumatic condition. This carries no little danger. So ask [the patient] if he is constipated, or has trouble passing urine, or if he only feels pain on one side, or if his sputum is changing in color: these are deadly signs. Therefore when these indications appear, you can know who will die, who will be cured, or who will be cured only with peril.

7. ECHOES OF METHODISM: "AURELIUS" ON RABIES

In the later Hellenistic and Roman period, Methodism was a popular and influential medical school. Although they were the principal target of Galen's On Sects *(doc. 3), Methodists claimed, with some justice, to be followers of Hippocrates. They nonetheless rejected humoralism in favor of the biological theories of Asclepiades of Prusa (Bithynia) (fl. 143 BCE). Asclepiades posited that the body was composed of sub-visible corpuscles that move through sub-visible channels. Health is simply the unimpeded flow of these tiny corpuscles through the channels. Disease could come about in two ways. Either the channels become blocked, causing excessive stricture, or the channels become slack and excessively wide, causing the body to become too lax. Stricture and laxness were readily* *apparent to the educated senses, and once the disease was categorized, the therapeutic choice was evident. Treatment followed a three-day cycle of fasting, recuperation, and treatment proper – for example, *evacuation in the case of a disease of stricture.*

The so-called Book of Aurelius *(a title that appears in only a few manuscripts of this widely diffused work) is the first of two parts of a manual of practical medicine created in the sixth or seventh century.* Aurelius *is about acute diseases; its companion,* Esculapius, *covered chronic conditions. This division echoes the structure of the most famous Latin handbook of Methodist medicine, Caelius Aurelianus's* Acute and Chronic Diseases *(fifth century), but while* Aurelius *retains Methodist therapeutics – notably the three-day treatment cycle (diatriton) – it has disposed of much of the theoretical framework. There is no reference to excessive stricture as the underlying condition of rabies, for example, and the therapies are not justified according to the category of disease. Methodism, it would seem, underwent much of the same kind of transformation as did Galenism: its doctrine faded in importance, and its treatments became more eclectic.*

Source: trans. Faith Wallis from the edition by Charles Daremberg, "Aurelius de acutis passionibus," *Janus* 2 (1847): 723–25. Latin.

Chapter 21. Hydrophobia (rabies)

The disease of hydrophobia is dangerous in many respects. The ancients say that it can come from the bite of a mad dog; others [say] that it comes from the bites of other wild animals and from the fear of water, whence it takes its name of "hydrophobia" from "fear of water." In Greek, *ydro* means "water" and *fobas* "fear." The old [writers] say that it comes from a waft of air without any bite, when foam is projected from the air into stone or into water, and if a man or any animal passes near it, he is suddenly filled with insanity or becomes mad. Thus hydrophobia itself is drawn out from the earth, or it is in a stone or in some other thing, or it comes from the fear of rain-storms, or from a blast of wind. For if a [mad] animal or human being is thrown into water, whoever enters the water or drinks it will immediately become insane and mad.

Signs of hydrophobia: this disease befalls those who are afflicted and who have drunk the poison, some sooner, some later. Those who [fall ill] sooner [do so] within fifteen days, or forty days, or in the third month; those who [fall ill] later, [do so] after a year. They suffer from the following symptoms: a craving for drink, combined with irrational movement; and they experience fear, as it were because they have been bitten by a dog. They are perturbed when they sleep and suffer when they are awake. After eating they feel heaviness in the stomach, tension in the limbs accompanied by trembling, and yawning. They are constantly hoarse and frequently sigh. The air seems greenish to them; they drink more than usual.... They experience a vehement craving for drink; their mouth gapes open, their tongue lolls out, they foam at the lips, their whole body together with the head is enfeebled, and their eyes are downcast as they walk. After a while they are debilitated in body, because the *nerves [are affected] when they are bitten. They desire neither food nor drink. Those who are bitten by a mad dog and only wounded by a bite from the teeth suffer no disturbance; but those who [are infected] with foam [from the mouth] of a mad dog fall into a rage. Even without any dog-bite they suffer from fear of water; or they take something to drink or suck and gulp it down. They suffer from *windiness in the stomach. They cannot lie down. Sometimes they cry out and shriek and roar. Some also break into a sweat with fear. Their eyes roll upwards. When they set out to walk, they fall down and injure themselves, losing consciousness. If their whole body goes into spasm, they die. They cannot pass stool. They do not lose their reason, but die with their wits intact.

They should be treated as follows. Let them not see what they are eating and drinking, for whatever they lay eyes on terrifies them greatly. If their strength and age permit, perform bloodletting for a three-day period. If age does not permit this, let them be treated with supporting therapies and cauterize the bite itself with a [hot] iron. At the outset, give a potion of gentian juice or oil, or roasted crayfish ground up in warm water, or the antidote *theriac. Treat the wound itself for a long time with wax salves. Let the patient's bowels be moved. [Foment] the chest and stomach with linseed and barley-flour and cooked mead; infuse in oil in which *castoreum has been cooked. You should provoke vomiting after [the patient has] ingested radishes. [A bowel movement] should be provoked with a *clyster. Contracted limbs should be *fomented with boiled fenugreek and anointed with a soothing salve or a wax-salve and with unguents made from *diasamsucum* and castoreum and wormwood. After forty days, they should take a potion of *asafoetida in hot water; and if their strength permits you must give them wild cucumber root in hot water, or castoreum and *oxymel, or green wormwood cooked in water, in order to provoke vomiting. The patient's food should be digestible, light and *hypnotica*, that is, conducive to sleep. Anoint the nostrils and forehead. After the remission, that is, after forty days, he can have wine and meat and visit the baths. Those who are left untreated through negligence die of epilepsy or possession, as the ancient writers say.

8. MEDICAL SELF-HELP FOR THE GENTLEMAN TRAVELER: THE *MEDICINE* AND *NATURAL REMEDIES* OF "PLINY"

In the fourth century, a writer who took the pen-name "Plinius Secundus Junior" assembled a medical recipe collection. The first two books followed a head-to-toe order, while the third dealt with ailments affecting the whole body. Much of the compiler's material was lifted from books 20–33 of the sprawling Natural History *of the Roman encyclopedist Pliny the Elder (Gaius Plinius Secundus, d. 79 CE), a vast storehouse of information on diseases, medical treatments, and the therapeutic properties of plants and animals. Plinius Junior's collection, the* Medicine of Pliny *(Medicina Plinii), was re-worked in the fifth or sixth century as the* Natural Remedies of Pliny *(Physica Plinii). Like many late-antique medical works, the* Natural Remedies *was an elastic text that was perpetually re-arranged and enlarged (for instance, with extracts from Gargilius Martialis's* Medicine from Vegetables and Fruits *– see doc. 9). The ostensible purpose of these collections was to provide the well-to-do traveler with the means to see to his own medical needs so that he could avoid the noxious, expensive, and frequently fraudulent treatments of local physicians. This pretext continued to be invoked by later compilers such as John of Mirfeld (see doc. 98), and since the opening chapter of* Natural Remedies *concerns the common head-cold, it has an air of plausibility.*

a. Prologue to the *Medicine of Pliny*

Source: trans. Faith Wallis from *Plinii Secundi qui feruntur de medicina libri tres*, ed. Alf Önnerfors, Corpus medicorum latinorum 3 (Berlin: Akademie Verlag, 1964), pp. 4–7. Latin.

While on my travels, I have often had occasion to experience various types of dishonesty on the part of doctors, either with regard to my own illnesses or to those of my entourage. Some of them sell the most appalling remedies at exorbitant prices and others, because of their greed, take on cases which they do not know how to cure. Indeed, I have encountered some people of this type who connive to prolong illnesses that they could repel in a few days or even hours, so that their patients will keep coming back and suffer more violently from these same diseases. For this reason, it seemed to me necessary to muster aids for health from wherever I could and collect them into summary form, so that wherever I go I may be able to avoid these traps and feel confident when I embark on a journey, knowing that if any illness befalls me, no money will go from my pockets to these people, nor will they be able to take advantage of me.

Above all, I think one ought to have ready at hand the things which one might need suddenly and which seem to be difficult to find, for example, aged oil. If not ready to hand, it may quickly be made. New oil which is boiled down exhibits the odor and powers of very old oil.

And if perchance the treatment demands that you seek out sea water in an inland region, this is no cause for worry. Two-thirds of a *sextarius* of salt dissolved in four *sextarii* of water will approximate temperate sea water, and a [whole] *sextarius* the most salty kind. If you add more, the salt cannot dissolve in the water.

We make *oxymel by dissolving two *cyathi* [*one twelfth of a sextarius*] of honey in a *sextarius* of vinegar.

We will describe how to make *thalassomeli* [*a purgative made of sea water, honey and rain water*] when we get to its use.

Sooner or later the question of porridge will arise, which should be made like this. Let barley which has been soaked in water dry out overnight. Then to twenty pounds of barley, three pounds of flax seed are added, half a pound of coriander, and an eighth of a pint of salt. In the morning, these are roasted and ground in a mill.

We recall that in all treatments, the honey which is most effective is that in which there are dead bees. If you happen to use it, it will be worth seeking out.

We also recall that unwashed wool from the neck [of the sheep] is best.

We are enjoined in some remedies to use ash made from birds, animals, or other things. Everything of this kind should be burnt to ashes in a new pot, with the lid sealed shut with clay, and in a very hot oven.

We take all gargles hot.

It is necessary to know medical weights and measures. A dram has three scruples. A dram is the weight of a silver penny and an *obolus* is one-sixth of a dram. A *cyanthus* has ten drams, a half-pint fifteen drams, a *cocleare* has a dram and a half, and a *mina* one hundred drams. A medical *sextarius* has 10 ounces.

These are things which should be observed in virtually every [illness]. Now we will apply remedies to particular parts of the body. In the following work we will treat *tertian [fevers], *quartan [fevers], and diseases of this kind, howsoever they occur, as they come to our attention. Let us begin, then, with the head.

b. Cures for the Common Cold from the *Natural Remedies of Pliny*

Source: trans. Faith Wallis from the edition by Joachim Winkler, *Physicae quae fertur Plinii Florentino-Pragensis Liber Primus* (Frankfurt: Peter Lang, 1964), pp. 51–70. Latin.

On *Catarrh or Abundance of *Humor in the Head

In cases of persistent headache, particularly when there is no *fever, it is necessary to extract the [morbid] matter through the nose or mouth, and this also helps in cases of prolonged earache or toothache. An infusion of cabbage juice *purges the head and mitigates the pain. Likewise, less than one-half a *cocleare* of juice of black beet root, mixed with a *cocleare* of honey and infused into the nostrils so that it passes through the palate and all the mucus runs out; if you want it to stop, take a mouthful of oil. Again, clover decocted in water and the water administered as a drink will extract the mucus. Again, you combine one ounce of mustard, one ounce of turnip seed, 20 grains of pepper, and equal parts of nasturtium seed, arugula, oregano and celery seed, and honey with hot water, and gargle with this for seven days....

Again, a gargle made as follows. Macerate two ounces of mustard seed in sweetened vinegar for a whole day; take 30 stems of stavesacre, and six ounces of hyssop heads, and crush them all up together; add six ounces of skimmed honey and grind it up with a sufficient quantity of sweetened vinegar. Gargle with this for three days under a clear sky and take moderately watered wine and sweet foods. It is very conducive to health to abstain both from wine and from clamor, from baths and wind and chills, so that you may have a bowel movement after a few days....

What Catarrh Is

Catarrh is humor flowing from the nostrils into the throat and lungs. "Catarrh" comes from [the word for] "morbid discharge," for the Greeks call a morbid discharge "catarrh." By some people – using other classifications and terms – catarrh is called *"rheum" when it is in the nose, "hoarseness" when it is in the throat, and *"consumption" when it is in the lungs. We detect catarrh in the nose from a sensation of oppression in the mouth and a narrowing of the nostrils and forehead, together with a morbid discharge of humor – thin, thick or green – accompanied by continuous sneezing and difficulty in smelling. There is a tickling in the throat from a sort of itching; the voice is muffled or irritated, and there is a sensation of choking and difficulty in swallowing, along with coughing. In the lungs, because of oppression of the chest, there is severe cough, with frothy or thick or purulent sputum.

9. A LATE ANTIQUE ESTATE-HOLDER'S MANUAL OF HOME REMEDIES

In his Institutes of Divine and Human Learning, *Cassiodorus commended Gargilius Martialis as suitable reading for monks, especially those not capable of tackling philosophical texts. Like other Latin authors of treatises on agriculture and husbandry such as Columella and Emilianus, Gargilius could be enlisted to teach lessons in practical charity, for he described how common foodstuffs could be used both to feed strangers who came to the monastery gate and to heal the sick (see doc. 21). The abbot was in many respects a* paterfamilias *who provided for the medical needs of his household and dependents from the resources of a substantial farm.*

Gargilius Martialis (d. 260 CE) was a member of the equestrian order and a local notable (decurion) of the colonia of Auzia in the Roman province of Mauretania in north-western Africa. He wrote a number of books on farming and estate management, including some of a medical nature. Only fragments of these have survived. The text conventionally entitled Medicine from Vegetables and Fruits *is found in manuscripts dating from the sixth to the sixteenth century, sometimes as an autonomous text and sometimes as book 4 of the Florence-Prague version of the* Natural Remedies of Pliny *(doc. 8). It is cited by several late antique and medieval writers, notably Odo of Meung ("Macer Floridus," eleventh century), author of the popular* Poem on the Powers of Herbs.

Gargilius's text frequently refers to his own experience with using vegetables, fruits, herbs, and nuts as medicine, and alludes to practical measures for preserving plants for ready use. On the other hand, Gargilius seems to have been able to read Greek, for he quotes Galen and Dioscorides; indeed, he may have composed Feminine Herbs *(De herbis femininis), a translation and adaptation of Dioscorides's great* Materia Medica. *Gargilius also drew heavily on Pliny's* Natural History.

Source: trans. Faith Wallis from Gargilius Martialis, *Medicina de oleribus et pomis*, ed. Brigitte Maire (Paris: Les Belles Lettres, 2002), pp. 14–15, 21–24, 28, 61–63, 72–74. Latin.

11. Lettuce (*lactuca*)

Lettuces are of a cold nature, but not so cold as to be harmful, for otherwise they would not be useful. They provide a mid-range, moderate coldness. They assuage the heat of summer, stimulate those who are weakened by loss of appetite to eat, and augment blood. They fill nursing women with abundant milk. They constrict the bowels, but in sufficiently large quantity will cause them to move. Dioscorides states that it is best to administer [lettuces] to people who have stomach trouble without washing them. Pounded up with salt, they cure burns, if they are applied before blisters appear. In the same way, they also cure *erisypelas. Cooked in a shallow pan and seasoned like other vegetables, they are of great benefit to those who suffer from *cholera. Some cook them in milk for the same purpose.

18. Garlic (alium)

Garlic has great strength, and that is why it is enormously useful. It vigorously wards off every harmful condition to which human beings are prey. By its smell alone it drives away snakes, scorpions, and other animals which lie in hiding. It heals the wounds which these animals inflict equally well whether it is applied to them, or taken in food or drink. When taken with honey, it heals the bite of a dog. Cooked in sweet vinegar, it kills tapeworms and other animals which infest the bowels and drives them out. Dried with its own leaves and mixed with oil, it treats all poisonous bites in an effective manner. Prepared in the same manner and used as an application, it soothes abrasions on the body and weeping ulcers of the head that have produced blisters. Travelers who eat [garlic] are not upset by change of water or locale. According to Hippocrates, *fumigating with garlic draws out a woman's after-birth. Some give it raw to those with impaired breathing; others give it mashed in milk. For patients with *dropsy, Diocles [of Carystus, d. ca 300 BCE] mixes it with centaury. This same Diocles also gives it boiled to patients with frenzy. Praxagoras [of Cos, fourth c. BCE] uses garlic as follows: for jaundice, with wine. Fresh and mixed with coriander and fig, it works to make the bowels move. Cooked with beans, it soothes coughing and suppurations of the chest. Boiled and applied to the temples, it helps a headache. Its juice, warmed with goose grease, is used as drops for earache. It soothes hoarseness when taken with peas or beans. It is held to be better cooked than raw, and juicy rather than dry. Cooked in porridge, it cures *tenesmus. With grease, it dissolves suspicious swellings.

19. Poppy (papaver)

The cooked heads and leaves of [the poppy] make *meconion*, a medication for illnesses that should be treated with moderate coldness. Mixed with oil of roses, its juice soothes earache. The leaves, cooked and mashed up with oil of roses, are excellent as an application for joint pain. A *fomentation of water in which poppy heads have been cooked is beneficial for those who suffer from insomnia due to illness or from *ophthalmia due to runny eyes. Poppy-seed crushed with vinegar and honey offers no little relief for swellings. The peel of its stalk, when ground to a powder and mixed with honey, is a good plaster for filthy wounds.

There is also a wild [poppy] with a small head and a stalk which is less tall. It is a wonderfully good cure for the windpipe when the throat is inflamed. A medication which the doctors call *diacodion* is made from this [poppy], so Chrysippus [*of Cindus, d. 277 BCE*] tells us.

22. Basil (*ocimum*)

There is no consensus among doctors about the virtues of basil. Influenced by Chrysippus, those who are critical of basil list its faults: it harms the stomach, weakens the eyes, causes madness, and damages the liver. That is why goats never touch this herb. They add that if it is crushed and placed under a rock, it engenders scorpions; if it is mashed up and placed in the sun, it produces worms and feeds lice. They think that Africans firmly believe that if anyone is stung by a scorpion on a day when he has eaten basil, he cannot be saved. But those who are of the opposite persuasion claim that these accounts are false. Quite the contrary: [basil] is beneficial for the stomach, because when it is cooked in vinegar, it relieves bloating by making one burp. It tightens up loose bowels. Its seed, crushed and taken as snuff, stops sneezing. It eliminates worms when taken with shoemaker's blacking [*blue vitriol, or copper sulfate*].

44. Peach (*persicum*)

Eating peaches is certainly deleterious to the stomach, because their juice can rapidly turn acidic and their flesh can also undergo harmful change in the course of digestion. But they are not too heavy if they do not remain in the bowels for a long time, and if they descend and are eliminated quickly. Moreover, early ripening peaches and those that come from Armenia are lighter. They cause fewer of the problems enumerated above than do the larger peaches. Again, early ripening peaches are better for the body than the Armenian ones. That is why they can even be given from time to time to sick people, but only insofar as their condition permits.

Doctors say that eating peaches does not nourish the body. Galen advises never, under any circumstance, to eat them after a meal, claiming that they will rot if they float on top of other foods. Crushed peach leaves kill and eliminate the animals that infest the bowels. Dried and powdered, these leaves close up fresh wounds which are bleeding. The pit of the peach, ground up with oil and vinegar, is applied for headache, although some prefer simply to rub [the head] with oil of roses. A drop of the gum that oozes from the trunk of the peach tree heals diarrhea. Mixed with wine, this [gum] also breaks up bladder stones. Ground up with vinegar, it stops scurf. Cooked with saffron, it soothes a swollen throat. It makes the windpipe smoother and is marvelously helpful to those who cough up blood. It opens up blocked passages in the chest and clears up affections of the lungs.

53. Almond (*amygdalum*)

Many people find that fresh almonds are heavy on the stomach. But Dioscorides thinks that they are also beneficial to the stomach, if they are swallowed whole without chewing. They make the head heavy, bring on impaired vision, and arouse sexual desire. When dried, they are effective against drunkenness, provided one consumes five of them before taking wine. They are known to provoke thirst, because (or so they say) a fox who has swallowed almonds without chewing them will die if there is no water nearby. [Almonds] make one sleepy, provoke urination, and bring on a woman's period. Ground up with starch and mint and then stirred into a drink, they help people who are coughing up blood. The oil in which almonds are cooked, spread on the head, revives epileptics and those who suffer from lethargy. Crushed with honey, they are good for ulcerated wounds and dog bites. A drink made of the water in which [almonds] are cooked, when mixed with a small amount of raisin wine (this counteracts the normal bitterness of this drink) eliminates pain in the liver and kidneys. Administered as an *electuary with terebinth gum, it breaks up bladder stones and frees the patient's blocked urinary tract. Crushed with sage and honey and taken in a quantity equivalent to a hazelnut, they are good for cough and colitis.

A medication which Dioscorides called *dia amygdalon picron* is made with bitter almonds; it is indispensable in diseases of the spleen and liver, especially jaundice. It is made as follows. Take two ounces of almonds, four of gentian, two of anise, one of Black Sea wormwood. Grind them all together and sift them. Give one spoonful of this powder in water. Those who are repelled by the strong bitter taste mix it with mead. I have tested the effectiveness of this medication on my household servants and it saved my wife's life.

The gum exuded by the almond tree, when mixed into a drink, is believed to be very good for those who spit up blood. When drunk with undiluted wine, it soothes a cough. It is said that this power is present in other parts of the tree, because the leaves or the bark, harvested at the appropriate time, are mildly cathartic, *purgative, and therapeutic.

10. THE DOCTOR AS CONNOISSEUR OF PULSES AND URINES

*This manual for diagnosing from pulse and urine is sometimes ascribed to Galen and sometimes to Alexander of Tralles (see doc. 5). Its real author, however, is unknown. As a medical handbook it is rather strange, though quite typical of late antique and early medieval writing. There is no information about diagnosing or differentiating *fevers: it is assumed that the practitioner knows that the disease he is confronting is (for example) an ephemeral fever. One can partially re-construct an *etiology of ephemeral fever (affections of the soul, inability to digest, exhaustion and so forth), but the particular pattern of pulse is not logically linked to these causes. When it comes to urine, the text is a straightforward catalogue of medical omens (not dissimilar, in this respect, to doc. 11). We might almost speak of a "connoisseurship" of urines, in that terms such as "delicate color" or "cloudy in an evil way" are not defined but taken to be understood. So how could a practitioner use such a text? Direct evidence is lacking, but we can infer that he acquired his connoisseurship through face-to-face training with a master; the text thus served as a mnemonic support. Notice that definitions of pulses are repeated from chapter to chapter, as if the author expected the reader to look up specific information rather than study the book from end to end. In any event, On Pulses and Urines is an eloquent example of how ancient medical knowledge could be stripped of theory and still be useful.*

Source: trans. Faith Wallis from the edition by Malte Stoffregen, *Eine frühmittelalterliche lateinische Übersetzung des byzantinischen Puls- und Urintraktats des Alexandros. Text – Übersetzung – Kommentar* (Diss., Freie Universität Berlin, 1976), pp. 72, 82–88, 104–5, 111–18, 120, 122. Latin.

Prologue

Learn what ought to be known about recognizing the fevers described above, which I have already spoken of at considerable length. First, we should acquaint ourselves with the causes, origins, species, and genera of fevers, so that we may know which are general and which are particular, that is, which are true and which are not true, or which are intermittent and which are acute, or which are simple and which are double, or which ones are twinned with other fevers, and of these as well, how they supervene and how they recede – that is, in what manner they are moved and in what manner they change direction and at what hours of day or night, or how long the paroxysm or agitation will persist, or when they will make their *anesis* or decline, what they really signify and where they will lead the patient. Also to be taken into consideration are the strength of the patient and the quality, the force of the illness and its magnitude, and from this, the signs of life and death, particularly so that you may be able to foresee the kind of fever from the pulse and from the examination of the urine (if one is assiduous in reading and very well instructed in practice) and also from other signs which our Hippocrates approved in his *Prognosis*, and by which he predicted the future before it arrived. For the patient's color, his eyes, face, voice, silence, the position in which he is lying, the attitude of his body, and his bearing will point [things] out to you, and as it were, will speak silently to you. All these things should be taken into consideration in patients, so that we may clearly know what we ought to persist with and what we ought to abandon, lest perchance by our ignorance of these things we do harm to our patients and delude ourselves as well. In addition, you should always and in every illness take into account the quality of the region, the location of its physical features, the temperament of the air, the change of season, the patient's age and habits, the nature of his body and soul, the cause and origin [of the disease], and also whether the sickness arose from a defect of the body or the soul, or whether it came about externally from food, drink, or corruption of the air. When you have well and truly investigated all these considerations by reason, you will do most satisfactorily whatever it is appropriate for you to do in all these [circumstances]. For the beneficial powers of medicine will be vanquished when assistance is not proffered at the right time, or when the body's nature, routed by disease, does not feel its benefits. Hence one who exercises forethought ought to observe all these things with diligence, and he should administer therapy at the right time, considering what is foreknown and from knowledge of causes, as I said.

1. Ephemeral Fevers

In ephemeral fevers, the pulse is simple, not very unequal, squalid (*sordidus*), or labored (*difficilis*). An "unequal pulse" is one in which the leaps and falls change in magnitude or intensity or speed or slowness or time or order. A "simple pulse" is one whose leaps and falls are properly ordered. You should know that patients who pass clear urine, drop by drop, and who have a headache, will succumb to stroke. If the fever is due to a sickness of the mind – that is, from sorrow or longing – the pulse is feeble and weak at the beginning, so that you would think they had been languishing for some time with a protracted illness. In these cases, the urine is more tawny than it is in other ephemeral fevers. But if the sickness arises from anger, it makes for a fever that is great and savage. It makes for a pulse that does not abate or slacken, as happens in the cases of those who suffer because of grief, sleeplessness or preoccupation. A pulse pertains to "greatness" and "savageness" when the motion of the arteries is extended in length, breadth, and depth. In cases where an inability to digest food has brought on fever, the urine is yellow, and the urine burns more than usual, and it is *choleric and stings when it passes out of the penis. Now in those who by working up a sweat from much labor succumb and take a chill, the pulse is diminished and more feeble. A pulse is "more feeble" which extends the artery in length for a short time and in depth with a feeble motion. The urine appears russet-colored and cloudy. If it suddenly becomes sharp and wine-colored and hot, it announces that a wasting-disease is in the offing. Or if it changes to a white color, it foretells pain in the joints or *apostemes of the ears, that is, inflammations of the parotid. If urine of the abovementioned color is abundant, but if the patient does not have the abovementioned pains, it shows that the disease will come to an end. Urine that is thick and white like a man's sperm signifies good health. But if the patient has urine of this color at the outset of his illness and yet does not have a headache, it foretells contraction of the body. Those who are exhausted by hard labor have a pulse that is feebler and bigger. A "bigger" pulse is one that generally by its leap extends the area surrounding the artery to the maximum length, breadth, and depth, so that when we investigate with the touch of our fingers, it is felt to be higher. In these people the urine is russet-colored and hot; in those whose pores are constricted, it passes out with more vehement force. Where inability to digest food has brought on fever, the pulse is more faltering and weaker in its beat when it was more energetic before, and the urine is not very russet-colored. In cases where pain in the groin brings on fever, the pulse is very big and with a great beat and rapid and swift. In these patients the urine is of a whitish color, and like [that of] the other ephemeral fevers....

5. Quartan Fevers

At the outset, a *quartan fever produces a pulse that is infrequent and sluggish and elevated. An "infrequent" pulse pulsates with a motion that is slight to the touch of the person inspecting it, accompanied by an interval of some kind. A pulse is "sluggish" that delivers its beat with a slow motion. When the disease is passing away, the pulse is found to be "squalid" and weary and sluggish and infrequent. A "squalid" pulse is one that goes from fast to slow and slow to fast. A pulse is "weary" that extends the artery longitudinally with a short, slow, weary motion. A pulse is "sluggish" that proceeds in its course with a torpid motion. In this case, when the time draws near, cold is diminished more than intense heat. In these [patients] the urine, mixed with diverse colors, appears especially pallid and dusky, for it appears undigested....

11. Pleurisy

In cases of pleurisy, the pulse is rapid. When the disease worsens, it becomes more rapid, and it is swift, strong, and (so to speak) fluctuating, and it feels like it is thrusting against the fingers of the person inspecting it. When this disease changes into pneumonia, the pulse becomes more rapid than the one described above. A "rapid" pulse is one that completes its leaps and falls in a short period of time. A "swift" pulse executes the movements of its course speedily. A "strong" pulse pulsates against the length of the inspector's [fingers] with a strong motion. A "fluctuating" pulse is one that flows more in its leap, like liquid enclosed [in a vessel]. The urine of these patients is thin and ichorous [*i.e., watery*]. If [this urine] arrives at the outset of the illness and lasts for many days, it foretells frenzy, particularly if there is dry cough and insomnia. If there is nosebleed and a great deal of sweat, it promises that the dissolution of the disease is at hand. Thick, tawny urine shows that death is at hand. Urine which is white and somewhat livid signifies death. Thin urine which has livid digested material like silt declares that death is at hand.

12. Pneumonia

In cases of pneumonia, the pulse is strong and rapid. When it reaches the danger point, the pulse becomes indistinct and seems to disappear and (so to speak) formicates. A "strong" pulse extends the surroundings of the artery to the greatest extent in its leap and pulsates against the parts of the fingers of the person inspecting it to the maximum degree of length, breadth, and depth. A "swift" pulse is one that speedily completes the movements of its course. "Ant-like" [*mirmizon*] pulse, because of weakness, is small and low because of its debility. Its movement is fast, and it derives its name from the movement of ants. Its pace is felt to be continuous and without quantity. Urine which is bloody and with the clouds described above shows that [the patient's] life is in danger. Undigested urine at the outset and before the *crisis declares that death is in the offing....

15. Hydrophobia

The pulse of patients with hydrophobia is restrained (*modicus*), attenuated and difficult to detect.

16. Pain in the Intestine

These people have a dense pulse. When [this disease] reaches the dangerous stage, their pulse becomes softer.

17. Discharge from the Penis

The pulse is condensed, that is, it is found to be stronger in one hand, forceful, full, dry, and swift....

18. Epilepsy

The pulse of epileptics who are not in spasm is huge (*ingens*), and by its leap extends the motion of the arteries to the maximum degree of length....

22. Nephritis

In patients with nephritis, the pulse is similar. A "weary" pulse is one that, wearied by a certain lowness, is not able to execute its leaps and falls. If these people's urine is tawny, it does not betoken good, and it says that the case will worsen. If these people's urine has the color of a man's sperm, it signifies death. Silt in urine signifies increasing pain....

25. Liver Conditions

When the urine of those suffering from liver trouble is white, thick, and thoroughly digested, it promises good signs of health. Thin, black urine with a viscous odor is deadly. Turbulent black urine with things like hairs or shavings in it signifies death....

29. Injury to the Kidneys

Urine that is thick and has what looks like [morsels of] flesh swimming on top of it signifies that severe pain is in the offing....

II. PROGNOSIS AND PROPHECY

In the genuine Hippocratic text entitled Prognosis, *the author recommends that physicians cultivate the art of foretelling the outcome of illness: a doctor who can make a prognosis seems to have the powers of a seer and will win the patient's respect. In fact, from a historical perspective, medical prognosis and religious divination have closely intertwined roots. The rational medical tradition associated with the names of Hippocrates and Galen always emphasized the logical connection between clinical signs and probable outcome; but late antique medical writing, with its strongly practical bent and its unspecialized readership, was more interested in straightforward formulas for forecasting. The two texts presented here were widely diffused in early medieval manuscripts. The first is called* The Ivory Casket, *or sometimes* The Secrets of Hippocrates *or* Prognostics of Democritus *or* The Indications of Illness. *It is a catalogue of diseases, comprising a few clinical signs followed by a bald declaration of the time that death will occur. The signs are often pustules that appear like tokens on the body. The absence of any causal explanation and the framework story of how these "secrets" were discovered lend an oracular air to the text. The "indications" all point to death, and this links* The Ivory Casket *to the second text below, the* Signs of Impending Death *ascribed to Galen. This text, and others like it, is found not only in medical manuscripts but also in prayer books and clerical compendia, particularly from the Carolingian period onwards. It has been argued that a new ritual focus on preparation for death prompted both parish priests and infirmary monks to learn to recognize its approach so that the proper rites might be performed.*

a. *The Ivory Casket*

Source: trans. Faith Wallis from the edition by Karl Sudhoff, "Die pseudohippocraktische Krankheitsprognostik nach dem Auftreten von Hautausschlägen, 'Secreta Hippocratis' oder 'Capsula eburnea' benannt," *Archiv für Geschichte der Medizin* 9 (1916): 88–102. Latin. The text is transmitted in two versions; Sudhoff's version I is translated here.

It has come down to us that when Hippocrates was nearing death, he ordered that the excellent things (*virtutes*) written in this book should be placed in an ivory casket and the casket itself placed with him in his tomb, lest someone should discover it. When Caesar wished to see the tomb of Hippocrates, he came and looked upon it. The tomb was very dilapidated, so he ordered that it be renovated and rebuilt and that [Hippocrates's body], if it were found intact, should be brought to him. When the tomb was excavated, this ivory casket was found within it, containing these excellent things. So it was brought to Caesar, who examined it and gave it to his friend and follower Misdos.

1. If [the patient] has pain or swelling of the face without cough and without other pain, and his right hand constantly scratches his chest or nostrils, he will die on the twenty-second day.

2. If both cheeks of someone suffering from frenzy are solid pink and swollen, and there is no digestion in the stomach, he will die on the ninth day. This disease begins with sweating and chills, cold ears, cold teeth.

3. There are three defects in the teeth: if [the patient's] mouth is in pain, if the veins of the neck bulge, and if he is asleep and just about deaf. And if he has hot pustules upon these veins and a little white stone appears there and if in his illness he desires hot baths or steam baths, he will die on the fiftieth day. This ailment happens to a person who desires hot baths.

4–5. Again, if pustules like small lentils appear under the tongue of someone who has a high *fever (causon), and if he desires baths or a steam bath, and the fever is in his inward parts, and if there is a small black swelling on his big toes, he will die on the seventh day.

6. Again, in a high fever, if a small pustule – not raised up, but flat – appears on the stomach or the sole of the right foot and [the patient] is full of the worst kind of *humor, and has no appetite, he will die on the twenty-first day.

7. Again, in a case of pneumonia, if blood comes out of [the patient's] thumb or a bloody pustule emerges from it, and if he sneezes frequently or latterly, he will die on the seventh day.

8. If [the patient's] liver hurts, and if two conjoined white pustules appear on his neck and throat, and the big toe of his right foot starts to itch a great deal, and later on he urinates and blood comes out, he will die on the seventh day.

9. Again, *cholera is an illness of a single day. If [the patient] does not improve on the same day, he will die on the third. These are the signs of cholera: if three pustules like scars appear next to the navel, to the left and right, one white, one somewhat livid, and the third pink, he will die on the same day.

10. If in [a patient] suffering from stomach pain, pustules like hazel-nuts appear on the eyebrows of the same color as the eyebrows, and he also feels pain, I know that he will die within four days.

11. If the spleen hurts and an odd number of white pustules appear on [the patient's] left hand and if rather foamy blood runs from his nose, he will die on the twelfth day.

12. If there is pain in the nose, and if on the left side there are thick red [patches] without pain, and if [the patient] consistently desires vegetables, he will die on the twenty-fifth day.

13. In a patient with dysentery, if a pustule resembling a plant appears behind his left ear, and if frequent thirst eventuates, he will die on the twenty-first day.

14. In those suffering from *lientery, if a hard white pustule appears on the left ear and abundant urine flows out, he will die on the twentieth day.

15. If *sanies exudes from any part of the body and if spots like Egyptian beans appear all over the body, he will die on the fifty-first day.

16. In one who is in pain from falling intestines, which the doctors call "hernia," should his right elbow become livid and he desire wine in his illness, he will die on the fifth day.

17. If there is pain in the bladder and a pustule like an apple appears in the arm-pit in the morning at the outset [of the disease] and [the patient] falls into a deep sleep, he will die on the fifteenth day.

18. When there is difficulty in urinating and many pustules like lentils appear on the left ear, and [the patient] in his illness rubs his eyes vigorously, he will die on the eleventh day.

19. If pustules appear on the soles of someone with hemorrhoids, he will die on the eighteenth day.

20. If in someone who is spitting up blood pustules like barley appear on the throat or saliva appears often on the chin, he will die on the twentieth day.

21. If in someone who has wounds or *fistulas or *rheumatic ulcers [?] or any kind of *aposteme, numerous solid white pustules appear on the neck or navel or next to the heart or near the vein that runs down the spine, he will die on the eleventh day.

b. Pseudo-Galenic *Signs of Impending Death*

Source: trans. Faith Wallis from the edition by Frederick S. Paxton, "Signa Mortifera: Death and Prognostication in Early Medieval Monastic Medicine," *Bulletin of the History of Medicine* 67 (1993): 649. Latin.

Galen took note of the signs in the body of impending death. In the human body, the forehead protrudes and the eyebrows slant downwards. The left eye becomes smaller. The tip of the nose turns white. The chin falls. The pulse slows. The feet grow cold. The belly loosens. A young man who is wakeful, and old man who sleeps. These are the signs of impending death.

CHAPTER TWO

CHRISTIANITY, DISEASE, AND MEDICINE

The Christian faith grew up in the age of Galen, and its historic fortunes intertwine with those of Galenism in a manner that is far from coincidental. Christianity held distinctive views on illness and healing, and these attitudes prevailed throughout the Middle Ages, though they were expressed in changing ways. Suffering was not something natural, but the unavoidable consequence of human sin; however, there was a distinction between one's own suffering, which was to be embraced with patience as a message or a test from God, and the suffering of others, which was to be relieved through Christian charity. Since God was the lord of nature, a disease could be at once natural and divine. One could treat it with secular medicine while at the same time acknowledging its moral meaning and adopting a suitable mental attitude of penance and submission. These avenues were not mutually exclusive. In fact, it was recommended that they be combined, but in the appropriate order: prayer first and foremost, then natural remedies. Strictly speaking, natural remedies were divine remedies: God the creator endowed plants with healing properties, and God was also the ultimate source of the physician's knowledge and skill. Christianity's process of coming to terms with Greco-Roman rational medicine was therefore one of conditional reconciliation. These conditions included privileging practical medicine, which could be appropriated for the work of charity, over theoretical medicine, which seemed either superfluous or potentially a threat to the notion of divine causes and cures.

*Much was at stake here, because Christianity was a religion of healing. It offered "salvation" – a word that in many languages, including Latin, is the same as that for "health" (*salus*). Acts of healing played an exceptionally important role in the revelation of the faith. In the Gospels, Christ's many miracles of healing were hailed as signs of salvation. Conversely, the salvation proclaimed by Christ's followers was destined to be consummated in a transcendent act of healing: the resurrection of the body at the end of time. Hence Christianity's principal rival in the world of late antiquity was not primarily the professional physician, but rather the healing god Asclepius. Asclepius, ancestor and divine patron of Hippocrates himself, treated his devotees with methods that were very like those of human physicians. But unlike the cures of his human counterparts, Asclepius's were immediate and exceptionally reliable. Over against Asclepius stood the Christian saint. Alive, the saint could through his merits receive the grace to replicate Christ's miracles of healing, which were also instantaneous and sure; dead, his relics served as a reservoir of sacred medicine, and his shrine, a sort of Christian Asklepion, became the resort of the sick. Like Asclepius as well, the saint healed within a framework of medical concepts and therapeutic expectations that were inherited from the pre-Christian world, though his power to heal came from the divine realm.*

Christianity continually asserted the primacy of spiritual healing through therapeutic rituals of prayer, anointing, and exorcism, but even these liturgical practices shared some important features with the medicine of classical antiquity.

I. SAINTS AS HEALERS

12. A SIXTH-CENTURY BYZANTINE SAINT DISPENSES MEDICAL ADVICE: THEODORE OF SYKEON

The cultural and religious landscape of late antiquity has come into much sharper focus over the past thirty years or so, thanks in large part to the remarkable work of the historian Peter Brown. According to Brown, the advent of Christianity signaled a crucial shift in the locus of divine power. Classical Mediterranean religion situated the divine in places (e.g., shrines or groves) or in impersonal channels such as oracles. Late antique religion, however, understood divine power as a force embodied in exceptional human beings: philosophers, mystics, wonder-workers, and, in the case of Christianity, martyrs and saints. Contact with a living "holy man" could result in physical healing, religious enlightenment, safety from danger, and even the resolution of social conflict. St Theodore of Sykeon was one such holy man. He lived in Anatolia, the central region of modern Turkey, at the end of the sixth century, a time when the eastern Roman Empire was under increasing attack from Persia. Some of the tension and uncertainty generated by this situation can be detected in the account of the saint's life. For the most part, however, Theodore's biography records the saint's exploits of healing, and these are quite typical of the range of early Christian medical miracles. The recipients include everyone from slave girls to the son of the emperor.

Source: trans. Elizabeth Dawes and Norman H. Baynes, *Three Byzantine Saints: Contemporary Biographies Translated from the Greek* (Oxford: Blackwell, 1948), pp. 146–48, 151–54, 156, 158, 181–82. Greek.

[St Theodore's "Holy Pharmacy"]

83. A woman living near Saint Theodore in the quarter of Sporacius brought her blind child of four years old to the saint who was lodging in the quarter of Varanas. He made the sign of the Cross over her eyes and blessed some water: with that she was to bathe her eyes every morning. This was done for three days and on the fourth day the child saw clearly. Her mother had previously been paralyzed, lying on her bed for seven months, but was cured by the saint's prayer.

[Exorcism of a Demon]

84. The slave girl of a magnate had been possessed secretly by a demon for twenty-eight years so that she was always ill and did not know what caused the malady. Her master brought her to the saint praying that either by death or a restoration to health she might be liberated from her sickness. Saint Theodore took hold of her head and prayed that the cause of her illness might be made known and driven away. Immediately the demon in her was disturbed and tore her, shouting: "You are burning me, ironeater, spare me, strangler of demons, I adjure you by the God who gives you power against me." Theodore bade the demon be silent and told the girl to return in a week's time. On the following Wednesday she came and once more the demon in her became excited and abusive: "Oh this violence that I suffer from this harlot's child! Twenty-eight years I have possessed this girl and none of the saints found me out, and now this harlot's son has come and has made me manifest and handed me over to dread punishment. Cursed be the day on which you were born and the day that brought you here!" Theodore rebuked the demon with the sign of the Cross: "Even if I am the harlot's son, nevertheless to the glory of our Lord Jesus Christ the Son of God I bid you in his name leave the girl and never take possession of her again." The demon shouted in reply: "I do your bidding and go out of her, but after three days she will die." The saint answered: "Come forth and the will of the Lord be done. For a God-fearing man may not trust you, since your words are vain and false." The demon tore the girl, threw her down at the saint's feet, and went out of her. And she, coming to herself, said: "It is through your holy prayers, father, that I have been healed, for I saw the demon coming out of my mouth like a foul crawling thing." Theodore prayed over her and dismissed her, bidding her remain in the church for seven days. And the word of the demon proved to be false, for after some days the girl and her master returned to the saint giving glory to God.

[Christian Therapy: Prayer and Anointing]

85. A woman who was paralyzed was brought to the saint by her attendants: he bade them put her on the ground: he seized hold of her head with his left hand, and stretching out his right hand to the East, he prayed to the God who gives healing and had cured the paralytic. He anointed her with oil, made the sign of the Cross over her, raised her up, and straightway she began to walk....

87. A sailor had been put under a spell by someone and was troubled by an unclean spirit: his limbs trembled and he suffered from many other symptoms

so that he was reduced to penury. The saint prayed over him and blessed oil with which he was to anoint himself and dismissed him. After some days the sailor returned cured to the saint: his affairs were prospering and "by way of fruitbearing and as a memento" he brought the tackle of his boat to Theodore, who was only induced to accept it after much insistence.

[St George Heals through a Dream]

88. A wrestler, wrought upon by an unclean spirit, suffered terribly in his head and all his limbs and came to the saint for healing. Theodore prayed over him and gave him wine and oil: "Go, my son," he said, "to your home and when you lie down to sleep on your bed in the evening anoint yourself with the wine and oil and whatever you see in a dream come and tell me." The next day the wrestler returned and said that in his sleep he had seen a young man wearing a cloak and "coming to me, as it seemed, from your holiness: he seized me by the hair of my head and drew me to himself and immediately all the pain was drawn off from my joints and bones and from all my limbs and through my hair there came forth, as it were, a violent wind." The man was cured and Theodore explained to him that the young man whom he had seen in his sleep was Christ's glorious martyr, George.

[The Saint Delivers a Prognosis]

The guardsman's wife, Theodora, besought the saint on behalf of herself and her husband to tell her which of them would die first. It was with great difficulty that the saint was persuaded to do as she wished; he prayed to God and received a revelation that her husband "would be short-lived in comparison with her." Day after day with many tears she besought Theodore to pray to God that he would quickly transport her from this present life. At last the saint was persuaded and prayed to his master Christ, who has a ready ear, to grant her desire. And assured by a divine revelation, he said to her: "God has granted your request; now look to yourself, for it will not be many days before you die." With great joy she set her affairs in order, and after forty days she departed from human life.

[Curing Sterility through "Christian Magic"]

93. Three men possessed by demons came to the saint. At that moment the Patriarch Kyriakus sent for Theodore, as he was accustomed to do. To two of the sufferers he gave relief at once, but the third he left to suffer terribly, for he was possessed by a demon who refused to yield. Theodore said to the

demon: "Since our most holy patriarch has sent for me and I am not free to deal with you at the moment, stand in the same place while you are being tortured and don't move from it until I come back." The saint then went to the patriarch and was with him for some hours. Sergius, deacon of the cathedral and attendant on the patriarch, had a daughter who had been married for three years but was still childless. So Sergius placed his daughter and her husband by the winding stairway of the crypt – the so-called "Side Door" – and he besought the saint's attendant, the subdeacon John, who was in the office of Thomas, the treasurer, to bring Theodore down that way when he was leaving the Patriarch. This was done, and Sergius brought husband and wife within the gates and all three knelt at his feet and begged him to give them a child. But he said to them: "Do not come to me, children, but to God and he will grant your request." But since they still remained beseeching him, he took the girdles of both of them and put one on one side of him and the other on the other and kneeling between them he made his prayer and gave them the girdles to wear. And by the grace of Christ a boy was born to them nine months later. And the saint having left by the so-called "Side Door," reached his lodging in the quarter of Euarane. John the subdeacon came with him to see if the demon had kept within the limit laid down for him. They found that he had not only kept the limit but was hanging above the ground. The demon swore by the Most High that he would go out – only let the saint spare him. But the saint lashed him on the chest saying: "Many a time have you agreed to this and have played me false. I will not give way to you." But the demon with many oaths promised to go out that same night when the wood was struck for service in the cathedral. And having received alleviation of his punishment, at the hour agreed upon the demon left the man and in the same way the other two sufferers having waited for three days with the saint were cured at the hour of the midnight service.

[Theodore Heals a Woman with an Issue of Blood]

96. A woman who had suffered for ten years from an issue of blood came for the saint's blessing, bringing an alabaster box with myrrh in it. Round Theodore she saw a great press of people and secretly mixed with the throng hoping to pour the myrrh on his feet. Knowing this, the saint gathered his feet up underneath him and called out to her: "Cease, woman; what do you intend to do? This is a grievous thing which you have planned to do to me," and in fear the woman gave him the myrrh and besought him to pray for her. And he prayed and said to her, "The Lord Jesus Christ, who knoweth secrets, will give effect to the mediation of the holy martyr George according

to your faith and he will fulfil your request." And immediately through God's grace the flow of blood was stayed and, declaring to all the miracle, she glorified God.

[Theodore Out-Performs the Doctors]

97. It happened that one of the children of the emperor Maurice fell ill of an incurable disease (for many sores had broken out on the child's body, so that it seemed to be a case of elephantiasis, a disease which some call "Paulakis," and others "Kleopatra") and, although the physicians had tried many remedies, nothing had done the child any good.

So the emperor sent for the holy man and had him fetched from the city to the palace at Hiereia (for thither the emperor had made a progress and there the child was lying); the servant of God said a prayer over the child and blessed some water; he bathed the child with it and left the rest for a further treatment; and through his holy prayer the child was cured of the disease and was restored to health. And at the invitation of the emperor and the augusta [*that is, the empress*] he dined with them and then he took his leave of them after giving them his blessing, and went his way, journeying to his own country, and thus reached his monastery.

[Healing through Relics of the Saint]

100. The blessed man greatly longed to find some relics of the glorious and victorious martyr George, and prayed to the latter to satisfy this longing. Now Aemilianus, the very holy bishop of Germia, had a piece of the martyr's head and one finger of a hand and one of his teeth and another small piece. So the martyr appeared to the bishop and exhorted him to give these relics to his servant Theodore for the church that the latter had built in his honor. The bishop sent to the monastery to the servant of God and invited him to come and offer up prayers in the venerable Church of the Archangel in order that he might welcome him and give him the much-desired relics of the martyr. Theodore was filled with joy by this promise and left the monastery and went to the town of Germia and offered up prayer in the Church of the Archangel. The very holy bishop, Aemilianus, welcomed him warmly, and then conducted him to the monastery of the Mother of God, called of Aligete....

102. In those days Stephen, the bishop of Cadossia (which is under the jurisdiction of Nicomedia) came in a litter; for he suffered from gout in his hands and was paralyzed in all his limbs and could not even convey his food

to his mouth with his own hands, but his attendants had to supply his every need. He was carried thus into the church of the Archangel and fell at the blessed Theodore's feet crying and saying, "Have pity upon me, servant of the most high God and amongst all the others grant that I, too, may have my share in your miracles; for I know that God will give you whatsoever you ask." When the servant of Christ heard that he was a bishop, he was grieved at his act of obeisance and implored him to rise; then standing in prayer he besought God to dispel the bishop's diseases. After the prayer he ordered him to be laid on the right hand side of the church of the holy martyr George, that is, in the adjoining oratory of the holy martyr Plato (where Theodore's own cage stood), and he said to the bishop, "Be of good courage, my lord, for I trust to the goodness of God to release you from this sickness shortly." He also blessed and gave to him some oil for anointing himself and in two weeks the bishop was restored to health and after he had received the blessing of Theodore he left the monastery "walking and leaping and praising God [Acts 3:8]."

13. THE MEDICAL WORLD OF GREGORY OF TOURS: PLAGUES, DOCTORS, AND SAINTS

Gregory of Tours (ca 538/539–594) was proud of his connections, both on earth and in heaven. As bishop of one of the most important cities in Merovingian Gaul, he was also the guardian and publicist of the kingdom's premier saint, Martin of Tours (ca 335–397). Gregory exploited his first-hand knowledge of the court and the clergy in the ten books of his Histories; *he celebrated his celestial patrons in numerous works of hagiography, notably in* The Life and Miracles of the Blessed Martin. *Martin's sanctity was definitely a kind of power, the spiritual equivalent of the social authority of a worldly grandee. For his clients, the saint was an advocate before God, a protector, and rescuer. He manifested his presence principally by healing the sick and afflicted; not infrequently, this healing also involved release from other more intangible kinds of oppression.*

In both his historiography and his hagiography, Gregory sought to convey a particular understanding of the relationship of sacred power to events in human life. The power of God and his saints, mediated by the Church and especially by bishops, was true, invincible, and benevolent. Good people acknowledged the supremacy of this power and comported themselves before it with perfect sincerity and reverence; bad people acted in defiance of this hegemony, or worse yet, behaved as if it did not exist. And yet Gregory himself often seems uncertain about the signs of divine power in the world; the bad apparently go unpunished, the good sometimes suffer, and even bishops cannot always read the meaning of events.

In this context, it is not surprising that Gregory's accounts of sickness and healing display all the complexity characteristic of the Christian attitude toward medicine. The plague of Marseilles described in book 9 of the Histories *occurred in 588. Typically, Gregory describes the plague as at once a spiritual and a natural event, a summons to penance and a communicable disease, and his account ends on an ambivalent note. In* The Life and Miracles of the Blessed Martin, *he paints the saint as a supreme physician whose acts of healing often mirror the therapies of secular medicine. Indeed, Gregory displays some rather detailed knowledge of medicine (one might compare the account of the cataract operation that Theudomer did not have to undergo with Benvenutus Grassus's description of the procedure in doc. 63). Hagiographers typically set up secular doctors as foils for saintly prowess, but Gregory takes a more nuanced approach. His accounts of his own illness and miraculous cures casually reveal the presence of secular doctors at his bedside. The doctor, of course, fails to cure Gregory, but he is neither mocked nor blamed.*

a. Plague in Marseilles

Source: trans. O.M. Dalton, Gregory of Tours, *The History of the Franks* (Oxford: Clarendon Press, 1927), book 9, c. 21–22, vol. 2, pp. 394–96. Latin.

21. At this time it was reported that Marseilles was ravaged by a plague affecting [that is, causing swellings in] the groin, which had rapidly spread to a village called Octavus near Lyons [*modern Saint-Symphorien-d'Ozon*]. The king [Guntram of Burgundy], like some good bishop providing the remedies to heal the scars of a people that had sinned, commanded every one to assemble in the great church and Rogations [*that is, fasting and petitionary prayers*] to be celebrated there with the utmost devotion; nothing was to be taken by way of nourishment but barley bread and pure water; all were to be constant in keeping the vigils. His orders were obeyed. For three days the largess of his alms much exceeded his wonted amount, and he was so anxious for the whole people that he might have been taken not merely for their king but also for one of the Lord's bishops. All his hope was now set on the Lord's mercy; all [his prayers] he threw upon God, through whose power he believed with a whole and perfect faith they should be brought to good effect. It was commonly told by the faithful that a certain woman, whose son was sick of a *quartan *ague and lay uneasily upon his bed, came up through the crowd immediately behind the king, and tore off by stealth some particles of the fringe of his royal mantle. These she steeped in water, which she gave her son to drink; and immediately the *fever was quenched, and he was made whole. I cannot doubt the story, since I myself have often heard evil spirits in

the hour of their possession invoking the king's name, and confessing their crimes, compelled by his miraculous power.

22. The city of Marseilles being afflicted, as I have just said, by a most grievous pestilence, I deem it well to unfold from the beginning how much it endured. At that time Bishop Theodore had journeyed to the king to make some complaint against the patrician Nicetius. King Childebert would scarce give ear to the matter, so [the bishop] prepared to return home. In the meantime a ship had put into port with the usual merchandise from Spain, unhappily bringing the tinder which kindled this disease. Many citizens purchased various objects from the cargo, and soon a house inhabited by eight people was left empty, every one of them being carried off by the contagion. The fire of the plague did not spread immediately through all the houses in the place; but there was a certain interval, and then the whole city blazed with the pest[ilence], like a cornfield set aflame. Nevertheless the bishop came back, and abode within the walls of the church of [St] Victor with the few who remained beside him; there throughout the whole calamity he gave himself up to prayers and vigils, imploring God's mercy that at last the destruction might have an end, and peace and quiet be granted to the people. After two months the affliction ceased, and the people returned, thinking the danger overpast. But the plague began once more, and all who had returned perished. On several other occasions Marseilles was afflicted by this [disease].

b. Healers Secular and Spiritual

Source: trans. Raymond Van Dam from the *Liber de virtutibus sancti Martini episcopi*, book 2, c. 1, 19–20, 56, 58, 60, in *Saints and their Miracles in Late Antique Gaul* (Princeton: Princeton University Press, 1993), pp. 228–29, 238, 256–59. Latin.

The Life and Virtues of St Martin, Bishop [of Tours], Book 2

1. How I Was Rescued from a Fever and Dysentery

One hundred and seventy-two years after the death of the blessed Bishop Martin and in the twelfth year of the reign of the most glorious Sigibert [in 573], I, although unworthy, received the burden of the episcopacy [at Tours] after the death of the bishop St Eufronius, not because of my merit, for I am morally very corrupt and bound by my sins, but because of the assistance of a devoted God who summons those [qualities] that do not exist as if they did. In the second month after my consecration I suffered from dysentery and a high fever while I was at a villa, and I began to suffer so badly that I completely gave up any hope of living, because death was imminent. Frequently my digestive system vomited undigested food that it could not absorb, and I was repelled by food; and as the efficiency of my stomach weakened from fasting, the fever was all the more sustenance for my body. Even expensive relief was unavailable. For there was a sharp pain that penetrated my entire stomach and went down to my intestines and that consumed me with its torment no less than the fever had distressed me. And when I reached the point that no hope of life was left, that all my thoughts were turned toward my funeral, and that the antidote of my doctor had no effect, I despaired about myself, because death had delivered me up for destruction. I called Armentarius, my doctor, and I said to him: "You have offered all the wisdom of your skill, and you have already tested the strength of all your salves, but the devices of this world have been of no use to me who am about to die. One option remains for me to try; let me show you a powerful antidote. Fetch dust from the most sacred tomb of lord [Martin], and then mix a drink for me. If this dust is not effective, every refuge for escaping [death] has been lost." Then a deacon was sent to the aforementioned tomb of the blessed champion. He brought back some of the sacred dust that they mixed [in water] and gave me to drink. As soon as I drank it, all the pain vanished, and I received my health from the tomb. The assistance available at that tomb was so effective that after this [cure] had occurred at the third hour, on the same day at the sixth hour I was healthy and went for a meal....

19. Theudomer, a Blind Deacon

... The deacon Theudomer suffered from a swelling on his head; when *cataracts developed, the openings to his eyes were painfully blocked for four years. Then he went to the cell at Candes in which the blessed man [Martin] had died. He knelt at his bed and spent the entire night [there] without moving; he moistened the ground with his tears and cherished the venerable wood of the railing with his sighs. When daylight came, the cataracts on his eyes were opened, and he deserved to see the daylight. What [cure] such as this one have doctors ever accomplished with their implements? Their efforts produce more pain than healing; and after stretching and piercing an eye with their needles they fashion the torments of death before they open the eye. If caution is lacking in this operation, the doctor is providing eternal blindness for the wretched patient. But the blessed confessor's implement is his affection, and his ointment is simply his power.

20. Desiderius, a Possessed Man

Desiderius was a possessed man who came from Clermont. After he had raved madly for an entire night in this cell [at Candes], at dawn he began to shout that the blessed Martin was burning him. As he was shouting, he coughed up an unfamiliar pus and blood; the demon was cast out, and he was cleansed. He left behind sand stained with his blood, and he departed from the cell as a healthy man....

56. The Woman Whose Fingers Were Bent into Her Palm and Who Came [to Tours]

In a similar fashion a woman from Poitiers next deserved to receive a remedy. Her fingers were bent into her palm, her fingernails were, if I may say so, piercing her bones, and her entire hand was already decayed. This pious woman came to the saint's festival [on 11 November, 580] and requested the medicine she hoped for. When the ceremonies were completed as usual, she said to her companions: "I came with a pure heart to request the assistance of the blessed [Martin], but because my sins were an obstacle, I did not deserve to receive what I sought. Now that my prayer is finished, let me return to my homeland still believing, through the goodness of my champion, that a prayer that is faithful to the heart might benefit a feeble body." After repeating these and similar words as if saying goodbye to the saint, she left. As the daylight was turning into evening, she took lodging along the bank of the Cher River. About midnight she was awakened and gave thanks to God because she still survived, because she was alive, because she was flourishing, and because she had touched the tomb of the blessed bishop. She offered her gratitude while weeping loudly, and then fell asleep again. And behold, a man stood before her who had hair that was white as a swan, who was dressed in purple, and who was carrying a cross in his hand. The man said: "In the name of Christ our Redeemer now you will be healed." Then he took her hand, placed his own finger among her fingers that were closed in her palm, moved them a bit, and straightened them. As she was seeing this in her dream, the woman awoke and, in praise of God, held up her hand that was healthy even though blood was still flowing from it. She returned to the church, gave thanks, and left rejoicing....

58. Another Boy Who Was Blind and Crippled

A boy from Paris had the skill of sewing clothes. Because he was attacked by *melancholy, that is, by a sediment of boiled blood, he suffered from a quartan fever; and as his swelling increased, his entire body was so afflicted with tiny blisters that he was thought by some to be a leper. He also suffered terrible pains in all his limbs, and he was deprived of sight in both eyes. After he heard about the reputation of the blessed bishop and his miracles that were publicized everywhere, this boy went to Tours. He came to the saint's church, and after fasting and praying for many days he recovered his sight and was restored to his earlier health. He was by birth free. But when Leudast, who was at that time count of Tours, heard that he was a talented tailor, he began to spread lies and said: "You have run away from your masters, and it will no longer be possible for you to wander about." Then he ordered that the boy must be bound and imprisoned at his own house. But the power of the angelic confessor was not lacking there. For when the boy was seized, immediately he was afflicted with the illness that he had just eliminated. Once the count saw that he could have no power over the boy who was suffering so badly, he ordered him to be released from his chains and to depart with his freedom. The boy returned to the church and was again healed....

60. The Pain in My Eyes and My Headache

... For after I had described fifty-nine miracles in this book [Book 2 of *The Life and Miracles*], and while I was still eagerly waiting for a sixtieth miracle, suddenly the temple on the left side of my head was contracted with pains. My veins twitched, tears flowed down, and such great agony afflicted me that I pressed hard on my eye to prevent it from bursting. I suffered from this pain for an entire day and night, and in the morning I went to the saint's church and knelt for prayer. At the conclusion of my prayer I touched the painful spot to the curtain that was hanging in front of the blessed tomb. As soon as this spot was touched, my veins stopped twitching and my tears stopped flowing. Three days later a similar pain attacked the right side of my head. My veins twitched and tears gushed down. Again I got up in the morning, touched my head to the curtain in the same manner as before, and left with my health. Ten days later it seemed best [that I should undergo bloodletting]; but three days after letting my blood I thought that my sufferings were due to my blood and that they would immediately cease if a vein was at once cut; I think that this idea was inspired by a deceiving [demon]. While I was considering and debating this idea, the veins in both temples twitched, and the pain that had existed previously was repeated and now attacked my entire head, not just one part. Because I was disturbed by these pains, I hurried to the church, requested forgiveness for my wicked idea, and touched my head with the shroud that covered the blessed tomb. Soon the pain was stopped, and I left the tomb with my health.

14. A RELUCTANT BISHOP-HEALER: JOHN OF BEVERLEY

Bede the Venerable (ca 675–735) passed almost all his life as a monk of the monastery of Jarrow in Northumbria, England. He was a prolific and versatile author of biblical commentaries, didactic treatises, and various genres of history. His Ecclesiastical History of the English People, *completed in 731, is the work for which he is best known today. It presents the story of the coming of Christianity to Anglo-Saxon England as a portrait gallery of saintly pioneers; their example was expected to inspire Bede's contemporaries but also to rebuke what he saw as the more tepid religion of his own day. One of these figures was John of Beverley (d. 721). Educated at Canterbury under the Greek archbishop Theodore of Tarsus and the deacon Hadrian, John became a monk at Whitby and in 687 was consecrated as bishop of Hexham. It was John who ordained Bede as both deacon and priest, and Bede's deep reverence for the man is evident.*

Bede explicitly regards John's acts of healing as miracles, and yet he portrays John himself as being somewhat reluctant to embrace this interpretation. The miracles certainly do not conform to hagiographic conventions. John's healing of the dumb boy begins with a prayer but quickly moves into speech therapy; moreover, the lad's scurf is treated in the ordinary way by a physician. Bede also reveals that John had acquired some knowledge of classical medicine at Canterbury; hence he considers the nun's inflamed arm to be the natural consequence of bloodletting when the moon was waxing (see doc. 57). Moreover, the nun's healing is not instantaneous or total, as is usually the case when a saint is the healer. These are, so to speak, rather natural miracles.

Incidentally, Bede devoted a chapter of his work The Reckoning of Time *(composed in 725) to the natural effects of the lunar cycle on all things fluid, from ocean tides to the inner *humors of living things. As this material is not found in his youthful* On the Nature of Things *or* On Times, *its inclusion in the later work may have been inspired by the miracle of John of Beverley.*

Source: ed. and trans. Bertram Colgrave and R.A.B. Mynors, Bede, *Ecclesiastical History of the English People*, book 5, c. 2–3, (Oxford: Clarendon Press, 1969), pp. 457–63. Latin.

Book 5, Chapter 2

At the beginning of Aldfrith's reign, Bishop Eata died and was succeeded as bishop of the church at Hexham by a holy man named John. Many miracles were told of him by those who knew him well and especially by the most reverend and truthful Berhthun, once his deacon but now abbot of the monastery called *Inderauuda* [Beverley], that is, "in the wood of the men of Deira." We have thought it fitting to preserve the memory of some of these miracles.

There is a remote dwelling, enclosed by a rampart and amid scattered trees, not far from the church at Hexham, about a mile and a half away, and separated from it by the river Tyne. It has an oratory dedicated to St Michael the archangel in which the man of God with a few others very often used to devote himself to prayer and reading when a favorable opportunity occurred, and especially in Lent. On one occasion, when he had come there to stay at the beginning of Lent, he told his followers to seek out some poor man who was afflicted by a serious disease or in dire need, to have with him during these days and to benefit from their charity; for this was his constant custom. There was in a village not far away a dumb youth known to the bishop, who often used to come to him to receive alms and had never been able to utter a single word. Besides this, he had so much scabbiness and scurf on his head that no hair could grow on the crown save for a few rough hairs which stuck out around it. The bishop had this young man brought and ordered a little hut to be built for him in the enclosure of their dwelling, in which he could stay and receive his daily allowance. On the second Sunday in Lent, he ordered the poor man to come in to him and then he told him to put out his tongue and show it to him. Thereupon he took him by the chin and made the sign of the holy cross upon his tongue; after this he told him to put his tongue in again and say something. "Say some word," he said, "say *gæ*," which in English is the word of assent and agreement, that is, yes. He said at once what the bishop told him to say, the bonds of his tongue being unloosed. The bishop then added the names of the letters: "Say A," and he said it. "Say B," and he said that too. When he had repeated the names of the letters after the bishop, the latter added syllables and words for the youth to repeat after him. When he had repeated them all, one after the other, the bishop taught him to say longer sentences, which he did. After that those who were present relate that he never ceased all that day and night, as long as he could keep awake, to talk and to reveal the secrets of his thoughts and wishes to others which he could never do before. He was like the man who had long been lame, who, when healed by the Apostles Peter and John, stood up, leapt and walked, entering the Temple with them, walking and leaping and praising God [Acts 3:2–8], rejoicing to have the use of his feet of which he had so long been deprived. The bishop rejoiced with him at his cure and ordered the physician to undertake to heal his scabby head. He did as he was bidden and, with the help of the bishop's blessing and prayers, his skin was healed and he grew a beautiful head of hair. So the youth gained a clear complexion, ready speech, and beautiful curly hair, whereas he had once been ugly, destitute, and dumb. So rejoicing in his new-found health he returned home, which he preferred to do though the bishop offered him a permanent place in his own household.

Chapter 3

Berhthun told another miracle which the bishop performed. The reverend Wilfrid was restored to the bishopric of the church of Hexham after a long exile, and the same John, upon the death of Bosa, a man of great holiness and humility, was made bishop of York in his place. He went on a certain occasion to a monastery of nuns in a place called *Wetadun* [Watton], over which Abbess Hereburh was at that time presiding. "After we had arrived," he said, "and had been joyfully received by them all, the abbess told us that one of the nuns, who was her own daughter, was afflicted by a grievous illness. She had recently been bled in the arm and, while still under treatment, was seized with a sudden pain which rapidly increased. Her wounded arm grew worse and became so much swollen that it could hardly be encircled with both hands. She was lying in bed and seemed likely to die through the violence of the pain. The abbess asked the bishop to deign to visit her and give her his blessing, believing that she would greatly improve if he blessed or touched her. Then he asked when the girl had been bled and, on hearing that it was on the fourth day of the moon, he exclaimed, 'You have acted foolishly and ignorantly to bleed her on the fourth day of the moon; I remember how Archbishop Theodore of blessed memory used to say that it was very dangerous to bleed a patient when the moon is waxing and the ocean tide flowing. And what can I do for the girl if she is at the point of death?' but the abbess entreated him still more urgently on behalf of her daughter, whom she loved greatly and had planned to make abbess in her place. At last she persuaded him to visit the sick girl. So, taking me with him, he went in to where the maiden was lying, suffering great pain as I have said, and with her arm so swollen that she could not bend her elbow. He stood by her, said a prayer over her, blessed her, and went out. Afterwards, when we were sitting at the table at the usual hour, someone came and called me out saying, 'Cwenburh' – that was the girl's name – 'asks you to come back to her at once.' I did so and as I went in I found her looking much more cheerful and apparently healed. As I sat by her she said, 'Shall we ask for something to drink?' I answered, 'Yes, indeed, and if you can drink I shall be delighted.' A vessel was brought and when we had both drunk she said to me, 'After the bishop had prayed for me, given me his blessing, and gone away, I felt better at once, and though I have not yet recovered my full strength, all the pain has entirely gone from my arm where it was most violent and from my whole body, just as if the bishop himself had carried it away, although the swelling still seems to persist in my arm.' After we had gone the dreadful swelling departed as the pain had done and the maiden, saved from suffering and death, gave thanks to her Savior and Lord, with all the other servants of his who were there."

15. A CAROLINGIAN THERAPEUTIC PASSION OF SAINTS COSMAS AND DAMIAN

The twin brothers Cosmas and Damian, doctors and saints, were allegedly martyred in Cilicia during the reign of Diocletian (284–305 CE). Their cult, which enjoyed enormous popularity in the early medieval West, illustrates both the willingness of Christianity to absorb the ancient tradition of professional medicine and its ambivalence about this act of appropriation. In his poem on the arrangement of a library, Isidore of Seville ranged Cosmas and Damian alongside Hippocrates and Galen as great medical sages; so does the poem on medical ethics included in the Lorsch Leechbook *(doc. 88). Their legend was copied into manuscript medical compilations, perhaps as a Christian substitute for the traditional pagan histories of medicine found in texts such as Isidore's* Etymologies *(doc. 1). In fact, in the ninth-century medical manuscript from which the text translated below is taken, the* passio *of the saints precedes a text entitled* Epitome perodeotecon, *which offers a religious account of the origins of disease and healing.*

However, this passio *focuses less on Cosmas and Damian's feats of healing than on their trial and grisly execution. Indeed, the text itself, if read over the bed of a sick person, was supposed to be therapeutic. The suffering patient could perhaps identify with the agonies of the martyrs, learn from their patience, and hope for their intercession. Our* passio *is preceded in the manuscript by a guide to recognizing the signs of impending death (see doc. 11b), which suggests that it was part of a ritual for the critically ill. But it is also hedged about with numerous medical tracts and recipes – further evidence of how sacred and secular therapies blended inextricably in the early medieval world.*

Source: trans. Faith Wallis from Paris, Bibliothèque nationale de France MS lat. 11218 (ca 800, Burgundy), fols. 2r–5v. Latin.

Here begins the passion of Saints Cosmas and Damian, doctors. The Lord will have mercy on anyone who is ill, when this passion is read over him.

In those days, there was a certain woman named Theodata who feared God all her life long from her childhood and who continued steadfast in all the laws of the Lord. She acknowledged God with alms and with a pure heart, steadfast in rectitude according to the law of the Lord, and by living a very holy life. She conceived and gave birth to two sons named Cosmas and Damian. She raised them with great care to live a righteous life. She taught them Holy Writ, but the servants of the Lord were taught the whole art of medicine by the revelation of the Holy Spirit. In accordance with the divine scriptures they treated every infirmity and every debility among the people and never demanded a fee. They cured not only people, but also animals. And among the sick they cured were the blind, that they might receive the light of Christ. They cured the weak and expelled demons.

Now at that time, there was a certain woman named Palladia, who was gravely ill and who had spent all her fortune on doctors. But she came to the blessed Cosmas and Damian, asking them in all confidence to visit her. Seeing the faith of this woman, they consented to her [request] and in the name of Jesus Christ, they cured her. Knowing that she was made whole by their intercession, the woman praised God. And hearing that they demanded absolutely nothing in the way of a fee, she offered St Damian only three eggs. The servant of God did not wish to receive them, but [God's] handmaid adjured him in the name of the Almighty to take them. When he heard the name of the Lord, he took the eggs; there were only three. When his brother Cosmas heard this, he was deeply grieved. And he gave an order to his household that after his death, they should not lay his body beside that of his brother Damian. And when he had delivered this order, on that same night, the Lord appeared to his servant Cosmas, saying "Why did you say such a thing about my servant taking three eggs? For he did not receive them as a fee, but because he was adjured in the name of God, and this is no sin."

At that time these two brothers came to a certain place. And an animal [called] a camel had a foot that had been broken by a devil. Putting medicines on it, they healed the camel and sent it on its way to its pasture.

When the blessed martyrs of God performed many mighty works and signs in the name of Christ, the emperors Diocletian and Maximinus heard of these miracles done in the name of Christ, and so did the governor Lysias whom they appointed over the tribunal in Aegae. [Lysias] was told by the priests of the [pagan] idols that the blessed brothers Cosmas and Damian were Christians who went about the cities and provinces healing the sick by the art of medicine and expelling demons. Seeing this [they said]; "They draw away worshippers of our gods ..." When he heard this, the governor ordered some of his officers to bring [Cosmas and Damian] before him. The holy brothers stood before the tribunal of governor Lysias.

Looking upon them, he said, "Why do you go about the cities and provinces and lure people away from our most sacred gods? If you do [not] worship these most sacred [gods], I will torture you with torments. But first, tell me what province you are from." They answered: "If you wish to know, we are from the province of the East. And these are our names: I am Cosmas and my brother is Damian; for we are Christians and from a prominent family. We have other brothers as well and if you want to know their names, we will tell you. The names of our brothers are Leoncius, Anthimius, and Euprepius." The governor ordered them to come before him.

When they had come, the governor said: "Think about what will procure your release. Come up here and sacrifice to our gods. Otherwise I shall torture you with hideous torments." The holy martyrs replied with vehemence: "You are mistaken, O governor. On the contrary, you blaspheme our Lord Jesus Christ, but your blasphemy will fall upon your head. We, however, are not afraid in the least of your torments nor are we frightened by your threats in any way. We will not adore your gods – deaf, blind, and mute idols of stone, wood, and lead." When he heard this, the governor ordered their hands to be bound and for them to be stoned until they confessed that the idols were gods. But the saints, when this was announced, said: "Lord thou has been our refuge from one generation to another; before the heavens were brought forth or ever the earth and the world were made, thou art God from everlasting and world without end [Ps. 90 (89):1–2]. Free us from the snare of the Devil and of Lysias his son. For in you we trust, O Lord, and yours is the glory forever." And the holy martyrs stood before Lysias, saying these prayers. When they threw stones upon them, the stones rebounded on those who cast them and they were slain, while the martyrs remained constant in their faith. They said "O most wicked governor, if you have torments even more cruel, then let us have them, that you may know that nothing can terrify us in the name of Christ; nor do we feel your torments, since you see your guards and executioners slain. For the glory of Christ aids us." The governor said: "I will persuade you with similar torments. I therefore order you to be cast into the sea bound in chains." God's martyrs, when they were led to the sea, rejoiced and sang psalms, saying: "I have delighted in the way of thy testimonies, O Christ most high, and in thy commands as if in all riches [Ps. 119 (118):14]. A spiritual table of salvation for our souls [are you] against those who trouble us, for yours is the power for ever and ever, amen." Singing these psalms, the holy martyrs came to the place. As they were commanded, the attendants threw them into the sea. Immediately, the angel of the Lord broke their chains and pulled them out of the sea unharmed. The attendants went to the judge and reported what they had seen. Then the judge ordered them to be put into a very dark dungeon. As they were led off, the blessed martyrs sang psalms, saying: "Sing unto the Lord a new song, for the Lord has done marvelous things. With his right hand and his arm has he saved us [Ps. 98 (97):1]. He has made us strong and saved us from the hand of the devil and his henchmen." Singing these psalms, they were sent into the prison. On the next day, the governor ordered that they be brought before him. When they were brought forth, they sang psalms thus, saying, "O Lord, give us help in our trouble, for vain is the help of man [Ps. 60:11 (59:13)]." When they came before the governor, he said to them, "You still persist in your madness." The holy martyrs answered, "Hear, you enemy of the truth: we are Christians to the end. In truth we say and will not deny that God is creator of all. So now, do whatever you wish to us, for we will never consent to worship an alien god." When he heard this, the governor was wild with rage. He ordered that kindling and wood be brought and a great fire lit. But the saints walked through the midst of the fire, exulting, and saying, "To thee O Lord we lift up our eyes, O you who dwell in the heavens, have mercy upon us [Ps. 123 (122):1]. Look upon us, Lord Jesus Christ, lest they say who are devoid of God and who do not know your name, 'Where is their God in whom they

II. RITUALS OF HEALING

16. ST SIGISMUND, PATRON OF SUFFERERS FROM FEVER

The cult of St Sigismund illustrates the fusion of saintly charisma with liturgical and para-liturgical rituals of healing. King Sigismund of Burgundy was a convert from Arianism to Catholicism, and founder of the powerful monastery of St Maurice at Agaune in the Valais (Switzerland). In 523, he was murdered by Chlodomer, one of the sons of the Frankish king Clovis; his remains were translated to St Maurice by the abbot Venerandus in 535/36. Gregory of Tours, in his Glory of the Martyrs, *says that people suffering from *fevers not only prayed to Sigismund, but offered a mass in his honor. Indeed, the mass of St Sigismund is one of the earliest examples of a votive mass — a Eucharistic celebration offered for a particular purpose of petition or thanksgiving. The mass is preserved in slightly different forms in a number of early liturgical manuscripts: some of these alternative versions are presented here.*

*The votive mass was a kind of surrogate pilgrimage or substitute relic, for it allowed the devotee access to the healing power of the saint in any place where the mass was sung. For those who could not arrange for (or perhaps afford) a votive mass, there was an even readier form of help: a Christian "charm" (*carmen*) invoking St Sigismund — half prayer, half conjuration — designed to be read over the body of the feverish patient. Though the idea of a Christian charm may seem shocking, such texts were not always considered problematic in the early medieval period. The difference between prayer and illicit magic lay not so much in the form of the words, but in the nature of the power invoked: if the words were addressed to God and his saints, they were acceptable. In this case, the charm contains quotations from the Gospels, a sort of litany, and formulas that resemble exorcism.*

a. The Mass of St Sigismund

Source: trans. Faith Wallis from *The Bobbio Missal: A Gallican Mass-Book (Ms Paris Lat. 13246)*, ed. E.A. Lowe, Henry Bradshaw Society 58 (London: Harrison and Sons, 1920), pp. 101–2, and from the sacramentary of Autun, *Liber sacramentorum Augustodunesis*, ed. O Heiming, Corpus christianorum: series latina 159B (Turnhout: Brepols, 1984), p. 269. Latin.

Lections for the Mass of St Sigismund (Bobbio Missal Version)
Epistle of the Apostle John to the Gentiles [1 John 2:15–16]. Brothers, love not the world nor the things which are of the world. [If any man love the world, the love of the Father is not in him. For all that is in the world, and the lust of the eyes] and the pride of life [is not of the Father, but of the world.]

A reading from the holy Gospel according to Matthew [4:23–24]. In those days the Lord Jesus traveled throughout Galilee teaching in their synagogues and proclaiming the gospel of the kingdom and healing every illness and every disease in the people. And his fame spread throughout all Syria, and they brought unto him all who were ill with various illnesses and torments and he cured them.

Mass of St Sigismund the King (Bobbio Missal Version)

Beloved brothers, let us beseech the almighty Lord, who through the apostles and martyrs bestows diverse gifts of health, that he may in his compassion cure this his servant N., who is burdened with the affliction of *quartan fever, through the prayers of his faithful servant Sigismund, conferring on us his merits, and on this man treatment (*medicinam*).

Secret. Incline, O Lord, your tender grace to the desires of those who supplicate you, and what they ask with devout heart, grant of your favor. In your compassion, receive the prayers of your faithful servant Sigismund on behalf of your servant N. who is tormented by the shaking of a quartan fever. Throw open [the saint's] merits to us, and confer upon the patient ready healing.

Preface to the Prayer of Consecration (Sacramentary of Autun Version)

Preface. It is meet and right, almighty and everliving God, to give you thanks always and everywhere, through Jesus Christ our Lord: for you smite your servants in the body so that they may grow in spirit, openly revealing the radiant salvation of your loving kindness, so that sickness itself may work health within us. For you, O Lord, are our God, in whom grace and mercy are equal, and who granted the triumph of martyrdom to your chosen one, King Sigismund. Yours are these gifts, Almighty Lord and Father, so that by the communion of the body and blood of your son Jesus Christ our Lord and in honor of your chosen one, King Sigismund, you may deign to drive away the storms of chills and repel the heat of fevers and recall this your servant to his former health, by him [through] whom you restored Peter's mother-in-law when she lay sick with a fever to full bodily health, [namely] Jesus Christ the savior of the world, through whom the angels offer praise.

b. The Sigismund Fever Charm

Source: trans. Faith Wallis, from Dijon, Bibl. municipale MS 448 (s. XI in.) fol. 181r, transcribed by Ernest Wickersheimer, *Les manuscrits latins de médecine du haut moyen âge dans les bibliothèques de France*, Documents, études et répertoires publiés par l'Institut de Recherche et d'Histoire des Textes, 11 (Paris: C.N.R.S., 1966), pp. 32–33. Latin.

Every day for three days [read this] three times over the fever-sufferer and he will be healed. Charm against fevers. In the name of the Father and the Son and the Holy Spirit. Amen. Behold the cross of the triune Lord. Christ was born: on. bon. jon. Christ suffered: don. ron. con. Christ rose from the dead: ton. son. yon. When the Lord Jesus had entered into the house of Simon Peter, he saw [Peter's] mother-in-law lying ill with a fever, and standing over her, he commanded the fever and dismissed it, and immediately she ministered to him [Matt. 8:14–15; Luke 4:38–39]. Syon. Syon. Syon. For the commemoration of St Sigismund, king: free your servant N., Lord God. In the name of the Father, I speak to you, O fevers. In the name of the Son, I speak against you. In the name of the Holy Spirit, I conjure you, O fevers. You are seven sisters. The first of you is called Lilia. The second, Restilia. The third Fugalia [*that is, "fleeing"*]. The fourth Suffoca [*"choking"*]. The fifth Affrica. The sixth Julia. The seventh Macha. If you are *quotidian, biduan, tertian, quartan or quintan or sextan or septiman or octavan or nonan or whatever kind you are, I conjure you and join issue with you by the Father and the Son and the Holy Spirit, and by the seat of the majesty and by the Hagia Sophia [*the Holy Wisdom*] and by the holy Trinity and by St Mary mother of our Lord Jesus Christ, and by St Michael the Archangel, and Gabriel, and Raphael who is called "medicine of God," and by the holy angels and archangels, the thrones and dominions, principalities and powers and virtues of the heavens, and by the cherubim and the seraphim. I conjure you and join issue with you by the Father and the Son and the Holy Spirit, and by the living Lord and the true Lord and the holy Lord, and the four evangelists, Matthew, Mark, Luke, and John and by the 144,000 Innocents, and by the Lamb of God, the Son of the Father, and by those powers which contain heaven and earth, and by St John the Baptist who baptized the Lord God in the River Jordan. I conjure you and speak against you by the majesty of the Father and the Son and the Holy Spirit, and by the Lord's annunciation, and by the Lord's advent and by the [Lord's] circumcision, by the baptism of the Lord, by the fasting of the Lord, by the Cross + of the Lord, by the death of the Lord, by the resurrection of the Lord, by the ascension of the Lord, and by the Holy Spirit, the Paraclete, and by the patriarchs and prophets, by the apostles, martyrs, confessors, and virgins, and all the saints who are crowned for the love of God. I conjure you, fevers, and join issue with you, that you be cast out of the servant of God N. Amen, amen, amen. Our Father.

17. "PRAYERS TO THE EARTH AND ALL HERBS"

Early medieval saints' lives provided riveting scripts for the dramatic confrontation of divine and demonic powers. However, one of the actors, the secular physician, played a rather ambiguous role. When the saint confronted pagan priests or enchanters, the doctor was often presented as an ally; his medicine was never as effective as that of the saint, but he belonged to the camp of those who placed their trust in the Creator. But the physician could also be the fall-guy for the saint. Quite apart from his proverbial greed, the doctor's narrow materialism was readily confounded by the holy man's more spiritual perspective on sickness and healing.

Rarely is the doctor himself accused of invoking non-Christian powers, yet that is what is implied in these prayers to the earth and to the herbs. There are, of course, Christian benedictions for medicines and prayers to accompany their administration; there are also numerous texts that advise gathering medicinal herbs at particular times, accompanied by prayers and sometimes gestures. But these prayers explicitly address the earth and plants as divine entities. Their date and place of composition are unknown, but they are preserved as a pair in manuscripts dating from the sixth to the thirteenth century, often in the company of a first-century CE Latin tract on the medical uses of the herb betony ascribed to Antonius Musa, physician to the emperor Augustus. In one manuscript (London, British Library Harley 1585, twelfth century, from the Meuse Valley), illustrations show the doctor supplicating the earth. The texts may have been considered mere works of literature, but their inclusion in medical compilations obliges us to leave open the question of how medieval readers understood them. The prayer to the herbs, which invokes the Creator, might have been spoken in good conscience by a Christian. "God created medicines from the earth" (Ecclus. 38:4), and some, at least, were not totally uncomfortable with the idea of addressing prayers to his creatures, in the interests of healing.

Source: trans. Faith Wallis from the edition by John I. McEnery, "Prayers to the Earth and to All Herbs," *Rheinisches Museum* 126 (1983): 175–76, 185. Latin.

a. A Prayer to the Earth

Holy goddess Earth, parent of the products of nature,
Who generates all things, and re-generates the stars,
Who alone bestows protection on the peoples,
Divine governor of all in the sky and sea:
Through you nature rests and takes her sleep,
And then you restore the light and drive off night.
You cover Pluto's shadows and the boundless chaos,
You hold winds, rains, and tempests in check,

And release them when you will, stirring the waves,
Banishing the sunshine; and then, when you wish, you bring forth
　　gladsome day.
With steadfast faithfulness you offer the food of life,
And when our soul departs, we find our refuge in you.
Worthy are you to be called Mother of the Gods,
For you outdo the powers of the gods in your dutiful care.
Truly, she is the divine parent of the nations,
Without whom nothing dies, nor can be born.
You, great goddess, you are the queen of the gods!
You, goddess, I adore and invoke your divinity
Grant with speed what I ask of you,
And I will give you thanks with the faithfulness you deserve.
Hear me, I pray, and favor my undertakings;
What I seek from you, goddess, grant me willingly.

Your majesty generates every kind of herb for the sake of healing, bestowing them on every race. Give to me this medicine of yours. Come to me with your powers. Whatever I do with this, may the outcome be good. May you grant healing to whomever I give [these herbs], and to whomever takes them from me. Now, goddess, I appeal to you; may your majesty grant to me what I, a supplicant, ask.

b. A Prayer to All Herbs

Here begins the prayer to all herbs.

Now I entreat you all, potent herbs. I address your majesty, you whom mother Earth generated and gave as a gift to all peoples. On you she conferred the medicine of health, and majesty, so that you might be a most useful aid to the whole human race. I, a supplicant, beseech and entreat. Come hither with your powers, because he who created you has given me leave to gather you; he also to whom medicine is entrusted shows his favor. As much as is in your power, grant good medicine for the sake of health. I implore you, bestow favor on me through your protection, that whatever I make from you with all your powers, and to whomever I give [this medicine], it may have a most speedy effect and a good outcome. I will offer fruits to you and give you thanks, in the name of the majesty which commanded that you be born.

CHAPTER THREE

MEDICINE IN EARLY MEDIEVAL COURTS
AND CLOISTERS

In 476, when the emperor Romulus Augustulus was deposed by the war-lord Odo-acer, few imagined that the western provinces would never again be under the direct government of the Roman Empire. A little over a century later, this was a fact tacitly acknowledged by all. But does that mean that the West was "medieval" in 600? Or was it transformed into a medieval society over decades, even centuries? And until that society was unquestionably medieval, what should we call it? "Barbarian kingdoms" no longer seems appropriate, but is "Sub-Roman Europe" any more satisfactory?

For a number of reasons — notably the birth of late antiquity as a special field of study, as well as new approaches to the history of the Germanic peoples who took control of the old western provinces — historians in recent decades have placed the accent on gradual transformation. Now the pendulum is swinging in the other direction: archaeology, economic and environmental history, and the resurgence of a catastrophic model of political history have made the period between Constantine and Charlemagne appear more discontinuous. These debates also affect the history of medicine. As we saw in chapter 1, there was considerable creative development in early medieval medical knowledge. But there was also loss, not just of medical theory, but of the whole frame-work of culture and education that sustained the ancient medical achievement. When we turn to the social history of medicine in this period, the picture is equally perplexing. In the textual record at least, lay physicians seem few in number, and overwhelmingly connected to the courts of kings and rulers. Other kinds of documents such as charters and legal decisions show that lay doctors were active in cities as well, particularly in Italy, but historians are only beginning to locate and evaluate these sources. By contrast, clerical involvement in medicine in the early Middle Ages has left abundant traces. This is to some extent the product of changes in education and patterns of literacy: schooling in the West, especially outside Italy, became to an overwhelming degree the responsibility of the Church. But it also signals a new identity for the clergy, and particularly for monks. In a sense, the Benedictine monastery was modeled on a Roman country estate, and the abbot was its paterfamilias. *The practical medicine of Pliny and Gargilius Martialis was as relevant in Carolingian St Gall as it was on the ancient farm. What was new and different was the monastery's investment in medical books. Manuscripts produced in convent scriptoria, like the* Lorsch Leechbook *(doc. 23), bear witness to the vitality of late antique and Christian traditions of practical medicine and to the commitment to preserving medical theory within Christian learning.*

The writings of the bishops who were the leaders of the early medieval church bear this out. The early medieval bishop was a pastor, of course, but he was also a great landlord, a busy administrator, and, whether he wished it or not, a man heavily involved in the affairs of kings. Bishops traveled and organized missions; they also collected books and oversaw the training of their clergy. Above all, they "networked" with other prelates and with lay grandees by giving and receiving medical aid and advice. To a large degree, these letters and gifts were part of the reciprocal exchange of obligations that fueled all pre-modern societies. But they are also evidence of how comfortable the Church had become with the idea that knowledge of medicine – even practical medical expertise – was part of what defined an educated cleric.

I. THE DOCTOR AT COURT

18. THE COURT PHYSICIAN IN OSTROGOTHIC ITALY

One of the many compliments that can be paid to Theodoric, the Ostrogothic ruler of Italy from 493 to 526, was that he attracted into his service civilian administrators of the caliber of Cassiodorus (d. 575). Cassiodorus came from an aristocratic Roman family with extensive estates in Calabria and a distinguished tradition of public service: his father held the post of Praetorian Prefect or chief civilian administrator of Italy. Cassiodorus served as Theodoric's secretary, turning his literary training to the drafting of laws and correspondence. He also wrote a history of the Goths in which he depicted the Goths and the Romans as two peoples destined to collaborate in preserving civilization. Cassiodorus continued to serve his Ostrogothic lords even after Theodoric's death. Thereafter, he retired to his family estate in southern Italy and founded the monastery of Vivarium (doc. 21).

A number of Cassiodorus's official letters, collected as Correspondence on Various Matters *(*Variae*), are technically letters from King Theodoric himself. Such is the case with the formula-letter for the appointment of the supervising physician of the royal household (*comes archiatrorum*) translated below.*

Source: trans. Faith Wallis from Cassiodorus, *Variae* 6.19, ed. A.J. Fridh, Corpus Christianorum: series latina 96 (Turnhout: Brepols, 1958), pp. 248–50. Latin.

Among the most useful arts which the Godhead has bestowed to supply the needs of human weakness, none seems to offer anything that can be compared to what medicine, our helpmeet, can confer. For with motherly kindness, she always comes to the aid of those who are imperiled by illness. She wages war against suffering on behalf of our weakness, and exerts herself to uphold us when no riches or honor will come to our aid. Those who have expertise in the law are deemed worthy of the palm of victory when they defend the private suits of individuals; but how much more glorious it is to cast out that which seemed to admit death, and to hold out to someone in mortal danger a means of rescue just when he was driven to the point of despair! This art, which finds out more about a man than he knows about his own self, gives strength to those in mortal danger and invigorates the afflicted. Foreseeing what is to come, it does not yield ground to the illness, even though the patient is distraught by his present weakness. It grasps more than can be seen and trusts more in interpretation than in the eyes, so that its judgment, based on reason, seems to the ignorant almost like an oracle.

If a judge lacked expertise, would this not be evidence of neglect for human concerns? And if there is an official in charge of licentious pleasures, does not [this art] deserve to have a top-ranking administrator? Therefore those to whom we commit our welfare should also have a supervisor; those who bear responsibility for human health should know to whom they are accountable. An art should not be something improvised, but rather, the fruit of learning; otherwise we are all the more exposed to danger, if we place ourselves at the mercy of unsettled whims. For if there are doubts, suddenly everything is called into question.

The health of human beings is something very difficult to understand, a balancing of contrary *humors: if any one of them exceeds its bounds, the body plunges into illness. Just as feeble health is built up again with a suitable diet, so also what is consumed without due consideration acts like poison. Therefore, for the sake of the safety of one and all, let the physicians have a teacher, even after they have left school; let them devote themselves to books and take delight in the ancient texts. To no one is diligent reading more appropriate than to him whose business is human health. Give up those quarrels which do harm to your patients, you craftsmen of healing; for when you do not wish to yield to one another, you seem to squander the discoveries you have made. You now have someone whom you can consult without jealousy. Every prudent person seeks out advice and he is reputed more diligent who shows more circumspection by frequently asking questions of others. When entering on the practice of this art, you are consecrated by certain oaths of a priestly character, for you promise your teachers that you will hate iniquity and love purity. Thus you are not at liberty deliberately to inflict harm – you who are given the right to bind the souls [of others] before the influence of your knowledge. Therefore, seek with diligence what will cure the injured, and strengthen the enfeebled with diligence; for a mistake will excuse an offence, but to err in the health of a human being is to be guilty of homicide....

So I bestow upon you the rank of *comes archiatrorum* from this time forward, that among the masters of health, you alone may hold that distinction, and that all may yield to your judgment who vex themselves in the vicious circle of mutual recrimination. Be the arbiter of this renowned art and resolve the conflicts of those who are normally judged only by the outcome [of their work]. You cure the ill among them, if you judiciously amputate their noxious quarrels. It is a great obligation to have prudent men under one's authority and to be put in a position of honor among those whom others reverence. Let your visit be therapy for the sick, a restorative for the enfeebled, a sure hope for the despairing. Leave it to clumsy practitioners when they visit their patients to ask if the pain has stopped, or if they slept; rather, let the patient ask *you* about his own illness and let him hear from you what he is really suffering from. For to be sure, you have your own most candid witnesses whom you can interrogate. To the experienced chief physician, the pulse of the veins proclaims what nature is suffering within; urines are held up to view, that it might be easier not to hear the voice of one crying out than to fail to perceive the least of such signs. Enter our palace whenever you wish; have the privilege of admission, which should be compared to the greatest rewards. For though others serve in a subaltern role, you must attend your lord with the zeal of an executive. You are allowed to tire us out with fasting. You are allowed to prescribe what goes against our desire and for our own good to dictate what gives us pain, for the joy of health. You know, then, that you have a power over us to do as you will – a power that we do not recognize ourselves to have over others.

19. DIETARY ADVICE FOR A MEROVINGIAN KING

Anthimus was a Byzantine doctor who lived as a political exile at the court of The-odoric the Great in Italy. Theodoric made use of both his medical services and his skill as an emissary. It was perhaps in the context of a diplomatic mission to the court of the Frankish king Theudoric or Thierry I of Austrasia (r. 511–533/534) that he composed On the Observance of Foods *(De observatione ciborum) for his host.*

Anthimus begins with some generalizations about the importance of diet for health. Moderation and balance are the keys to good regimen, so it is the wealthy and powerful, with their access to a great variety and quantity of foods, who run the greatest health risks. The treatise differs from later medieval regimens of health in that the author focuses not only on the choice of food and its quantity, but also on the details of how it should be cooked. Cooking food is an absolute necessity and a marker of civilized life. On the other hand, Anthimus is prepared to take into account local resources and foodways; his chapter on that Frankish delicacy, raw bacon, is a case in point.

Source: trans. Mark Grant, *Anthimus, On the Observance of Foods* (Totnes: Prospect Books, 1996), pp. 47–51, 55–57. Latin.

Here begins the letter of Anthimus, a distinguished gentleman [*vir inlustris*], count and legate to his excellency Theuderic, king of the Franks, concerning the observance of food. Or: how all food should be eaten so that it may be properly digested and promote health, rather than cause stomach problems and persistent infirmity of the body.

I have taken care, to the best of my ability, following the directions of medical writers, [to devise] a plan of diet for your Reverence which will be of benefit to you, because in men excellence of health corresponds to the suitability of food. By that I mean: if food has been prepared well, it helps towards good *digestion, but if it has not been cooked properly, it causes a heaviness in the stomach and bowels. It can even engender undigestible fluids, together with smelly hiccoughs and violent belching. Following on this, a *vapor rises into the head, as a result of which sudden dizziness and unpleasant exhalations can often arise. This type of indigestion can lead to violent diarrhea, or at the very least to vomiting, because the stomach is unable to digest raw food. But if food has been well prepared, the ensuing digestion is good and agreeable, and useful humors will be nourished. To such a degree does excellent health depend on this, that anyone who is prepared to take care over his food in the way which I shall set out will have need of no other medicine.

Drink should be treated in the same way, for as much should be taken as will harmonize with the food. If too much is drunk and at too low a temperature, the stomach grows chilled and loses its efficacy, so that there ensues diarrhea and the other conditions that I mentioned above. Let me give you an analogy: if someone is constructing a wall of a house, he should mix the lime and water in the correct proportions to ensure that the mortar is thick, for then it is both useful for the building and it sets; but if too much water is added, then it is no longer useful. In a similar way proportion ought to be observed in food and drink, for as we said above, excellence of health corresponds to food that has been properly cooked and properly digested.

But let us suppose that someone asks how anyone can take this sort of care when engaged in military maneuvers or a long journey. I would say that if a fire can be lit and if there is time, what has been suggested ought to be possible. However, if force of circumstance compels one to eat meat or anything else raw, then eat sparingly rather than to excess. What I am arguing can be summed up by the ancient motto: "Everything in excess is harmful." As far as drink is concerned, if someone drinks too much before riding his horse or hurrying about his business, then he will suffer pain when jolted on his horse, and what will be produced in his bowels will be worse than if he had taken food.

Perhaps there will be asked the question of how it is that other peoples eat raw and bloody meat and yet are healthy. The answer is that these people may not really be healthy, because they make themselves remedies; for when they feel ill, they burn themselves on the stomach and the belly and in other places in the same way that untamed horses are burned. My explanation for all this is as follows: these people just like wolves eat one sort of food rather than a variety of foods, since they possess nothing but meat and milk, and whatever they have they eat, and they appear to be healthy because of the restricted nature of their diet. Sometimes they have something to drink, and sometimes they do not, and this lack of abundance seems to be responsible for their state of health. By way of contrast, we who excite ourselves with different food and different delicacies have, by necessity, to govern ourselves in such a way as not to be aggravated by excess, so that by living more frugally we may maintain our health. If pleasure is taken from eating food of whatever kind, then the food that is eaten first should have been properly prepared, and anything else taken more sparingly, in order that what is eaten may not only be of benefit but also be digested well.

With this in mind, everyone should steadfastly observe what has been put forward by me through the help of our divine majesty and lord Jesus Christ, by whose bountifulness we may have a longer life and excellent health. I therefore present, to the best of my knowledge, a scheme of how different foods should be used according to the instructions of a number of writers....

Chapter 14. Bacon

At this point I will explain how bacon may be eaten to the best effect, for there is no way I can pass over this Frankish delicacy. If it has been simply roasted in the same way as a joint of meat, the fat drains into the fire and the bacon becomes dry, and whoever eats it is harmed and is not benefited; it also produces bad *humors and causes indigestion. But if bacon that has been boiled and cooled is eaten, it is more beneficial, regulating constipated bowels and being well digested. But it should be boiled well; and if of course it is from a ham, it should be cooked more. None of the rind should be eaten, because it is not digested. Bacon fat which is poured over some foods and vegetables when oil is not available is not harmful, but frying brings absolutely no benefit.

As for raw bacon which, so I hear, the Franks have a habit of eating, I am full of curiosity regarding the person who showed them such a medicine as to obviate the need for other medicines. They eat it raw, because it is very beneficial and as a remedy is responsible for their health. Its effect is akin to that of a good medicine for their internal organs, and if they have any difficulties with their bowels or intestines, it cures them. Stomach and gnawing worms are expelled by this medicine as soon as they are born. It regulates the bowels and, what is so good for them, they are healthier than other people because of this food. Let me give a good example so that what I am writing may be believed: thick bacon, placed for a long time on all wounds, be they external or internal or caused by a blow, both cleanses any putrefaction and aids healing. Look at what power there is in raw bacon, and see how the Franks heal what doctors try to cure with drugs or with *potions.

20. ALCUIN ON THE DOCTORS AT CHARLEMAGNE'S COURT

The English scholar, poet, and educator Alcuin of York (d. 804) arrived at the court of Charles, king of the Franks, in 782 and remained there as one of the principal agents of the king's religious and educational reforms until 794 when he was appointed abbot of the monastery of St Martin in Tours. For reasons both personal and political, he missed the life of the court, which he invokes in this verse letter to Charles. Alcuin pictures the court as a hierarchy, almost a procession. First come the clergy and, directly after them, the physicians, followed by the palace school and chancery. The doctors' relatively lofty rank is striking, particularly as they are consistently represented as working with their hands. Their work is holy by association, but only as long as they do not descend to selling it for a fee.

Source: trans. Faith Wallis from the edition by E. Dümmler, Alcuin, *Carmina*, 26, *Monumenta Germaniae Historica. Poetae latini aevi carolini* 1 (Berlin: Weidman, 1881), p. 245. Latin.

The letters of Your Piety arrived from court,
O dearest David [*that is, Charles*], beloved of God,
Bearing to us, Flaccus [*that is, Alcuin*], the pious gifts of your health,
Which I hope almighty God may ever increase.
You are praise and hope to your people,
You, the joy of the entire realm,
You, the ornament of the Church, its ruler, defender, and cherisher.
You have sent forth ministers worthy of their rank
In holy orders to their accustomed places in the chapel.
See, the priests of Christ uphold his laws,
Ministers give their seemly service in due form,
And prophets rejoice under their steadfast prince.
Forthwith flock in the doctors, disciples of Hippocrates:
This one opens veins, this one mixes herbs in a pot,
That one cooks up a poultice, another offers *potions.
And yet, O doctors, dispense to all without a fee
So that Christ's blessing may be upon your hands....

II. MONASTIC MEDICINE IN THE EARLY MEDIEVAL WEST

21. THE CARE OF THE SICK AT THE MONASTERY OF VIVARIUM

After a long career as secretary to the Ostrogothic rulers of Italy (see doc. 18), Cassio-dorus began to plan his retirement. Initially, he thought that he would collaborate with the pope in setting up a Christian academy in Rome, but when the emperor Justinian's campaign of re-conquest in Italy began in earnest, he decided instead to retire to his family estate in Calabria. There he founded in 539 a monastery called Vivarium (The Fish-Pond) with himself as abbot. The aim of the monastery was not only to share a common life of prayer and asceticism, but also to make copies of important books, both Christian and classical, especially classical works that would be useful for the study of the Bible, such as works on grammar. Cassiodorus described the program of Vivarium in his Introduction to Divine and Human Readings. *The book is divided into two sections, covering sacred erudition and secular erudition – that is, the ancient "liberal arts." It is interesting that medicine is included in the section on sacred erudition, as part of a group of chapters on the organization of the monastery.*

Source: trans. Leslie Webber Jones, Cassiodorus, *Institutes of Divine and Human Learning* 1.31, trans. Leslie Webber Jones, *An Introduction to Divine and Human Readings* (New York: Columbia University Press, 1946), pp. 135–36. Latin.

Part 1. Divine Letters

1. I salute you, distinguished brothers, who with sedulous care look after the health of the human body and perform the functions of blessed piety for those who flee to the shrines of holy men – you who are sad at the sufferings of others, sorrowful for those who are in danger, grieved at the pain of those who are received, and always distressed with personal sorrow at the misfortunes of others, so that, as experience of your art teaches, you help the sick with genuine zeal; you will receive your reward from him by whom eternal rewards may be paid for temporal acts. Learn, therefore, the properties of herbs and perform the compounding of drugs punctiliously; but do not place your hope in herbs and do not trust health to human counsels. For although the art of medicine be found to be established by the Lord, he who without doubt grants life to men makes them sound [Ecclus. 38:1–15]. For it is written: "And whatsoever you do in word or deed, do all in the name of the Lord Jesus, giving thanks to God and the Father by him [Col. 3:17]."

2. But if the eloquence of Greek books is unknown to you, you have first of all the *Herb Book* of Dioscorides, who has treated and portrayed the herbs of the fields with remarkable accuracy. After this read the Latin translations of Hippocrates and Galen (that is, the *Therapeutics* of Galen, addressed to the philosopher Glaucon) and a certain anonymous work, which has been compiled from various authors. Finally, read Caelius Aurelianus's *On Medicine*, and Hippocrates's *On Herbs and Cures* [*an unknown, probably pseudonymous work*], and various other works written on the art of medicine; with God's help, I have left you these books, stored away in the recesses of our library.

22. MEDICAL INJUNCTIONS IN THE *RULE OF ST BENEDICT*

St Benedict (ca 480–547) was born at a time when the western Roman Empire had just about come to an end, and he died shortly after the end of the devastating wars in which the Byzantine Empire tried to re-establish control over Italy following the death of King Theodoric. He came from a prosperous provincial family and was sent to Rome for advanced education, but he left school to become a hermit. As disciples began to gather around him, Benedict came to the conclusion that life in community was, for the average monk, a better and more humane way. Eventually he migrated some 80 miles south of Rome to Monte Cassino, where he established his monastery. The Rule of St Benedict was composed for Monte Cassino. Its keynotes are obedience of the monks to their abbot; discipline, order, regularity, and simplicity in the organization of communal life; humaneness, moderation, and fraternal charity rather than heroic individual asceticism; and a daily routine balanced between prayer and work. The monastery, as a self-contained and self-supporting community (not unlike a Roman estate) takes care of its own sick (see doc. 24). But medicine also figures in the Rule as a symbol of the abbot's duty to heal the spiritual diseases of his monks, and the relationship of the patient to the caregiver is understood in mystical terms.

Note that Benedict allows baths for sick monks. These are Roman style bathhouses, with hot and cold pools, a steam room, massages, etc. The medical purpose of a bath is to open the pores and *evacuate *corrupt *humors. They are quite distinct from the ordinary facilities for daily washing.

Source: trans. Leonard J. Doyle, *St Benedict's Rule for Monasteries* (Collegeville, MN: Liturgical Press, 1948), pp. 45–47, 54–55. Latin.

Chapter 27. How Solicitous the Abbot Should Be for the Excommunicated [Brethren]

Let the Abbot be most solicitous in his concern for delinquent brethren, for "it is not the healthy but the sick who need a physician [Matt. 9:12]." And therefore he ought to use every means that a wise physician would use. Let him send *senpectae*, that is, brethren of mature years and wisdom, who may as it were secretly console the wavering brother and induce him to make humble satisfaction; comforting him that he may not "be overwhelmed by excessive grief [2 Cor. 2:7]," but that, as the apostle [Paul] says, charity may be strengthened in him [*cf.* 2 Cor. 2:8]. And let everyone pray for him....

Chapter 28. On Those Who Will Not Amend after Repeated Corrections

If a brother who has been frequently corrected for some fault, and even excommunicated, does not amend, let a harsher correction be applied, that is, let the punishment of the rod be administered to him.

But if he still does not reform or perhaps (which God forbid) even rises up in pride and wants to defend his conduct, then let the abbot do what a wise physician would do. Having used applications, the ointments of exhortation, the medicines of the Holy Scripture, finally the *cautery of excommunication and the strokes of the rod, if he sees that his efforts are of no avail, let him apply a still greater remedy, his own prayers and those of all the brethren, that the Lord, who can do all things, may restore health to the sick brother.

But if he is not healed even in this way, then let the abbot use the knife of amputation, according to the apostle [Paul]'s words, "Expel the evil one from your midst [1 Cor. 5:13]," and again, "If the faithless one departs, let him depart [1 Cor. 7:15]," lest one diseased sheep contaminate the whole flock.

Chapter 36. On the Sick Brethren

Before all things and above all things, care must be taken of the sick, so that they will be served as if they were Christ in person; for he himself said, "I was sick, and you visited me [Matt. 25:26]," and, "What you did for one of these least ones, you did for me [Matt. 25:40]." But let the sick on their part consider that they are being served for the honor of God, and let them not annoy their brethren who are serving them by their unnecessary demands. Yet they should be patiently borne with, because from such as these is gained a more abundant reward. Therefore the abbot shall take the greatest care that they suffer no neglect.

For these sick brethren let there be assigned a special room and an attendant who is God-fearing, diligent and solicitous. Let the use of baths be afforded the sick as often as may be expedient; but to the healthy, and especially to the young, let them be granted more rarely. Moreover, let the use of meat be granted to the sick who are very weak, for the restoration of their strength; but when they are convalescent, let all abstain from meat as usual.

The abbot shall take the greatest care that the sick not be neglected by the cellarers or the attendant; for he is also responsible for what is done wrongly by his disciples.

23. A MONASTIC DEFENSE OF MEDICINE AGAINST RIGORIST CRITICS: THE *LORSCH LEECHBOOK*

The Lorscher Arzneibuch − *"Lorsch Book of Remedies" or "Lorsch Leechbook" (Bamberg, Staatsbibliothek med. 1) − is a manuscript volume compiled in the German monastery of Lorsch around 800. Most of its pages are taken up with drug recipes and dietary advice, but it opens with an interesting defense of human medical intervention against charges of impiety. The "fundamentalists" opposed by the author of the defense are strict supernaturalists who reject any human intervention in illness as presumptuous. The author's position is closer to that found in a tract found in two Carolingian codices and entitled* Medical Order *(*De ratione medicinae*).* Medical Order *argues that a good doctor should know how to prevent disease through dietary regimen and how to predict outcomes, but he ought not to boast that he can cure through medications. Real cures come from God, and despair is the lot of those who rely on drugs. Indeed, ascribing therapeutic efficacy to God alone, and not to the physician or the herbs, marks the frontier between licit and illicit medicine − a frontier that separates practical techniques of diagnosis, prognosis, patient management, drug lore, dietetics, and surgery from two zones of danger: ancient medical naturalism and pagan magic. If not placed in proper religious context, healing treatments could appear to be magical or superstitious: applying a poultice, after all, is not visibly very different from binding on a* ligatura *or amulet (see doc. 5). In sum, suspicion might fall on medicine not only because it was rational, but because it could come perilously close to the irrational. For these reasons, the author of the defense is at pains to point out that God the Father and Jesus Christ both made use of physical means, including compounds and manual applications, in performing divine cures.*

Source: trans. Faith Wallis from *Das 'Lorscher Arzneibuch'. Ein medizinisches Kompendium des 8. Jahrhunderts (Codex Bambergensis medicinalis 1). Text, Übersetzung und Fachglossar*, ed. Ulrich Stoll, Sudhoffs Archiv, Beiheft 28 (Stuttgart: Franz Steiner, 1992), pp. 48−63. Latin.

I am obliged to respond to those who say that I have been foolish to write this book and that very little of what is written in it is true. But like a deaf man, I did not listen to their words [Ps. 38 (37):14], because I gave more heed to the necessity of those in need than to the carping of enemies against me. For this reason, I shall answer them, not with my own words, but with the words of Holy Scripture, that human medicine (*humana medicina*) is not to be utterly rejected, since it is evident that it is not unknown to the divine books. Thus, with the Lord's help, let us set forth what is found there.

For in many books it is written (and it was true before it was written) that God made heaven and earth, the sea, and all that therein is [Ps. 146 (145):6]. And because the earth is the Lord's and the fullness thereof, the whole world and all that dwells therein [Ps. 24 (23):1], the Psalmist yet again cried out to the Lord, "Yours are the heavens and yours the earth; thou hast founded the circle of the world and its fullness [Ps. 89 (88):12]." Therefore if all things on earth are created and founded by God – and far be it from anyone to believe otherwise – then without doubt all things are good. For God does not make what is evil; but if anything is evil, it was itself the author of its own evil, and not God, of whom it is written, "And God saw all that he had made, and it was very good [Gen. 1:31]." For the almighty God, to whom [belongs] supreme power, since he is the supreme good – a fact even infidels admit – could in no wise permit any evil to exist in his works.

If therefore everything that God created is very good, wise men everywhere in the world were good by nature. But through pride and faithlessness they became evil; and therefore they were good because they were men and evil because they were proud. Nonetheless their wisdom and learning (*doctrina*), because it was given by God, seems to be worthy of imitation. As the Lord said in the Gospel, "Everything which they say, do." By which we should understand that we should preserve and do everything in their sayings that pertains to the necessities of life, present and future. I do not wish ([Christ] says) that you should act according to their works [Matt. 23:3], [but rather] so that you should do for the glory of almighty God what these men did for their own sake, and not for God's sake. Therefore when something useful is found in their writings, it is just like gold [which] is often found in a dung heap. As a certain man of God observed when he was asked why he was reading a pagan book, "I am seeking for gold in a dung-heap."

The ancients called the wisdom of these men "philosophy," that is, the knowledge (*scientia*) of all things human and divine. And they said that this philosophy was divided into three parts; namely *physica, logic, and ethics. Ethics pertains to instruction in morals, and is divided into the four cardinal virtues, namely prudence, justice, fortitude, and temperance. Let him who wishes to know what distinguishes them read the book of the homilies of

St Gregory on Ezechiel [book 3, no. 8]. Logic consists of dialectic and rhetoric; the abovementioned [Gregory] is known to have devoted attention to this discipline, for by the mouth of Bede the priest he is called "the orator." For orators follow the methods of logic. But *physica* is divided into seven disciplines. Of these, some are compatible with religion, but some are very foreign to it in many ways. The first of these is arithmetic, the second geometry, the third music, the fourth astronomy, the fifth astrology, the sixth mechanics, the seventh medicine. Whoever wants to know what realm of knowledge these pertain to, let him read the book of the *Etymologies* of Isidore, bishop of the church of Seville. Here, it is enough for me to speak of medicine.

Medicine is the knowledge of treatments (*scientia curationum*). It was discovered for the tempering and well-being of the body and is also not unknown to the divine books, so that words are found there which are derived from [medicine]. For it is said by Isaiah [1:6]: "Every festering wound is not bound up, nor cured with medicine, nor soothed with oil." And in the book of Exodus [21:19] it is commanded that if anyone wound a stranger, he should compensate him for his injury and for the expenses of the doctors.

We know that not only is [medicine] mentioned in the divine books, but also from time to time the names of drugs. We read in Jeremiah [8:22], "Is there no balm in Gilead, and is there no physician there? Why then has the scar not been removed?" And again, the same prophet says, "Though you wash yourself with lye and heap soapwort upon yourself, yet are you stained [Jer. 2:22]."

In all these things, at least according to the literal meaning, we can see that balm is suitable against the hardened scar of wounds and that lye and soapwort are very effective for remedying filthy stains. The apostle Paul also explicitly describes medicine as the gift of the Holy Spirit, saying, "To another, the knowledge of treatments (*curationum*) is given by the Spirit [I Cor. 12:9 and 28]."

It is not for nothing that that which restores a man to the exercise of good works is called the gift of the Holy Spirit. For diseases happen to the body for three reasons; namely because of sin, because of a trial [of faith], and because of the intemperance of the passions. However, human medicine can be of help only for the last kind of illness, and for the others, only the compassion of the divine mercy. But in fact, even these will sometimes not be cured without human relief. We will demonstrate this better if we produce evidence.

It was indeed because of sin that Saul [*that is, St Paul, prior to his conversion*] was smitten with the loss of his eyes, but nevertheless he was not cured without the laying on of a man's hands [Acts 9:8–18]. [One can fall sick] as a trial, like Tobit when he lost the use of his eyes, even though he walked in the way of justice. Yet the angel Raphael (which means "medicine of God") cured him, not personally, but through his [Tobit's] son, by means of a medicine made from a fish [Tob. 11:10–14].

[One can fall sick] from intemperance of the passions, like the man whom the apostle commands, "Let him who is weak eat vegetables [Rom. 14:2]," and like that disciple of the Apostle whom he exhorts, saying, "Take a little wine for your stomach's sake, and because of your frequent infirmities [1 Tim. 5:23]." In all this, it is evident that human relief and human medicine are not to be rejected utterly, because if they deserved to be condemned, the Lord would never have commanded Paul to receive his sight back by the imposition of the hands of Ananias, nor would he have commanded his disciples to lay their hands upon the sick, as long as there was something better [Mark 16:18, Luke 9:2]. Neither would Tobit have been cured through his son by means of the medicine that the angel pointed out. And if wine (in which lies luxury, if it is consumed beyond what is necessary) did not, for the most part, do good to the body, that renowned preacher [St Paul], who elsewhere says, "It is good not to consume meat and wine [Rom. 14:21]," would never have commanded his disciple to relieve his infirmities with a little wine. Therefore when he said, "It is good not to eat meat and drink wine," he was speaking to people who were healthy and in good condition. But when he said, "Take a little wine for your stomach's sake," he was showing compassion for the sick, and those who were not in good condition. For he does not say, "Take wine for the sake of enjoyment," but, "Take wine for your stomach's sake, because of your frequent infirmities."

But some are in the habit of saying, "What need have we to be cured by physicians, we who cast our cares upon [God] who is able to care for us [1 Pet. 5:7]? Can he not vouchsafe us health without medicines, who by his word alone can restore all things?" To be sure, these people evidently speak the truth. Far be it that anything should be said to be impossible for God. But it is necessary that they have faith in the words of him in whose care for them they do not lack trust. For he says, "The healthy do not need a physician, but rather those who are sick [Mark 2:17]." Now they should know that no one, however righteous he is, can escape this present life without affliction. For blessed Job, who was so perfect that even though he was not immune from the lighter sins (from which an infant one day old is not free) nonetheless had no crime upon his conscience, so that he was heard to say, "My heart has not reproached me in all my life [Job 27:6]," who also was so commended by the divine voice that [God] said that there was none on earth like him [Job 1:8], [even he] was said to have been smitten by a very grievous ulceration so that he scraped the flowing pus and the teeming mass of worms with a potshard [Job 2:8]. But the apostle Paul also often declared that he had an infirmity in his flesh, when he said, "When I am weak, then I am strong [2 Cor. 12:10]," and again, "Willingly will I glory in my infirmities, that the power of Christ may abound in me [2 Cor. 12:9]." O how desirable is that tribulation of the flesh, which causes the power of the Redeemer to dwell within man.

We do not read that these men were cured with any medicine. But our Lord Jesus Christ, who left us an example that we might follow in his footsteps [1 Pet. 2:21], deigned to indicate very clearly in the Gospel that in his view, medicine and human means of relief ought not to be refused. For when he was reclining in the house of the Pharisee and the prostitute approached him, took an alabaster box full of precious ointment, and poured it over his head as he lay reclining, he took no offence, but praised her devotion highly, so that he said to the Pharisee, "Amen, I say unto you, her many sins are forgiven [Luke 8:47]." But the disciples complained about her, saying, "What was the purpose of wasting this unguent?" The Lord said to them, "She has done a good deed for me; for in anointing my body with this unguent, she prepared me for my burial [Matt. 26:6–12]." Why, then, should a pure man despise what the God-Man showed ought not to be despised?

The apostle Paul imitated [Christ's] example in saying (as we mentioned earlier), "Let him who is weak eat vegetables." But other people, and very many holy men, also emulated him, whom we know to have relieved their own illness with medicine and who entered the gate of the heavenly kingdom. But it would serve our purpose to recall them here.

When Germanus, bishop of Capua, suffered severe physical distress, the doctors told him that for the health of his body he should wash at the neighborhood baths. And he took care to carry this out as often as he could. He even mentioned these baths to Paschasinus, deacon of Rome. Later the venerable man, abbot Benedict, looking through a window in the dead of night, saw the soul of the same bishop Germanus borne up to heaven by angels in a fiery sphere. The deacon Servandus also witnessed this, so that the witness of two men might validate the account. But Pope Gregory as well (who related these things which I said concerning Germanus [*Dialogues* 2.35]), sometimes suffered such great torment that he could scarcely speak. He recounts this in his homily on the Gospels [22:1], saying: "My stomach, racked with chronic distress, forbade me to speak of the explanation," and again, "The summer season, which greatly disagrees with my body, forbade me for a long time to speak about the explanation [*Homily* 54.1]." We learn beyond doubt that he made full use of medicaments, if we read his *Homilies* and the book of the *Dialogues* carefully. For he says in the *Homilies* [4.3], "By the bitter draught of medicine one arrives at the joys of health." And again in the *Dialogues* [4.55]: "A certain monk named Justus was steeped in the art of medicine, and he was wont to tend me in my monastery with great diligence and to watch over my unremitting illnesses." Bishop Isidore as well, whom we mentioned earlier, indicated that he suffered in these words: "Have mercy, Lord, upon poor Isidore, who does unworthy deeds and suffers things which he deserves, ceaselessly sinning and daily bearing your torments." These torments can be understood to pertain to the mind as well as to the body. For God does not withdraw his mercy from the just man or the impious man, for he either judges good men in this life through affliction and rewards them in the next life with mercy, or else he rewards the wicked with temporal clemency in this life and punishes them in the next with eternal justice. Sickness which detaches the mind from intransigency is very salubrious, but health which leads a man into disobedience is pernicious. The person who is loved by God is reproved more, as Solomon says: "For the Lord reproves whom he loves; he chastens every son whom he receives [Prov. 3:12, Heb. 12:6]." And as the prophet Amos says, "You only have I known of all the families of the earth; therefore I will punish you for all your iniquities [Amos 3:2]." The Psalmist cries out for this visitation, saying, "Visit us in thy salvation [Ps. 106 (105):2]." Likewise the Lord himself says in the Apocalypse, "Those whom I love I reprove and chasten [Rev. 3:19]." For it is very necessary for them to be attacked by vices and smitten by affliction in this life, so that when they are assailed by vices, they are not proud of their virtues, [and] when they are indeed ground down by suffering of mind or body, they may be withdrawn from the love of the world. For this reason, everyone who is reproved by illness should take heed lest he fall into the evil of complaining. For he who complains at scourging irritates God all the more. But let him take care to remember that one must enter the kingdom of God through many tribulations [Acts 14:22]. The Apostle says, "The sufferings of this present time are not worth comparing with the glory that is revealed in us [Rom. 8:18]." Therefore, according to the Lord's command, you ought to possess your souls in patience [Luke 21:9] however long we must remain in this world, in order that we may bear scourges and suffering, as it is written, "Six days shall you plough; on the seventh you shall cease [Exod. 34:21]." What else should be understood by the number six save the total time of this present life, in which we are commanded to plow, that is, to bear tribulation? And what is symbolized by the seventh day, in which we are enjoined to cease plowing, save the repose of eternal life, in which all the suffering of those who patiently suffer will be rewarded with perennial respite? O how desirable is the plowing of the tribulation of the six days, which will be rewarded by a rest of days without number!

For this reason, human medicine is not to be rejected but to be used with thanksgiving for suffering; for no one should hate his own flesh because it is created, but because it readily falls into sin, he ought not to give it free rein in pleasure. Although Paul says, "Make no provision for the flesh, to gratify its desires [Rom. 13:14]," he evidently permits in need what he prohibits in desire.

And now we should ask whether the Lord can rightly be called a physician, or if it can be said that he performed any action in a medical fashion (*medicinali more*). Why cannot the Lord be called a physician, who healed the whole world when it was oppressed in the languor of infidelity? Therefore when the people of Israel, having departed from Egypt, came to the bitter waters and could not drink them, they began to murmur against the Lord. But the Lord, taking pity on their exhaustion, commanded that Moses take wood and put it in the water. When he put it in, the water was made drinkable [Exod. 15:23–25]. Again, in order to heal the sterile and malignant waters at the request of the inhabitants of Jericho, he ordered Elisha to take a new earthenware bowl, put salt in it, and throw it into the river, and immediately the waters were made wholesome [2 Kings 2:19–22]. To whom would this deed not seem to be done, in the literal sense, in a medical manner, when even now doctors are wont to act in this way? For when they encounter something bitter and repugnant, they mix it with honey or garlic, by which (in their view) the bitterness or repulsive taste is tempered. But if you are not reluctant to inquire into the mystical meaning, you will find the symbol of the physician in these events.

Therefore, just as Moses sweetened the bitter water for the faithful people by putting wood into it, so also almighty God by introducing the confession of the wood of the Cross into the water of baptism, converted the bitter letter of the Old Testament into the sweetness of the Holy Spirit for all believers. And just as Elisha cured the sterile and diseased waters of Jericho by putting into them salt in the earthenware bowl, so also the almighty Father liberated the whole world from sterility and disease by putting his wisdom into a human body. Wisdom is symbolized by salt. For Christ is called the power and the wisdom of God [1 Cor. 1:24].

When [Christ] appeared in the flesh, he confessed that he was a physician, saying, "Those who are well have no need of a physician, but those who are sick [Luke 5:31]." That he was referring to himself in these words is attested by the following statement, "I have come not to call the righteous, but sinners [Matt. 9:13]." And he deigned to show this by his deeds. For when he saw a certain man who had been blind from birth, he spat on the ground and made mud from his spittle and daubed his eyes, and said to him, "Go and wash in the pool of Siloam," and when he washed, he immediately received his sight [John 9:1–7]. It is no wonder that the Lord restored the sight of the blind man by daubing with earth, for he ordains that medicine (*medela*) come from [the earth] for all mortals. As was said by a certain wise man, "The

Lord created medicines from the earth [Ecclus. 38:4]." So it is fitting that at God's dispensation, man, who is formed of earth, should receive relief of his infirmity from the earth. For the earth brings forth nothing without cause, but all by necessity; as the Psalmist says, "The earth is satisfied with the fruit of thy work, bringing forth grass for cattle and plants for man to cultivate [Ps. 104 (103):13–14]." For this reason, no one should spurn earthly medicine where he knows that it will do him good and not inflict harm, when holy men have not condemned it.

Indeed it is evident that Luke, an apostolic man who wrote down the acts of the Apostles (which he saw) and the life of Christ (which he heard), was expert in the art of medicine; for Paul said, "Luke my beloved physician salutes you [Col. 4:14]," and he is said to be well-known in all the churches for [preaching] the Gospel [2 Cor. 8:18 (*which does not in fact refer to Luke*)]. And there are martyrs of renown who were said to practice medicine and to pursue it with diligence, namely Cosmas and Damian. Therefore we should give honor to physicians that they may help us when we are sick. You should remember what the wise man says: "Honor the physician according to your need, for the Lord created him [Ecclus. 38:1]." And what they proffer you as medicine, you should take with confidence. "The Most High," says that same wise man, "created medicines from the earth, and a sensible man will not despise them [Ecclus. 38:4]." Someone who does not seek medicine in time of need will be called foolish and lacking in sense. For this reason, I say give the physician his due as is right, while you are healthy, so that if you fall ill you will be able to obtain his benefits, lest perchance if you spurn him when you are in sound health, no one will come to your aid in time of need.

For God desires to be honored in the miracles which he performs through human beings, for whatever good is done by man is brought to perfection by God, as Isaiah testifies, saying, "The Lord hath wrought for us all our works [Isa. 26:12]." And in the Gospel [God] himself says, "Without me you can do nothing [John 15:1]." And so when one falls sick, one respectfully requests from the physician a medication appropriate to the illness and implores a healthful remedy for the disease from God with humility. One asks for a healthful remedy when one desires to become healthy in order to do good. For when one strives to become healthy for other reasons, one loses the result of one's prayer, and hence it happens that one does not receiving healing. For when we in our ignorance ask for ourselves things that are harmful and contrary, our Lord out of his goodness refuses. It is just as if someone burning with fever were to beg for cold water from the doctor, saying, "Take pity on me and give me what I ask," and he were to respond, "I know at what time I ought to give you what you are asking for. I will not take pity on you now, because such pity is cruelty, and because what you want is contrary to what is good for you." Therefore no one should ask from the Lord what he thinks would not be his will, because if it is requested, he will not deign to grant it. But let him ask that it may befall him as [God's] will has decreed, for he desires that all men should be saved [I Tim. 2:4]. And if one who is being treated with medicaments does not regain his health, he should ascribe this to his guilt, or to [God's] testing, and not to the physician's lack of expertise. Nor should he for this reason cease to take care of his body, but he should strive to care for it as much as he is able, not for the sake of fleshly desires, but for the sake of the good works that are in him, "so that he may be able to give to those in need [Eph. 4:28]." And if his effort is to no avail, then let him fall back on the medicine of patience, and he shall not fail to win everlasting well-being (*salutem*) not only for his body, but also for his soul. Thus in vintage-time grapes are trodden underfoot so that later they may appear at royal banquets, and without their blood there is no power to rule. Thus wheat is ground at the mill, that pure bread might be made and placed upon the table of the great king. So the more one is ground by tribulation here, the purer one will be found in the realm to come, if one is patient despite everything.

But now I address you, beloved brethren, who treat the health of the human body with painstaking care and fulfill the duty of blessed compassion towards the sick – you who are saddened by the suffering of others, grieving for those whose lives are in danger, pierced through by the pain of those in their care and always absorbed in another's calamities, to your own grief. You should serve the sick with sincere effort as the skill of your art teaches. For this you will receive a reward by which things eternal can repay things temporal. And so, learn the natures of herbs and the differences between drugs, and carry out the mixing of medicine with careful attention. Do not, indeed, put your hope in herbs, nor your security in human eyes. For although medicine, we read, is created by God, still it is he who grants life and who makes one healthy, without a doubt. For it is written, "Whatever you do, in word or deed, do everything in the name of the Lord Jesus, giving thanks to the Lord and Father through him [Col. 3:17]," saying, "Not unto us, O Lord, not unto us, but to thy name give glory [Ps. 115:1 (113:9)]," and what we said earlier on, "The Lord has wrought for us all our works [Isa. 26:12]." Therefore be not slothful to help those who languish, for the grace of God. For whatever you do for the sick you do for Christ the Lord, who on the Day of Judgment says, "I was sick and you visited me [Matt. 25.36]," and "whatsoever you do for the least of these, you do for me [Matt. 25.40]." Do not neglect, then, to visit Christ. Moreover, you should know – and I would that you would act in accordance with what you know – that Christ is to be visited primarily in the poor, for the very wealth of the rich compels doctors to visit them [*Rule of St Benedict* c. 53]. Remember the deeds of the Lord, who did not refuse to go to the centurion's slave when he was oppressed with sickness [Luke 7:2–10] and who nevertheless refused to go in person to the official's son [John 4:46–53]. Here is our pride subdued, who honor in men not their nature (in which they are made in the image of God), but their titles and wealth. Lo, he who came from heaven did not disdain to visit a slave on earth, while we, who are dust and ashes, refuse to go to the sick poor. Do not, then, look to what kind of reward you will receive in this world, but to what kind of reward you will receive in the world to come. Blessed shall you be, if you devote your treatment to those whom you know cannot repay you. You should ask nothing from them, if you wish to find a reward in eternal rest, because it is more blessed to give than to receive. Visit, then, those who seem to you to be poor and regard those whom you perceive are despised by the world because of their external circumstances as friends of God. For why should you be slothful, when what you offer to one lying upon the earth, you give to the one enthroned in heaven? Learn then to show pity for the poor so that the Lord will also have pity on you. "Blessed are the merciful, for they shall obtain mercy [Matt. 5:7]." So if in doing this you seek not your own glory, but Christ's, you will deserve on the Day of Judgment, in the company of those at his right hand, to hear, "Come, O blessed of my Father, inherit the kingdom prepared for you from the foundation of the world [Matt. 25:34]."

But if the eloquence of Greek letters is unknown to you, you have the book of herbs of Dioscorides, who has described and portrayed the herbs of the field with marvelous accuracy. After these, read Hippocrates and Galen in Latin translation; that is, Galen's *Therapeutics* addressed to the philosopher Glaucon, and a certain anonymous compilation from various authors. The *On Medicine* by Caelius Aurelianus and Hippocrates's *On Herbs and Cures*, and various other works on the art of healing. So read these, and in accordance with what they say, confect medicine and so give help to the sick. You will receive a reward from Christ, who will not fail to reward in the eternal kingdom a cup of cold water given in his name [Matt. 10:42], where he lives and reigns together with the Father and the Holy Spirit, world without end. Amen.

24. *THE PLAN OF ST GALL*: MEDICAL FACILITIES WITHIN AN IDEAL MONASTERY

The so-called Plan of St Gall is the ground plan of a model Benedictine monastery. It was made around 820–833 and is a copy traced from a lost original. Its purpose is unknown, though it has been plausibly suggested that it was connected with a monastic reform program initiated by the emperor Louis the Pious (814–840). The Plan projects the idea of the monastery as a self-contained community open to guests and pilgrims from the world, but also carefully protecting the monks' privacy. The abbot lives in his own house, strategically positioned beside the hostel for important secular visitors, and guarding the approach to the church and cloister. Within the monastic zone, there are two smaller cloisters. One is for the novices – Carolingian rulers and their ecclesiastical advisers gave close attention to the schooling of candidates for the monastic life – and the other is for the sick. This "health services area" is remarkable for its detail and reveals much about Carolingian and monastic ideals of medical care, but it raises almost as many questions as it answers. Are we to assume that only the brethren of the house were to be treated in this infirmary space? Were the doctors who cared for them monks themselves?

Source: Illustrations from Laura Price, Walter Horn and Ernest Born, *The Plan of St. Gall in Brief* (Berkeley and Los Angeles: University of California Press, 1982), pp. 32, 33, 36. Commentary on the illustrations by Faith Wallis.

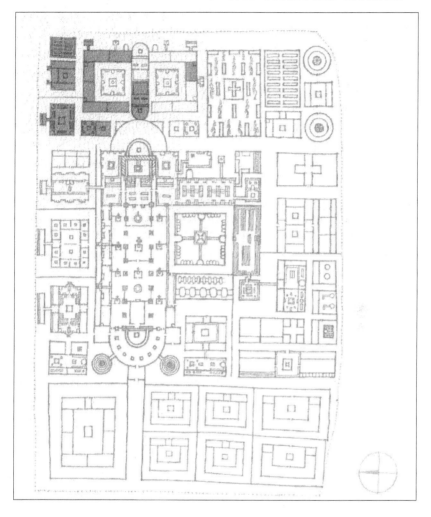

Fig. 1. The Plan of St Gall, and Its "Health Services Area"

This is a schematic rendering of the Plan. The great monastery church dominates the center, with the cloister and its surrounding dormitory, refectory, and cellars to the right of the church. Above the cloister is the monastic cemetery with an orchard and circular henhouses to the right. To the right of the main cloister are kitchens and other food preparation areas, and below it is a hospice for poor travelers. To the left of the church and below the shaded area are the abbot's quarters and a hospice for distinguished guests. Just above the main church is a smaller church flanked on either side by cloisters. The upper half of this church and the cloister to the right belong to the novices; the shaded area, including the lower half of the church and the cloister to the left, is the "health services area."

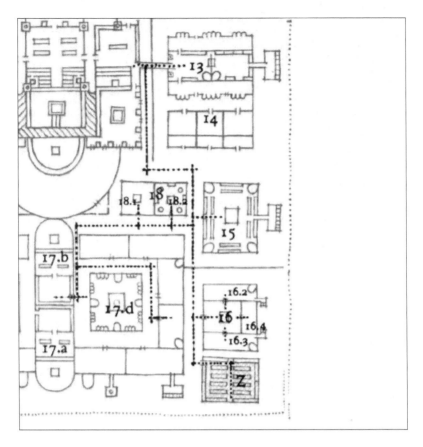

Fig. 2. The Health and Medical Facilities

This image is rotated 180 degrees from fig. 1 and shows details of the shaded "health services area." Numbers 13 and 14 mark the abbot's house and its private kitchen. Note that the pathways allow the abbot access to the health services area.

The sick have their own chapel (17b) which abuts, but is strictly walled off from, the chapel for novices (17a). Each of the two parts of the chapel can be accessed only from one of the adjacent cloisters. The cloister for the sick (17d) is surrounded by an infirmary building. Medical treatment is carried out in three purpose-built structures: a bath-house for the sick (18.2), a bloodletting facility (15), and a house for the physicians, which doubles as a pharmacy and "intensive care unit" (16). This last is discussed in detail below.

The floor plan of the bloodletting building shows the beds around the walls, the adjacent privy, and no fewer than four corner chimneys. A person undergoing bloodletting would be weakened by the procedure and so needed to be kept warm; but medical instructions for bloodletting often advised as well that the body part where the vein was to be opened be warmed up in advance of the procedure. Bloodletting was also carried out *as a routine preventive measure and was built into monastic calendars and rituals. This serves to remind us that the care of the body was inseparable from the global project of reforming monastic life, so that it could incarnate the virtues of "rule" and "regularity."*

Finally there is the medicinal garden (labeled Z). On the original plan, the individual beds are inscribed with the names of the herbs grown in them: lilies, roses, climbing bean, pepperwort, costmary, fenugreek, rosemary, mint, sage, rue, iris, pennyroyal, watercress, cumin, lovage, and fennel. The medicinal uses of many of these plants are described by Walahfrid Strabo in his poem The Little Garden *(doc. 25).*

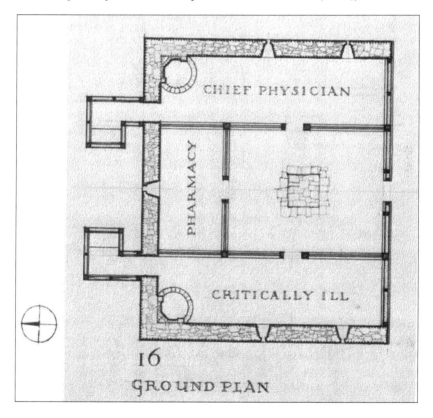

Fig. 3. The Physicians' House

*The physicians' house (*domus medicorum*) comprises a common-room and three adjacent rooms. The physician's living quarters (*mansio medici ipsius*) faces an infirmary for the critically ill (*cubiculum valde infirmorum*) with a storeroom for drugs (*armarium pigmentorum*) between. The first two rooms have corner chimneys for heating and toilet facilities en suite. The arrangement of the physicians' house would allow the doctors access to the medicinal plants in the garden and permit them to keep a constant watch over the acutely ill.*

25. MEDICINE, MORALITY, AND MEDITATION IN A MONASTIC HERB-GARDEN: WALAHFRID STRABO'S *THE LITTLE GARDEN*

Walahfrid Strabo (d. 849), sometime tutor to Louis the Pious's youngest son Charles the Bald, became abbot of Reichenau on Lake Constance in southwestern Germany in 838. Driven from his post in the political upheaval of 840, he was reinstated in 842. It was around this time that he composed his poem The Little Garden *(Hortulus). It is an apt companion piece – almost a key – to the images from the* Plan of St Gall *presented in the preceding document. Coincidentally, it is dedicated to the abbot of St Gall, Grimald, and, like the famous* Plan, *projects an ideal of both monastic spirituality and monastic medicine. Beneath its guileless surface,* The Little Garden *is a tissue of intriguing allusions and layered meanings. Though modeled to some degree on Virgil's* Georgics, *Walahfrid's poem is novel in its emphasis on medicinal herbs. With the exception of the gourd and the melon, every item in his catalogue has an explicit medicinal use that includes details about the preparation and administration of the relevant plant part. This information derives from Walahfrid's own wide reading in medical literature. For example, his personal commonplace book, MS St Gall 878, contains pseudo-Hippocratic tracts, medical recipes, and extracts.*

But the garden is also an allegory of the cloister and the habits and virtues of the plants can also be read as moral or mystical symbols. The Little Garden *starts with a Virgilian allusion to Paestum, the southern Italian city famous for its roses (the flower of Venus), and to Priapus, the Roman guardian-spirit of gardens, represented in sculpture with a huge erect phallus. The poem ends with the rose, emblem of Christ's passion, the blood of martyrdom, and divine love. The movement from carnal to spiritual love is marked by a chapter devoted to the lily, symbol of purity, which is strategically positioned in the middle of the poem. The* envoi *addressed to Grimald pictures the abbot reading* The Little Garden *in his own garden with his pupils about him, and so hints at the poet's didactic purpose. Is Walahfrid instructing the children of the cloister in* medicina, *as mandated by Charlemagne's Capitulary of Thionville (805), or in the moral remedies for sin, or both?*

Source: trans. R. Payne, excerpts from Walahfrid Strabo, *Hortulus. De cultura hortulorum* (Pittsburgh: Hunt Botanical Library, 1966), pp. 25–65. Latin.

1. On the Cultivation of Gardens

A quiet life has many rewards: not least of these
Is the joy that comes to him who devotes himself to the art
They knew at Paestum, and learns the ancient skill of obscene
Priapus – the joy that comes of devoting himself to a garden.

For whatever the land you possess, whether it be where sand
And gravel lie barren and dead, or where fruits grow heavy
In rich moist ground; whether high on a steep hillside,
Easy ground in the plain or rough among sloping valleys –
Wherever it is, your land cannot fail to produce
Its native plants. If you do not let laziness clog
Your labor, if you do not insult with misguided efforts
The gardener's multifarious wealth, and if you do not
Refuse to harden or dirty your hands in the open air
Or to spread whole baskets of dung on the sun-parched soil –
Then, you may rest assured, your soil will not fail you.

This I have learned not only from common opinion
And searching about in old books, but from experience –
Experience of hard work and sacrifice of many days
When I might have rested, but chose instead to labor.

2. The Difficulty of the Undertaking

Winter, image of age, who like a great belly
Eats up the whole year's substance and heartlessly
Swallows the fruit of our unstinted labor,
Had gone into hiding deep below the earth.
For Spring had arrived and driven him under. Spring
Source of the world's life and glory of the year,
Had returned, and was wiping away the ugly traces
Of greedy winter and restoring to ailing fields
Their former loveliness.

A purer air was now beginning to herald
Fine weather. Plants stirred in the zephyr's path
Thrusting out from their roots the slender tips
Which had long lain hidden in the earth's blind womb,
Shunning the frost they hate. Spring smiled
In the leaves of the woodland, the lush grass on the slopes
And the bright sward of the cheerful meadows.

But this little patch which lies facing east
In the small open courtyard before my door
Was full – of nettles! All over
My small piece of land they grew, their barbs
Tipped with a smear of tingling poison.

What should I do? So thick were the ranks
That grew from the tangle of roots below,

They were like the green hurdles a stableman skillfully
Weaves of pliant osiers when the horses' hooves
Rot in the standing puddles and go soft as fungus.
    So I put it off no longer. I set to with my mattock
And dug up the sluggish ground. From their embraces
I tore those nettles though they grew again and again.
I destroyed the tunnels of the moles that haunt dark places,
And back to the realms of light I summoned the worms.
    Then my small patch was warmed by winds from the south
And the sun's heat. That it should not be washed away,
We faced it with planks and raised it in oblong beds
A little above the level ground. With a rake
I broke the soil up bit by bit, and then
Worked in from on top the leaven of rich manure.
Some plants we grow from seed, some from old stocks
We try to bring back to the youth they knew before.

3. The Gardener's Perseverance and the Fruit of His Labor

    Then come the showers of Spring, from time to time
Watering our tiny crop, and in its turn
The gentle moon caresses the delicate leaves.
Should a dry spell rob the plants of the moisture they need,
My gardening zeal and fear that the slender shoots
May die of thirst make me scurry to bring fresh water
In brimming buckets. With my own hands I pour it
Drop by drop, taking care not to shift the seeds
By too sudden or lavish a soaking. Sure enough,
In a little while the garden is carpeted over
With tiny young shoots. True, that part there
Below the high roof is dry and rough from the lack
Of rain and the heaven's benison; true, this
Part here is always in the shade, for the high wall's
Solid rampart forbids the sun to enter.
Yet of all that was lately entrusted to it, the garden
Has held nothing enclosed in its sluggish soil
Without hope of growth. What is more, those plants that were
More dead than alive, to the newly dug furrows are now
Green again; our garden has brought them back
To life, making them good with abundant growth.

Now I must summon all my skill, all
My learning, all my eloquence, to muster
The names and virtues of this noble harvest,
That this my lowly subject may receive
The highest honor that my art can give.

4. Sage

There in the front grows sage, sweetly scented.
It deserves to grow green for ever, enjoying perpetual youth;
For it is rich in virtue and good to mix in a *potion,
Of proven use for many a human ailment.
But within itself is the germ of civil war;
For unless the new growth is cut away, it turns
Savagely on its parent and chokes to death
The older stems in bitter jealousy.

5. Rue

Here is a shadowed grove which takes its color
From the miniature forest of glaucous rue.
Through its small leaves and the short umbels which rise
Like clusters of spears it sends the wind's breath
And the sun's rays down to its roots below.
Touch it but gently and it yields a heavy
Fragrance. Many a healing power it has –
Especially, they say, to combat
Hidden toxin and to expel from the bowels
The invading forces of noxious poison.

6. Southernwood

Admire too the tall bushes of southernwood
With their bloom of down, and the sharp spikes
Which grow on its wealth of branches like finest hair.
It is good to mix the scented sprigs, plucked
With the supple stem, into healing medicines.
It has power against fevers, banishes stitch, and if
Your limbs ache with the elusive and mysterious
Pain of gout, it will bring relief. Indeed
As many virtues it has as strands of foliage....

8. Melon

In the same patch at the bottom of the garden where this fine crop
My humble lines have just described is planted,
You will see something else which looks like an eager vine creeping
Over the dusty ground and nursing a rounded fruit.
This one commonly lies on the dry ridges of earth
And the growth it makes is beautiful – until the time when,
Yellow and ripe with summer sun, it fills the gardener's basket.
    Some you will see are completely round and even;
Others you'll find with a drooping oblong belly, the shape
Of a nut or an egg –
                    Or like a soap bubble. You know how it is
When you hold up a cake of soap: it gleams in your upraised hands
As the slippery wetness runs over its surface, until by pouring
More water on it you wash the fresh froth off.
But when the fingers work on it, kneading and rubbing purposefully
This way and that, it softens; and then, with your hands together
And only a crack between, if you blow through narrowed lips
Gently, gently, your breath will make the hollow suds
Swell like blown glass, and the curve of the vaulted skin
Meets to form a slippery center at the bubble's base.
    When a knife-blade finds the guts of a melon a gush
Of juice comes out, and many seeds with it. Then
Your lucky guest can divide by hand the hollow body
Into several pieces and thus enjoy the luscious delicacy.
Its freshness and savor delight the palate; nor can this food
Defeat a man's teeth, for it's easy to eat and its natural
Properties cool and refresh his whole inner body.

9. Wormwood

The next bed grows bushes of bitter wormwood. Its supple stem
Resembles the Mother of Herbs [that is, mugwort], but the leaves have a
    different color.
The smell of its downy branches is different too, and the brew
It makes has a bitterer taste by far.
    Its powers are famous,
Its effectiveness proven. It tames a raging thirst; fever
It banishes. If, besides, your head should suddenly start to
Throb and throb with pain, if fits of fainting worry you,

Seek its help:
   Boil the bitter stem of a plant
In leaf, tip the brew into an ample basin
And pour it over the top of your head. Then having bathed
Your soft hair with the liquid make a garland of leaves
(Do not forget this) and put it on, so that the bandage
Gently binds your hair and holds the warmth in it.
A few hours later – not many – you will be marveling
At this yet further proof of the healing powers of wormwood.

10. Horehound

Horehound comes next, and what shall I say of this
Powerful worker? A precious herb, though biting
And sharp on the tongue where it tastes so unlike
Its scent: for whereas the scent is sweet, the taste
Is not sweet at all. Yet taken in a draught,
For all its nastiness it assuages pain
In the chest, and most when drunk still warm from the fire
And ladled out quickly to close the meal.
   If ever
A vicious stepmother mixes in your drink
Subtle poisons, or makes a treacherous dish
Of lethal aconite [*wolfsbane or monkshood, a powerful narcotic*] for you, don't
   waste a moment –
Take a dose of wholesome horehound; that
Will counteract the danger you suspect.

11. Fennel

Let us not forget to honor fennel. It grows
On a strong stem and spreads its branches wide.
Its taste is sweet enough, sweet too its smell;
They say it is good for eyes whose sight is clouded,
That its seed, taken with milk from a pregnant goat,
Eases a swollen stomach and quickly loosens
Sluggish bowels. What is more, your rasping cough
Will go if you take fennel-root mixed with wine....

14. Chervil

Come, holy Muse, thou who in sacred song
Canst stablish monuments of mighty wars
And mighty deeds – come, scorn not to touch with me
The humble riches that my garden yields.
   Now chervil, though it splits and divides itself
In flimsy branches and gives but a paltry seed
In its thick clusters of ears, yet flourishing
All the year through gives largesse to the poor
And comfort.
   A draught of this, so easy to take,
Will counter and check internal bleeding. Again,
When mixed with pennyroyal and poppy leaves
It makes a poultice which will prove effective
For a stomach that's upset and racked with pain.

15. Lily

Now the lily, and ah! what lines can my simple Muse,
Lean and meager as she is, find to praise
The shining lily. Its white is the white of glistening snow,
Its scent the scent of sweetest frankincense.
Not Parian marble in whiteness, nor spikenard in fragrance
Surpass our lily.
   If a snake, treacherous and wily
As it is by nature, plants with deadly tongue its parcel
Of venom in you, sending grim death through the unseen wound
To the inmost vaults of the heart – then crush lilies with a weighty
Pestle and drink the juice in wine. Now place the pulp
On the top of the livid spot where the snake's tongue jabbed;
Then indeed you will learn for yourself the wonderful power
This antidote has. Nor is that all: this same pulp
Of crushed lily is good for limbs that are twisted awry.

16. Poppy

Here in this tale of trifles let me speak of Ceres' poppy –
Hers it is because, mourning the loss of her stolen daughter [Persephone],
She is said to have eaten poppy to drown her sorrow, deep
Beyond measure – to forget, as she longed to forget, her grief of mind.
　　The poppy will often help to check that dark ulcer,
Deep in the chest, which sends to the mouth the foul and acid
Belch. Its head, loaded with tiny grains, is held high
On a long delicate neck and, like the Phoenician pomegranate,
Under the broad mantle of a single skin it holds
A mass of seeds of remarkable power. The sound of chewing
(From a Latin word (*papare*)) gave it the name (that is, *papaver*) we know
　　it by now....

19. Pennyroyal

The humble scale of my song will not allow me
To embrace in fleeting verse the many virtues
Of pennyroyal. They say that Eastern doctors
Will pay as much for it as we pay here
For a load of Indian pepper. Since such a people,
Rich as they are, blessed with gold and ebony,
Who give to an eager world a wealth of marvels –
Since they will buy at such a price, so greedily,
Our pennyroyal, who can doubt its power
To allay a host of troubles?
　　Oh, how wise,
How good is God! Let us praise him as we ought.
From no land he withholds his bounty; what is rare
Beneath this sky, under another lies
In such abundance as the cheapest trash
We have among us here: some things we scorn
Rich kingdoms pay great prices for. And so
One land helps another; so the whole world,
Through all its parts, makes one family.
　　Believe me, my friend, if you cook some pennyroyal
And use it as a potion or a poultice, it will cure
A heavy stomach – that you can take for truth.
Some things are only hearsay, but custom and usage
Allow us to blend them in with lofty truth – like this:

When the sun is blazing down on you in the open
To prevent the heat from harming your head, put a sprig
Of pennyroyal behind your ear ...
    Ah me!
If my impatient Muse were not now forcing me
To take in sail and make at last for harbor,
Many another flower could I gather for you.

20. Celery [or Parsley]

    Celery is not held cheap in our gardens and many think
Taste is its only merit. But it has its virtues
And offers quick help in many remedies. If you grind
The seeds and take them, they are said to banish the racking pains
Of a troubled bladder. If you chew them together with the tender bud
It helps digest the food as it moves through the inmost parts
Of the system. And if the stomach, that king of the body, is sick,
Hurry to take a draught of water and sour vinegar
With celery: the discomfort will pass, routed and quickly cured.

21. Betony

    In the mountains and woods, in the meadows and depths of the valleys,
Almost everywhere, far and wide, grows the precious abundance
Of betony. Yet I have found it too in my garden, and there
It learns a softer way of life in the tended soil.
So great is the honor this genus has won for its name
That if my Muse wished to add to it she would find herself
Defeated at last, overwhelmed; and soon she would see
She could add nothing more to the value it has already.
    Perhaps you pick it to use it green, perhaps
To dry and store away for the sluggish winter.
Do you like to drink it from cloudy goblets? Or do you
Prefer to enjoy what it gives after long and careful
Refining? Whatever your fancy, the wonderful powers
Which this herb has will supply all your needs.
Indeed some men I know rate it so highly
That, hoping to find protection from every harm
That assaults the inner body, day after day
They drink a dose of this harsh but soothing tonic.
    Again, if your head is cut and the wound turns septic,

Crush some sacred betony, make of it dressings
And apply them frequently: you will be amazed
How quickly its powerful influence closes the wound.

22. Agrimony

And here in handsome rows you can see my agrimony.
It clothes all the fields with its profusion; it grows
Wild in the woodland shade. Much honor it has and many
Virtues – among them this: if it's crushed and drunk
The draught will check the most violent stomach-ache.
    And if an enemy blade happens to wound us
We are accustomed to try its aid, pounding
The shoots and putting them on the open place.
    If we remember to add to the dressing some sharp
Vinegar, our full strength will soon be restored ...

24. Catmint

Among the herbs my garden is always renewing
The sprigs of catmint grows as brisk as any.
Its leaves are like the nettle's, but the scent it casts
So lavishly round its tall head is passing sweet.
    It has long been known as a cure for many ailments
And ranks high among herbs. Mixed with oil of roses,
The juice makes an ointment which, they say, can clear
The hurt of a wound and the unsightly marks of a scar,
Restoring the bloom of the skin and renewing the hair
Which the blood and pus of the gaping sore had eaten away.

25. Radish

Here, in the last row of all, the radish
Roots itself strongly and raises its leaves in a broad
Canopy. Chew the root – though it's rather hot –
To check a spasm of coughing; the troublesomeness
Of that same complaint can also often be cured
If you grind the seed in a potion and swallow it down.

26. Rose

I am tired. To travel further this road would exhaust
My failing strength; the rough path of untried song
Frightens me. Else, as I ought, I should
Crown my precious roses with gold from the [River] Pactolus
And the sparkling jewels of Araby.
    Since Germany
Yields no tint of Tyrian purple and the wide realm
Of France cannot boast the proud glow of murex,
For us the rose from year to year renews in abundance
The yellow stamens of its crimson flower.
Far and away the best of all in power and fragrance,
It well deserves the name "the Flower of Flowers."
It colors the oil which bears its name. No man can say,
No man remember, how many uses there are
For Oil of Roses as a cure for mankind's ailments.
    Over against it grows the famous lily;
Its flowers breathe a scent that hangs
Long in the air; but he who crushes the gleaming buds
Of its snow-white flowers will find to his amazement
That the heavenly perfume, sweet as a scattering of nectar,
Vanishes in a moment.
    For in this flower,
Shines Chastity, strong in her sacred honor.
If no unclean hand disturbs her, if
No illicit passion does violence to her,
The flower smells sweetly. But should her pride of innocence
Be lost, the scent turns foul and noisome.
    These two flowers, so loved and widely honored,
Have throughout the ages stood as symbols
Of the Church's greatest treasures; for it plucks the rose
In token of the blood shed by the Blessed Martyrs;
The lily it wears as a shining sign of its faith.
    O Holy Mary, Mother from whose womb was born
The Son, Virgin of purest faith, though bride
In name of Joseph, O Bride and Queen and Dove,
Our refuge and our friend for ever – pluck thou
Roses for war, for peace the shining lily!
To thee came a flower of the royal stem of Jesse,
A single Son to restore the ancient line.

By his holy word and life he sanctified
The pleasant lily; dying,
He gave its color to the rose.
Peace and war he left for his church on earth,
And the virtues of peace and war are joined in Him;
In him their triumphs eternal reward.

27. Dedication

This small gift, the worthless labor of an easy service,
Is offered to you, most learned Father Grimald,
By your humble servant, Strabo. A thing of no weight,
But the heart that gives is sincere ...
   I can picture you
Sitting there in the green enclosure of your garden
Under apples which hang in the shade of lofty foliage,
Where the peach-tree turns its leaves this way and that
In and out of the sun, and the boys at play,
Your happy band of pupils, gather for you
Fruits white with tender down and stretch
Their hands to grasp the huge apples ...
   So I see you,
And I offer you this, that as you read what I gladly
Dedicate to you, you may know of my labors. And, please,
As you read, prune the faults and approve what is good.
   God give you the crown of eternal life, the palm
That is green for ever. To this my prayer may the Father,
The Son, and the Holy Ghost grant their Amen.

III. THE MEDICAL NETWORKS OF MISSIONARIES AND BISHOPS

26. THE MEDICAL NETWORKS OF EIGHTH-CENTURY ANGLO-SAXON MISSIONARIES

The Anglo-Saxon missionaries who evangelized the German lands in the eighth century also participated in spreading the teachings and techniques of ancient medicine. On at least three occasions, St Boniface (ca 672–764) received gifts of precious imported medicinal spices and resins from high-ranking members of the Roman clergy. But as the letter of Bishop Cynehard of Winchester to Boniface's collaborator and successor Lull (710–786) indicates, the English missionaries gave as well as received.

Willibald (ca 700–789) was a kinsman of Boniface, who induced him to take up missionary work. Before going to Germany, however, Willibald journeyed with his father and brother to the Holy Land, probably in 721–727. His memoir, written down by an English nun living in Heidenheim named Huneberc, is the only western narrative of a pilgrimage to the Holy Land in the eighth century. Given that Willibald later became bishop of Eichstätt in Bavaria, it is perhaps surprising to read that he was guilty of smuggling drugs. "Balsam" is a term that covers the aromatic oily or gummy resins of a number of Asian trees and shrubs. The balsam that Willibald acquired in the Holy Land probably was balsam of Mecca or opobalsamum *– the Biblical "balm (that is, balsam) of Gilead." It is made from the gum of* Commiphora gildeadensis, *a tree native to the southern Arabian peninsula, and was much prized in both pharmacy and perfumery. The customs officials in Tyre would certainly have confiscated such a valuable substance.*

a. Bishop Cynehard of Winchester Asks Lull for Drugs and Medical Books

Source: trans. Faith Wallis from the edition by Michael Tangl, *Die Briefe des heiligen Bonifatius und Lullus, Monumenta Germaniae Historica, Epistulae selectae* (Berlin: Weidman, 1916), Letter 114, pp. 246–47. Latin.

… And we beseech you, if you have access to sources of consolation that are either needful for us, or unknown to us, be they in ancient books of spiritual learning which we do not have, or through other forms of ecclesiastical assistance, do not neglect to share them generously with us. As well, if you should come into the possession of any books of secular learning unknown to us, for example, concerning medicines – of which we have a goodly quantity here, but nonetheless drugs from overseas which we find written about in these [books] are unknown to us and difficult to come by – or if you were to see to other purchases or spices [*i.e.,* drugs] which we are in need of, you might consider sharing them [with us], as you did by sending the towel.

b. Willibald Smuggles Balsam Out of the Holy Land

Source: trans. C.H. Talbot, extract from the *Hodeporicon* of Willibald *The Anglo-Saxon Mision-aries in Germany* (London: Sheed and Ward, 1954), p. 170. Latin.

When Bishop Willibald was in Jerusalem on the previous occasion he bought himself some balsam and filled a calabash with it; then he took a hollow reed which had a bottom to it and filled it with *petroleum and put it inside the calabash. Afterwards he cut the reed equal in length to the calabash so that the surfaces of both were even and then closed the mouth of the calabash. When they reached the city of Tyre the citizens arrested them, put them in chains and examined all their baggage to find out if they had hidden any contraband. If they found anything they would certainly have punished them with death. But when they had thoroughly scrutinized everything and could find nothing but one calabash which Willibald had, they opened it and sniffed at it to find out what was inside. And when they smelled petroleum, which was inside the reed at the top, they did not find the balsam which was inside the calabash underneath the petroleum, and so let them go.

27. BISHOP PARDULUS OF LAON DISPENSES MEDICAL ADVICE

*By the Carolingian period, the cathedral library in the city of Laon, north-east of Paris, possessed a remarkable collection of books on medicine. Along with Chartres, it appears to have been the gate through which texts by Mediterranean writers such as Alexander of Tralles (doc. 5) passed into the Frankish world. It was also an important center of scholarship and education, with strong links to Ireland that went back to the Merovingian period. Pardulus, bishop of Laon from 848 to 865, may well have consulted some of these medical books before writing to an ailing friend, Archbishop Hincmar of Rheims. Pardulus diagnoses Hincmar's problem as excessive *phlegm and tailors his dietary advice accordingly. He ends with a recipe for a "dessert" of broad beans in oil, which he coyly identifies as a laxative.*

Source: trans. Faith Wallis from the edition by John J. Contreni, "Masters and Medicine in Northern France in the Reign of Charles the Bald," in *Charles the Bald: Court and Kingdom. Papers based on a Colloquium held in London in April 1979,* ed. Margaret Gibson and Janet Nelson, BAR International Series 101, 2nd ed. (Aldershot: Variorum, 1990), pp. 281–82. Latin.

... For this reason, if you in your usual way show contempt [for your illness] and take little care for the health of your body, you ought to remember [your friends] and studiously preserve the health which has been restored to you by divine grace. And you should abstain completely from everything which seems to be contrary to your ailment – namely, from much fasting and from small fish, which you are accustomed to devour freely, and also from all foods which are quite fresh, that is, [fish] which are taken from the water on the same day that they are to be eaten; or if we are talking about fowl or four-footed animals, those which are consumed on the day they are slaughtered. It is necessary that these first be gutted, and the *humors carefully dried out with salt, and then afterwards he who desires health may eat them to his advantage. But never abstain from bacon or four-footed animals, for without these it will be difficult to reinvigorate your stomach. Besides this, one should abstain from everything which can be eaten raw, and even from celery, which you often eat, until it is quite certain that the Lord has restored your health. And one should return to the dry, spare, and rather bland diet of the monks. Finally, when rising from table, one should take a measure of beans that have been thoroughly purged and cooked with very clear fat. Although according to the philosophers this is said to dull the senses, it is nonetheless believed to *evacuate and dry out phlegm. It stirs up the rest of the food, which is, as it were, sleeping; and it teaches it the way it should go – and not silently! – as if [it were teaching] one who does not know how to find a way of escape through winding courses and circling paths. And therefore one should not lack familiarity with what promotes health – the *hygeia* of the Greeks. One should drink wine which is neither very strong, nor weak, but in the middle range. It should be grown not on the mountain tops, nor yet from the valley floors, but on the mountain-sides.... But other [wines] which are quite strong or very weak also nourish the humors....

28. ELIAS OF JERUSALEM SENDS A PRESCRIPTION TO KING ALFRED OF WESSEX

King Alfred the Great of Wessex is a paradoxical figure: the hero of English resistance against the Vikings, he was also a man beset with chronic health problems. Kings do not usually broadcast their physical weaknesses, yet Alfred was not reticent about his ailments. His official biography as well as his public regimen of devotion indicate that suffering was central to his identity as a Christian monarch. It bound him in a mystical way to his afflicted people and actually constituted proof of divine favor, since he succeeded in spite of his handicaps. Alfred is justly famous for his patronage of and personal involvement in the translation of a number of Latin works into Old English.

Some of these translations introduce medical allusions into the original text; these digressions may represent the king's private interests. Alfred has also been linked to Bald's Leechbook *(see doc. 30). The unique manuscript of this encyclopedia includes a fragmentary excerpt or summary of a letter from the Patriarch of Jerusalem, Elias, conveying medical advice to the king.*

Source: trans. Faith Wallis from Bald's *Leechbook*, book 2, c. 64, ed. Thomas Oswald Cockayne, *Leechdoms, Wortcunning and Starcraft of Early England*, Rolls Series 35 (London: Longman [et al.], 1864–66), vol. 2, pp. 288–90. Old English.

[*The beginning of the recipe is missing.*] ... to the weight of a penny and a half. Grind it fine, and add the white of an egg, and give it to the person to drink. It is also very good in this manner for cough and *carbuncle; apply this herb, and the person will swiftly be healed. Anoint with this balsam for all infirmities of the human body: against *fever, apparitions, and every delusion. *Petroleum is also good to drink straight in cases of internal tenderness, and to anoint the exterior of the body on a winter day, because it abounds in heat. For this reason one should drink it in winter. If anyone has lost the power of speech, let him take [petroleum] in his mouth, make the sign of Christ under his tongue, and then swallow a little of it. Again, if a man is out of his wits, let him take a dose of [petroleum], and make the sign of Christ on every member, except for the cross on the forehead, which should be made with balsam, as well as the one on the top of the head. *Theriac is a good drink for internal tenderness. The person who does what is written here will do himself much good. On the day when he is to drink [theriac], he should fast until midday and stay out of the wind that day. Then let him go to the bath and sit there until he sweat. Then he should take a cup, and put a little warm water into it, and take a small amount of theriac and stir it into the water. Strain it through fine cloth, and drink it. Then let him go to bed and cover himself warmly and lie there until he sweats profusely. Then let him get out of bed, sit up and put his clothes on. He should have his meal at nones [*3 p.m.*] and he should take care to stay out of the wind that day. This will help the man greatly, as I believe in God. The white stone is effective against the stitch and against flying poison and every untoward calamity. You should grate it into water and drink a substantial amount, and grate into it some red earth. In *potions, stones are all very effective against every untoward thing. When a spark is struck from a stone, it is effective against lightning and thunder and against every kind of delusion. Should a traveler lose his way, he should strike a spark in front of him, and he will soon be going in the right direction. The lord Elias, patriarch of Jerusalem, ordered that all this be conveyed to King Alfred.

29. LETTERS OF MEDICAL ADVICE FROM BISHOP FULBERT OF CHARTRES AND HIS CIRCLE

Bishop Fulbert of Chartres (d. 1028) enjoyed a reputation during his lifetime and long after as a man of learning, a saintly personality, and a charismatic teacher. His diocese was in a politically sensitive position, being technically a royal bishopric but actually in the domain of one of King Robert the Pious's most ambitious vassals, Count Odo of Blois. A collection of Fulbert's letters assembled by his student Hildegar after his death reveals the networks, clerical and secular, that the bishop of Chartres needed to manage and maintain. They also provide insight into the many meanings, practical and spiritual, of medicine amongst the clerical elite, for one way in which Fulbert sustained his friendships with his fellow bishops was by offering them remedies and medical advice. The letter to Bishop F. reveals that prior to becoming a bishop himself, Fulbert actually compounded medicines. Moreover, when he sent some rather sophisticated compound medicines to Bishop Adalbero of Laon for the use of one Ebalus, he casually assumed that Adalbero could consult an *antidotarium to learn how they ought to be administered. Nonetheless, Hildegar, Fulbert's closest disciple, subdean and scholasticus of Chartres, saw fit to send detailed instructions to Ebalus on how to take the *hiera.

Because Fulbert was marginally involved in a dispute between King Robert and Count Odo over certain lands in Champagne, some letters relating to this event are included in his collection. King Robert's ally, Count Fulk of Anjou, recruited Bishop Hubert of Angers to attack Tours. Hugh, archbishop of Tours, excommunicated the two men. Hubert's protest against this sentence elicited Hugh's response in the letter below. In this letter, Hugh freely employs a conventional analogy between sin and sickness, penance and therapy.

Source: trans. Frederick Behrends, *The Letters and Poems of Fulbert of Chartres* (Oxford: Clarendon Press, 1976): letters 24 (pp. 45–47), 47–48 (pp. 83–85), and 71 (pp. 119–29). Latin.

Letter 24. Fulbert to Bishop F.: Sending Him Some Ointment (1006–28)

To his father and fellow bishop, F. from F(ulbert).

Believe me, father, I have not prepared any ointments since I was raised to the bishopric. But the little that is left of what a doctor (*medicus*) gave to me I am sending as a gift from me to you with the prayer that Christ, the author of good health, may make it help you. Farewell.

Letter 47. Fulbert to Bishop Adalbero of Laon: Sending Him Some Medicines (before 12 March 1021)

To Bishop A(dalbero), by whom virtue is possessed rather than professed, from F(ulbert).

As your friend we rejoice to hear that you are in good health; and as for the illness of your faithful servant and our good friend Ebalus [*Adalbero's secretary; see letter 48 below*], we have taken steps to give him all the help in our power, if God in his mercy approves, by sending three doses of Galen's *hiera and three of the four-in-one [*theriac]. What these are good for and how to take or to administer them can easily be found in your *antidotaria. We are also sending the wild nard that you asked for, though we do not advise a man of your age to weaken himself by using this as a *purgative, but rather, if it is necessary to be relieved, to stimulate sluggish bowels with *oximel and radishes (which can be done frequently and without danger) or indeed, as is more suitable for an older man, with laxative pills. We are taking the liberty of sending you about seven and a half dozen of them, and please consider as your own whatever else we have that might help you. Farewell.

Letter 48. Hildegar to Ebalus: Directions for Taking a Laxative [*the hiera of Galen*]

To his lord, E(balus), whom he cherishes with sincere love and affection, from H(ildegar), with many greetings.

Take the dose of *hiera* which the bishop is sending you with warm water before twilight. On the evening when you are going to take it, do not eat supper. On that evening put the *hiera* in the vessel in which it is to be mixed and sprinkle it with a crystal of salt or, if this is not available, with one twenty-fourth of an ounce by weight of clarified salt. After you take it, sit in front of the hearth, away from any excitement, and guard yourself completely from the cold. If you lie down for a little while, it will not hurt you, but I do not want you to go to sleep. As soon as you feel your bowels moving, walk slowly and go to the privy. If you should become thirsty because of the purging, do not drink anything except a little vinegar mixed with warm water so as to wash out and refresh the stomach. (You can do this, even if you are not very thirsty, when the purging is almost over.) Do not eat until you feel that the purgative has stopped acting. When you sit down at the table, see to it that you observe moderation and eat nothing sharp or more salty than average. I would set down more about how to take this save that a few words are enough for a wise man. But I am writing this much at the bidding of charity, which cannot be feigned, so that you may feel a good effect from this medicine and remain in continual good health. Farewell.

Letter 71. Archbishop Hugh of Tours to Bishop Hubert of Angers: Answering His Charge That He Had Rashly Excommunicated Him and Admonishing Him as Regards the Health of his Soul (before 10 June 1023)

To Bishop H(ubert) of Angers from Archbishop H(ugh) of Tours, with his greetings.

Although the letter that you recently sent me ought to be answered in kind, I have thought it better for the time being to refrain from answering you as your arrogance deserves and instead to attend to my duty as regards your salvation and while doing this to make a reasoned and humble reply to certain passages in your letter. It is a physician's duty to offer those who are suffering from depression (*melancholia*), insanity (*mania*), or other illness what he has learned in the exercise of his art and to apply himself with all diligence to the task of curing them even if they are ungrateful and insult his skill. Similarly it is my duty – though I do not claim to be even the most unskilled of physicians, but only somehow to have advanced to where I have an obligation as your archbishop to correct you if you go astray – to administer to you, ungrateful as you may be, the remedies I have acquired from the holy fathers and to apply myself to the task of curing you whether you want me to or not....

I can tell from what you are doing, brother, that your soul is fostering various disorders. If these are not counteracted by some remedy before they grow to full strength, they will result in your soul's dying a miserable death. But the proper remedy for each disorder cannot be known unless their origins and, as it were, their roots are examined with care and discernment. All disorders of the soul have the same source and origin, but each has its own proper name in accordance with the nature of the part of the soul which is diseased. This is also shown by the diseases of the body. If a harmful *humor should attack the head, the illness is known as a headache; if it should attack the feet, it is known as gout-of-the-feet (*podagra*); if the hands, it is called gout-of-the-hands (*ciragra*). Thus it is that a disease caused by a single humor has as many different names as the parts of the body that it attacks. Moving from the realm of the visible to the invisible, we think that the power of each vice dwells in different parts of the individual soul. Now philosophers distinguish three faculties in the soul: the rational, the irascible, and the concupiscible; and it is in accordance with the nature of the diseased part that each *infection receives its name. If it should infect the rational part, it will produce the vices of vainglory, self-elation, envy, pride, insolence, scorn, heresy. If it should afflict the irascible part, it will bring forth anger, impatience, depression, spiritual sloth, faint-heartedness, and cruelty. If it should infect the concupiscible part, it will engender gluttony, fornication, greed, avarice, and harmful and worldly desires.

So, brother, as I have said I can tell from what you are doing that your soul is fostering that which will kill it. In showing such monstrous pride, scorn, and insolence toward me, your especial master, you reveal that the rational faculty of your soul is dreadfully diseased. That you possess these three vices is clearly proven: pride, by the haughtiness of your answer to the archbishop; scorn, by your having no regard for his injunctions...; insolence, by your having ventured to celebrate mass when you were excommunicated.... These three vices are clear proof, as I have said, that the rational part of your soul is diseased. As to whether the other parts of your soul have fostered any vice, you must see to it yourself; for to this part, which I see to be so horribly diseased, I shall, as I have promised, administer one of the remedies acquired from the holy fathers so as to restore it to health. But what I administer will not do you any good unless the remedy of penance is first applied to heal that wound which will lead to your death. As soon, I say, as this has been healed by penance, use the scalpel of prudence to cut away the tumors of pride, scorn, and insolence, which I have reason to believe have already become hardened in your soul. Then *cauterize the raw wounds that this produces with the hot iron of holy fear so as to prevent their fostering some other disorder; and keep the places you have cauterized warm with the fire of charity and the oil of mercy that they may not be chilled by the touch of impiety. When you have done this and have destroyed that pride which moved you to assail me with such savage replies, that scorn which prompted you to have no regard for my injunctions, and that insolence which led you to venture to celebrate mass when you were excommunicated, the rational part of your soul will in large part be restored to good health. Then take the virtues of humility, patience, and obedience, and mix them with the honey of the divine word, and carefully store this remedy in the cupboard of your mind. By eating some of this daily, not only will your soul never foster these same disorders, but it will shine forth untarnished by any others....

CHAPTER FOUR

A REGIONAL CASE STUDY: MEDICINE IN ANGLO-SAXON ENGLAND

Up to this point, we have been concentrating on medical knowledge conveyed through texts in Latin. Indeed, medicine in the Carolingian period benefited from the effort of rulers and clerical leaders to shore up and improve Latin literacy. So successful was this revival that in the Romance zone, Latin continued to be the primary written language well after French, Italian, and Spanish had emerged as distinctive vernaculars.

But there were parts of Europe where the spoken language was not Latin-based: the German-speaking parts of the Carolingian empire, the Slavic and Celtic lands, and Anglo-Saxon England. The vernacular languages of these regions evolved written forms in the early medieval period not only to record their native literatures, but also to convey didactic, religious, and administrative information. In the case of Anglo-Saxon England, vernacular writing extended to medicine.

The unique manuscript of the first Leechbook *presented here (the word* leech *means "doctor" in Old English) was commissioned by a man named Bald, who may or may not have been a medical practitioner. It was "written" (though whether in the scribal or in the literary sense is unclear) by a certain Cild. The manuscript dates from about 950, though the text itself may have been composed as early as 900. Bald's* Leechbook *comprises two parts: book 1 covers external diseases, arranged in head-to-toe order, and book 2 deals with internal ailments. The work is heavily dependent on classical Mediterranean sources – the chapter on pain in the side bears some resemblance to the account of pleurisy in the* Liber tertius *(doc. 6) – though there is evidence that it was carefully edited for use in northern regions, where Mediterranean drugs were rare and costly. In short, it is both a scholarly and a practical manual. Reproduced below are some representative extracts from both sections.*

The anonymous Leechbook III *is medieval Europe's oldest vernacular medical text. Though for the most part organized in the classical head-to-toe order, its contents reflect an Anglo-Saxon medical practice that is less closely tied to Mediterranean influences. Most of its ingredients are native, and there are a number of treatments that modern readers might consider magical. It is worth remembering that the definition of magic in the Middle Ages was quite precise: it denoted an intention to harm or control another person through the invocation of pagan or demonic spiritual forces. If the intention was to do good, and the spiritual power invoked was the Christian God, it was not "magic."* Leechbook III *also has a number of treatments for a mysterious condition called "elf-sickness," apparently a debilitating or wasting disease of sudden onset and often fatal course. The underlying idea was that elf-sickness was caused by an invisible wound from a supernatural weapon – an arrow shot by an elf.*

30. *BALD'S LEECHBOOK* AND *LEECHBOOK III*

Source: trans. M.L. Cameron, *Anglo-Saxon Medicine* (Cambridge: Cambridge University Press, 1993), and Michael Swanton, *Anglo-Saxon Prose* (London: Dent, and Totowa, NJ: Rowman and Littlefield, 1975). The source of each excerpt is indicated in the editorial title. Old English.

1. Bald's Leechbook, Book 1. External Disorders

[*Surgery for Limbs Which Have Lost Circulation (1.35; Cameron, pp. 170–71)*]
About blackened and deadened body. The disease comes most often from *erysipelas; after the inflammation of the disease has gone away, the body sometimes becomes blackened. Then, from the original inflammation, the disease is to be cooled and treated with cold things, and when the disease comes from outside without obvious symptom, then you must first cool the heat with pounded coriander, with bread crumbs moistened with cold water, or with the juice itself of the coriander, or with white of egg, or with wine, or with other things which have the same properties. When the inflammation and the heat are gone away and the part of the body has turned either somewhat pale or livid or something like that, then *scarify the place (then you will improve it), and dry with a poultice such as is made with a *cerote and warm barley and such things. He is not to be let blood from a vein but rather shall be tended with *purgative *potions, either *emetic or diuretic, with which you can cleanse the *corrupt *humor and its red *bile sickness. Indeed, even though the harm does not come from the inflammation of *erysipelas the sharp potion is good for such patients. If the inflammatory livid or red condition come from outside, from wounds or from cuts or from blows, immediately treat the conditions with scarifying and poultices of barley; according to the way which physicians well know you will amend it. If the livid body is so deadened that there is no feeling in it, then you shall at once cut away all the dead and unfeeling part as far as the living body, so that there be nothing of the dead body left, nor of that which before felt neither iron nor fire. After that let the wound be treated as you would the parts which still may have some feeling and are not altogether dead. With frequent scarifyings, sometimes with many, sometimes with few, wean and draw off the blood from the deadened place. Treat the scarifyings thus: take bean or oat or barley meal, or of such meal that you think it will accept, add vinegar and honey, cook together and lay on and bind on the sore places. If you should want the salve to be stronger add a little salt, bind on at times and wash with vinegar or with wine. If there is need, give at times a herbal potion and at all times observe when you give the strong medicines what is the power and nature of the body, whether it is strong or hard and easily can

stand strong medicines, or is soft and tender and thin and cannot stand the medicines. Apply the medicines according to how you see the bodies, for there is a great difference between man's and woman's and child's bodies and in the constitution of a daily laborer and of the idle, the old and the young, and of one used to suffering and of one unused to such things. Also, pale bodies are softer and weaker than the dark and the red. If you wish to carve or cut off a limb from a body, then observe what sort of place it is and the power of the place, because some places putrefy if one tends them carelessly, some feel the medicines later, some earlier. If you must carve or cut off a diseased limb from a healthy body, then cut it (not) on the boundary of the healthy body, but much rather cut or carve on the healthy and living body, so that you may cure it better and sooner. When you set fire on a patient, then take tender leek leaves and pounded salt, lay over the places; then the heat of the fire is the sooner drawn away.

[Jaundice (1.42; Cameron, p. 14)]

From bile disease, that is from the yellow one, comes great misery. It is the most powerful of all diseases; then an excess of humor grows internally. These are the symptoms: that his body all becomes bitter and turns yellow like good silk and under his tongue strongly black and bad veins and his urine is yellow. Let him blood from the lung vein, give him often a stirring potion, stone baths [that is, saunas] frequently. Prepare for him then a calming drink of dock in wine and water, and every morning in the bath let him drink a mulled drink; it will alleviate the bitterness of the bile.

[Pains in the Side (1.46–50; Cameron, p. 15)]

If these symptoms continue for a long time, then the ailment is too dangerous and the patient cannot be cured. Nevertheless, ask the one who suffers this whether he ever was struck in the side or stabbed or whether some time before he had fallen or got a fracture. If it were that, then he will be easier to cure. If it comes from cold or from harmful internal humors it will be because of that harder to cure. Then if he had earlier suffered from pain in the liver or in the lungs and the pain in the side comes from that then it is very dangerous. If it had been earlier in the spleen then it is easier to cure. Then if he had earlier been wounded in the lung and the pain in the side comes from that, then that is very dangerous. If it had been earlier in the spleen then the pain comes in the left side, that also has serious danger; ask him whether his spleen is sore or whether he has a sore throat. Thus you may understand that pain in the side comes from harmful humors and is very dangerous.... By these symptoms you may understand where the man is to be treated and where not.

[*A Sampler of Recipes, with Some Advice about Bloodletting (1. 68–72; Swanton, pp. 181–82*]

1. 68. In case a poisonous spider – that is the stronger one – should bite a man, cut three incisions close to and running away from it; let the blood run into a green hazel-wood spoon, then throw it away over the road so there will be no injury. Again; cut one incision on the wound, pound a plantain, lay it on; no harm will come to him. For the bite of a weaving-spider, take the lower part of *æferthe* [*an unidentified substance*] and lichen from a black-thorn; dry it to powder, moisten with honey; treat the wound with that. For the bite of a poisonous spider: black snails fried in a hot pan and ground to powder, and pepper and betony; one is to eat that powder, and drink it and apply it. For the bite of a poisonous spider: take the lower part of mallow; apply it to the wound. Again: cut five incisions, one on the bite and four around about; in silence, cast the blood with a spoon over the wagon-road.

1. 69. For the bite of a mad dog: mix agrimony and plantain with honey and the white of an egg; treat the wound with that. For a wound from a dog: boil burdock and groundsel in butter; anoint with that. Again: bruise betony; apply it to the bite. Again: beat plantain; apply it. Again: seethe two or three onions; roast them on ashes; mix with fat and honey, apply it. Again: burn a pig's jaw to ashes; sprinkle on. Again: taken plantain root; pound it with fat; apply it to the wound so it casts out the poison.

1. 70. If a man be over-virile, boil water agrimony in Welsh ale; he is to drink it at night, fasting. If a man be insufficiently virile, boil the same herb in milk; then you will excite it. Again: boil in ewe's milk water agrimony, alexanders, the herb called Fornet's palm; so it will be as he most desires.

1. 71. For the dorsal muscle: seethe green rue in oil and in wax; anoint the dorsal muscle with it. Again: take goat hair; let it smoke under the breeches against the dorsal muscle. If a heel-sinew be broken, take Fornet's palm, seethe it in water, *foment the limb with it, and wash the limb with it; and make a salve of butter; anoint after the fomentation.

1. 72. At which time bloodletting is to be avoided, and at which to be allowed. Bloodletting is to be avoided for a fortnight before Lammas [*August 1*] and for thirty-five days afterwards, because then all poisonous things fly and injure men greatly. Those doctors who were wisest taught that no one should drink a [medicinal] potion in that month, nor anywhere weaken his body, unless there were great need for it – and then to stay inside during the middle of the day, since the air is most infected then. Therefore the Romans

and all southern people made earth-houses for themselves because of the air's heat and poisonousness. Doctors also say that flowering herbs are then best to work, both for potions and salves and powder.

How one should avoid bloodletting on each of the six "fives" of the month [*every day which is a multiple of five*]; and when it is best. Doctors also teach that no one should be let blood at a five-night old moon, and again at a ten-night, and fifteen and twenty and twenty-five and a thirty-night old moon, but between each of the six "fives." And there is no time so good for bloodletting as in early spring when the evil humors which are imbibed during winter are gathered together, and best of all in the month of April, when trees and plants first sprout, when the bad pus and the bad blood increases in the cavities of the body....

1. 87. If a man's hair fall out, make him a salve; take great hellebore and viper's bugloss, and the lower part of burdock, and gentian; make a salve from that plant and from all these, and from butter on which no water has come. If hair fall out, boil the polypody fern, and foment the head with that very hot. If a man should be bald, the great doctor Pliny [*i.e., the* Physica Plinii*: see doc. 8*] prescribes this remedy: take dead bees, burn them to ashes – linseed also – add oil to it; seethe very long over the coals, then strain and wring out; and take willow leaves, pound them, pour into the oil, boil again for a while over the coals, then strain; anoint with it after the bath....

2. Bald's Leechbook, Book 2. Internal Disorders

[*Liver Diseases (2.17–18; Swanton, pp. 183–84)*]
2. 17. For all liver diseases, their origins and consequences, and concerning the six things which cause pain in the liver; and remedies for all those, and plain symptoms respecting both urine and lack of appetite, and their color. The liver extends on the right side as far as the pit of the stomach; it has five lobes and cleaves to the loins; it is the blood's material, and the blood's dwelling and nourishment. When foods are 'digested and attenuated, they come to the liver; then they change their color and turn into blood; and then it casts out the impurities which are there and collects the pure blood and sends it through four arteries; chiefly to the heart, and also throughout the whole body to the furthest members.

Respecting six things which cause liver-pain: first swelling, that is, a tumor of the liver; second is the bursting of the swelling; third is a wound of the liver; fourth is surging heat with sensitiveness and with a sore swelling; fifth is a hardening of the stomach with sensitiveness and with soreness; sixth is a hardening of the liver without sensitiveness and without soreness. You may discern a swelling or tumor of the liver thus: the swelling in the liver occurs first under the soft rib on the right side, and there the man first feels heaviness and pain; and from that place the pain ascends over all the side as far as the collar-bone and as far as the right shoulder; and his urine is blood-red, as if it were bloody; and he is afflicted with lack of appetite and his color is pale, and he is somewhat feverish and constantly feels cold, and trembles as one does with typhus; he cannot keep food down; the liver enlarges and one cannot touch the pain with the hands, so severe is it; and when it is most severe one has no sleep. When the swelling bursts, then the urine is purulent like pus; if it runs out the pain is less.

[*Surgery for Liver Abscess (2.21; Cameron, p. 172)*]
The description of the symptoms of liver abscess in Bald's Leechbook *strongly suggests that it is caused by the parasite* Entemoeba histolytica, *which is responsible for dysentery. When it invades the liver, this parasite can cause abscesses that discharge into the colon, pleural cavity or body wall. The operation closely resembles one described in the Hippocratic corpus for removing pus from the pleural cavity.*

Yet if the swelling and the pus rise so that it seems to you that it can be lanced and let out, then prepare for him first a salve of dove's dung and such like, and beforehand bathe the place with sprinklings with the water and herbs that we wrote about before. When you consider that the swelling is becoming soft and subsiding, then touch him with the iron lancet and cut a little bit and skillfully so that the blood can come out lest a harmful pocket descend in thither. Do not release too much blood at any time, lest the sick man become too exhausted or die, but when you pierce or lance it then have a linen bandage ready so that you may bind up the wound at once, and when you wish to let out more afterwards remove the bandage; let it out thus little by little until it dries up, and when the wound is clean enlarge it so that the opening is not too narrow. Moreover, every day syringe it with a tube and wash with those things; afterwards lay on what may clean the wound. If it discharge very uncleanly, cleanse with honey and draw it together again.

[*Hemiplegia (Paralysis on One Side of the Body) (2.59; Cameron, p. 16)*]
The disease comes on the right side of the body or on the left; there the sinews are relaxed and have a slimy and thick humor, harmful, thick and plentiful. The humor must be removed with bloodlettings and potions and medicines. When the disease first comes on the patient, then open his mouth, look at his tongue; then it is whiter on the side on which the disease will be. Then treat him thus. Carry the patient into a very well enclosed and warm chamber, let him rest there very well sheltered and let warm coals be

brought in frequently. Then unwrap him and look at his hands carefully and whichever one you find cold, at once bleed him on the cold vein.

3. Leechbook III

[Headache (III.1; Swanton, p. 184–85)]

In case a man ache in the head: take the lower part of crosswort, put it on a red fillet; let him bind the head with it. For the same: take mustard seed and rue, rub into oil, put into hot water; wash the head frequently in that water; he will be healthy. For an old headache, take pennyroyal, boil in oil or butter; with that anoint the temples and over the eyes and on top of the head; even though his mind be turned, he will be healthy. For a very old headache, take salt and rue and bunches of ivy berries; pound all together, put into honey, and with it anoint the temples and the forehead and on the top of the head. For the same: look for little stones in the stomachs of swallow chicks; take care that they do not touch earth or water or other stones; sew up three of them in whatever you wish; put them on the man who is in need; he will soon be well; they are good for headache and for eye pain and for the Devil's temptations, and goblins, and typhus, and incubus and herbal seizure and bewitching and evil enchantments; it must be big chicks in which you will find them. If a man ache on one side of his head, thoroughly pound rue, put it into strong vinegar, and with that let the head be anointed right on top. For the same: dig up plantain, without iron, before the rising of the sun; bind the roots around the head with a moist red fillet; he will soon be well.

[Pregnancy and Childbirth (III.37, Cameron, p. 175)]

In case a woman cannot bring forth a child, take wild parsnip, the lower part, boil in milk and in water, put equal amounts of both, give the roots to eat and the juice to sup. For the same, bind on the left thigh, up against the genitalia, the lower part of henbane or twelve grains of coriander seed, and that shall be done by a boy or a girl; when the child is delivered remove the herbs lest the innards come out. If the natural afterbirth will not go out of the woman, boil old fat bacon in water, [and] with it foment the vulva; or boil in ale brooklime or mallow leaves, give it to drink hot. If there be a dead child in a woman, boil brooklime and pennyroyal in milk and in water, give to drink twice a day. A pregnant woman is to be earnestly warned that she should eat nothing salty or sweet, nor drink beer, nor eat swine's flesh nor anything fat, nor drink to intoxication, nor travel by road, nor ride too much on horseback, lest the child be born before the proper time. If she bleeds too much after birthing, boil the lower part of *clote [unidentified herb]* in milk, give to eat, and the juice to sup.

[*Charms against Various Ills (III.57, 61, Swanton, p. 185)*]

Against a woman's chatter: eat a radish at night, while fasting; that day the chatter cannot harm you.

Make thus a salve against the race of elves, goblins, and those with whom the Devil copulates; take the female hop-plant, wormwood, betony, lupin, vervain, henbane, dittander, viper's bugloss, bilberry plants, cropleek, garlic, madder grains, corn cockle, fennel. Put those plants in a vat; place under an altar; sing nine masses over it; boil it in butter and in sheep's grease; add much holy salt; strain through a cloth; throw the herbs into running water. If any evil temptation come to a man, or elf or goblin, anoint his face with this salve, and put it on his eyes and where his body is sore, and cense him and frequently sign him with the cross; his condition will soon be better.

[*Elf-Sickness (III.62–63; Cameron, pp. 138–39, 154)*]

For elf-sickness, take bishopswort, fennel, lupin, alfthone the lower part and lichen from a hallowed crucifix and frankincense, put a handful of each, tie up all the herbs in a cloth, dip in consecrated font-water three times, let sing over them three [votive] masses: one, *Omnibus sanctis* [*in honor of all the saints*], another *Contra tribulationem* [*against tribulation*], the third, *Pro infirmis* [*for the sick*]; then put coals in a brazier and lay the herbs on them, then cense the man with the herbs before tierce [*9 a.m.*] and at night and sing the *Litany* and *Creed* and *Pater noster* [*the Lord's Prayer*] and write a Christ's cross for him on every limb, and take a little handful of herbs of these same kinds similarly consecrated and boil in milk, drip holy water on them three times and let sup before his meal; he will soon be well....

If he has the *elfsogoþa* [*literally, "elf-sucked"*], his eyes are yellow where they should be red. If you wish to treat the man, consider his behavior and observe which sex he is: if it is a male and he looks up when you first examine him and his face is dark yellow, that man you might cure completely if he has not been too long in it; if it is a woman and she looks down when you first examine her and her face is dusky red, you may treat her also. If it is longer by a day than twelve months and the appearance be like this, then you can improve it for a while, and yet cannot cure completely. Write this writing: *Scriptum est rex regum et dominus dominantium. byrnice. beronice. luslure. iehe. aius. aius. aius. Sanctus. Sanctus. Sanctus. dominus deus Sabaoth. amen. aleluiah.* [*It is written: King of King and Lord of Lords. byrnice. beronice. luslure. iehe* [*In Greek*] *Holy. Holy. Holy.* [*In Latin*] *Holy. Holy. Holy. Lord God of hosts. Amen. Alleluia.*] Sing this over the drink and the writing: *Deus omnipotens pater domini nostri ihesu christi. per inpositionem huius scriptura expelle a famulo tuo N. omnem impetum castalidum, de capite, de capillis, de cerebro, de fronte, de lingua, de sublingua, de guttore, de faucibus, de dentibus, de oculis, de naribus, de auribus, de manibus, de collo, de brachiis, de corde, de anima, de genibus, de coxis, de pedibus, de compagnibus omnium membrorum intus et foris, amen.* [*Almighty God, Father of our Lord Jesus Christ, by the imposition of this writing cast out from your servant N. every elfish assault, from the head, from the hair, from the brain, from the forehead, from the tongue, from under the tongue, from the throat, from the gullet, from the teeth, from the eyes, from the nostrils, from the ears, from the hands, from the neck, from the arms, from the heart, from the soul, from the knees, from the hips, from the feet, from the joints of all the members within and without. Amen.*] Then make a drink: font water, rue, sage, cassock, dracontia, smooth plantain the lower part, feverfew, dill blossoms, three cloves of garlic, fennel, wormwood, lovage, lupin, all of equal amounts; write three times a cross with oil of extreme unction [*oil used for the ritual anointing of the dying*] and say: *Pax tibi* [*Peace be with you*]. Then take the writing, with it write a cross over the drink and sing this over it: *Deus omnipotens pater domini nostri ihesu Christi per inpositionem huius scripture et per gustum huius expelle diabolum a famulo tuo N.* [*Almighty God, Father of our Lord Jesus Christ, by the imposition of this writing and by this drink, cast out the devil from your servant N.*] Wet the writing in the drink, and write a cross with it on each limb and say: *Signum crucis Christi conservate in vitam eternam amen.* [*Preserve the sign of the cross of Christ to everlasting life. Amen.*] If you do not wish to, bid the patient himself or one who is most closely related to him, and let him cross him as best he can. This treatment is good for every temptation of the devil.

III. 63. If one is in the water elf-sickness, then his fingernails are livid and his eyes watering and he wishes to look downward. Do this for him as a treatment: boarthroat, cassock, the lower part of iris, yewberry, lupin, elecampane, marshmallow heads, fen mint, dill, lily, attorlothe, pennyroyal, horehound, dock, elder, centaury, wormwood, strawberry leaves, comfrey. Pour over with ale, add holy water, sing this charm over three times:

> For wounds I have bound on the best of battle-bandages,
> so that the wounds may not burn or burst,
> nor expand, nor multiply, nor skip about,
> nor wound grow, not lesion deepen;
> but to him [I] myself hold out a cup of health,
> nor may it pain you more than earth *on eare* [*meaning unknown*] would
>   pain.

Sing this many times: "Earth bear on thee with all her might and main." This charm may be sung on wounds.

PART II.

PHYSICA: THE ADVENT AND IMPACT OF ACADEMIC MEDICINE (1100–1500)

Between the turn of the millennium and the beginning of the thirteenth century, certain fundamental conceptions of medicine began to change in western Europe. So did the words used to denote medicine. Medicina *retained all its traditional meanings of "medication," "medical treatment," or "medical knowledge." But now there was a new synonym for medical knowledge:* *physica. Physica's *primary meaning was "natural philosophy." Hence, equating medicine with* physica *shifted the epistemological status of medical knowledge toward what modern doctors call basic sciences: anatomy, physiology, and pathology. Medieval medical writers called this "theory."*

Medicine's theoretical turn first emerges into view in the writings associated with the city of Salerno in south-central Italy (chapter 5). Salerno's achievement was to braid together three strands of cultural innovation. One strand was the translation into Latin, largely from Arabic, of texts that expounded medical theory, as well as of encyclopedic and specialized medical literature with an explicit theoretical framework. The second strand was the emergence of formal academic teaching of medicine, based on the analysis of texts and the logical solution of doubtful and contradictory points. This teaching was, apparently, accompanied by anatomical demonstrations. The third strand of the braid was the impetus to recast medical practice into a more systematic, rational form. Together, these formed the fabric of a new style of learned medicine that called itself physica.

Because physica *was synonymous with natural philosophy, it supported medicine's claim to a place in the new universities. The documents in chapter 6 illustrate how that claim was made good. Depending on where the university was located, medicine's niche would be carved out in different ways, but all medieval medical faculties adopted and adapted the common intellectual style of the academy, scholasticism, as its own "way of the schools" (*via scolaris*). The methods of analysis and debate that were nurtured in Salerno were now applied to a much larger corpus of texts. These included the great medical syntheses of the Arab-Islamic world and an expanded selection of the writings of Galen. Learned doctors would rediscover the core argument of Galenic "rational" medicine, namely, that only the practitioner who understands the* cause *of a disease can safely and effectively treat it. Chapter 7, "Theory and Practice in Scholastic Medicine," shows how the new learned medicine rose to the challenge of translating theory into practice – or restating practice in terms that harmonized with theory. In the university environment, medicine also came face to face with other sciences that claimed to be based on rational knowledge of natural processes and promised to enhance medicine's practical efficacy. Astrology and alchemy (chapter 8) seem superstitious to the modern mind, but* *they were considered rigorously natural by scholastic thinkers. That did not, however, mean that the claims of these "power sciences" were always accepted as plausible, practical, or licit. From this contested frontier, we can begin to map the relationship of medicine and medieval society: this will be the subject of Part III.*

CHAPTER FIVE

SALERNO: MEDICINE'S "THEORETICAL TURN" AND THE RATIONALIZATION OF PRACTICE

In antiquity, the region around the city of Salerno in southern Italy was colonized by Greeks, and a Greek-speaking culture persisted into the medieval period; it is also close to Sicily and north Africa and in consequence was exposed to Arab-Islamic civilization. Salerno had a reputation as a health resort that produced and attracted skilled doctors. By the beginning of the twelfth century, that reputation had taken on a more scholarly coloration. Salerno, however, was not the only place where a new style of academic medicine was emerging. Indeed, in this chapter "Salerno" will stand for a whole constellation of developments in eleventh- and twelfth-century medicine, whether physically situated in Salerno or elsewhere. The stars in this constellation are translation, medical theory, academic instruction, and the textualization of medical practice.

One symptom of western European society's growing confidence and complexity in this period was its self-conscious and deliberate project to locate and appropriate ancient knowledge. Medical learning played a rather large role in this project. This involved translating texts into Latin, either directly from Greek or via Arabic translations. The Arabic translations, moreover, arrived with traveling companions – commentaries, encyclopedias, and specialized treatises that were to enlarge Europe's library of medical learning substantially. Both a cause and a consequence of this translation project was a significant change in how medicine was defined and conceptualized. As early as the end of the tenth century, one begins to notice an emerging distinction between practical medicina *and a kind of medicine grounded in textual scholarship and concerned with broader scientific questions about anatomy, physiology, and pathology (doc. 31). Under Arab-Islamic influence, this dimension of medicine was baptized "theory." Texts on theory translated and commented on in the milieu of Salerno bear the unmistakable marks of an academic setting. They are didactic and analytical – not manuals for reference but textbooks for classroom study (docs. 33–34). Nowhere is the atmosphere of formal instruction more vividly evoked than in a group of innovative texts on dissecting animals (doc. 35). This new theoretical way of thinking and writing about medicine could shape more practical kinds of medical knowledge as well. Pharmacy, therapeutics, and surgery were recast into textual forms that are quite unlike those of the early medieval period (docs. 36–38). Above all, these texts are eager to emphasize that every practice has a rationale that ties it to theory.*

Salernitan medicine was unquestionably part of the wider cultural effervescence commonly called the "Renaissance of the Twelfth Century," but it was also closely connected to movements for religious reform and to developments in theology and spirituality.

The great Benedictine monastery of Monte Cassino was the final home of Constantine the African (doc. 32) and an important force in both the diffusion of medical writing and the Gregorian Reform of the Church. The combination is not coincidental. The equation of health and salvation was an old one; what was new in the twelfth century was the way in which religious reformers exploited the language of medical theory to articulate their vision of humanity's role in creation, and its spiritual destiny.

31. TENTH-CENTURY MEDICINE: THE TESTIMONY OF RICHER OF RHEIMS

In one sense, little seemed to be happening in western European medicine in the tenth and eleventh centuries. There were no changes in the way it was taught, few additions to the library of medical texts (until the second half of the eleventh century), and no evident alterations to practice. In another sense, this was the period when something very significant was changing: Europe itself. Medicine was one of many elements of western culture that began to mutate in the decades on either side of the millennium.

The direction of this shift is illustrated in the history of his own times composed by Richer, a monk of Saint-Rémi in Rheims (d. after 998). Rheims was an important ecclesiastical center in northeastern France, and in Richer's day its cathedral school was presided over by a charismatic teacher, Gerbert of Aurillac, later Pope Silvester II. As a young monk, Gerbert traveled to Catalonia, where (in Richer's words) he engaged in "deep and rewarding studies in mathematics." Returning to France, he taught as scholasticus or master of the cathedral school of Rheims for ten years, specializing in rhetoric, dialectic, and the mathematical sciences of the quadrivium *(i.e., arithmetic, geometry, music, and astronomy). Gerbert's efforts to flesh out the curriculum of the liberal arts with new materials were carried forward by his many pupils. This ensured that scientific knowledge would have a secure place in the cathedral schools of the eleventh century; it was within that scientific niche that learned medicine eventually found an intellectual home.*

Richer was intensely interested in medicine and recorded a number of medical anecdotes in his Historia. *Two are reproduced here. The first describes Richer's own medical studies. Notice that Richer was interested in reading medical texts as part of his "program" in the liberal arts. He was not pursuing practical training, and the diagnostic and prognostic maxims of Hippocrates's* Aphorisms *initially attracted him as* logica, *or texts about reasoning. The second anecdote contrasts the medicine of a learned and literate bishop with the practical skill of a doctor from Salerno. Richer's point is that the best medical practice is based on a thorough knowledge of "the nature of things," grounded in book learning. It is Derold's mastery of language and logic that marks him as the most accomplished doctor. Ironically, text-based medicine grounded in "the nature of things" would shortly become the hallmark of Salerno.*

Source: trans. Faith Wallis from Richer, *Histoire de France,* ed. Robert Latouche (Paris: Les Belles Lettres, 1967), vol. 2, pp. 224–30, and vol. 1, pp. 222–26. Latin.

a. Richer's Study of Medicine (book 4, chapter 50)

While I was deeply immersed in the study of the Liberal Arts and eager to master the *logica* of Hippocrates of Cos, I met one day in Rheims a man of horseback from Chartres. I asked him who he was, whom he served, why and from whence he came. He replied that he had been sent by Heribrand, a cleric of Chartres, and that he wished to speak with Richer, monk of St Rémi. I immediately recognized the name of my friend and the reason why he sent the messenger, so I indicated to him that I was the one he was looking for. I greeted him with a kiss and we went inside. He then produced a letter inviting me to [travel to Chartres and] read the *Aphorisms* [with Heribrand]. I was overjoyed, and taking a servant along with the horseman, I made ready to depart for Chartres....

[*Richer describes at length his dangerous and uncomfortable journey from Rheims to Chartres.*]

[Arriving at Chartres], I applied myself with diligence to the *Aphorisms* in the company of Master Heribrand, a man of great generosity and learning. But all I learned from it was the prognosis of diseases; simple knowledge of diseases like this was not enough for me and so I begged to read the book entitled *The Harmony of Hippocrates, Galen, and Soranus* [*an unidentified work*] with him. I got my wish, for the secrets of the action of drugs, pharmacy, botany, and surgery were not hidden from this man, so well versed in the Art was he.

b. Bishop Derold and the Doctor from Salerno
(book 2, chapter 59)

At this time Bishop Derold of Amiens died, a distinguished man, a courtier, a great favorite of the king, and very well versed in the art of medicine. They say that when he was still in the king's service at court, he was deceived by a doctor from Salerno, but that he deceived [the Salernitan] in turn. Both men were very accomplished in the art of medicine, but the king [Louis IV of France] preferred Derold, while the queen thought that the Salernitan exhibited greater expertise. By a subterfuge of the king, it was revealed which of the two knew more about the natures of things.

[The king] invited them to dine with him, carefully concealing the reason. He frequently posed questions to them; each resolved them as best he was able. Derold, who was deeply learned in those sciences conveyed through the study of texts (*litterarum artibus*) gave convincing explanations of the subjects proposed. As for the Salernitan, although totally lacking in any book learning (*litterarum scientia*), he nonetheless had considerable practical experience thanks to his innate intelligence.

At the king's command, they sat every day at the royal table and drank together. One day the discussion turned to the particularities of drug action and they talked at length about what drugs, surgery, and botany did. The Salernitan, unfamiliar with these strange terms, blushed and declined to explain them. Thus he became very jealous [of Derold] and pondered how to make a poison that would kill him; meanwhile he cunningly feigned goodwill.

When the poison had been prepared and when they were all together at dinner, the Salernitan dipped the nail of his middle finger, which he had impregnated with the poison, into the pepper sauce with which they were seasoning their food. All unawares, Derold ate it, and when the poison started to worm its way [into his body], he began to feel weak. His people carried him away and he drove off the power of the venom with *theriac.

Three days later he came back and rejoined the Salernitan. When questioned about what had happened to him, he said – to give the impression that he was unaware of the crime – that he had been mildly indisposed, due to cold from *phlegm. In this way he put his enemy off guard. When they were at table once again, Derold sprinkled some poison which he had concealed between his ring and his index finger on the food which [the Salernitan] was about to eat. Spreading swiftly through the veins, [the poison] put the vital heat to flight; [the Salernitan] was carried off by his people in agony. He tried to expel the poison, but his efforts were of no avail. So praising Derold and proclaiming him to be the very summit of medicine, he earnestly begged him to treat him.

Yielding to the king's command, [Derold] administered antidotes to the poison, but he deliberately did not *purge it completely. For when [the Salernitan] took the theriac, the power of the poison was lodged in his left foot; in this way (as he told his close companions) the poison, climbing up the vein from his foot like a chick-pea, was pushed back into the foot when it met with the antidote. Because these reactions went on for a long time, the skin on his foot became ulcerated. This brought on illness, and after that the surgeons performed a painful amputation.

32. CONSTANTINE THE AFRICAN: THE ROMANCE OF TRANSLATING ARABIC MEDICINE

Constantine the African's translations and adaptations of Arabic medical writings were the foundation of the expansion of European medical learning in the twelfth century. We know very little about him, save that he was of north African origin, possibly from Kairouan in Tunisia. Many of the works he translated were by physicians from this region. He came to Salerno before 1077 and died as a monk in Monte Cassino sometime between 1085 and 1098. Under the patronage of Archbishop Alfanus of Salerno and Abbot Desiderius of Monte Cassino, Constantine translated encyclopedias such as the Pantegni *(the* Whole Art of Medicine *composed ca 977 by 'Ali ibn al' Abbas al Majûsi, known in the West as Haly Abbas), works of practical medicine such as the* Viaticum *(Medicine for Travelers, an adaptation of* Provisions for the Traveler and the Nourishment of the Settled *by Abu Ja'far Ahmad ibn Ibrâhîm ibn alî Khâlid al-Jazzâr, d. 979), and the works on regimen, 'fevers, and urine inspection by Isaac Judaeus (Ishâq ibn Sulaymân al-Isrâ'îlî, d. ca 932). His translation of the* Isagoge *of Hunayn ibn Ishâq (doc. 33) became the standard introductory textbook on medical theory and the cornerstone of the new* Articella *anthology.*

Constantine's early life and education, as well as the motives for his migration to Italy and his translation project, spawned a number of more or less romantic legends. These tales reveal conflicting views about the value of Arabic medical learning, the relative strength or weakness of western medicine, and the dynamics of cultural transmission. The principal medieval source for the career of Constantine is Peter the Deacon's biographical notice in On Distinguished Men *(De viris illustribus, composed ca 1130–40). It is paralleled by an entry in the* Chronicle of Monte Cassino *(Chronica Cassinense), a work begun around 1099 by Leo Mariscanus (d. 1115), which Peter himself revised and continued. This account of Constantine depicts him as the conduit of exotic eastern scientific and medical lore to the Christian West. Peter also includes an extensive bibliography of Constantine's translations, though there are some omissions, such as* On Melancholy *(a translation of a work by Ishâq ibn 'Imrân) and, rather surprisingly, the* Isagoge. *Later in the twelfth century, a certain "Master Matthaeus F." (probably Matthaeus Ferrarius) incorporated a different biography of Constantine into a marginal gloss on Constantine's translation of Isaac Judaeus's* Universal Diets. *Matthaeus claims that he obtained his information from one "Johannes" – possibly Johannes Afflacius, Constantine's fellow monk and collaborator. Constantine is now a merchant, not a scholar or doctor, and his interest in medicine is sparked by a visit, not to the Orient, but to Rome. Nor did the tales stop here: yet a third account, which may have originated in Montpellier (Salerno's rival as a center of medical learning), paints Constantine as a fugitive from Spain and a dangerous incompetent who nearly killed a royal patient.*

a. Peter the Deacon: Constantine the Oriental Sage

Source: trans. Faith Wallis from Peter the Deacon, *De viris illustribus*, c. 23 (with supplementary material from *Chronica Monasterii Casinensis* III.35), ed. Francis Newton, *Montecassino in the Middle Ages* (Cambridge, MA: Harvard University Press, 1986), vol. I, pp. 126–29. Latin.

The Chronicon Monasterii Casinensis's *account roughly parallels Peter the Deacon's but begins with the following additional information:*

At the time of this abbot [Desiderius] Constantine the African came to this place and took the holy habit, and with great devotion he donated [to

Monte Cassino] the church of St Agatha in Aversa, which Prince Richard had granted him. So that these things may be remembered by those who come after us, it behooves us to convey how much and what kind of things he wrote.

Constantine the African – a monk of this monastery, highly learned in all philosophical studies, master of East and West, a new Hippocrates – left Carthage, his birthplace, and went to Babylon [*Cairo*], where he learned grammar, dialectic, rhetoric, geometry, arithmetic, mathematics, astronomy, necromancy, music, and the medicine (*physica*) of the Chaldeans, Arabs, Persians, and Saracens. Departing thence, he went to India and devoted himself to study there. And when he had learned all the arts, he went to Ethiopia and there learned the Ethiopian disciplines. When he was replete with their knowledge, he went to Egypt, where he learned all the Egyptian arts to the fullest extent. Having spent thirty-nine years in all these studies, he returned to Africa. When the Africans saw that he was so learned in all the knowledge of the nations, they conspired to kill him. When Constantine found out about this, he secretly took ship for Salerno and hid there for some time as a poor man. Then he was recognized by the brother of the king of Babylon, who had come there, and he lived in great splendor with Duke Robert. Then Constantine left and went to the monastery of Monte Cassino, and was warmly received by Abbot Desiderius and became a monk. In this monastery, he translated many books from different foreign languages, of which the most important are:

The [*Theory of the*] *Pantegni*, which he divided into twelve books, which expounds what a doctor should know

The *Practice* [*of the Pantegni*], in which he set forth how a doctor should preserve health and cure illness, and which he divided into twelve books

The *Book of* *Degrees*

Diets [that is, Isaac Judaeus, *Universal Diets* and *Particular Diets*]

Book of Fevers, which he translated from the Arabic [of Isaac Judaeus]

Book of Urine [of Isaac Judaeus]

On Internal Members

On Sexual Intercourse

Medicine for Travelers [*Viaticum*], which he divided into seven parts: the first concerning illnesses which arise in the head; then on illnesses of the face; of the instruments [of sensation]; illnesses of the stomach and intestines; illnesses of the liver, kidneys, bladder, spleen, and gall bladder, and those which arise in the organs of generation; and all which arise on the surface of the skin

The commentary on the *Aphorisms* [of Hippocrates, by Galen]

The Art of Medicine [*unidentified: perhaps the Isagoge?*]

Megategni [*an abbreviated version of Galen's Therapeutic Method*]

Microtegni [*Galen's Tegni or Art of Medicine*]

Antidotary [*an expanded version of Book 10 of the Practice of the Pantegni*]

The Debate of Plato and Hippocrates concerning their Opinions

On *Simple Medicines

On Women's Diseases, that is, on the organs and bodies of women

On pulses

Prognosis [by Hippocrates]

On Tried and True Remedies

Glosses on Herbs and Spices

Surgery [*part of Book 9 of the Practice of the Pantegni*]

Book of Medicine for the Eye

This man spent forty years in the study of the sciences of various peoples. He died at the age of ninety, an old man and full of days, at Monte Cassino. He lived in the times of the abovementioned emperors.

b. Master Matthaeus's Notice: Constantine the Autodidact

Source: trans. Faith Wallis from the edition by R. Creutz, "Die Ehrenrettung Konstantins von Afrika," *Studien und Mitteilungen des Benediktiner Ordens* 49 (1931): 40–41. Latin.

This work is not by Constantine, but by Isaac, as we said; however, Constantine translated it. But because Constantine never said how he came here and translated the books, we have obtained this information from Johannes [Afflacius]. Constantine was a Saracen. He was a merchant, and he came here in the course of business, and brought much merchandise with him which he peddled on the street. He went to the court of St Peter [in Rome], in which there was a very distinguished *medicus*, the brother of a prince, and who was called "the abbot" by the curia. Constantine, watching him judge urines and not knowing our language, paid some Saracen servants to translate the judgments for him. Learning through the interpreters that [the *medicus*] was quite competent in medicine, [Constantine] inquired through the interpreters concerning the color and texture of the urine. And in all matters concerning urines, [the *medicus*] answered well. [Constantine] asked him, through the interpreters, whether there were many books in Latin concerning *physica*. [The *medicus*] answered that he had none, but that he had learned through much diligence and drill. So Constantine, returning to Africa, devoted himself to the study of *physica* for three continuous years; then he came back, bringing with him many books. When he approached Palermo, he met with a storm which swamped the ship and caused him to lose part of the *Practice of the Pantegni*. But when he came here, he learned the Roman and Latin tongue, and became a Christian and a monk at the monastery of St Benedict at Monte Cassino. And he translated those books into our language. But of the practical part of the *Pantegni* he only translated three books, because it was damaged by the water. A certain Stephen of Pisa went to [Arab lands] and learned the language and translated them, so that the *Practice of the Pantegni* is now ascribed to Stephen. But in [Monte Cassino] Constantine composed the *Book of Simple Medicines* and the *Book of Degrees*, and on his own wrote a book on the stomach which he dedicated to Archbishop Alfanus, who had done him great service. Archbishop Alfanus wished to cover his expenses for the completion of the *Pantegni*.

33. MEDICAL THEORY AND THE FORMATION OF THE *ARTICELLA* (1): THE *ISAGOGE* OF JOANNITIUS

It is curious that none of the biographical notices of Constantine the African mentions the Isagoge, *even though it proved to be one of his most influential translations. The* Isagoge *(Introduction) was adapted from* Masâ'il fi-tibb *(Questions about Medicine), a summary in question-and-answer format of Galen's* Art of Medicine, *also known in the West as the* Tegni *(from the Greek* techne, *"art"). Its author was Hunayn ibn Ishâq (809–887), a Nestorian Christian who contributed enormously to the translation movement of early ninth-century Baghdad. Hunayn was the student of another famous Nestorian physician, Yûhannâ ibn Mâsawayh (d. 857), known in the West as Mesue. Hunayn's name means "John, son of Isaac," so Constantine Latinized it to "Joannitius." Constantine also changed Hunayn's book rather significantly by eliminating the dialogue, cutting the sections on pulse and urine diagnosis, and concealing the Arabic origin of the text under a Greek title. These changes may have been imposed by Constantine's patron, Archbishop Alfanus of Salerno, for the* Isagoge *rapidly joined some new translations of Hippocrates (apparently commissioned by Alfanus), and two Byzantine tracts on pulse and urine by Philaretus and Theophilus, to form the* Articella, *an anthology designed for teaching "Greek" medicine. The* Articella *was the backbone of the theoretical component of the new medical curriculum associated with Salerno, but the* Isagoge *remained in use as a standard text even after more detailed and critical expositions of Galenic theory became available, notably through translations of the major Arabic medical writers such as Avicenna.*

The catalogue-like structure of the Isagoge *made it an ideal framework for lectures, and helped facilitate memorization. On the other hand, there are some passages in the translation that are compressed to the point of obscurity, or frankly confusing (for example, the chapters on the "powers" and "spirits"). One really had to know what Galen was saying in the* Art of Medicine *to understand Hunayn's summary. This stimulated teaching commentaries on the* Isagoge *and eventually the inclusion of the* Art of Medicine *itself in the* Articella. *Moreover, Constantine did not always grasp the technical philosophical meaning of the terms used by Hunayn. The phrase translated below as "with a physical reaction" (in Latin:* cum effectu) *has an Aristotelian meaning in the original: "in act," as distinct from "in potency." This nuance was lost on Constantine, but it would not be long before western students of medicine were engaging directly with Aristotle's natural philosophy and its implications for their subject.*

Source: trans. Faith Wallis from the edition by Gregor Maurach, "Johannicius. Isagoge ad Techne Galieni," *Sudhoffs Archiv* 62.2 (1978): 148–74. Latin.

1. Medicine is divided into two parts, namely, theory and practice. And of these, theory is further divided into three, that is to say, the consideration of things that are natural, and of things that are non-natural (whence comes knowledge of health, disease, and the neutral state), and when these natural things depart from the course of nature – that is, when the four humors increase beyond the course of nature; and from what cause and symptoms disease may arise.

[The *Naturals]

2. **Natural things.** There are seven natural things: the elements, the mixtures [of qualities] (*commixtiones*), the *humors (*compositiones*), the members [of the body], the *powers (*virtutes*), the faculties (*operationes*), and the *spirits. Some people add to these four others: namely, the ages of life, the colors, the shapes, and the distinction between male and female.

3. **The four elements.** There are four elements: fire, air, water, and earth. Fire is hot and dry; air is hot and moist; water is cold and moist; earth is cold and dry.

4. **The mixtures [of qualities].** There are nine mixtures [of qualities]. Eight are unequal and one equal. Of the unequal, four are *simple: namely, hot, cold, moist, and dry. And from these come four composite [mixtures], namely, hot and moist; hot and dry; cold and moist; cold and dry. [A mixture is] equal when the body is brought to a state where it is sound and intact through a balance [of all four qualities].

5. **The humors.** There are four compound [humors]: blood, *phlegm, red
*bile, and black bile. Blood is hot and moist, phlegm is cold and moist, red
bile is hot and dry, black bile is cold and dry.

6. **Phlegm.** There are five varieties of phlegm. There is the salty phlegm,
hotter and drier than the other kinds, and tinged with red bile. There is the
sweet phlegm, associated with warmth and moisture, and tinged with blood.
There is the acrid phlegm, associated with cold and dryness, and tinged with
black bile. There is the glassy phlegm, caused by great coldness and coagulation, such as occurs in old people who are destitute of natural warmth. And
there is one which is cold and moist; it has no savor, but retains its characteristic coldness and moisture.

7. **Red bile.** Red bile exists in five kinds. There is red bile which is naturally
and substantially clear, and it originates in the liver. There is another which
is lemon-colored; it originates from the watery humor phlegm and from red
bile, and therefore it is less hot. There is a bile which is like egg yolk, which
originates from the mixture of coagulated phlegm and clear red bile, and
which is less hot. 8. A fourth kind of bile is green, like *prasius* [*a light green
semi-precious stone*] and it generally originates in the stomach; and there is
another bile that is green like verdigris and it burns like a poison. It comes
from too much *adustion and it possesses its own innate heat and innate
harmful quality.

9. **Black bile.** Black bile comes in two kinds. One kind is natural – the
dregs of the blood and its perturbation, so to speak. It is known from its
black color when it flows out of the body from below [through the bowel] or
above [from the mouth], and this kind is truly cold and dry. The other kind
is unnatural and its origin is from the adustion of the *choleric mixture, and
so it is rightly called black (that is, black bile). It is hotter and lighter than the
abovementioned kind, having in itself a vigorous action and a quality which
is extremely deadly and pernicious.

10. **Kinds of members.** There are four kinds of members. Some of them
are principal – the foundations and material, so to speak. These are four: the
brain, the heart, the liver, and the testicles. Other members serve the aforesaid
principal members, such as the *nerves, which minister to the brain, and the
arteries which minister to the heart, and the veins, which minister to the liver,
and the spermatic vessels which convey sperm to the testicles. Some members
have their own inherent power that governs these members and comprises
their quality – for example bones, all the cartilages or the membranes that are

between the skin and the flesh, the muscles, fat, and flesh. 11. There are other [members] that originate from their own innate power and derive vigor from the fundamental [members], for example, the stomach, kidneys, intestines, and all the muscles. By their own proper power, these members seek out food and transform it, and they perform their actions according to nature. They also have other inherent powers that derive from the fundamental principal [members]; sensation, life, and voluntary motion come from these.

12. **The *powers.** The powers are divided into three. There is the natural power, the spiritual power, and the animal power. One natural power ministers, and another is ministered to. Sometimes it generates, at another time it nourishes, and at another time it feeds. But the power that ministers sometimes seeks out, retains, *digests, and expels the things that minister to the feeding power, just as the feeding power ministers to the nourishing power. 13. The other two serve the generating power, one by altering food, the other by re-fashioning it. These differ from one another in that the first power alters, and it serves the generating power through the activity of re-fashioning. But the operations of the re-fashioning power are five: assimilation, hollowing out, perforating, roughening, and smoothing.

14. **Spiritual power.** From the spiritual power, two others proceed: one is operative and the other is operated upon. The operative power is that which dilates the heart and arteries and then contracts them. From the one which is operated upon come anger, indignation, triumph, domination, astuteness, and anxiety.

15. **Animal power [*the power of* animus *or* mind].** Animal power encompasses three things. One animal power arranges, discriminates, and assembles; a second one moves with voluntary motions; the third is called "sensing." From the ordering, discriminating, and assembling power come these things: imagination in the front part of the head, cognition or reasoning in the brain, and memory in the occipital region. The [second animal] power moves with voluntary motion. And the sensing power consists in sight, hearing, taste, smell, and touch.

16. **Faculties.** Faculties are of two kinds. There are faculties of which each accomplishes on its own what pertains to it, such as appetite for food [which works] by means of heat and dryness; digestion [which works] by means of heat and moisture; retention [which works] by means of cold and dryness; expulsion [which works] by cold and moisture. There are also composite faculties which are composed of two [faculties]: such are desire and expulsion.

For desire is compounded of two powers: one longs for something and the other senses, for the stomach senses its emptiness. Expulsion is composed of two or more powers, one which expels and the other which senses.

17. *Spirit. The spirits are three. First, the natural spirit takes its origin from the liver; second, the vital spirit, [originating] from the heart; third, the animal spirit, from the brain. Of these three the first is diffused throughout the whole body in the veins which have no pulse; the second is transmitted by the arteries; and the third by the nerves. These are considered in the seventh division of the seven natural things, that is, the spirit.

18. **The ages [of life].** There are four ages; namely, youth, prime of life, maturity, and old age. Adolescence is of a hot and moist *complexion; in adolescence the body increases and grows up to the twenty-fifth or thirtieth year. The prime of life follows, which is hot and dry, preserving the body in a perfect state, with no diminution of its powers, and it ends at age thirty-five or forty. After this comes maturity, which is cold and dry, in which the body begins to decline and decrease, although its power is not abated, and it lasts to the fiftieth or sixtieth year. After this comes old age, abounding in phlegmatic humor, cold and wet, in which it is apparent that there is a decline of power, and it ends with the end of life.

19. **Skin color.** The colors of the skin are two kinds: those due to internal causes and those due to external. The internal causes again are two in number; namely excess or equality of humors. From equality comes that tint which is composed of white and red; from inequality proceed black, yellow, red, greyish (*glaucus*), and white. Red, black, and yellow signify that heat dominates in the body: yellow alone signifies reddish bile; black alone, black bile; red alone, an abundance of blood. White and greyish signify abundant cold; but greyish shows that the cause is black bile, white shows it is phlegm. 20. Colors also arise from external circumstances: for example, from cold among the Irish; from heat among the Ethiopians; and from many other incidental factors. There are also spiritual colors, originating in fear, or anger, or other disturbances of the mind.

21. **Hair color.** There are four colors of hair – black, red, grey, and white. Black is due to an excess of scorched bile or to a great burning of blood; red to an abundance of heat that is not scorched – this is always the cause of reddish hair; grey arises from an abundance of black bile, and white from a deficiency of the natural heat and the effect of *putrid phlegm (this is mainly found in the elderly).

22. **The tunics of the eye.** The eye has seven coats and three humors. The first coat is called the retina, the second the secundine, the third the sclera, the fourth the web [*choroid*], the fifth the uveal, the sixth the cornea, and the seventh the conjunctiva. The first humor is the vitreous, the second the crystalline, and the third the albugineous.

23. **The colors of the eyes.** The colors of the eyes are four: back, whitish, varied, and grey. Black color is due to a defect of the *visual spirit, because it is clouded, or from a lack of crystalline humor, or because most of the crystalline humor remains on the inside [of the eye], or from abundance of the humor that is like the white of an egg [*the albugineous humor*], or because it is perturbed, or from the high quality of the uveal humor. 24. Whitish [color] comes from seven things which are the opposite of those just mentioned, namely from an abundance or clarity of the visual spirit, the magnitude and prominence of the crystalline humor, a reduction in the quantity and clarity of the albugineous humor, and a deficiency in the quality of the uveal humor. Varicolored and grey come about when the circumstances which result in black and white converge. Variable color signifies by its variety that the visual spirit is more abundant and brighter; grey color signifies by its greyness that the visual humor is less abundant, and somewhat darkened.

25. **The qualities of the body.** The qualities of the body are five in number; namely, obesity; thinness; emaciation, atrophy, and the mean state. Fatness of flesh arises from lack of heat and overabundance of moisture; thinness arises from heat and intense dryness. Emaciation arises from cold and intense dryness; atrophy from cold and intense moisture. And a mean state arises from a mean proportion of the humors. These are the shapes of the body.

26. **The difference between male and female.** The male differs from the female because he is hotter and dryer; she, on the contrary, is colder and more moist.

[The *Non-naturals]

27. **Changes of air.** Changes of the air come about in five different ways; from the seasons, from the rising and setting of the stars, from the winds, from the lands, and from the vapors that arise from them.

28. **The four seasons of the year.** The seasons of the year are four: spring, which is hot and moist; summer, which is hot and dry; autumn, which is cold and dry; winter, which is cold and moist. The nature of the air is changed by

the stars, for when the sun approaches a star or a star the sun, the air becomes hotter. But when they separate the coldness of the air is increased.

29. **The winds.** There are four winds: the east wind, the west wind, the north wind, and the south wind. Of the latter two, the nature of the first [that is, the north wind] is cold and dry and of the second [the south wind] is hot and moist. The two others are of an equal nature, for the east wind is hot and dry and the west wind is cold and moist. The south wind is slightly hotter and moister and the north wind colder and dryer.

30. **Modalities of terrain.** There are four modalities of terrain: namely, height, depth, nearness to mountains or to the sea, and the level quality of places or terrains. How do terrains differ from one another? In height and depth, for height produces cold and depth the contrary; in nearness to mountains, for if the mountains are to the south, the locality will be cold because the mountains block the hot winds, and so the north winds seek it out with their cool blasts. 31. But if the mountains are to the north of the locality, the reverse is the case. As regards proximity to the sea, a south [-facing coast] will make the terrain hot and dry, the north will make it cold and dry. Moreover, terrains differ amongst themselves by their nature. Stony terrain is cold and dry; thick and heavy terrain is hot and moist; clay is cold and moist. Exhalations from marshy terrain or other places where decay is going on also change the air and give rise to disease and pestilence in human beings.

32. **Exercise.** Exercise produces change in the body. When it is moderate, it causes a moderate amount of heat; when it is increased, it warms it to a greater degree and afterwards cools it down.

33. **Rest.** Rest produces change in the body; if excessive, it increases cold and moisture.

34. **Baths.** Baths are either of fresh water or of water which is not fresh. A fresh-water bath softens the body, a hot bath warms it, a cold bath cools it. But a fresh-water bath dries out the body, while baths of salt or bitter or sulphurous waters heat and dry the body, and alum or alkaline baths cool and dry it.

35. **Kinds of foods.** Foods are of two kinds. Good food generates good humor and bad food generates an evil humor. That which produces a good humor is that which generates good blood; namely, that which is in a balanced state as regards mixture [of qualities] and operation, such as clean bread [with

bran removed] and the flesh of yearling lamb or kid. Bad food brings about the contrary state, for example old bread, or bread with bran in it, or the flesh of old rams or goats. Foods producing good or evil humors are of two kinds, heavy or light. Pork and beef are heavy; chicken or fish are light. And of the latter, the flesh of the middle-sized and more active kinds is better than that of the fatter and scaly varieties. 36. Some kinds of vegetables produce an evil humor of red bile; for instance, nasturtium, mustard, and garlic. Lentils, cabbage, and the meat of old goat's flesh or beef produce black bile. Suckling pig, lamb, purslane, and mountain spinach beget phlegm. Moreover, heavy foods produce phlegm and black bile, and light food produces red bile; in either case, this is bad.

37. **Kinds of drink.** Drinks are of three kinds. First, there is drink which is nothing but a drink: for example, water. Secondly, there is drink which is both drink and food, such as wine. Thirdly, there is drink which is both of these, and this is the *potion which is given to counteract the harm from a disease, such as melicrate [*honey and water*], mead, or spiced tonic. Food is useful because it restores the integrity of the body in its proper order. Drink is useful because it distributes food throughout the body. But that kind of drink which we called "potion" is useful because it changes the nature of the body into itself.

38. **Sleep.** Sleep changes the nature of the body in that it cools it on the outside and warms it on the inside. If it be prolonged, it cools and moistens the body.

39. **Wakefulness.** Wakefulness also changes the body, for it warms it on the outside while it cools and dries it on the inside.

40. **Sexual intercourse.** Sexual intercourse is beneficial for the body; it dries the body and diminishes the natural power and so cools it down, although oftentimes the body is warmed by a good deal of vigorous motion.

41. **Incidental states (*accidentia*) of the soul.** Some incidental states of the soul have an effect on the body, such as those which bring the natural heat from the interior of the body to the surface of the skin. Sometimes this happens suddenly, as with anger; sometimes gradually and agreeably, as with sensations of delight. Some affections, again, contract and suppress the natural heat – either suddenly, as with fear and terror, or gradually, as with anguish. There are some which disturb the natural energy both in the interior [of the body] and on the exterior, for instance, sorrow.

[The *Contra-naturals]

42. *Fever. Fever is unnatural heat, exceeding the normal course of nature, proceeding from the heart into the arteries; and it inflicts harm by its effect. There are three kinds: the first is in the spirit (*animus*), and it is called "ephemeral"; the second arises from humors which *putrefy, and it is called "putrid"; and the third damages the members of the body, and this one is called "*hectic." Of these, the ephemeral variety arises from incidental causes, and putrid [fever] also, [which arises] from things that are putrefied. 43. Some of these are simple and not combined with others, and these are four. The first is that which arises from the putrid state of the blood, scorching both the interior and exterior of the body; for instance, a continued fever. The second is that which arises from the putrid state of red bile; for instance, *tertian fever. The third arises from the putrid state of phlegm; for instance, *quotidian fever. And the fourth arises from the putrid state of black bile; this attacks the sick man after an interval of two days, and this is called *quartan [fever].

44. **Kinds of fever.** In addition there are three kinds of fevers that follow on a state of putridity. There is the fever which diminishes day by day, and there is the one that increases until it departs; and there is the one which remains in a constant state until it departs. Continuous fever arises from putridity in the veins, and when it is declining, it is outside the veins in certain parts of the body. Goose-flesh in fevers comes about from an infusion and superfluity of putrid matter in sensitive members, gnawing and chilling them. Therefore, goose-skin occurs in these fevers which are characterized by remissions, because [the sensitive members] are outside the veins.

45. **Swellings (*apostemata*).** There are four simple kinds of swellings: those which arise from the blood and are called *phlegmons; or those which arise from red bile and are called *erysipelas; those which arise from phlegm which has coagulated and are called *zimiae*; or those that arise from black bile and are called cancers. The signs of phlegmon from blood are these: redness, hardness, throbbing, pain, heat, and swelling. The signs of those arising from red bile are these: heat, redness mixed with a yellow color, great pain, and rapid growth. The signs of those arising from phlegm are these: white color and softness, so that if you press your finger into it, it makes an indentation, and it has no color. The signs of those arising from black bile are these: great hardness, black color, and absence of sensation.

46. **What produces health.** If each of the natural things in the human body preserves its proper nature, health is maintained. If any should lose its

proper nature, this will make either for illness or the neutral state. There are three classes of illness: similar, universal, and official. 47. A [similar disease] is one affecting the *similar members and they have a similar name when the type of suffering is the same, for example, an *aching* head. An [official disease] befalls *official members such as the feet, hands, tongue, or teeth. This takes its name from the infirmity incident to them, for instance podagra [in the foot] or chiragra [in the hand]. And finally there is a universal disease, which is linked to the other two, for example dislocation of the members.

48. **Similar diseases.** There are eight diseases that attack the similar parts. Four are simple, that is, [they are] hot, cold, wet, and dry. The four composite [diseases arise] from the combination of these: cold and moist, cold and dry, hot and moist, hot and dry. Each of the eight kinds comes in two types, for either it arises from a simple quality or from combination with another humor. 49. A disease arising from a simple quality and which affects the members, is what the Greeks call "hectic." A hot disease arising from a humor is a fever that comes from putridity, as has been said above. A "chill" is a cold disease that occurs without any humor, from very cold air or snow, and it is a simple cold disease without admixture of any humor. But paralysis, either complete or partial, is a cold disease with an admixture of humor. 50. A cold wound or one that is open and very fetid and accompanied by wasting, like the puffy flesh of *dropsy patients that languishes in open filth, is the type of moist disease that arises from itself and does not need moisture from another humor. A moist disease is one that attracts humor to itself, like dropsy. A dry disease is one without humor, like a seizure caused by weakness. A hard, dry cancer is a dry disease with an admixture of humor.

51. **Diseases of official members.** There are four diseases in official members: those that occur in the substance and form of the creature, in the size of the members, in a superfluity of unnatural number, and in the position of the members. 52. There are five types of diseases affecting the human form: a lack of harmony in the members, for example, ugly elongation of the head; in the hollow parts, as when the hollow of the hand or foot is filled with flesh; constriction or dilation of the pores; roughness, for instance of the throat or roughness of the channels in the lungs; smoothness, for example smoothness of the uterus.

53. **Diseases of size in members.** Diseases in the size of members happen from excess when they grow larger than is fitting (as we see in a big head or a thick tongue) or from disproportionate and unseemly smallness (for example a small head, stomach, or liver).

54. **Diseases of number in members.** Diseases in the number of members arise from augmentation or diminution. Those due to augmentation are either according to the course of nature, such as an extra finger, or outside the course of nature, such as round worms, thread worms, warts, and hanging warts. Those due to diminution are either universal, such as loss of all the fingers, or particular, such as the loss of one [finger]. 55. Diseases in the position of members happen either because the member is removed from its proper place or from the disposition of a neighboring part, such as fingers and lips which are fused or adhere together and do not separate, or which are separated and not fused together. 56. Separation of a fused member happens in both similar and official members – in similar members such as the bones, the nerves, the flesh, the veins, the muscles and the skin. If it happens to a bone, it is called a fracture; when it happens to the flesh and is fresh, it is called a wound. But if it is old, it is not called simply a wound, but a putrid wound. When it happens in veins, nerves, or arteries, it is sometimes called by one name and sometimes by the other. 57. If it occurs in the middle of a muscle, it is called a contusion or a crushing wound. If it occurs in the skin, it is called excoriation; but if it is of long standing, it is called a putrid wound. Separation occurring in the official members becomes permanent, for example, when a hand or foot is amputated.

58. **The quality of the body.** The qualities of the body are three in number: namely, health, sickness, and the neutral state. Health is a balanced condition (*temperamentum*) that composes the natural things according to the course of nature. Sickness is an imbalanced condition outside the course of nature from which harm results. The neutral state is that which is neither healthy nor diseased. But there are three kinds of neutral state: when health and disease co-exist in different parts of the same body; [a state] such as obtains in the body of an elderly person, where not a single member remains that is not causing trouble or suffering; 59. and [a state] such as obtains in the body of a man who is sometimes healthy and sometimes sick – for instance, those who are sick in the summer and healthy in the winter. People who are of a cold nature are sick in the winter and healthy in the summer; those who are of a moist nature are sick in childhood, but well in youth and old age, while those of a dry nature are healthy in childhood, but sick in youth and old age. 60. Health, sickness, and the neutral state are found in three things: in the body in which any one of the three qualities occurs; or in the cause which produces and establishes these [qualities]; or in the signs which signify them.

61. **Types of causes.** There are two kinds of causes: either what is natural or what is outside the course of nature. Natural causes either produce health

or preserve it. The causes that preserve, pertain to health; and the causes which produce, pertain to illness. Some of the causes that transgress nature pertain to illness, and others to the neutral state. But sickly causes produce sickness and also the things that maintain sickness. Those that pertain neither to health nor to sickness, preserve or constitute the neutral state. 62. There are six types of causes that are associated with health and sickness. The first is the air which surrounds the human body, [then] food and drink, exercise and rest, sleep and waking, fasting and fullness, and incidental conditions of the mind. All these preserve health from accidents, if used with appropriate moderation as to quantity, quality, time, function, and order. But if anything is done contrary to this, diseases occur and persist.

63. **The types of causes that produce disease.** There are three types of causes that produce disease: some are called "primitive" and happen to the outside of the body, such as cold and heat; some are "antecedent" and act within the body, such as repletion or starvation; while yet others are called "conjoint," because when they are present, the disease is present, and when they depart, so does the disease, such as putridity in fevers.

64. **The distinction of causes.** According to another division, there are two kinds of disease: either common or proper. Those that occur commonly occur either by necessity, or accidentally – accidentally, such as a blow, a burn, a bite, a tear, or some other harm, and the other things mentioned above, which are (as we said) associated with health and sickness. Truly proper sicknesses occur and persist either in the similar members, or in the official members, or in permanent division.

65. **Types of diseases.** There are five kinds of disease arising from heat. The first is either from agitation of the spirit or from agitation of the body – from an agitation of the spirit such as anger, from an agitation of the body such as pain. The second is from the convergence of visible heat with a physical reaction, as in sunstroke. The third is from heat which comes upon the body with violence, as when it receives heat from eating sharp foods. The fourth is from closure of the pores, as from cold in the winter. The fifth is from putridity as in fevers.

66. **Cold diseases.** There are eight causes of cold disease. The first is the incursion of visible frigidity with a physical reaction, as from the coldness of snow. The second is the coldness of opium, which overwhelms the human body. The third is excess [of food], which overwhelms the body, fills it up,

and extinguishes the natural heat. The fourth is from scanty food, which extinguishes the natural heat; the fifth, from abundance of cold humor blocking the pores, so that the natural heat is diminished; the sixth, from looseness of the bowels and opening of the body, so that the natural heat is dissolved and *evacuated. The seventh is from agitation and much exercise, whence come great dissolution of the humors, and evacuation, and sweating, by which the body is weakened. The eighth is caused by much rest and idleness.

67. **Dry diseases.** There are four causes of dry disease. The first cause is external, visible dryness, with an evident reaction – for example, the dryness of poison. The second is the violent intrusion of something dry in the body, for instance, vinegar, salt, or mustard. The third is scantiness of food or drink. The fourth is excessive agitation and exercise.

68. **Moist diseases.** There are four kinds of moist disease. The first is an encounter with a source of heat that produces a physical response, such as a bath. The second in the ingestion into the body of something moisture-bearing, together with [its natural] virtue, such as fresh fish. The third is excess of food or drink. The fourth is sleep and leisure.

69. **The unnatural type of diseases.** There are four kinds of disease that flow to weakened members from an unnatural evil, together with a certain humor. The first is the power of the expulsive member and the weakness of the retentive member. The second is a great quantity of humor. The third is weakness of the power of nutrition. The fourth is expansion of the pores.

70. **The evil quality of diseases.** The evil quality of a disease attacks and overcomes a similar member in five different ways: either it happens in the mother's womb, or at the time of birth, or from tight swaddling, or from bad feeding, or from any disease occurring before or after. 71. If debility of a similar part happens at the time of conception in the uterus, this is caused by overabundance of sperm, or from scantiness and defect in the appropriate quality of the sperm, which may be gross and thick, or watery and thin. When the child is born, a member may be injured if [the child] does not come out in the proper way, but in a bad way, for example with face upwards or with the knees bent. If it be too tightly swaddled with inappropriate swaddling, it is doubly injured. 72. When it is badly and inappropriately fed in taking milk or suckling, it is enfeebled. And at these times or afterwards, when sickness occurs, evil befalls the similar member by the cutting of some sinew. Or some accident may occur, or a wound, or a swelling. 73. Sickness

may affect a similar member in seven different ways: either from a midwife who makes a mistake when she holds the child or allows the child to walk before the appropriate time; from a physician if he sets and bandages broken or bruised limbs unskillfully; from the patient, if he moves [a limb] after it has been set by the doctor but before it has properly consolidated or healed; from a fracture, as when the tailbone is twisted by the muscle of the vertebra which is in the thighbone; from a blow as, for instance, if the nose be driven in and a splayed nose results; or from the evil humor that affects lepers; or from the deficient humor that affects those with *consumption.

74. **Constriction of the pores.** Constriction of the pores has three causes: from limited constriction; or from fleshiness; or from narrowing. Constriction is caused by an excess of retentive power, or by deficiency of expulsive power, or by much cold, or by tight constriction of some part of a limb, or by much dryness, as often happens from a tight ligature. 75. The pores are also constricted due to fleshiness, as when there is an *aposteme and fleshiness is created, or if there was a wound there beforehand. [It happens] because of narrowing when there is something in the pore such as humor, or a stone, or a blood clot, or something concealed in [the pores] such as superfluous flesh or scabies.

76. **Dilation of the pores.** There are four causes of dilation of the pores: from excessive agitation of the expulsive power, or deficiency of the retentive power; from excessive heat and humor; or from taking *aperient medicines. Smoothness happens in two ways, either internally or externally; if internal it is due to viscous humor, and if external it is caused by liquefied wax, combined with an ointment. Roughness likewise happens in two ways: internal and external. Internal [roughness] comes from superfluous and sharp humor, external from smoke and dust.

77. **Superfluity of members.** An excess in the number of members happens in two ways: either the excess is natural in which case it is due to an excess of the natural and good humor, or it is from excess of vital power. If it is outside the course of nature, it will be because of an unnatural and discordant humor or from excessive vital power.

78. **Diminution of the members.** Diminution of the number of the members is likewise of two types, either internal or external. Internal [diminution] is due to diminution of humors; external to burning, cold, putridity, or cutting. Putridity is caused either by a potion which causes mortification and putrefaction, or by constriction and retention of the humor, which then breaks down.

79. **Largeness and smallness of the members.** Largeness of the members occurs in three ways: either from a great deal of humor, or from an excess of the natural power, or from agitation of both. Smallness likewise occurs in three ways: from deficiency of vital power, from reduction of natural humor, or from an external injury such as cutting, burning by fire, or from cold and snow.

80. **Disturbance of a member.** Disturbance of a member from its place happens in two ways: either from a voluntary disturbance, or when a humor that is close to the quality [of the member] dissolves the member and makes it slippery.

81. **Dislocation of a member.** Likewise, a member or bone is removed from its proper joint and altered in two ways: either from a joining in which the separation is not as it ought to be, or from a separation in which the joining is not as it ought to be. If this happens from joining without separation, it will be due to the humor of the patient or the inflicting of a wound, or a spasm. If it happened from a separation in which the joining was not as it should be, it happened either because of a thick humor, or because a wound was inflicted, or because of a spasm.

82. **Separation of joints.** Separation of things that are joined together has two causes: either intrinsic or extrinsic. The intrinsic [cause] is either from a sharp and cutting humor, or from a thick *windiness that distends and dissipates. The extrinsic cause is either from ablation, fracture, excessive exercise, a cut (for example, with a sword), or from something that stretches (such as a rope), or that bruises (such as a stone).

83. **The genera of signs.** There are three genera of signs: some signify health, others sickness, and others the neutral state. Each genus is divided into two; for there are those that signify concerning the official members, and there are also those which signify concerning the similar members. Signs relating to similar members are of two kinds: some are substantial and others accidental. The substantial ones are heat, cold, dryness, and moisture. Some accidental ones signify either by touch, as hardness or softness, or by sight, such as color; others signify by perfection, for example, full and complete functioning. 84. Signs in official members are likewise divided into substantial and accidental. There are four substantial signs: skill (*ars*), arrangement, number, and position. There are likewise four accidental [signs]: namely, good, bad, perfect, and imperfect. 85. There are three genera of sign that bring their own genus into full view. There are some that signify something in the past which has already gone away, and these are called "cognitive" or "perceptual." For instance,

when we see that the body is wet, we *perceive* that sweating has preceded. Others signify a present condition and are perceived through signs, as when the pulse is found to be large and rapid and we understand that it signifies a dominant fever. Then there are those that signify the future and perception anticipates this, as when we see the lower lip trembling and apprehend that vomiting will occur. After the event, this is called a "signifying precedent." 86. But there is a distinction between signs and accidents, for there is a division between them which gradually widens. If you wish to investigate any one of these divisions, they have a single physical appearance. However, to the patient these are accidents, while to the doctor, they are signs.

87. **Significant accidents.** There are three significant accidents: one is altered function (for example, indigestion); another is a quality of the body (for example, jaundice); and another is something emitted by the body (such as black urine). Altered function is threefold: either total as in indigestion; or partial as in cloudy vision or slow *digestion; and from one quality to another – for example, from good [digestion] to smoky and acidic [digestion], or when specks and lines appear before the eyes.

88. **Altered quality of the body.** A sign of a change in the quality of the body happens in four ways: either by sight as in jaundice, morphew, a blackened tongue and the like; or by smell, such as fetid breath or sweat [that smells like] a lobster or a he-goat or the like; or by taste – for example, salt, bitter or acidic; or by touch, as in soft and hard. 89. What comes out of the body signifies in two ways: either with or without sound. With sound: as in burping from the mouth or rumbling of the guts or breaking wind from the anus. What is without sound is unnatural in three ways: either in quantity, as in *lientery; or in quality, as in black urine; or in both, as in bloody diarrhea.

90. **Signs of alteration of the parts.** A sign of alteration in the members belongs in one of two categories, namely, intrinsic and extrinsic. Intrinsic [signs] are six in number: some are from change in the functional power in a member; others are from changes in the body's excretions; others are from pain which is close to the member in question; others from the place itself; others from unnatural removal from the place; others from what the patient discloses. And intrinsic [signs] are three in number: either by sight, as whiteness or blackness; or by touch, as hardness or softness, heat or cold; or by both, as greatness or smallness, increase or decrease.

91. **Causes.** There are three causes of sickness: alteration of the nature [of the body]; unsuitable condition of an official member; separation of a joint.

92. **The functioning of medicine.** The functioning of medicine has a threefold result: either it preserves health in accordance with its likeness, or it produces health from either sickness or from its contrary.

93. **The supervision (*regimen*) of health.** There are three categories of healthy people who should receive supervision: those who are prone to fall ill, those who are just beginning to be sick, and those who are in a weakened state. We supervise those who are prone to illness by suitable moderation of the six [non-naturals] discussed above. We apply a twofold treatment to those who are beginning to be sick: for we either withdraw the superabundance of *chyme, or by way of repairing a defect in nature we prescribe observance of the aforementioned six necessary things. Of those who are in a weakened state, some are infants, others elderly, and others are convalescing from an illness. 94. All medicine is either universal or particular. Universal medicine is the right ordering of the aforementioned six [non-naturals]; [particular medicine] is concerned either with the similar members, the official members, or with separation of things that are joined. 95. We restore altered similar members to their kind and we restrain them in their proper quality by bandaging. If hollow parts are excessively dilated, we bring them back to their proper size and keep them at rest. If they are too small, we do the contrary. Likewise in large members, something is applied which is contrary to the cause of the defect. If the orifices be tighter than normal, [and] if there be a defect of the retentive power, we soften [the member] with *fomentations and a poultice. If there be any defect of the expulsive power, we use *diaphoretics and strengthening medicine: if the cause is something *styptic, [we deploy] softening; if it is something dry, moistening; if it is something constricting, loosening. 96. We restore to its proper place whatever has changed from its natural position. If [the change is] by morbid swelling, we cure the swelling by *"ripening" it. If there is an unnatural adhesion, we disconnect it either by an aperient medication or through surgery. If there is some new growth, we remove it – if it is smooth, by roughening, and if it is rough, by smoothing.

97. **Superabundant quantity.** We remove a superfluity in quantity either partially, as in the case of scrofula, or in its entirety, as in the case of cancer. If excessive quantity is caused by an abundance of blood, we cure it at any age; but if it is caused by sperm [*that is, during conception*], only in childhood. We significantly increase small members by exercise and fomentation; we shrink large ones by bandaging and by rest.

98. **Changes of members.** We return displaced members to their proper place in two ways: either we join what is separated or we separate what is joined. Four things are necessary to join what has been separated: to join the separated parts; to keep the joined parts together; to prevent them from coming apart again; to maintain the natural condition of the place.

99. **The division of medicine.** All medicine [consists] either in the harmonious maintenance of the six [non-naturals] mentioned above, or in drugs, or in surgery. The practice (*operatio*) of medicine is either on the exterior or on the interior [of the body]. The interior concerns those things which are administered through the mouth, the ears, the nose, or the anus. The exterior [concerns] external applications, poultices, and plasters. Medicine administered internally acts in three ways; either it loosens like a [laxative] drug, or it binds like figs, or it alters the quality, as cold does in a fever. Its action is fourfold: either it reduces excess, like a laxative, or supplies deficiency, as for instance, flesh or blood; or it binds what is loosened, like a styptic; or it changes a quality, as cold water in a fever. Surgery is twofold: on the flesh or on the bones. On the flesh, [it consists of] cutting, sewing, and *cautery; on the bones, [it consists of] consolidating and restoring the joint.

100. **Judging drugs.** Judgment about drugs has five aspects: distinguishing quality, quantity, timing, and order [of administration], and distinguishing good [drugs] from bad.

34. MEDICAL THEORY AND THE FORMATION OF THE *ARTICELLA* (2): BARTHOLOMAEUS OF SALERNO COMMENTS ON THE *ISAGOGE*

Bartholomaeus of Salerno (fl. ca 1175) composed one of the first commentaries on all five parts of the original Articella *anthology (Joannitius's* Isagoge, *Hippocrates's* Aphorisms *and* Prognosis, *Theophilus's* On Urines, *and Philaretus's* On Pulses) *as well as on a new addition to the* Articella, *Galen's* Art of Medicine *(Tegni). His commentaries were the first to make prominent use of some recently translated works of Aristotle, especially the* Physics. *The text below is an excerpt from the beginning of his commentary on the* Isagoge. *The* accessus, *a conventional series of "who, what, when, why" topics that opened all learned commentaries (see, for example, doc. 2), offered the master an opportunity to explain the place of medicine in the wider world of learning, and the underlying principles governing the subject. Those principles, for Bartholomaeus, are framed by Aristotle's notions of nature and natural change.*

Source: trans. Faith Wallis from Bartholomaeus of Salerno's commentary on the *Isagoge*, MS Winchester, Winchester College 24 (ca. 1200), fol. 22v. Latin.

In every discipline, the proper order of teaching (*ordo doctrinae*) follows the order of the subject matter underlying the discipline, for the memory retains more readily material in which the sequence of reading harmonizes with the natural order of the subject matter. Hence Galen, in whom alone the integral and orderly teaching of the art of medicine is found, elicited the order of teaching from the order of the subject. For just as in the body of an animal the elements are prior to everything else, with the *complexions coming second, and the *powers third, and so forth, so [Galen] proposes that we read a book about the elements first, and then secondly one about complexions, and thirdly one about powers, and thereafter other books, arranged according to the order and sequence of the subject-matter.... Among the Latins, no authority has definitively established the proper order in which books should be read. Nonetheless the book entitled *Isagoge* by Joannitius the Alexandrian serves as an introduction to all the other books, and so deserves to be read first. At its outset, the following merit consideration: the author's intention, the cause of the work, the usefulness of the book, what part of philosophy it belongs to, what type of teaching it employs, what the division or order of the book is, and what its title is.

In this work, the intention of the author is to gather together in brief chapters the principles of the medical art with a view to introducing the *Tegni* of Galen and other books about this art. We term "the principles of the art" those things that are encountered first in the course of teaching or learning, in the absence of which one cannot accede to the other books of this art – for example, the introductory knowledge concerning the elements, complexions, *humors, members, powers, and the other things that are contained in this book.

The cause of the work is the difficulty of Galen's *Tegni*. For he wrote this book after composing 159 volumes on the art of medicine and in it he collected chapters on the entire art and a summary of all the other volumes. Because it included the entirety of the art, this book was entitled *Art*. This is its inscription: "Here begins the *Tegni* of Galen, that is, the *Art* of Galen." Hence *Pantegni*, that is, "the whole art," *Megategni* [*the medieval title for Galen's Therapeutic Method*], "long art," for *megalon* means "long," *Microtegni* [*the alternate title for the Tegni*] "shorter art." And because [the *Tegni*] is inaccessible due to its brevity and difficulty, Joannitius wrote this book as an introduction to the *Tegni* of Galen, so that through it one might have easier access to the *Tegni* of Galen. It is useful for knowing about things that are natural, non-natural, and against nature....

This work pertains through medicine to *physica, and through *physica* to natural science, and through natural science to philosophy. The division of philosophy will make this more evident. For philosophy is divided into three parts: natural philosophy, moral philosophy, and rational philosophy, or as the Greeks divide it: *theorica, ethica, logica.* And because this work pertains to *theorica,* the definition and division of *theorica* is in order, so that it may be evident through which kind of *theorica* this book pertains to *physica.* *Theorica* is the knowledge (*scientia*) which considers nature or the principle of nature. Because the word "nature" has come up in this definition, it is useful to know what "nature" is…. In his *Physics,* Aristotle defines nature as follows: nature is the principle of motion and rest in a thing that possesses an inherent capacity for motion. By "motion," Aristotle understands the six kinds of motion that he himself distinguishes in his book of *Categories,* that is: generation, corruption, growth, diminution, alteration, and change of location. And he is right to define nature by motion. For nature is the efficient cause of everything that happens or has happened in time. Without the motion of nature, nothing exists. [Motion] is necessary in order for anything to be generated. The principle of motion is twofold: an efficient cause and a material cause. In order for motion to take place, two necessary [factors] concur: what moves and what is moved – that is, that which effects the motion, and that which receives the motion of the efficient cause. Now although both the efficient and the material cause can be called the principle of motion, nonetheless the efficient cause is termed the first principle of motion, because it precedes so to speak the material [cause]. For something that acts is naturally prior to something that suffers action. Because the principle of motion is twofold, in the description of nature this is understood to be the efficient cause. This principle – that is, the efficient cause – is of two types: extrinsic and intrinsic. Extrinsic motion is defined as the principle that, while existing outside and around the thing, nevertheless moves it with some mediation of the intrinsic principle, which will be explained in what follows. This extrinsic principle is divided into two: one with motion and the other without motion. The latter is unique, and is the first cause of everything, which is God. For God, while remaining unmoved, is the principle and cause of every movement. Boethius says: "And remaining stable, you give all things motion [*Consolation of Philosophy* 3, met. 9]." The extrinsic principle with motion is manifold, for example the heavenly bodies, the stars, which by their movement and irradiation of the air effect the aforementioned movement in earthly things. The principle of their motion is attributed to the sun and moon, some of whose operations are manifest and others of which are hidden…. The intrinsic principle of motion is the form or collection of forms. I call them "forms" from the properties of things, such as heat, cold, wetness, and dryness, and thus lightness, heaviness, obtuseness, and sharpness. Of these, some by themselves and others in conjunction produce the aforementioned motion. For form lends motion to matter, as heat and lightness do to fire. Hence Aristotle says in the *Physics*: "It is a moot point whether form or matter should be said to be the principle of motion, but more likely form." The nature of matter proves that the forms and qualities are the principles of motion. For the complexions proceed from the qualities, and the powers from the complexions. From the powers come the operations and the motion of the body, such as appetite, retention, generation, corruption, and so forth....

35. SALERNITAN ANATOMY: THE *SECOND SALERNITAN DEMONSTRATION*

The style of medical teaching associated with Salerno introduced a significant innovation: the use of dissection to teach anatomy and physiology. As in Galen's day, these early medieval dissections were performed on animals rather than humans, most commonly on pigs. The earliest anatomical texts, such as Anatomy of the Pig *(composed between 1100 and 1150, and sometimes ascribed to Copho, author of a manual of medical practice), follow the order in which the organs would become visible during the demonstration but pause to remark on how the form of the organ reflects its function and to comment on its characteristic diseases. The main challenge was to match up terminology with the visible structures. Isidore of Seville furnished a basic vocabulary, but the translations by Constantine the African introduced new Arabic words as well.*

All these features are prominently displayed in the Second Salernitan Demonstration. *It is possible, though by no means certain, that this text is by Bartholomaeus of Salerno (doc. 34). The author refers to his own commentaries on two works in the* Articella *anthology: the* Aphorisms *of Hippocrates, and Philaretus's* On Pulses. *Bartholomaeus composed commentaries on the entire* Articella *suite and frequently cross-referenced his own writings. The* Demonstration *author claims to have discussed the branching of the vena cava in his gloss on Aphorisms 5.68, and indeed Bartholomaeus's commentary does mention this subject, although certainly not "fully." However, the other principle commentaries of the twelfth century do not mention the branches of the vena cava at all. The reference to Philaretus is too vague to be helpful. The* Demonstration *includes a lengthy introduction that lays out important elements of Galenic physiology, as summarized in the* Isagoge *(doc. 33) and in the medieval adaptation of Galen's* On the Usefulness of Parts, *translated by Bartholomaeus's collaborator Burgundio of Pisa. One also detects the influence of the new translations of Aristotle's works, particularly the* Posterior Analytics, *in the author's discussion of*

*efficient and final causes; there are also echoes of Aristotle's concern with the "animal"
as an overarching category in which to situate human life. The structures of the body are
still important, as are the diseases to which they are subject, but now they are situated
within a hierarchy of organs, each with its distinctive functions and powers. Nonetheless, this is still the record of a dissection unfolding in time. The author narrates what
he is doing as he moves along, and even interjects the students' questions.*

Source: trans. George W. Corner, *Anatomical Texts of the Earlier Middle Ages* (Washington, DC: Carnegie Institute, 1929), pp. 54–66. Latin.

In frame and fabric the animal body is composed of members various and diverse; for Nature, the first and foreknowing cause, greatly to be revered in all
her works, constructed the animal body of many members differing in quantity and quality, in order that the animal kingdom might be the culmination
of all created things. Therefore each kind of animal has bodily members
appropriate to serve its spirit and nature. The lion, for example, since he is of
bold and angry spirit, has a body perfected to these qualities and is provided
with suitable weapons in the shape of claws upon his feet and very sharp teeth
in his mouth. The hare, on the other hand, being the timidest of beasts, possesses members which by their lightness are adapted to swift retreat, and its
forelegs are shorter than its hind legs, that it may easily run uphill. Because of
these diversities in the endowment of nature and spirit, the great Creator and
Father of all things formed organs adapted to various functions, such as the
human hand, in which the fingers are several and distinct, in order to grasp
objects both large and small. He suffused the liver with redness to promote
the formation of blood and with foreseeing discretion endowed the breasts
and testicles with whiteness for the making of milk and sperm.

There are also three general operations, with three corresponding instru-
mental members, namely, ˙animal, spiritual, and natural. The animal members are created for sensation and voluntary motion in all animals; also in
some animals for imagination and memory. The spiritual members are for
protecting the channels of breath and natural heat. The natural members are
nutritive and generative. The nutritive are for the reintegration of bodily loss
and waste and for the alteration of materials permuted from evil to good. The
generative organs are made for the specializing of general substance and for
the individualizing of special substance. In each of these systems there is one
principal organ with others protective, expurgative, and adjuvant or accessory.

Among the animal organs the brain is principal, because the animal force
is principally located in it, and from it arise the other structures such as the
nerves; and it is provided with others protective, expurgative, and adjuvant
or accessory. The protective are the pia mater, which, by enfolding the brain

like a devoted mother, protects it from the harshness of the dura mater; the dura mater, which protects the brain and pia mater from the hardness of the cranium; and the cranium, which protects all of these from outward harm. The skin in turn protects the cranium from external injury. The expurgative and adjuvant organs are the ears, eyes, nostrils, and the tongue [together] with the palate. The ears drain the brain of *biliary excess, the eyes of *melancholic, the nostrils of *sanguineous and *phlegmatic; the palate drains away excess of phlegm. These organs are also adjuvant, for hearing is established by mediation of the ears, sight by the eyes, smell by certain [fleshy structures] which hang like udders in the ends of the nostrils; taste is mediated by the tongue. The nerves are accessory, because they receive animal spirits from the brain and transport them throughout the body to endue it with sensation and voluntary motion.

Among the spiritual members one is principal, namely, the heart, because the spiritual force is principally located in it and because other parts, such as arteries, arise therefrom: and it is provided with other structures, protective, expurgative, or adjuvant and accessory. The protective parts include that membrane surrounding the heart which is called [the capsule of the heart], the diaphragm, and the ribs outside. The expurgative and adjuvant parts are the lung, the muscles of the chest, and some of the membranes, because by their motion air is drawn in to temper the natural heat, to restore the *vital spirit, and to *evacuate excess of *vapors. The accessory parts are the arteries, which receive the vital spirits from the heart and convey them throughout the whole body to conserve the natural heat.

Among the nutritive members the liver is principal, because the nutritive force is principally seated in it, and because other parts, such as veins, arise therefrom; and it is also provided with organs protective, expurgative, and accessory. The protective organs include a certain membrane delicate as a spiderweb, and also a certain fatty structure, and much flesh on the outside. Expurgative are the lung and brain, from which excess phlegm is drained by the liver, black *bile by the spleen, yellow bile by the gall-bladder, urine by the kidneys and urinary bladder. Several organs are accessory, for some prepare the food for alteration in the stomach, as, for instance, the teeth; others, such as the stomach and upper small intestines, *digest and alter it preparatory to conversion into *humors by the liver. Others, namely, the mesenteric veins, convey it to the liver; still others, the small intestines, attract to themselves the excess of moisture generated in the stomach. Finally, other organs receive the four humors from the liver, together with the *natural spirits, and transport them throughout the body; in this way they deliver nutriment to the whole organism.

Among the generative members the testicles are principal, because the generative force is principally located in them and because other parts arise therefrom; and they possess organs protective, expurgative, and accessory. In the first place, the testicles are protected by a covering called [the scrotum]. The expurgative parts are the seminal ducts, which receive sperm from the testicles and deliver it to the penis. The accessory parts are those vessels that deliver sperm to the testicles, the uterus, and the breasts.

Knowledge of all these things is gained in many ways; from anatomy we learn their position and differences of structure and we get a simple and clear demonstration of their form. The word "anatomy" is derived from *ana*, or equal, and *tomos*, a division; hence an anatomy is an orderly dissection and it is to be done as follows:

The pig is killed by cutting the throat; not as some do, by putting a knife into the heart, for thus a great quantity of blood is drawn to the vital members and they can be less easily examined. When the throat has been cut, the pig is suspended by the hind feet with the head downward, so that all the blood may remain and not be shed; otherwise when the pig grows cold, there will be a constriction of the arteries and veins, and they cannot well be distinguished. The ancients held various dissonant opinions on the subject of dissection; some said that anatomy should be studied from dead animals, others after due consideration declared that living animals were more useful for dissection, and the latter opinion prevailed on the authority of Galen, because the various passages are more easily visible when the living heat is still in them.

[Organs of the Neck Region]

The pig is next placed on its back. When the lower jaw is partially separated from the upper, one sees the tongue, which is the organ of taste and speech; it is composed of soft flesh and is put together like a sponge, clothed by certain membranes which cover it entirely on the upper side, but which cover the lower surface only as far as the ligaments by which it is attached to the jaw. In some persons these ligaments are too far from the end of the tongue and the tongue is therefore too long and lax, so that it cannot be moved upward for the production of semi-vowels nor downward for the production of consonants, and this is one cause of impediment of speech. But this varies in different men; in others the ligaments may be too near the end of the tongue, and the latter thus being unable to move in diverse directions, speech is impossible. In such cases the ligament should be cut, in order to allow motion of the tongue over the whole mouth and palate. At the sides of the ligament and membranes are certain veins, as you have well seen, which conduct saliva to the tongue. Next there are passages leading to the vital parts and to the brain, by which air drawn in through the nostrils passes in part to the brain and in part descends to the spiritual organs, as does also that air which is inspired through the mouth; thus occurs the collision and repercussion of spirits and vapors descending from the brain and arising from the spiritual organs, and this is the cause of sneezing.

By making an incision in the fauces there appear certain rather large, loose, and spongy glands [*possibly the thyroid*], which some call *faringes*, but I do not give assent to this usage, because I have not found it written in any book, nor have I heard it from any teacher. The word *faringes* is properly applied to the projections of the gullet. There are also certain other masses which are smaller and firmer. These are all placed here for the purpose of gathering moisture from the brain and thus of preventing loss of motion by drying of the nerves and muscles. When abnormal humors gather here they cause [throat tumors] and scrofula.

[Respiratory Organs]

Now let a small incision be made over the gullet. Certain muscles are seen by which voluntary motion is produced. When a similar incision is made laterally, other muscles appear between skin and flesh, and there are still others all the way to the joints of the leg-bones; in all these voluntary motion is produced. In swine they are all fleshy in the middle and cord-like and ligamentous at the ends. By means of a deeper incision the gullet is seen; this is the extremity of the passages of the lung, placed and formed here for a double purpose. Its first and chief function is to inhale air and to emit gross and vaporous superfluities; the second is to produce the voice, of which it is the chief instrument. It is formed of three cartilages. The first is convex inwardly and concave outwardly; in some men it can be palpitated. The second cartilage is placed posteriorly near the esophagus, wherefore some say (and this seems to be in agreement with the truth) that the second is relaxed at the beginning of the esophagus when a man speaks, but the first covers the beginning of the trachea when he drinks; therefore, if anyone while drinking suddenly attempts to begin speaking, the food finds an open passage through the trachea and passes downward; thus by irritating the vital spirit it sets up coughing. The third cartilage has a cavity continuous with the organs of [the] vital spirits. It is to the projections of this gullet that the term *faringes* properly applies. To it the esophagus is joined; in the beginning of this junction, which is called [the] isthmus, there is a place as it were between two beginnings, that is, between the trachea and the esophagus. When fluid gathers here it causes the first kind of *quinsy; but if partly outside and partly inside it causes the second kind; if entirely outside it makes the third kind. If fluid gathers between the esophagus and the spine – for the esophagus is attached to the spine at the posterior aspect – it causes either a gathered swelling of the vertebra from within, if the gathering be in the middle, or torsion of the neck if it be lateral. Afterward look at the end of the third cartilage, where at its lower and inner side the esophagus is joined to it; you will find there the beginnings of the recurrent nerves, which are also instruments of speech. Next to them is another and larger nerve, descending from above, which enters the mouth of the stomach, below the diaphragm. This is called *tornabilis* [*the vagus nerve*]. When you have studied over these things, let a straight incision be made as far as the diaphragm. When the ribs are separated from the vertebrae, all the spiritual organs will be plainly discernible; first you will observe the [trachea], composed of many round cartilages in the form of rings, attached each to the other; on the inner side, to which the esophagus is attached, the cartilages are bound to each other by membranous ligaments. The [trachea] begins at the gullet; it descends the whole length of the neck as far as the lung, and divides at the beginning of the lung into two large branches that descend through the two great lobes of the lung. You may see clearly that the substance of the lung is distinct from the branches of the [trachea], as we have actually shown to many by dissection. Next observe that the lung is composed of a delicate substance of slight density; it is cavernous, and formed of various lobes, so that the lung when expanded may receive air from the outside into these chambers and spaces, and may, when contracted, discharge the gross and vaporous superfluities; this you may see by blowing air in through the throat, for the lung is thus inflated to a large size. Fluid collecting above its lobes causes peripneumonia; if such matter were constantly collected within the lung it would end in *phthisis, from ulceration of the lung tissues. Whenever fluid is abundant in the lung, it gathers and causes *sansugium*, which is difficulty of inspiration. When matter occurs about the lung and weighs upon it and impedes its dilation, it causes *anhelitus*, which is difficulty of respiration. When matter occupies the passages and inner spaces of the lung and resists its constriction, it causes *ortomia*, which is a combination of both difficulties caused by fluids inside and outside.

Next look between the two great wings of the lung, which are seen to comprise other lobes bulging on the posterior side; there you will plainly see a passage going to the heart [*the pulmonary vein*], through which air is drawn from the lung to the heart and vaporous superfluities are transmitted from the heart to the lung. Clearly visible between these two organs there is a large branch of the vena cava ascending through the middle of the diaphragm, which is plainly seen to bifurcate before reaching the heart. One of the branches passes upward; I have spoken fully about its division and distribution in my gloss on the *Aphorisms* [of Hippocrates], when discussing the passage "Posteriora capitis dolentia," etc. [*Aphorisms 5.68: "When there is pain at the back of the head, some help may be given by dividing the vessel which runs vertically in the forehead."*] Another branch reaches the heart and there divides; one of its branches courses through the substance of the heart, chiefly superficially; the other, entering the right auricle from below, takes on another coat and becomes an artery. This passes out alongside the left [side of the heart] and not through it; therefore, if you find "through the left" it is to be understood "alongside the left"; it is called *adorthi* [*aorta, though the description of the vessel suggests confusion with the pulmonary artery*]. This again divides and the larger branch passes downward along the middle of the spine; we shall speak of this again at the end of this address. The other branch passes upward and divides into various branches, as may be read in the *Pantegni* [of Constantine the African]. We have also referred to it when commenting upon Philaretus.

[The Heart]

Next examine the heart in its position on the left side, bordered laterally by the lung, and covered everywhere by a kind of membrane which is called the capsule of the heart. An abscess can easily occur in the capsule, though in the heart itself never, or with difficulty. Oftentimes abnormal humors gather here in great abundance and cause *syncope. The substance of the heart is composed of villous and nervous parts variously placed, and of firm flesh, being thus arranged because of the motions of dilation and constriction, which are so diverse, extensive, and rapid that if the heart were of weak structure it might easily be damaged. Its form is that of a pine-cone, broad below and pointed above, and hollowed out into various chambers, both to permit of ready motility and to avoid angles which might do harm by retaining superfluous material.

[The Diaphragm]

Below all these organs is the diaphragm, which begins at the front where the chest wall is soft and reaches to the twelfth vertebra, where it is attached by cord-like ligaments from all sides; matter which gathers above it, in the membrane of the ribs, causes pleurisy.

[Digestive Organs]

Having demonstrated and gone over all this, let us proceed to the examination of the digestive organs. Some of these are above the diaphragm, namely, the esophagus and opening of the stomach; the others are below it. That which is called *os ventris* [*"mouth of the belly"*] in Latin is *stomachus* in Greek; for *stoma* is translated "mouth" and *cusis* "belly"; therefore *stomachus* is the mouth of the stomach, but in Arabic it is called *meri*. Although according to Constantine, *meri* includes under the one term both *os ventris* and esophagus, actually it may be divided into these two structures. The part that is thicker and reaches about four fingers' breadths above the diaphragm is the *os stomachi*; the remainder, which is more slender and goes all the way to the throat, is the esophagus; the *os stomachi* is nervous [*that is, sinewy*], in order that appetite may develop there as a result of frigidity.

Now let a deep longitudinal incision be made downward from the diaphragm, penetrating to a certain delicate membrane resembling a spider's web, which according to Constantine is called in Arabic *siphac* [*peritoneum*] (not *asiphac*, as someone, not in a Hippocratic spirit, but from his own deep and searching knowledge, has recently borne witness, against whom I would have written something on this and other points were it not that it might be set down to pride). This membrane envelops all the nutritive organs and gives off the membrane which encloses the testicles.

Upon enlarging the incision, the *zirbus* [*Arabic word for omentum*] appears, composed of two layers and resembling a net; it almost entirely covers the digestive organs. That part of it which covers the fundus of the stomach is called omentum from *operio operis* [*"I cover over, you cover over ..."*], because it covers the fundus of the stomach; but it is not the omentum – a certain person to the contrary – but a kind of fatty material, commonly called *axungia* [*lard*]. To tear it out is impossible or at least very difficult.

Next note the fundus of the stomach sloping toward the right, embraced by the liver with its five lobes; the stomach is fleshy, in order to promote the first digestion. Its lower orifice is called *porta* [*gate*] both by Constantine and by Isaac [Judaeus] in his book *De urinis* [*On Urines*], because it remains closed until in the necessity of nature food is to be passed out of the stomach, but opens when it begins to pass out.

[The Intestines]

Next observe the intestines, which Constantine in the *Pantegni* divides into six. Of these, the first is not the *portanarium* (because, as we have said, the *porta* is the inferior opening of the stomach), but the duodenum, which has a length of [twelve] digits. Next to it is the jejunum, so called because in the dead animal it is found to contain no fluid; from it, according to Isaac, the purer part of the juice formed in the stomach is drawn off through the mesenteric veins; but according to Constantine, this juice is drawn off from the *subtile* [*lower or descending part of the duodenum*]. Yet these writers are not averse to one another, but diverse; for Isaac means by jejunum that organ which begins at the duodenum and extends to the *orbus* [*probably caecum*], but Constantine applies the term jejunum only to the upper part of that which I have described, and distinguishes by the term *subtile* the lower part, which, as you have seen, is more delicate than the upper; thus Constantine divides the structure into two parts. This portion of the intestine is the seat of strophic [*i.e., twisting*] pain. The *intestinum subtile* ends in the *orbus*, which is also called *saccus* because it is made like a sack. An excess of bile going down to this intestine through the lower fork of the gall-bladder causes sickness. At the *orbus* begins another intestine, which is thick, called [ileum]. The iliac pain caused by retention of coarse refuse and by other causes often mentioned in the books is, according to Constantine, located here and not in the "lateral intestines," which I have never discovered in animals, nor have I found anything written about them except in a recent booklet. Lowest and last of all is the *longaon* or *extale* or [rectum]. This is called *extale* or *longaon* because it extends along the spine from the lower extremity of the pudendal region. This intestine is the seat of colic pain.

[The Liver]

Next comes the liver, which is situated in the right hypochondrium and is shaped like a Greek sigma [*like the letter C*]. On the upper side, where with its five lobes it is joined to the diaphragm, it is convex. If matter gathers here it causes *dyspnea and cough, as Galen says, in the passages beginning "Per species disniae" and "Tussis quaeque fiunt etc." [in *Tegni* 20.4]. On that side on which it is attached to the stomach, it is concave, and, as we have said, its five lobes surround the stomach. Although the number of lobes varies in different animals, there are five in the pig, as I have recently shown you, and certainly the same number occur in man. Upon one of the larger lobes is the gall-bladder, which gives the appearance of having but one duct. There are, however, two ducts, one above the other, so adherent and joined together that they seem but one; but while you have been watching I have separated them. The one which is uppermost appears larger. The larger one lies under the liver and is attached to it, and the lesser descends to the intestine, conveying excess bile to serve the function of the stomach. But the upper, which is larger, is continued to the fundus of the stomach, as I have clearly demonstrated to you; for while I had the liver separated thus from the stomach, somebody inquired how and where the branch in question continued to the stomach, and I made it known while you all looked on. One opening was cut in the fundus of the stomach; and in case someone who is anxious to criticize seems to find it missing, because it corrodes [*the translator notes that* *the meaning is unclear and text possibly corrupt*], I say that the branch of the gall-duct which goes to the stomach is larger in the pig because of the smoothness of the stomach, for the stomach of the pig is smooth and not villous. Nature, therefore, in her providence, instituted the said branch, in order that food may quickly and without long retention by the stomach be brought to a great ebullition and alteration by means of mild bile reaching the stomach in large quantity through the larger branch. Moreover, the passage by which the liver transmits excess bile to the gall-bladder is continued to the larger branch, a fact you will easily understand by placing a quill inside the passage; for above it goes into the fundus of the stomach and then by [a] somewhat transverse course it enters into the substance of the liver from below. And note that the stomach of the pig is not villous for two causes, one final and the other efficient. The efficient cause is moisture, for the pig is moister in its digestive organs than other animals and from this overflowing moisture comes smoothness. The final cause is the nature and substance of the pig; for in order that anything may be nourished, it is necessary that the nutrient material shall be similar to the substance which is dissolved from the body. Now the substance and nature of the pig is somewhat cold and moist, and for this reason the pig's stomach ought not to be villous and long retentive of its foods, for these do not require a long time for ebullition.

[Blood Vessels of the Liver]

When these things have been committed to memory, observe the mesenteric veins in the concavity of the liver, in which is also the *lactea porta* [*milky gate*] or *vena ramosa* [*branching vein*] (which is called *lactea* because moisture generated in the stomach enters it as white as milk, *porta* because it is like a gate, *vena ramosa* because all the branches of the veins arise from it. You will find it about the middle of the concave side of the liver, where there is a certain whiteness of those membranes that unite the concave aspect of the liver to the fundus of the stomach. Below this in some recently killed animals I have seen those little narrow vessels [that are] red and full of blood. If they are not visible easily and at once, divide and separate the membranes before mentioned and you will find many such vessels, as you have already seen.

Next you will find hair-like veins in the convexity of the liver, where the vena cava is, in this way. Near the beginning of the vena cava break off a bit of the liver substance and rub it between your fingers and the veins will appear; they are small, round, and narrow like hairs. Somebody who wanted to criticize, last year after we had done a dissection, said these were *nerves – a statement which we did not refute at the time. To confute his opinion we now exhibit, before you all, these vessels [that are] red and full of blood, with their beginnings at the origin of the vena cava.

[The Spleen]

The spleen is oblong and is located in the left hypochondrium; it readily presents itself for observation. On its inner side it is attached lengthwise to the *zirbus*; on this side you will see, all the more easily because of the whiteness of the *zirbus*, three vessels full of black biliary blood. Since they are colored by these substances they are easily visible amid the whiteness. There is one about the middle of the upper end of the spleen through which part of the excess black bile is sent to the stomach to promote appetite; another about the middle of the lower end through which part is sent to the stomach; a third between the others, through which the liver drains off excess black bile. In some animals these black or red vessels full of black biliary blood do not course as described and therefore are not so easily recognized. Carefully separate the *zirbus* from the substance of the spleen and the channels alone will remain because of their toughness; or put a quill in the middle of the spleen where it is joined to the *zirbus*, and insert it lengthwise, and you will find these channels.

[The Kidneys]

When all this has been completed, let the organs which have been examined be removed from the pig, so that the rest may be better seen; and first observe the kidneys, situated on either side of the spine, fleshy and round. They are venous within, and contain corpuscles after the fashion of hairs; and they are hollow, which is the cause of stone. From them descend two vessels called [*emunctories] by physicians, one of which descends to each side of the neck of the bladder. Also, there are fleshy masses on each side of the spine, called *lumbi* [*loins*].

[The Bladder]

In males the bladder is situated above the rectum (that intestine which, as I have said, is called [the colon]) and therefore these organs are much bound together and become involved in the same lesions (see Hippocrates, the *Aphorisms*: "Ex stranguria, etc." [*probably Aphorisms 6.44*] and elsewhere "In ano flegmonem patientem," [*Aphorisms 5.28*] etc.). Stone occurs in the fundus of the bladder, and if it reaches the neck it interferes with the passage of urine and causes *strangury and *scunia* [*unidentified condition*]. Also, there is in the neck of the bladder a certain constricting muscle that does not permit the urine to pass without volition. Around the fundus are nerves and muscles, which you have clearly seen; when *animal spirits flow down to these they are compressed and contracted, so that urine passes out through the neck of the bladder. How the neck of the bladder is continued into the penis you may see by putting a long quill through the neck.

[Blood Vessels of the Abdomen]

The large artery which descends from the heart, about which I promised I would speak, descends along the middle of the spine as far as the kidneys and there bifurcates. One branch proceeds to each kidney; and from other branches, which pass downward, two branches are separated, one going to each testicle to give it *vital spirits. The remainder of the descending branches are distributed in various ways to the thighs and other members.

The venous branches from each side of the spine descend to the inferior regions and give off two branches, one of which goes to each testis to convey blood. The remaining branches are distributed in diverse fashion throughout the lower members; some of them descend to the pudendal ring and there undergo multiple division. These give rise to hemorrhoids, as we have made known to you.

[The Testicles]

The testicles, which are the instruments of the sperm, are formed of glandular, white, soft, and spongy flesh, in order that sperm may be generated in them. Each is covered by a membrane, which is derived from the *siphac*. The substance of the sperm before it comes to the testicle is received in a certain follicle, in which it is altered and whitened, and this membrane is below the kidneys and above the testicles; in some animals there is found in the said membrane a great quantity of that moisture which is the material of the sperm; in other animals little is found, and in others none; and as we have shown you, there are two passages, one on each side of the membrane, through which this material descends to the testicles. Proceeding from the inferior part of the testicles are two vessels called [seminal], through which the sperm passes from the testicles to the penis, and these vessels are long, white, and hard like muscular flesh; they are long, so that the testicular excretion may better undergo *coction as it passes along, and broad, that the sperm may pass quickly from these vessels into the penis and from the penis into the female pudenda. In your presence I have incised one of these ducts and have shown you the sperm.

[The Penis]

The penis is fleshy, nervous, round, and hollow, beginning at the two [pubic bones]; and is formed of two cords placed side by side transversely, which is necessary for a double cause. First, that it may eject the sperm into the vulva; for this reason it is made nervous, in order that by virtue of its great sensitiveness there may be intense pleasure even in so unseemly an act as emission of the sperm. It is hollow, in order that in the presence of ardent desire it may be extended and erected with the greatest possible rigidity by means of much spirit in its large cavity and in the muscles placed at its sides; and thus it is not readily deflected, but may be inserted directly into the vulva. The second necessary cause is that it may expel the urine passing through it from the neck of the bladder without interruption and without harm, as we demonstrated very clearly in the dissection by means of a quill inserted through the neck of the bladder.

[The Uterus]

The uterus is a hollow and nervous organ placed lengthwise, beginning at the umbilicus and descending into the region of the female genitals. It is placed above the [rectum], which as we have said is called *longaon*, and the bladder in turn is above the uterus; so that when enlarged and distended by the bulk of the foetus the intestine and the bladder form as it were cushions and cover it on both sides. It has two orifices, one external, which is properly called *collum matricis* [*literally* "neck of the uterus," *vagina*], in which coitus is completed; the other internal, which is properly called *os matricis* [*literally* "mouth of the uterus," *cervix*] and this closes, according to Hippocrates, after the seventh hour of conception, and will not thereafter admit the point of a needle. The os itself is nervous and somewhat sensitive, in order that much delectation may be caused in intercourse by contact of this organ with the male member, and it is moderately firm, in order that it may easily be distended for the entrance of the sperm and closed when the sperm is received; for if it were not so – if it were over-hard or over-soft – it would be inextensible through hardness or for softness could not be shut. The [uterus] is villous inside, that it may better retain the sperm and the fetus when conceived. For it is constructed for this special purpose, namely, the generation of the fetus from sperm conceived within it. The superfluities formed in it are discharged by the menses. There are two large cavities in the uterus, one right and the other left, but both of these unite in one, which is properly called *collum matricis*; and there are certain pits in them from which the menstrual flow originates and in which by conception of sperm generation occurs as follows.

[The Process of Conception]

Acting upon the mass composed of male and female sperm, the natural force and heat cause solidification in the liquid and more subtle parts as well as in the superabundant and more consumable grosser elements and alters them into a kind of membrane, just as a crust forms on dough when a hot iron is brought near it. Then when the rest of the mass is coagulated throughout by similar action of force and heat and becomes transmuted into the essence of the organs, its swelling bursts the middle of the crust. Veins and arteries emerge and are united with the veins and arteries of the uterus to form the *secundines* [*placenta*], or membranes of the fetus; and through these veins the four humors, the *natural spirit, and the vital spirit are borne for nourishment and vivification of the fetus. The sources of the veins and arteries of the uterus, to which the veins and arteries are joined, are called cotyledons. By these veins and arteries, as if by ligaments, the fetus is suspended and is retained in the uterus, but they are broken when the fetus departs at birth, and after the waters have been discharged the midwife ties them with a thread at a distance of three or four fingers' breadths from the umbilicus. It often happens that due to pain from the ligature humors are drawn thither and cause suppuration of the umbilicus.

[The Ovaries]

After considering this, note the two testicles situated at the summit of the *collum matricis*, one right and the other left. You will find them by a long straight incision above the *collum matricis*. The testicles are smaller than in men, round, superficially somewhat flattened, glandular, and harder than in men. To each of them comes a single vein from the kidneys, and they lie under the trumpet-like extremities of the uterus. From each testicle there goes a stem-like cord, through which the testicle ejects sperm into the spermatic vessel. Observe, moreover, that the female organ, which as we have said is called *collum matricis*, is different in different women according to varying times, ages, and natures; for in pregnant women it is greater than in the non-pregnant because of the enlargement caused by conception; it is never so large in those who have never been pregnant as in those who have borne children; and moreover it increases in size during the course of pregnancy. In girls and elderly women this organ is smaller than in adults, and in ardent women it is larger than in those who are not passionate.

[The Head]

Concerning the anatomy of the head, we may say that it is of rounded form, but tapering before and behind. It is round in order that it may not be subject to injury; for if there were angles tending to retain superfluities, they would be the source of harm. It is tapering in front because of the chamber of imagination and the sensory nerves, which proceed to the organs of sensation; and it tapers behind because of the chamber of memory and the motor nerves, which run to the organ of locomotion, and also because the spinal medulla makes its exit at the rear. Let the cranium be centrally incised, above and below, down to the dura mater; it is found to be rough on its inner surface, hollowed out in one part, jagged in the other, and composed of many bones interlocked. The purposes of this arrangement are several; it makes the head an efficient outlet of the great ascending vapor which is resolved from the triple digestion; it permits freer entrance and exit of the veins and arteries of the brain; finally it causes firmer adhesion of the cerebral membranes and thus if perchance any one part of the skull is fractured the whole need not collapse. Immediately under the cranium there is a membrane called [the] dura mater, which protects the brain and pia mater from the hardness of the cranium; when this is incised there is found another membrane like a network of veins; this is called [the] pia mater and protects the brain from the hardness of the dura mater. Under the pia mater is the brain, which is white, soft, and chambered. It is made white and soft in order that it may fully respond to the diverse qualities of sensations. From the forepeak of the brain proceed all the sensory nerves, among which is a large one called [optic] or [ocular], from *obtalmo* (that is to say, eye), which descends as far as the crystalline humor, which is in the middle of the eye.

[The Eye]

The eye is composed of four humors and seven tunics, which are recognizable as follows. One tunic, which begins at the center of the eyes and lines the whole inner surface, is called the conjunctiva. The outermost superficial layer is the cornea; a bit of it cut off appears bright and clear like very translucent horn. When this is cut away still more, a very black layer is found beneath it, and this is called uvea; under it is a very black delicate membrane called *tela aranea* [*"spider's web"*] or pupil. There are three others on the cranial side; the first is retina, the second *secundine*, the third sclerotic.

After you have seen these things, cautiously make a deep incision in the center of the eye and compress it slightly at the sides. The first humor that emerges, resembling [the] white of [an] egg, is called *albugineus*. After that, a clear, translucent, and rather firm humor escapes; this is called [crystalline]. The third, which escapes from about the crystalline humor, but which is softer than the crystalline, is called vitreous. The before-mentioned optic nerve, which descends from the brain to the eyes, passes through the center of the eye as far as the crystalline humor; through it comes the *visible spirit, and as it emerges through the uveal tunic and the cornea it is mingled with the clear air and transports its rays to the body, and thus sight is brought about, as we have said in our commentary on Joannitius.

36. THE PRACTICE OF PHARMACY RATIONALIZED

The elaboration of medical theory in the twelfth century went hand in hand with a concerted effort to write about medical practice in a new way. The shape of practice laid down by the Isagoge — *diet therapy first, followed by *purgative drugs and surgery (comprising *evacuative surgery such as bloodletting, as well as wound treatment) — situated therapy in relation to the overarching principles of medicine. Early medieval therapeutic literature was abundant and creative, but it rarely tried to articulate a rational basis for the doctor's action. The new therapeutic writing of the twelfth century set out not only to do this, but also to produce works on medical practice dressed in the academic robes of* doctrina. *In two domains, pharmacy and surgery, the transformation was particularly impressive.*

The literature on pharmacy falls into two basic genres: works that deal with ma-teria medica or "simples," and works on compounding medicines from a number of ingredients, called antidotaria. *The two most widely diffused works of Salernitan pharmacy are a pair of texts often found as companions in medieval manuscripts: the* Circa instans, *which deals with simples, and the* Antidotarium Nicolai.

Circa instans, like many reference manuals, was subject to amplification and re-arrangement throughout its long medieval career. It was also adapted into numerous vernacular languages. The translation below comprises two entries from a version that scholars have identified as fairly close to the original. One concerns the exotic spice car-damom, and the other is about white lead, a substance used in ointments and cosmetics.

The Antidotarium Nicolai *ascribed to Nicholas of Salerno (fl. ca 1150) is a col-lection of recipes for compound remedies culled from an eleventh-century compendium, the* Great Antidotarium (Antidotarius magnus). *Each entry contains an explana-tion of the drug's name, followed by its therapeutic indication, ingredients, mode of preparation, dosage, and form of administration. Nicholas also equipped his manual with an index of synonyms for drug names. All these innovations made the* Antidot-arium Nicolai *the bible of medieval practical pharmacy. In some places, it became the official formulary. A commentary was composed in the third quarter of the twelfth century, possibly by the Salernitan master Matthaeus Platearius. The passage from the* Antidotarium *reproduced here describes the compound medicine called* *"*theriac.*" *Theriac (from which comes our modern word "treacle") was the universal antidote to poison and an all-purpose panacea. It was the ultimate compound drug, and in the extract from his commentary below, Matthaeus Platearius explains why compounding drugs enhances their efficacy.*

a. Extracts from *Circa instans*

Source: trans. Faith Wallis from Hans Wölfel, "Das Arzneidrogenbuch Circa Instans in einer Fassung des XIII. Jahrhunderts aus der Universitätsbibliothek Erlangen. Text und Kommentar als Beitrag zur Pflanzen- und Drogenkunden des Mittelalters" (Diss., Berlin, 1939). Latin.

Cardamom

Cardamom is hot and dry in the second *degree. It is the fruit – or rather, the seed – of a certain tree. In spring, the fruiting tree produces certain protuberances that look like the seeds of rue and resemble grapes; the seed is contained in these. There are two kinds: the greater and the lesser. Greater cardamom is better because it is more aromatic, so one should choose the larger kind. It has some sharpness and sweetness mixed together. When it is added to medicines, the little pits should be removed and ground up in a cloth.... It will keep for ten years. It has strengthening virtue thanks to its aromatic quality, as well as the virtue of dissolving and consuming [morbid matter] in quantity.

Against fainting and conditions of the *cardia* [*region of the solar plexus*] due to cold, make a *decoction [of cardamom] in fragrant wine, add rose water, and give to the patient.

For weakness of the stomach and to strengthen *digestion, powdered cardamom and powdered anise should be given in food.

To stimulate appetite and also for vomiting due to cold, offer [the patient cardamom] powder compounded with mint juice and stirred into food. Powdered cardamom with mint – green or dry – should be cooked in vinegar and water which is sour and salted, and a sponge soaked in this should be placed on the upper end of the stomach.

Against weakness of the stomach and brain, powdered [cardamom] should be applied to [the patient's] nostrils. If there is *rheum, put the powder, mixed with musk oil, into an eggshell and heat it in ashes until its boils; then anoint the head.

Ceruse [*white lead*]

Ceruse is cold and dry in the second degree. Ceruse is called "flower of lead" or *gersa*. It is made like this. Take sheets of lead, weighing a pound, and put them in a glass container which is narrow at the top and a foot wide. But first fill the container with very strong vinegar. Then place poles over the opening of the vase and from one end to the other hang the pierced lead sheets on strings [so that they are] four fingers' breadth from the vinegar. Then cover over the opening and the container very well; put it in a dark place and leave it for four months. At the end of four months, open the seal so that the power of the vinegar is exhaled and you will find certain protuberances and muci-laginous materials around the lead (which you will find to have diminished in size). Scrape these off with a knife and put them in a large container and after adding water, tread it with the feet. Afterwards draw off the water and place the remaining substance into a somewhat concave container. Add water and expose it to sunshine until the water has evaporated; add more [water] and continue doing so until [the ceruse] is very white. Take it out of that concave container and make the ceruse into a ball. Note that people who manufacture ceruse sometimes incur stroke, epilepsy, paralysis, and arthritis because of the coldness of the vinegar, which dissolves and bites. Ceruse has the virtue of cleaning and extracting superfluities. Hence some women use it this way: first they wash their face and then they apply a fine powder of ceruse. Others improve on this, for they mix the ceruse, which has a rather bad smell, with rose-water and leave it out in the sunshine, particularly in summer. When [the rose-water] has evaporated they add more, and they do this until it is very white and somewhat perfumed. Afterwards they make pills and apply these to the face. Others apply powdered borax or camphor or both, and little [pow-dered] sea-side flowers, and they improve it. Those who wash with ceruse for a long time suffer tooth-ache, or stinking and rotting in the mouth.

b. The *Antidotarium Nicolai* on Theriac

Source: trans. Michael R. McVaugh in *Sourcebook in Medieval Science*, ed. Edward Grant (Cambridge, MA: Harvard University Press, 1974), pp. 788–89 (no. 110.2). Latin. The recipe is translated by Faith Wallis.

The Great Theriac of Galen

Theriac is called the chief of the Galenic medicines, since it was compounded by him. It is good for the most serious afflictions of the entire human body: against epilepsy, catalepsy, *apoplexy, headache, stomach ache, and migraine; for hoarseness of voice and constriction of the chest; against bronchitis, asthma, spitting of blood, jaundice, *dropsy, pneumonia, colic, intestinal wounds, ne-phritis, the stone, and *choler; it induces menstruation and expels the dead fetus; it cures leprosy, smallpox, intermittent chills, and other chronic ills; it is especially good against all poisons, and the bites of snakes and reptiles, although the dose varies according to the quantity and quality of the different ailments, as is written at the end; it clears up every failing of the senses, it strengthens the heart, brain, and liver, and makes and keeps the entire body incorrupt.

Recipe

Pills of squills: 2 drams, 2 scruples; long pepper: 2 drams less 7 grains; pills of viper's flesh, and *diacoralli*: 2 drams each; balsam wood: 2 scruples, 7 grains; opium, agaric, rose, *scordion* [*either ramsons or bluebell*], wild turnip seed, cinnamon, balsam: 1 scruple 14 grains each; rhubarb, crocus, spikenard, costmary, camel's hay, ginger, cassia wood, calamite gum, myrrh, terebinth, male frankincense, calamint, dittany, lavender, pentaphylon root, parsley, white pepper: 1 scruple 7 grains each; gum arabic leaves, sweet flag, *chalacanthi usti* [*possibly burnt colocynth*], *sagapeni* [*unidentified: possibly sweet marjoram*], *terra sigillata* or [*Armenian*] bole, juice of hypocist, *celtica* [*probably* Valeriana celtica], wall-germander [*chamadreos*], gentian, dill, Balm of Mecca [*carpobalsami*], amomum [*an eastern spice plant*], celery, fennel, wild caraway, cicely, nasturtium, anise seed, St John's wort: 1 scruple each; mummy, *castoreum, opoponax, asphalt, galbanum, lesser centaury, long aristolochia, wild carrot: 1 scruple each; skimmed honey as needed. Grind up those [ingredients] which require it, and mix the gums, dissolved in wine, with this powder and sufficient honey, or else grind them up with the spices.

It is given in a pill the size of a hazelnut with warm [water?] for apoplexy, dizziness, headaches, hoarseness of voice, and constriction of the chest; with honey or tragacanth [*an aromatic gum*], so that it is held in the mouth, to asthmatics; with a decoction of wild sage, to those spitting blood from the chest and for failings of the lungs with a ptisan; it is given for chronic illness with an elixir of hyssop; for jaundice, with a decoction of hazelwort; for dropsy, with *oxymel or *oxysaccharum; for pneumonia, with henbane or a decoction of [horehound]; for colic, with an elixir of celery; for those suffering from intestinal wounds, with a decoction of sumach; for those with kidney trouble, the stone, and biliousness, it is given with an elixir of gromwell and wild or cultivated celery; for bronchitis, with henbane or a decoction of rue; for use against poison, or for expelling the menses or a fetus, it is given with hot wine, or with honey mixed with water in which mint has been cooked, or basil, and for intermittent chills and all illnesses, with warm [water?].

c. The Commentary on the *Antidotarium Nicolai* Ascribed to Mattheus Platearius: Why Compound Medicines Are Superior

Source: trans. Michael R. McVaugh in *Sourcebook in Medieval Science*, ed. Edward Grant (Cambridge, MA: Harvard University Press, 1974), p. 787 (no. 110.1). Latin.

Some medicines are *simple, others compound. A simple medicine is one which is as nature produced it, or which has been artificially prepared without anything else added: examples are pepper, *scammony, and many others of this sort. Since medicinal virtue is present in these simples in the highest degree, it may properly be asked, What is the reason for compounding medicines? The reasons are manifold. The first and principal one is for greater efficacy; the second for action against a combination of illnesses, of which one may be quite the opposite of another; the third is for the repression of harmful properties; the fourth is for the preservation of the medicine; the fifth [to disguise] the horrible taste.

Greater efficacy is a reason [for compounding medicines], since some illnesses are compound and cannot be cured with one medicine alone; and because the lesser virtue of one medicine can be increased by the greater virtue of another; it can then do twice as much, which it could not by itself. Combination of illnesses is a reason, since some illnesses are hot, others cold, yet both can exist together in the human body; but one medicine is unable to have different effects on different imbalances. A compound medicine can be useful as a laxative when it contains scammony, which primarily purges hot, but secondarily cold, humors. Opposition of illnesses relates to the members. Sometimes the afflicted member is noble, such as the liver, which (being porous) is responsive to dissolution; for if it is chilled, it needs *solutive medicines to purge it, so that the pores may be opened and the cold material dissolved. But because violently solutive materials are harmful to the substance of the liver, *styptic medicines are to be mixed with the solutive ones, and this will strengthen the weakness of the liver. [Compounding is needed] in order to repress harmful properties, since some medicines, such as the solutive ones, are harmful and sharp, and cannot be taken internally by themselves unless they have previously been mixed with others to repress their sharpness and harmfulness: for example, mastix, scammony, hellebore, and gariophyllus – for black hellebore and scammony cannot be given by themselves. Compounding is necessary to preserve medicines, since some are naturally humid and quickly decay, so that unless they are mixed with others they cannot be used; examples are ginger, jujubes [*fruit of the plant* Zizyphus spina-Christi], and *myrobolans. Green jujubes have greater efficacy, and lest they decay they are administered with *syrups and other things. Compounding is necessary because of a horrible taste, for some medicines, like aloes, are so loathsome that the sick cannot take them, and if they manage to take them, they do not have the required effect: therefore sweet things must be mixed with them to repress their abominable, horrible taste, such as honey and sugar.

Antidotum means "given against," from *anti* which means "against" and *dosis*, which means "a giving." Those compound medicines are called *antidota* which are compounded from selected medicines, chosen with great care, so that all medicines can really be called *antidota*.

37. THE PRACTICE OF THERAPEUTICS RATIONALIZED: THE *PRACTICE OF MEDICINE* BY BARTHOLOMAEUS OF SALERNO

In Richer of Rheims's day, "Salerno" was synonymous with expert medical practice, not book learning. By the twelfth century, Salernitan medicine meant medical theory as conveyed in the Articella *and its early commentaries, or the texts translated by Constantine the African, notably the* Pantegni. *Yet it is notable that two of the earliest commentators on the* Articella *– Archimatthaeus (doc. 78) and Bartholomaeus of Salerno (doc. 34) – also composed substantial works on therapeutics; so did Bartholomaeus's student and editor Petrus Musandinus, Platearius (doc. 36c), and the anatomist Copho. Bartholomaeus's* Practice of Medicine *(Practica) circulated in at least two versions. The long version, represented in the passage translated below, is notable for its theoretical explanations, including some passages that seem to echo the debates of the schools (for example, where a question is posed and the author "responds"). The* Practica *is in two parts. The first is a treatise on medicines and their actions. The second discusses diseases and therapies, and is in turn divided into two sections: "universal" or whole-body diseases (fevers, followed by diseases like leprosy, jaundice, etc.) and diseases particular to different members of the body, in head-to-toe order. The passage on headache below opens this latter part of the book.*

Source: trans. Faith Wallis from Bartholomaeus of Salerno, *Practica Bartholomaei*, ed. Salvatore De Renzi, *Collectio salernitana* 4 (Naples: Filiatri, 1856), pp. 372–73, collated with Cambridge, Gonville and Caius College MS 159, fol. 17r. Latin.

Now that we have discussed universal diseases, it is time to speak about particular diseases. Let us begin first with the head. Headache can be accompanied by fever, and we have discussed the kind that comes with fever above [in the section of the *Practica* on fevers]. The kind that is without fever comes either from the head itself, [in which case] the pain is continuous, or from the stomach. If it originates from some defect of the head, it is from matter in which one of the four *humors is in excess. This happens particularly when the condition of the body exhibits excess in relation to its habitual condition, for example, if the head suffers from hot humors and the rest of the body is hot. If it comes from the stomach, the heat is intermittent. If it originates from some defect of the head itself, it is either from blood, or from red *bile, or from *phlegm, or from *melancholy. If it comes from red bile, these are the signs: urine which is constrained [in its passage] and somewhat thin; the color of the face [will be] yellow; and the saliva in the mouth will seem salty. Give them the decoction described above, made from cassia bark, yellow *myrobolans, and violets, and make it up as described above. Let [the patient] be *purged with Saracen tryphera [*a mild purgative*]; and then provoke sneezing with woman's milk, and with a feather dipped in oil of roses or in that milk, anoint his nostrils within. Bathe his feet as well with a decoction of lettuce, poppies, and red roses. If [patients] suffer from insomnia, their temples should be anointed fore and aft with opium mixed with a woman's milk. Let their nostrils be anointed on the inside, or their temples, and let them rest. It also helps to give an opium preparation in the evening; blend it with hot water and administer it. If the headache is caused by blood, the urine will be constrained [in its passage] and thick, the face red, moist and bloated, and the taste in the mouth will be sweet. The first treatment is to let blood from the head vein. Provoke sneezing with oil of violets, and anoint the head with oil of roses or unguent made from poplar buds, and anoint the temples with vinegar and egg white mixed together. Or take *nitre and white salt, reduce them to powder, [add] barley flour and powdered incense and mastic, blend with egg white and apply like a plaster to the temples where the artery pulses; it will reduce the pain immediately. Wash the feet as specified above. If [the headache] is caused by phlegm, these will be the signs: urine which is thick and free-flowing, a face white and bloated. You will first treat it thus: let the patient be purged with sharp *hierapigra and cooked *scammony if his liver is weak, for raw scammony damages a weak liver, though not a healthy one, provided it is *tempered in an *electuary for fifteen days. Let the head be anointed with oil of camomile, dill, bay, and *marciaton* [*an ointment*]. The signs of headache that comes from melancholy are these: urine which is thin and free-flowing; a face livid and lean; a bitter taste in the mouth. If they suffer much from aversion to food, but not due to phlegm, they should be purged with hierapigra, *hieralogodion, *theodoritum anacardium* [*a compound purgative*], strong *hiera*, *paulinum* [*a compound purgative*], gilded pills, and cooked pills. It is a great help to them and to those who suffer from phlegm to have their feet washed in water with a decoction of mint, calamint, pennyroyal, oregano, and things of this kind. They benefit from whey of goats with opium added, from *mithradatum, from "Alexander's gold" [*a drug made with opium and gold*], and especially from *sotira* or *diacastoreum. A plaster made from euphorbia, pyrethrum, and mustard, or from mustard alone, is beneficial. It helps those who suffer from red bile or phlegm if they can vomit after dinner. Also beneficial for headaches from hot humors is a plaster made from galbanum and opium blended with cold water and applied to the pulse. The diet of the patient should be thus: well baked bread, white wine which is refined and not too strong; meat which is easy to digest, such as that of yearling lamb and yearling pig, hens and their chicks, partridge, pheasant and the like. Beware of beef, veal, and things that generate *windiness, and especially of beans, and of fried and roasted foods; but boiled foods may be used.

38. THE PRACTICE OF SURGERY RATIONALIZED: THE *SURGERY* OF ROGER FRUGARD

Most early medieval surgical texts were mere memoranda or lists, but from the twelfth-century "Salernitan" milieu sprang a tradition of comprehensive and detailed Latin treatises that would transform this branch of medical learning. The most important of these was the Surgery *of Roger Frugard, sometimes called Roger of Salerno (fl. ca 1170). Roger may not have actually lived or taught in Salerno, but his book was almost certainly read and glossed there. A revised version by one Roland of Parma appeared around 1200. Though many other, more sophisticated surgeries followed in its wake, it retained its popularity and was translated into several vernacular languages. Roger "textualizes" surgery, first, by emphasizing the causes of the conditions that the surgeon is called on to treat; surgical cases are thus comparable to medical cases. Second, he furnishes a detailed differential diagnosis. Third, he expounds each procedure step by step, leaving nothing to implicit knowledge or assumed craft expertise. Such descriptions were perhaps not of immediate practical benefit to the surgeon, but they lent surgery itself a rational aspect.*

The illustration reproduced here is from a thirteenth-century manuscript of a French translation of Roger's Surgery. *The upper register shows the Annunciation, Visitation, and Nativity, but the two lower ones show, frame by frame, the stages of the operation described in the excerpt translated below. It is instructive to match the pictures to the parts of the operation and to reflect on how images like this might relate to the text.*

Source: trans. Michael R. McVaugh in *Sourcebook in Medieval Science*, ed. Edward Grant (Cambridge, MA: Harvard University Press, 1974), pp. 795–96 (no. 112). Illustration from London, British Library MS Sloane 1977, fol. 2r (*Chirurgia* of Roger Frugard, 14th c.), reproduced in Peter Murray Jones, *Medieval Medicine in Illuminated Manuscripts* (London: The British Library, 1988), p. 83 (fig. 75).

On Injuries to the Head

Chapter 1

The head may suffer several kinds of injury. Sometimes the injury involves fracture of the skull, sometimes not. Sometimes such a fracture associated

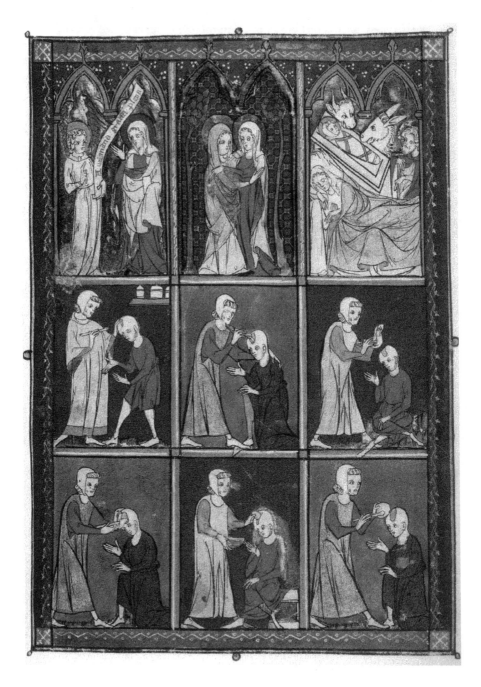

with the injury is considerable and obvious; sometimes it is small. Both large and small fractures may occur with a large, wide wound; or they may occur with a small and narrow one. But whatever sort of fracture of the skull is involved, we must always be alert for injury to the cerebral membranes; sometimes the pia mater is injured, and sometimes the dura mater. Injury to the dura mater is known by these symptoms: the patient suffers pain in the head, is red of face with inflamed eyes, is deranged, and has a blackened tongue. Injury to the pia mater can be recognized by these symptoms: a failing of strength, loss of voice, appearance of pustules on the face, flow of blood and pus from the nostrils, constipation, and chills three or four times a day, which [last] is a certain sign of death. If all or most of these symptoms are to be seen, death will follow or can be expected during the next hundred days at most. And in particular, if there is injury to the cerebral membranes, it usually happens that the patient dies at the next full moon. Thus, since there is considerable danger from fracture of the skull, we will proceed to explain systematically how we can treat it.

Chapter 2

When the fracture of the skull is considerable and obvious, with a broad, long wound, as if made with a sword or something similar, and bone has to be withdrawn (unless there would be a great gush of blood, or unless something else interferes), the bone to be withdrawn is removed and a very fine linen cloth is carefully introduced as it were obliquely between the skull and the dura mater, using a feather. At the opening of the fracture, a linen or silk cloth, preferably long enough for both ends to pass under the head, will prevent corrupt matter from flowing from the outside onto the dura mater, which would bring about still greater harm to the brain. A clean, dry marine sponge is also used, for this thirstily soaks up the corruption deriving from the surface. The external wound should be carefully packed with linen soaked in egg-white and slightly pressed out, a little feather placed on top [for drainage], and the whole bound up carefully, following the contour of the head. The dressing should be changed twice [a day] in winter, three times in summer; the patient should be placed to lie with the injured part downward [for drainage]. This treatment is to be maintained until the skull is fully healed....

Chapter 4

If the fracture of the skull is large, but the wound small in area, so that you cannot fully determine the extent of the fracture, introduce your finger into the wound and carefully probe it; for there is no better way to determine the nature of a skull fracture than by your sense of touch. After you have generally determined the extent of the fracture, cut the narrow wound with a razor in the form of a cross, and with a scraper – that is, an iron instrument – separate the flesh from the skull. And unless a large quantity of blood, or something else, should prevent it, bone or anything else which has to be taken out should be removed with forceps. But if there is an efflux of blood, wait until it ceases, although it means postponing your treatment; just remove it as soon as you can. Then carefully introduce a cloth between the dura mater and the skull with a feather, and pursue the treatment of the skull that we have outlined above. The four quarters of the incision then having been drawn tightly together, the whole wound is to be bound up with a linen cloth soaked in white of egg, together with a little feather, and wrapped according to the contour of the head; let it be unbound from morning to evening, or vice versa. If on coming back to the wound you find the four corners swollen, it is a good sign; while if they are shrunken and show signs of mortification, it is a bad one. Continue this external treatment until you know that the skull is fully healed, and then you can reduce the bandage and bring the quarters back to their proper place; you should not use lint, or another cloth, until the very end. For in wounds involving fracture of the skull we only use one cloth, unmoistened [by egg-white] after the second or third day. Indeed, we entirely avoid using an ointment or anything greasy; but we do put some of the surgical *apostolicon on the skin at the end.

If you want to apply something of your own, make up the following ointment, which you can safely put on the external lips of the wound: take saffron and put it in water, and let it stand long enough for the water to become well colored; then strain it, and add wheat flour to the strainings, and mix it in well. Boil this briefly over a fire, stirring continually. This [ointment], kept for use, eases pain and soothes.

Chapter 5

It may happen that the skull suffers a hairline fracture, so that one side seems neither higher nor lower than the other; and it cannot be told whether such a fracture runs through to the inside or not. In order to tell, let the patient hold his mouth and nostrils shut, and exhale strongly, and if he forces something out through the crack, the skull is split down to the brain itself. We cure this in the following way. If the wound is narrow, enlarge it, and unless there is too much blood, make a space on either side of the crack. Then, with a trepan [an iron instrument that functions like a drill], using the greatest care, make as many holes as you think necessary, and with a chisel cut the skull itself from one hole to another, so that the incision runs to the end of the crack; by this means you can carefully withdraw the *putridity that has collected above the brain, using cotton or a very fine cloth inserted with a feather between the brain and the skull. To treat the wound from this point on, follow those instructions that we have given above. If the skull is so fractured that one side is slightly depressed, so that you cannot easily remove a fragment from the side where it adheres, you should begin to cut; make as many openings as seem necessary to you; then treat as described above, with the chisel and other instruments.

39. THE SALERNITAN TRADITION OF GYNECOLOGY: *THE TROTULA*

Trotula *is not the name of a person, as is commonly thought, but the title of a text assembled at the close of the twelfth century by the amalgamation of three Salernitan tracts on health care for women:* On the Conditions of Women, Treatments for Women, *and* Women's Cosmetics. *The second of these tracts is by Trota or Trocta, a female physician of Salerno, who also composed a general treatise on medical practice. Trota was the "author" of* Treatments *in the sense that she was the source and author-ity for its contents. She may not, however, have actually put the text onto parchment, or at least not in its entirety. Indeed, there are clues suggesting that its editor was from England, perhaps one of the numerous scholars, clerics, and health-seekers who journeyed from the British Isles to Salerno in the eleventh and twelfth centuries (doc. 105).* Conditions *and* Cosmetics *were almost certainly written by men. But such was the reputation of Trota that the whole ensemble came to bear her name:* Trotula *means "Little Trota," a title probably meant to distinguish this book from Trota's larger* Practica.

The Trotula *rapidly became the premier text on gynecology in the emerging world of academic medicine because it articulated a new style of* Galenic *gynecology. Pre-Salernitan Latin literature on women's health was predominantly based on Methodist, and to some degree Hippocratic, sources. Galen himself wrote very little on gynecol-ogy, but his Arab readers, as part of their larger project to systematize his medicine, reframed non-Galenic material about women's disorders within a Galenic explanation of female *humoral physiology. Women were colder and wetter than men; this both explained their disorders and justified particular therapeutic interventions.* Conditions *in particular draws heavily on Constantine the African's* Viaticum, *itself an adapta-tion of an Arabic encyclopedia.* Treatments, *on the other hand, is a miscellany of therapeutic instructions that assumes knowledge of Galenic theory but rarely alludes to it in an explicit manner. Both texts, however, bear the imprint of a southern Italian milieu. Salerno's place within a Norman kingdom that included a substantial Muslim population explains the numerous references to "Saracens" and "Saracen women" as the source of medical practices. The recipes for restoring the appearance of virginity also* *speak to a Mediterranean culture that equated female honor with chastity.*

The passages presented here are from the "standardized" edition of The Trotula *ensemble, as it took shape in the thirteenth century. This version circulated widely in the later Middle Ages; it was the basis of translations and adaptations into medieval Dutch, French, German, and English. Though female readers usually read vernacular rather than Latin works,* The Trotula's *owners and readers, regardless of the language of the text, were overwhelmingly men.*

Source: ed. and trans. Monica Green, *The Trotula: A Medieval Compendium of Women's Medicine*, (Philadelphia: University of Pennsylvania Press, 2001), pp. 71–73, 85–87, 125–27, 145–47. Latin.

a. The Learned Tradition: Excerpts from *On the Conditions of Women* on Female Physiology, and "Suffocation of the Womb"

Because she is cold and wet, a woman cannot fully concoct or "cook" the food she eats. She therefore accumulates more superfluities of digestion *than does a man, and requires a special additional mechanism – menstruation – to evacuate these superfluities before they putrefy and generate disease. Much of* The Trotula *is concerned with regulating menstruation, any disruption or unnatural cessation of which would constitute a serious threat to health.*

[1] When God the creator of the universe in the first establishment of the world differentiated the individual natures of things each according to its kind, he endowed human nature above all other things with a singular dignity, giving to it above the condition of all other animals the freedom of reason and intellect. And wishing to sustain its generation in perpetuity, he created the male and the female with provident, dispensing deliberation, laying out in the separate sexes the foundation for the propagation of future offspring. And so that from them there might emerge fertile offspring, he endowed their *complexions with a certain pleasing commixtion, constituting the nature of the male hot and dry. But lest the male overflow with either of these qualities, he wished by the opposing frigidity and humidity of the woman to rein him in from too much excess, so that the stronger qualities, that is the heat and the dryness, should rule the man, who is the stronger and more worthy person, while the weaker ones, that is to say the coldness and humidity, should rule the weaker [person], that is the woman. And [God did this] so that by his stronger quality the male might pour out his duty in the woman just as seed is sown in its designated field, and so that the woman by her weaker quality, as if made subject to the function of the man, might receive the seed poured in the lap of Nature.

[2] Therefore, because women are by nature weaker than men and because

they are most frequently afflicted in childbirth, diseases often abound in them especially around the organs devoted to the work of Nature. Moreover, women, from the condition of their fragility, out of shame and embarrassment do not dare reveal their anguish over their diseases (which happen in such a private place) to a physician. Therefore, their misfortune, which ought to be pitied, and especially the influence of a certain woman stirring my heart, have impelled me to give a clear explanation regarding their diseases in caring for their health. And so with God's help, I have labored assiduously to gather in excerpts the more worthy parts of the books of Hippocrates and Galen, so that I might explain and discuss the causes of their diseases, their symptoms, and their cures.

[3] Because there is not enough heat in women to dry up the bad and superfluous humors which are in them, nor is their weakness able to tolerate sufficient labor so that Nature might expel [the excess] to the outside through sweat as [it does] in men, Nature established a certain *purgation especially for women, that is, the menses, to temper their poverty of heat. The common people call the menses "the flowers," because just as trees do not bring forth fruit without flowers, so women without their flowers are cheated of the ability to conceive. This purgation occurs in women just as nocturnal emission happens to men. For Nature, if burdened by certain humors, either in men or in women, always tries to expel or set aside its yoke and reduce its labor.

[4] This purgation occurs in women around the thirteenth year, or a little earlier or a little later, depending on the degree to which they have an excess or dearth of heat or cold. It lasts until the fiftieth year if she is thin, sometimes until the sixtieth or sixty-fifth year if she is moist. In the moderately fat, it lasts until the thirty-fifth year. If this purgation occurs at the appropriate time and with suitable regularity, Nature frees itself sufficiently of the excess humors. If, however, the menses flow out either more or less than they ought to, many sicknesses thus arise, for then the appetite for food as well as for drink is diminished; sometimes there is vomiting, and sometimes they crave earth, coals, chalk, and similar things.

[5] Sometimes from the same cause pain is felt in the neck, the back, and in the head. Sometimes there is acute *fever, pangs of the heart, *dropsy, or dysentery. These things happen either because for a long time the menses have been deficient or because the women do not have any at all. Whence not only dropsy or dysentery or heart pangs occur, but other very grave diseases.

Though it was also called "hysteria" (particularly after the sixteenth century), suffocation of the womb was understood to have a physical and not a psychological basis. Some Hippocratic texts appear to claim that the uterus can overheat, dry out, and develop a violent craving for moisture. It then flies upwards, latches onto the liver (because it is moist), and generates alarming symptoms such as choking and fainting. Post-Hippocratic medical writers explicitly refuted the notion that the womb could wander (doc. 47) but continued to describe and prescribe for the condition they called suffocation. In spite of these new explanations, old therapies grounded in the notion that the uterus had to be lured or driven back into place by attractive or repulsive smells persisted.

On Suffocation of the Womb

[45] Sometimes the womb is suffocated, that is to say, when it is drawn upward, whence there occurs [stomach] upset and loss of appetite from an overwhelming frigidity of the heart. Sometimes they suffer *syncope, and the pulse vanishes so that from the same cause it is barely perceptible. Sometimes the woman is contracted so that the head is joined to the knees, and she lacks vision, and she loses the function of the voice, the nose is distorted, the lips are contracted and she grits her teeth, and the chest is elevated upward beyond what is normal.

[46] Galen tells of a certain woman who suffered thus and she lost her pulse and her voice and she was as if she had expired, because no exterior sign of life was apparent, though around her heart Nature still retained a little bit of heat. Whence certain people judged her to be dead. But Galen put some well-carded wool to her nose and mouth, and by its motion he knew that she was still alive. This [disease] happens to women because corrupt semen [*female "seed"*] abounds in them excessively, and it is converted into a poisonous nature.

[47] This happens to those women who do not [have sexual relations with] men, especially to widows who were accustomed to carnal commerce. It regularly comes upon virgins, too, when they reach the age of marriage and are not able to use men and when the semen abounds in them a lot, which Nature wishes to draw out by means of the male. From this superabundant and corrupt semen, a certain cold fumosity is released and it ascends to the organs which are called by the common people the "collaterals," because they are near to the heart and lungs and the rest of the principal instruments of the voice. Whence an impediment of the voice generally occurs. This kind of illness is accustomed to originate principally from a defect of the menses. And if both the menses are lacking and the semen is abundant, the illness will be so much the more menacing and wide-ranging, especially when it seizes the higher organs.

[48] The best remedy is that the hands and feet of the woman be rubbed moderately with laurel oil and that there be applied to the nose those things which have a foul odor, such as galbanum, opoponax, *castoreum, pitch, burnt wool, burnt linen cloth, and burnt leather. On the other hand, their

vaginas ought to be anointed with those oils and hot ointments which have a sweet odor, such as iris oil, chamomile oil, musk oil, and nard oil. For these things attract and provoke the menses . Let *cupping glasses be applied to the inguinal area and the pubic area. The women ought also to be anointed inside and out with oils and ointments of good smell. Likewise, in the evening let her take *diaciminum with the juice of wild celery or with a *syrup of calamint or catmint, or with the juice of henbane or juice of catmint. Or take one dram each of castoreum, white pepper, costmary, mint, and wild celery; let them be ground, and let them be mixed with white or sweet wine. And give one dram of it in the evening.

[49] The physician Justinus prescribed for this illness that cumin be dried and given in a *potion [in the amount of] one dram or two spoonfuls. He also prescribed that the penis of a fox or roebuck be taken and made into a powder and inserted by means of a *pessary.

b. The Empirical Tradition: Excerpts from *Treatments for Women* on the Dangers of Childbirth, and on Cosmetic Procedures to Restore the Appearance of Virginity

The Trotula devoted considerable attention to promoting conception and dealing with the complications and consequences of childbirth. By contrast, there is no discussion of normal childbirth, which was not seen as a medical problem. The treatment for torn perineum recorded here is unique in Salernitan medical literature.

On the Dangerous Things Happening to Women Giving Birth

[149] There are some women for whom things go wrong in giving birth, and this is because of the failure of those assisting them: that is to say, this is kept hidden by the women. For there are some women in whom the vagina and the anus become one opening and the same pathway. Whence in these women the womb comes out and hardens. We give aid to such women by repositioning [the womb]. We put on the womb warm wine in which butter had been boiled, and diligently we *foment it until the womb has been rendered soft, and then we gently replace it. Afterwards we sew the rupture between the anus and the vagina in three or four places with a silk thread. Then we place a linen cloth unto the vagina to fill the vagina completely. Then let us smear it with liquid pitch. This makes the womb withdraw because of its stench. And we heal the rupture with a powder made of comfrey, that is, of bruisewort, and daisy and cumin. The powder ought to be sprinkled [on the wound], and the woman should be placed in bed so that her feet are higher [than the rest of her body], and there let her do all her business for eight or nine days. And as much as necessary let her eat; there let her relieve herself

and do all customary things. It is necessary that she abstain from baths until she seems to be able to tolerate them. Also, it is fitting that she abstain from all things that cause coughing and from all things that are hard to *digest, and this especially ought to be done. In [subsequent] birth we should aid them thus. Let a cloth be prepared in the shape of an oblong ball and place it in the anus, so that in each effort of pushing out the child, it is pressed into the anus firmly so that there not be [another] *solution of continuity of this kind.

A Good Constrictive

[190] A constrictive for the vagina so that they may appear as if they were virgins. Take the whites of eggs and mix them with water in which penny-royal and hot herbs of this kind have been cooked, and with a new linen cloth dipped in it, place it in the vagina two or three times a day. And if she urinates at night, put it in again. And note that prior to this the vagina ought to be washed well with the same warm water with which these things were mixed.

[191] Take the newly grown bark of a holm oak. Having ground it, dissolve it with rainwater, and with a linen or cotton cloth place it in the vagina in the above-mentioned manner. And remove all these things before the hour of the commencement of intercourse....

[193] Likewise, there are some dirty and corrupt prostitutes who desire to seem to be more than virgins and they make a constrictive for this purpose, but they are ill counseled, for they render themselves bloody and they wound the penis of the man. They take powdered *natron and place it in the vagina....

[195] What is better is if the following is done one night before she is married: let her place leeches in the vagina (but take care that they do not go in too far) so that blood comes out and is converted into a little clot. And thus the man will be deceived by the effusion of blood.

CHAPTER SIX

VIA SCOLARIS: MEDICINE IN THE UNIVERSITY

Salerno's emphasis on medical theory prepared the way for medicine to be taught in universities. This was a step fraught with consequences, not only for the Middle Ages, but also for the history of medicine in the West: medicine would henceforth be insepara-bly associated with "science." In the Middle Ages, scientia meant knowledge that was formally ordered (and therefore teachable) and exceptionally reliable or certain, because it was based on reason. The great authorities of the past constituted a heritage of rea-soned knowledge, but that heritage could be refined, extended, and even critiqued using the tools of logic. The paradigmatic scientia of the medieval university was philosophy.

But medicine's entry into the university was not inevitable, nor did the university constitute the only locus of medical training. Even after the establishment of faculties of medicine and doctoral colleges, much medical instruction was still given by the informal method whereby a master instructed his socius *(apprentice). Medical texts were created and disseminated outside the schools as well as within. Nonetheless, academic medicine rapidly became the accepted model that all medicine, even most "alternative" medicine, sought to emulate, and it was eagerly digested into the mainstream of medieval learned culture (doc. 49).*

The earliest universities began by amalgamating smaller "boutique schools" run by individual masters into an umbrella organization called a studium generale. *A* studium *was a facility for advanced study; a* studium generale *taught the basic arts course, plus one or more of the advanced disciplines of law, theology, and medicine. Certification (a "degree") from a* studium generale *was a* licentia ubique docendi – *a "license to teach anywhere." A* studium generale *was therefore essentially a place that trained master teachers. The word* universitas, *on the other hand, means "guild," and it refers to the fact that the members of the university were a self-governing, legally constituted, publicly recognized corporate body.*

Regional variations in medieval universities had an impact on how medicine was taught. In the north (notably in Paris), the dominant faculty was the undergraduate faculty of arts. It was historically the first to be formed, it was always the largest faculty, and its masters were the most active in university government. Teachers were normally clerics (though not necessarily priests), and they were supported by ecclesiastical benefic-es – income from parish tithes, or the endowment of a major urban church. In the south (notably in Bologna), the premier faculty was law. Medicine entered the university as a learned profession analogous to law and brought arts teaching along with it (doc. 40). However, all universities and all faculties shared the common intellectual culture of "scholasticism," the method of the schools, a way of tackling intellectual problems that derived from classroom experience. Its core activities were analyzing authoritative texts and arguing about questions. Most of its products were formal genres of scholarly writing: the commentary on the authoritative text (the "lecture," lectio or lectura), the discussion of doubtful points through logical debate (the "disputed question": quaestio disputata), and the summa, or synthesis.

The first part of this chapter presents documents that illustrate how medical knowledge was organized into a curriculum of authoritative texts for scholastic teaching (docs. 40–42). The pedagogy of medicine was also a means to extend and rationalize medical knowledge itself. A key role in this process was played by Galen's Art of Medicine or Tegni. From the mid-twelfth century onwards, this book was part of the Articella, and in the universities of the thirteenth and fourteenth centuries it was required reading. Galen began by declaring that medicine is essentially about thinking: it has three methods, namely analysis or deduction, synthesis or induction, and definition. Its subject matter was a spectrum of abstractions: the sick, the healthy, and what is neither sick nor healthy, or else in between the two states. This spectrum could be applied to the body itself (anatomy, physiology), the signs it displays (medical semeiotics), and the things that can cause health or disease (hygiene and pathology). It also determined the shape of practical medicine, which comprised preventive medicine to maintain health ("regimen") and therapeutic medicine to restore it (diet, drugs, and surgery). All of this lay in germ in the Isagoge of Joannitius, but it was Galen's stature as an authority that transformed this schema into the foundation of a reformed medical curriculum, notably in Montpellier (doc. 41). This reform introduced a number of newly translated works by Galen (the "new Galen") designed to provide a knowledge base for every category named in the Tegni's analysis.

In this chapter and the next, the Tegni schema will be used to situate the documents on scholastic medicine. In this chapter, the focus will be on "body," and notably the appearance, for the first time since the Hellenistic age, of dissection of the human cadaver for the purpose of learning about anatomy (docs. 47–48).

Scholasticism was based on the fundamental axiom that truth was discovered through reason. Where views differed, logical argument would decide the case. Scholastic medicine found itself fighting these logical battles on many fronts. First, it had to uphold its dignity as scientia, particularly against philosophy, while at the same time defending its distinctive styles of reasoning (docs. 43–45). Second, its authority in the field of the sciences of life was at once bolstered and challenged by Aristotle, whose writings were the foundation of the arts curriculum. But if Aristotle and Galen disagreed (doc. 46), whose authority would prevail?

I. FACULTIES AND CURRICULA

40. FROM PHILOSOPHY TO PHYSIC: PARIS FROM THE LATE TWELFTH CENTURY TO THE LATE THIRTEENTH CENTURY

In his memoirs of his student days in Paris in the 1140s, John of Salisbury lamented that many abandoned the study of the arts for careers that promised higher incomes. Those who wanted to study law decamped to Bologna, while those who had medical ambitions left for Montpellier. By the mid-1170s, the situation in Paris had changed. Alexander Nequam (1157–1217), in his own reminiscences of the Paris schools of his youth, described how the philosophy master Adam of the Petit Pont incorporated the Articella *as a textbook of natural philosophy or* physica. *In Adam's school, medicine came directly after the preparatory liberal arts and preceded moral philosophy (ethica, represented by law) and theology, the Christian equivalent of metaphysics.*

Not long after Alexander left Paris, Adam's student Gilles of Corbeil arrived (doc. 50), fresh from his medical studies in Salerno. It was Gilles, apparently, who first lectured on medicine as a distinct subject in Paris, though the details are difficult to reconstruct. The earliest reference to a separate medical faculty dates from 1251, and in 1270–74 formal statutes were drawn up. These included a curriculum of works to be studied, as well as a syllabus of "ordinary" lectures (given in the mornings by the senior professors) and "cursory" lectures (given in the afternoons by bachelors, who read through the assigned texts in a cursory fashion with the students). Requirements for graduation were also laid out: these included "responding" or presenting a reply in proper logical form to disputed questions arising from the authoritative texts. The contents of the medical curriculum at Paris do not seem to have changed much in the century between Alexander Nequam and the 1270–74 statutes. The methods and goals of teaching, on the other hand, were significantly transformed.

a. Alexander Nequam: Adam of the Petit Pont's Reading List in *Physica*

Source: trans. Faith Wallis from Nequam's *Sacerdos ad altare*, ed. Charles Homer Haskins, *Studies in the History of Mediaeval Science* (Cambridge, MA: Harvard University Press, 1927), pp. 374–75. Latin.

Whoever desires to undertake the study of medicine – so very useful to the needs of the children of Adam – let him hear [lectures on] Joannitius, and both the *Aphorisms* and *Prognosis* of Hippocrates, and the *Tegni* of Galen and the *Pantegni*. The author of this book is Galen, but the translator is

Constantine. He should also read the *Particular Diets* as well as the *Universal Diets* of Isaac, as well as the *Book of Urines* [of Isaac?] and the *Viaticum* of Constantine, along with the *Book of Urines* [of Theophilus] and the *Book of Pulses* [of Philaretus], and Dioscorides and Macer, who discuss the natures of herbs, and the books of Alexander [of Tralles].

b. The Curriculum of the Paris Medical Faculty in 1270–74

Source: trans. Faith Wallis from H. Denifle and E. Chatelain, *Cartularium Universitatis Parisiensis* (Paris: Delalaine, 1889–1897), vol. I, nos. 452–543, pp. 516–17. Latin.

452. *Concerning [Bachelors] Who Wish to Begin to Teach a Course*

Be it known that bachelors in the Faculty of Medicine who wish to begin teaching a course for the first time are sworn to uphold all the following [regulations]. They will swear to preserve such ordinances, statutes, privileges, and customs of the faculty as shall be made known to them by the dean, the dean's delegate, or by the faculty as a whole. They shall swear to the dean or the dean's delegate or before the whole faculty that they have attended lectures in medicine for [three] years, and that they are in their fourth year, having attended lectures for five months. And if the bachelor has not studied medicine for nine months of each of these years, the license to lecture (*licentia legendi*) may nonetheless be granted provided he has diligently studied this subject in Paris by attending the ordinary lectures for thirty-two months (not counting vacations). Also, they shall swear that they have "responded" to a question twice, in the classrooms of two masters (meaning in the course of a formal disputation, not in the course of a lecture), or at least once in a general disputation. Fourthly, they shall swear that the book on which they will deliver a cursory lecture is one on which they have heard the ordinary lectures. Also, they shall give the four purses [of money] which are required from a bachelor who wishes to begin teaching a course, before any oath is taken; as well, one purse at least [shall be given] to the beadle [*the officer in charge of maintaining order during lectures, ceremonies, etc.*]. They shall also swear that for as long as they are lecturing, they shall attend mass every Saturday like the masters, or be fined two pence.

453. *Concerning Those Who Wish to Receive the License in Medicine at Paris, and the Books They Shall Study*

This is the format for licensing bachelors in medicine. First, the master who is supervising the bachelor shall swear to the chancellor [of the university], in the presence of the masters who have been summoned for this purpose, that the bachelor is fit to receive the license. The time that he has spent in attending lectures should be attested by at least two witnesses, and the duration of attendance at lectures should be five and a half years if he taught or was a licentiate in Arts, or six years if he was not. The form for studying the texts is that he should have attended [1] the ordinary lectures on the *Art of Medicine* [*that is, the Articella*] twice, and the cursory lectures once, except for [lectures on] the *Urines* of Theophilus, on which it suffices to have attended either the ordinary or the cursory ones once; [2] the ordinary lectures on the *Viaticum* [of Constantine the African] twice; [3] the ordinary lectures on the other books of Isaac [Judaeus] once, and the cursory lectures twice, except for *Particular Diets*, on which it suffices to have heard either the ordinary or the cursory lectures; [4] the lectures on the *Antidotary* of Nicholas once. The verses [on urines] by Gilles de Corbeil are not compulsory. Also, he should have read one book of the *Theory* [*of the Pantegni*] and one of the *Practice* [*of the Pantegni*]. He should take an oath to this effect; if anyone is convicted of perjury or lying, he can be deprived of the license.

41. MONTPELLIER AND THE "NEW GALEN"

The medical school at Montpellier, a vibrant commercial city on the Mediterranean coast of southern France, had already established a European reputation by the middle of the twelfth century. It is somewhat surprising, then, that we know so little about the organization and content of medical instruction at this school prior to the middle of the thirteenth century. By this time, Montpellier was fully constituted as a university, and its medical teaching was poised to undergo an important transformation. A second wave of translations of the works of Galen (the so-called New Galen), combined with the adoption of Avicenna's Canon *as a core text, not only solidified the dominance of theory but greatly expanded the quantity and scope of medical knowledge. It also stimulated more sophisticated and ingenious medical thinking. The figures of Arnau of Vilanova (doc. 44) and Bernard of Gordon (doc. 55) dominate the period from 1280 to 1320, when Montpellier medicine was at its apogee. The text below was the final product of a process of curriculum reform spearheaded by Arnau and his colleagues: the letter of Pope Clement V granted new statutes to the medical faculty and spelled out the revised reading list.*

Source: trans. Faith Wallis from *Cartulaire de l'Université de Montpellier*, ed. Conseil général des facultés de Montpellier, 2 vols. (Montpellier: Maison Richard Frères, 1890–1912), pp. 219–21. Latin.

Bull of the lord Pope Clement concerning the manner of proceeding to the promotion of bachelors for the license, together with statutes to be observed in the course of studies.

Bishop Clement, servant of the servants of God, to his beloved sons, all the masters of the Faculty of Medicine located at Montpellier in the diocese of Maguelone: greeting and apostolic benediction. In order to feed the Lord's sheep committed by the divine disposition into our care in sound wisdom and doctrine, we survey the lofty summits of rich and verdant pastureland, so that when they are stationed upon those same summits under our management they may be refreshed in that same pasture with health-giving instruction. We seek out gushing streams of sweet water for them to drink so that, drinking deeply of these waters, they may joyfully imbibe from them a copious flow of manifold knowledge as from the fountains of the Savior. But we both desire to gather into the bosom of Mother Church her more expert sons in the praiseworthy Faculty of Medicine, and to bestow the favor of more ample honor upon those whom we have gathered – and all the more so, the more frequently their activity is demonstrated to be necessary and useful for the salvation of the bodies of mortal humanity.

The petition which you very properly submitted to us contained this as your particular desire, namely: that the bachelors who are recognized as belonging to this faculty in the University at Montpellier in the diocese of Maguelone and who have been found competent and qualified at the present time, and no others, should be admitted to the rank of master in the aforementioned faculty for the sake of the public welfare and in order that they may have the reward they deserve. We, therefore, assenting with the favor of paternal benevolence to your worthy desires in this matter and wishing that the qualifications and competent expertise of these bachelors be fully established, by apostolic authority, on the advice and appeal of our beloved sons, masters Guillelmo of Brescia and Jean d'Alès, physicians and our chaplains, as well as of Master Arnau of Vilanova, physician, for the benefit of this same university, do decree that every bachelor in this faculty who is a candidate for promotion to this rank within this university should be obliged to possess, at the time of his promotion [the following books]: the commented books [of the *Articella*]; Galen's [books entitled] *On Complexions, The Vices of Different Complexions, On Simple Medicine, On Disease and Accident, On Crisis and Critical Days,* and *Therapeutic Method;* the books of Avicenna, or failing him, Rhazes, and also of Constantine and Isaac [Judaeus]. Furthermore, they are expected to have read [*studied and lectured on*] two commented and one uncommented [works], namely the *Art of Medicine* [of Galen] and the *Prognosis* or *Aphorisms* of Hippocrates (the latter up to part 5), and *Regimen* [*in Acute Diseases*] and Joannitius and the book on *fevers by the same Isaac or the *Antidotary* [*of Nicolas*] or [Galen's] *On Disease and Accident* and *Therapeutic Method* up to book 8. They should "respond" at least once to questions which you will put to them publicly in the schools of the said faculty by expounding their arguments and resolving problems.

And in reputable places, they shall attend lectures in medicine at the same faculty for five years if they are qualified masters of Arts, and otherwise for six years, for not less than eight months in each year. And in similar places, for a minimum of eight months or two summers, they shall practice [medicine]. Notwithstanding, at the time of their promotion to the aforementioned rank of master, they shall deliver two lectures, one on theory and the other on practice, at the summons of the chancellor of the university or his deputy in your presence, being assembled as is customary at the hour of vespers in the church of Notre Dame des Tables or in the church of St Firmin in Montpellier. And let them answer the questions posed by you concerning the said lectures, with modesty and due order being observed in these [transactions], so that you can test their knowledge by means of the lecture, the response, and the solution [of the questions]. Thereafter, when the bachelors have withdrawn from your presence, and when you have, under oath, come to a judgment of the truth concerning the competence or lack of competence of these bachelors, if these bachelors are by you or by a report of this kind considered and found qualified to be promoted to this honor, and after they have sworn an oath in person to observe the statutes of the university, let them be promoted to the honor of the master's degree by him or by them, to whom the promotion of such people is recognized to pertain. For we have from this time forth declared null and void any assault upon the admission to the said rank of master which is against the tenor of this our statute, notwithstanding any privileges or custom which may contradict it. Therefore let no one at all be permitted to infringe this charter of our statute and constitution, or to act against it with audacity. Should anyone presume to thus attack it, let him know that he will incur the wrath of Almighty God and of his apostles, the blessed Peter and Paul. Given at Avignon on the 8th of September, in the fourth year of our pontificate.

42. THE "UNIVERSITY OF ARTS AND MEDICINE" AT BOLOGNA

Students in Paris studied Aristotle's natural philosophy and Ptolemy's astronomy as undergraduates before proceeding to medical studies as a graduate course. In Italian universities, on the other hand, medicine and arts were often joined in one faculty. Many professors taught in both fields, and arts and medicine could be studied simultaneously or consecutively. This distinctive arrangement originated in the career of the first recorded professor of medicine at Bologna, Taddeo Alderotti (d. 1295).

Taddeo Alderotti of Florence started out as a successful practitioner before moving into medical education. His expertise in medicine was complemented by an interest in literary culture and particularly in Aristotelian philosophy. He taught both logic and medicine and had close connections to the Dominican and Franciscan schools in Bologna. Taddeo and his school, as pioneers in developing the Bologna medical curriculum, helped to establish the characteristic features of Italian learned medicine in the Middle Ages and the early modern period. First, he fostered scholastic-type instruction through the study of texts. Teaching continued to be based on the Articella, but Bologna also adopted the "new Galen" discussed in doc. 41. Some of the earliest commentaries on the Canon of Avicenna were also written in Bologna. The second feature was the use of "material demonstration" in the teaching of anatomy. This was implicit in the Salernitan anatomy lessons on animals (see doc. 35) but was reinforced by the strong Bologna tradition of surgical education. Taddeo's circle introduced dissection of human cadavers for purposes of instruction (doc. 47). Finally, Taddeo succeeded in establishing Bologna's earliest regulations governing medical study. This Bologna model of the "University of Arts and Medicine" was imitated by other Italian universities such as Padua and Florence.

Translated below is the curriculum laid out in the Bologna statutes of 1405, followed by the regulations for conducting a dissection. The philosophy or arts program is covered first. Then follows the four-year sequence of lectures in medicine, and finally a calendar of astronomy/astrology lectures. Notice how Aristotle dominates the arts curriculum, and how in the medicine lectures the "new Galen" and the Arab encyclopedists have pushed the old Articella into the background. The exceptional space devoted to astronomy and astrology is a distinctive feature of the Italian universities. The importance of these subjects for medicine is discussed in chapter 8.

As in Paris, the calendar is divided into "ordinary" morning lectures delivered by the professors, and "extraordinary" lectures given in the afternoon, usually by junior lecturers. Lectures often repeated material studied in previous years – a pattern followed in medical schools well into the nineteenth century. The following summary will clarify the structure of the medical portion of the curriculum:

Lectures in Medicine

Ordinary	Extraordinary
First year	
1. Avicenna, *Canon* book 1 (with omissions)	Avicenna, *Canon* book 4 *fen* [*that is, section*] 2; book 2
2. Galen, *On Distinguishing Fevers* Galen, *On Complexions* Galen, *On the Bad State of the Complexion* Galen, *On Simple Medicine* except book 6 Galen, *On Critical Days* book 1	Galen, *On Affected Parts* except book 2 Galen, *Hygiene* Galen, *On Critical Days* book 2 Hippocrates, *Aphorisms* except pt. 7

Second year

1. Galen, *Tegni*
   Hippocrates, *Prognosis*
   Hippocrates, *Regimen in Acute Diseases* except book 4
   Avicenna, *The Powers of the Heart* in part
2. Galen, *On Accident and Illness*
   Galen, *On Crises*
   Galen, *On Critical Days* book 2
   Galen, *Therapeutics to Glaucon* tract on fevers
   Galen, *On Wasting*
   Galen, *On the Utility of Breathing*

1. Avicenna, *Canon* (as under first year)
2. Galen, *Distinguishing Fevers*
   Galen, *On the Bad State of the Complexion*
   Canon book 4, *fen* 2
   Galen, *On Simple Medicine* except book 6
   Galen, *On Critical Days* book 1

Third year

1. Hippocrates, *Aphorisms* except pt. 7
2. [Galen] *Therapeutics* books 7–13
   Averroes, *Colliget* in part
   Galen, *On Natural Faculties* in part
   Galen, *On Critical Days* book 2

1. Galen, *Tegni*
   Hippocrates, *Prognosis*
   Hippocrates, *Regimen in Acute Diseases*
   Avicenna, *The Powers of the Heart* in part
2. Galen, *On Accident and Illness*
   Galen, *On Crises*
   Galen, *On Critical Days* book 3
   Galen, *Therapeutics to Glaucon* tract on fevers
   Galen, *On Complexions*

Fourth year

1. Avicenna, *Canon* (as under first year)
2. *Canon* book 4, *fen* 1 and book 2
   Galen, *On Affected Parts* except book 2
   Galen, *Hygiene* book 6
   Hippocrates, *The Nature of Man*

1. Hippocrates, *Aphorisms* except pt. 7
2. [Galen] *Therapeutics* books 7–13
2. Averroes, *Colliget* in part
   Galen, *On Natural Faculties* in part

Source: trans. Faith Wallis from *Statuti delle Università e dei Collegi dello studio bolognese*, ed. Carlo Malagola (Bologna: Nicola Zanichelli 1888), pp. 274–77 and 289–90. Latin.

88. The Lectures and the Order of Books to be Read

[*The Arts Curriculum*]

Therefore they have ordained, since it is useful and necessary to give attention to the reading [*lectura*] of books by scholars for their advantage, that this sequence shall be observed in the lectures and concerning the books to be read both in medicine as well as in philosophy and astronomy: namely, that after the manner laid out below and for the twenty-five years to come, and in the order laid out below, the whole of [Aristotle's] *Physics* shall first be read in the philosophy [course]. After this has been read, book 1 of [Aristotle's] *On Generation and Corruption* shall be read. In the extraordinary lectures, book 2 of *On Generation and Corruption* shall first be read. [Aristotle's] *On Sleep and Wakefulness* shall be read, and when this has been read, [pseudo-]Aristotle's book *On Physiognomy* shall be read.

In the second year [Aristotle's] *On the Heaven and the Universe* shall first be read, and when it has been read, [Aristotle's] book on *Meteorology*, and when that has been read, his book *On Sense and Sensation*. In the extraordinary lectures, [Averroes's] *On the Substance of the Heavenly Sphere* shall first be read; and when this has been read, [Aristotle's] *On Memory and Reminiscence* shall be read; and when this has been read, his book *On Breathing and Respiration* shall be read. After that has been read, let the book *On Death and Life* be read.

In the third year following, [Aristotle's] *On the Soul* shall be read first, except for the errors in book 1; and when this has been read, let the prologue of [Aristotle's] *Metaphysics* be read, but no more from book 1. When this has been read, book 2 of the same work should be read, and when this has been read, books 5, 6, 7, 8, 9, 10 and 12. In the extraordinary lectures, book 4 of the *Metaphysics* should be read [to the end of part 3] up to where it says "for it is the starting point for everything else." When this has been read, let [Aristotle's] *On Length and Shortness of Life* be read; and when this has been read, [Aristotle's] *On the Cause of Movement of Animals* should be read. And the extraordinary lectures should always begin at Easter.

[*The Medicine Curriculum*]

In medicine, in the first year, the first book of [the *Canon*] of Avicenna should be read first, except for [the chapters] on anatomy, and the chapter on the nature of the seasons of the year in *fen* [*that is, section*] 2, and the whole of *fen* 3 apart from these chapters: chapter 1 "On the necessity of death," the chapter "On illnesses which befall children," the chapter "On regimen with regard to eating and drinking," the chapter "On regimen with regard to water and wine," and the chapter "On sleep and wakefulness." For the second lecture in the morning, [Galen's] *On Distinguishing Fevers* should be read; and when that is read, his *On Complexions* should be read; and when that has been read, let his *On the Bad State of the Complexion* be read; and when that has been read, his book *On Simple Medicine* should be read, except for book 6. When that has been read, let book 1 of [Galen's] *On Critical Days* be read. At nones [*3 p.m., during the extraordinary lectures*] book 4, *fen* 2 of the *Canon* [on prognosis] and book 2 [of the *Canon*, on medicines] should be read. When these have been read, [Galen's] book *On Affected Parts* should be read, except for book 2; and when that has been read, let his *Hygiene* be read; and when that has been read, book 2 of his *On Critical Days*. And when that has been read, the book of the *Aphorisms* [of Hippocrates] should be read, except for part 7.

In the second year, for the first lecture in medicine in the morning, let [Galen's] *Tegni* [*that is, Art of Medicine*] first be read. And then [Hippocrates's] *Prognosis* should be read, without the commentary; and when this has been read, let his *Regimen in Acute Disease* be read without the commentary, and omitting book 4. When this has been read, [Avicenna's] book *On the Powers of the Heart* should be read, only up to where the text says "afterwards we said." For the second lecture in the morning, [Galen's] *On Accident and Illness* should be read. When that has been read, his book *On Crises* should be read. When that has been read, let book 3 of [Galen's] *On Critical Days* be read; and when that has been read, the section on fevers in the first part of his [*Therapeutics*] *to Glaucon*. When that has been read, [Galen's] *On Wasting* and *The Utility of Breathing* should be read. At nones [during the extraordinary lectures], the first book of Avicenna's [*Canon*] should be read, except for [the chapters speci-fied above].... For the second lecture, [Galen's] *On Distinguishing Fevers* should be read. When that has been read, let [*Canon*] book 4, *fen* 2 be read; and when that has been read, [Galen's] *On the Bad State of the Complexion*; and when that has been read, his *On Simple Medicine* should be read, omitting book 6. When that has been read, book 1 of *On Critical Days* should be read.

In the third year, for the first lecture in the morning [Hippocrates's] *Apho-risms* should first be read, omitting part 7. For the second lecture, let [Galen's] *Therapeutics* [*that is, Therapeutic Method*] from 7 to 13; and when that has been read, [Averroes's] book *Colliget* – the prologue of book 1, chapter 2 of book 1 and all of book 2 [on physiology]. When this has been read, one should read from book 5 up to that chapter where he begins to expound on *simple medicines, and after that, the last chapter in book 5, where he expounds on the necessity of compound medicine, up to the end of book 5. When that has been read, [Galen's] book *On Natural Faculties* should be read in the first [lecture] up to chapter 7 of book 1, which begins "therefore it is necessary for it to resemble what it has." When this has been read, book 3 should be read. When this has been read, Galen's *On Critical Days* book 2 should be read. At nones [during the extraordinary lectures], the *Tegni* should first be read.

When this has been read, [Hippocrates's] *Prognosis* should be read, without the commentary. When this has been read, let his *Regimen in Acute Diseases* be read, without the commentary, and omitting book 4. When this has been read, [Avicenna's] book *On the Powers of the Heart* should be read, only up to where the text says "afterwards we said." For the second lecture, [Galen's] *On Accident and Illness* should first be read. When that has been read, his book *On Crises* should be read. When that has been read, let book 3 of [Galen's] *On Critical Days* be read; and when that has been read, the section on fevers in the first part of his [*Therapeutics*] *to Glaucon*. And when this has been read, [Galen's] *On Complexions* should be read.

In the fourth year, for the first lecture in the morning the first book of Avicenna's [*Canon*] should be read, except for [the chapters specified above].... For the second lecture, book 4, *fen* 1 should first be read, and when this has been read, the canons of book 2 of Avicenna. When these have been read, [Galen's] *On Affected Parts* should be read, omitting book 2; and when this has been read, book 6 of his *Hygiene* should be read. When this has been read, Hippocrates's *On the Nature* [*of Man*] should be read. At nones, for the first lecture, let [Hippocrates's] *Aphorisms* be read, omitting part 7. For the second lecture, let [Galen's] *Therapeutics* from books 7 to 13 be read; and when that has been read, [Averroes's] book *Colliget* – the prologue of book 1, chapter 2 of book 1 and all of book 2. When this has been read, one should read from book 5 up to that chapter where he begins to expound on simple medicines, and after that, the last chapter in book 5, where he expounds on the necessity of compound medicine, up to the end of book 5. When that has been read, [Galen's] book *On Natural Faculties* should be read in the first [lecture] up to chapter 7 of book 1, which begins "therefore it is necessary." When this has been read, let book 3 of the same work be read.

[*The Astronomy/Astrology Curriculum*]

In astronomy in the first year, let [John of Sacrobosco's (d. ca 1244–56)] *Algorism on Integers and Fractions* be read first; and when this has been read, the *Geometry* of Euclid with the commentary of Campanus [of Novara (d. 1296)] should be read. When this has been read, let the *Alfonsine Tables* with their instructions be read. When these have been read, the *Theory of the Planets* [*a composite textbook of Ptolemaic astronomy*] should be read.

In the second year, [Sacrobosco's] *The Sphere* should be read first, and when that has been read, the second book of Euclid's *Geometry*, after which should be read the *Canons on the Tables* by John of Lignières [fl. 1320]. After these have been read, let the treatise on the astrolabe by Messahala [*Masha'allah, ninth-century Jewish-Persian astronomer*] be read.

In the third year, Alchabitius should be read first [*The Introduction to the*

Art of Judgement from the Stars by Abû al-Saqr al-Qabîsî, d. 967], and when this has been read, the *Centiloquium* of Ptolemy with the commentary by Haly [*that is, 'Ali Ridwan, 998–1067*]. When this has been read, let the third book of [Euclid's] *Geometry* be read, and when this has been read, the *Treatise on the Quadrant.*

In the fourth year, the whole *Quadripartitus* [*the astrology treatise of Ptolemy*] should be read, and when this has been read, read *On Urine which has Not Been Seen* [*by William of England, fl. 1219, a tract on astrological uroscopy*]. When this has been read, let book 3 of [Ptolemy's] *Almagest* be read.

When all the said years are over, and the said books completed in this order, go back to the beginning, and repeat the lectures of the first year, and then the lectures of the second year, and so on in order. For the required lectures on practice, proceed in the manner laid out below, namely, that in the first year, book 3, *fens* 1, 2 and 3 of the *Canon* of Avicenna shall be read. For the second year, read book 3 of Avicenna's *Canon*, *fens* 9, 10, 11 and 12. For the third year, read book 3, *fens* 13, 14, 15 and 16 of Avicenna's *Canon*. For the fourth year, read book 3, *fens* 18, 19, 20 and 21 of Avicenna's *Canon*. The remaining *fens* are to be read in the second lecture, or in the extraordinary lecture, as the Rector and members of the Council shall determine.

96. Concerning the Anatomy Which Is to Be Made Every Year

Because it is relevant and pertinent to the activity and benefit of students to do anatomy, and because many disputes and rumors habitually arise over finding and asking for the bodies from which, or on which, the anatomy shall be made, [the university authorities] legislate and ordain that no doctor or student or any other person shall dare or presume to acquire for himself any dead body for performing the said anatomy without prior license from the lord rector in office at the time. The rector is obligated, in according the license to the students and doctors, to observe the manner and order in which the said license is requested. Also, no more than twenty people may attend any anatomy of a man, and no more than thirty of a woman. And no one may see any anatomy except he be a student who has studied medicine for two whole years, and who is in his third year, even if he had studied during an interdict. And anyone who has seen the anatomy of a man once may not see it again in the same year. He who has seen it twice may not see it again at Bologna, except if it is the anatomy of a woman, which can be seen only once and not again, whether he has seen the anatomy of a man or not. The aforesaid twenty or thirty who can see and attend the anatomy are selected and chosen in the following way: for the anatomy of a man, five from the Lombard Nation, four from the German Nation, four from the Roman

Nation, three from the Ultramontane Nation, and three from Bologna. And for the anatomy of a woman there should be chosen eight from the Lombard Nation, seven from the German Nation, seven from the Roman Nation, five from the Ultramontane Nation, and three from Bologna, except that the lord rector with one companion may be present at any anatomy, over and above the number specified above, without being obliged to pay the fee, and notwithstanding [the rule] that one who has seen an anatomy may not see another in the same year. Let it be in the discretion of the person who has the license from the lord rector to choose those whom he wishes, as long as the form of this statute is observed. Also, let no one dare to petition the lord rector for an anatomy at the time of his election in [the Church of] St Francis, under penalty of five pounds Bolognese. And the lord rector immediately after taking office is obliged to publish in the schools [the names of those] to whom he has given the license for an anatomy, that everyone might be notified; and if the rector does not observe and cause to be observed these things, he shall be fined ten pounds Bolognese, and any student contravening [these rules] or who acts against the aforesaid [rules shall be fined] one hundred shillings Bolognese. Also, any doctor who is petitioned by his students is obligated to conduct this anatomy in the aforementioned manner and form, notwithstanding that he has done others in the same year, and he shall have for his salary one hundred shillings Bolognese. The abovementioned expenses and any others which are incurred in the aforementioned or which are to be paid for the aforementioned, shall be borne in common and proportionally by the students who attend or see [the anatomy], save that for the anatomy of a man no more than sixty pounds Bolognese shall be spent, and for the anatomy of a woman not more than twenty pounds Bolognese, with the doctor's compensation being one hundred shillings Bolognese. Nonetheless the individual who thus had taken the oath and seen to the payment of the expenses, with one companion whom he shall name, shall be completely exempted from the said expenses. And before the anatomy begins, the lord rector shall summon the student to whom he has given the license for the anatomy, and shall cause him to swear an oath that the expenses were paid in good faith and without fraud, and that among the students viewing the anatomy he will distribute ten pounds Bolognese, under penalty from the rector then in office.

II. MEDICAL SCHOLASTICISM IN ACTION: AUTHORITATIVE TEXTS AND ACADEMIC COMMENTARIES

43. IS MEDICINE A SCIENCE? (1): AVICENNA AND HIS COMMENTATOR GENTILE OF FOLIGNO

Medieval academic medicine was keenly aware of the influence – at once stimulating and disquieting – of Aristotle. Aristotle dealt with a number of scientific issues pertinent to medicine (see Bartholomaeus of Salerno's commentary on the Isagoge *in doc. 34), but some doubted that medicine itself could qualify as a* scientia *in the Aristotelian sense. Was medical knowledge based on first principles, and arrived at by logical deduction? Was medicine a "speculative"* scientia, *that is, knowledge concerned with establishing truths; or was it a practical* scientia *that tried to achieve a certain outcome? Galen and Hippocrates called medicine an* ars *or "art," but did that mean that it was just a set of intellectual – or even manual – skills?*

Medical masters could no longer evade this question after the middle of the thirteenth century, when the Canon *of Avicenna (Abû Alî al-Husain ibn 'Abdallâh ibn Sîna, 980–1037) became part of the reformed medical curricula. This comprehensive encyclopedia of medicine was written by a man who was both a great philosopher and a physician, and its opening chapter is a challenging discussion of the question of whether medicine is a science in Aristotle's sense. Here we will see how one medieval commentator responded to the challenge. Gentile of Foligno (d. 1348) was educated in medicine at the University of Bologna under Taddeo Alderotti. His brilliant and productive academic career was spent largely in Perugia, and it was there that he composed the work for which he was most famous, a comprehensive commentary on the* Canon. *This commentary engaged a wide spectrum of contemporary medical thinking, from the Bolognese school of Taddeo's followers Dino del Garbo (ca 1280–1327), Bartolomeo of Varignana (d. after 1321), Torrigiano de' Torrigiani (d. after 1319), and Guglielmo of Brescia (d. 1326), to the radical Padua Aristotelian Pietro d'Abano (ca 1250–1315/16). It also made extensive use of the Aristotelian commentaries and medical writings of Averroes (Abû-l-Walîd ibn Ahmad ibn Muhammad ibn Rushd, 1126–98). To his medieval readers, Gentile was "the soul of Avicenna" and "the Theoretician (*Speculator*)." His commentary continued to be studied and printed well into the sixteenth century.*

In the translation of Gentile's commentary below, the passages from the Canon *that he is expounding are printed in bold type, as in doc. 3.*

Source: trans. Faith Wallis from *Praesens maximus codex est totius scientie medicine principis Aboali binsene cum expositionibus omnium … interpretum eius … Expositores … gentilis de fuliginio, Auerrois cordubensis, Jacobus de partibus, Matheus de gradi, Dinus florentinus, Thadeus florentinus, Ugo senensis, Gentilis florentinus* (Venice: a Philippo Pincio Manuano, sumptibus Luceantonij de Gionta, 1523), fols. 1r–2r. Latin.

[Avicenna's Text: *Canon* Book 1, *Fen* (*i.e.*, section) 1, Doctrine 1, Chapter 1]

Medicine is the science by which we learn the dispositions of the human body when it is healthy and when it deviates from that state, so that present health can be preserved and lost health can be recovered. Some divide medicine into theory and practice, but when you say that medicine is a science, you have assumed that it is theory. But we respond and say that some arts are both theory and practice, and that philosophy is both theory and practice, and it is said of medicine that it is both theory and practice. In each of these fields, we mean one thing by theory and another by practice. However, we need to explain the difference only in the case of medicine. So when we say, in the case of medicine, that it has a theory, and that practice proceeds from [theory], we do not mean to say that there is one division of medicine that is knowing, and another that is doing, as many who have examined this issue suppose. Rather, you should know that we mean something different, and that neither of the two divisions of medicine is anything other than science. But one of them is directed towards the principles that should be known, and the other towards knowing how to put [these] into operation. To the former we apply the term "science" or "theory," and to the latter, "practice." By "theory" we mean that which, when we have knowledge about it, allows us to form a judgment, apart from any question of how it will be executed. Thus it is said that there are three types of *fever and nine *complexions. And by "practice" we mean, not the work that is carried out, or the exertions of bodily movements, but the division of the operation of medicine that, when we know it, helps us to form a judgment (*sententia*), and this judgment will be directed towards how to carry out the treatment. Thus it is said in medicine that in a case of hot *apostemes, the first agents to employ are those which repel, cool and coagulate. Then we *temper the *repellents with *solvents; and after the *stasis and in the recovery stage softening *solvents will suffice, save in the case of apostemes which arise from material expelled by the principal members. Here systematic, rational instruction (*doctrina*) helps one to acquire knowledge, and this knowledge proclaims the basis of the choice of intervention. Once the character of the two divisions [of medicine] is understood, you can become skilled in both the science of what is known, and the science of what is done, even if you never actually practice.

[Gentile of Foligno's Commentary]

The question arises whether medicine is a science or an art, and it would seem that it is not a science: see the commentary [of Averroes] on [Aristotle's] *Metaphysics* 5: "Science is not the genus of medicine." It would appear that it is an art from the first aphorism [of Hippocrates], and in the *Law* [of Hippocrates]. And Averroes in his commentary on [Aristotle's] *On the Soul* book 1, c. 17, and in *Colliget* in the seventh chapter on the cure of cold apostemes says that medicine is one of the necessary *arts*. Besides, a science which considers its subject with a view to action is not worthy [of the name], if we take "science" as it is understood in the commentary on the second book of the *Metaphysics*, c. 3. But this is precisely what medicine is like.

Avicenna holds the opposite opinion, as can be seen in the third *fen*. Bartolomeo [of Varignana] says that medicine, when considered with respect to its principles, is a science and [when considered] with respect to its goal, which is a way of taking action, is an art. The *Conciliator* [of Pietro d'Abano] in distinction 4 says that medicine is a science with respect to theory and an art with respect to practice. Dino [del Garbo] and Torrigiano de' Torrigiani say that medicine can be considered a habitual condition (*habitus*) of the speculative intellect by means of which we consider certain conclusions which are necessary and eternal – for instance, that there are four complexions and three types of illness; in this sense, medicine is a true science. In another way, [medicine can be taken] as a certain habitual condition in the practical intellect which results from these propositions, by which habitual condition one is guided in action; in that sense it is an art. Nonetheless medical thinking is more correctly said to be that art which is a habitual condition created in the intellect or cogitative [faculty], which results from frequent action, just as other arts are constituted from frequent actions. Habitual conditions arising from actions are not teachable, but rather are acquired by application.

These statements, put this way, may be retained as true. But we say that when it is asked whether medicine is a science, one can answer such as Galen does in the *Tegni*: if the term "science" is taken in the strict sense, then medicine is not a science, because a science in the strict sense is purely speculative and does not exist for the sake of action, as [is said] in the commentary on the second book of the *Metaphysics*, c. 3. But if the term "science" is taken in the ordinary sense – that is, loosely, as designating a term directed to an action (*noticia termini in opus directa*) – then medicine can be called a science, and the other arts can be called sciences. But the art of medicine differs from the other arts, because many of the other arts like tailoring and tanning and the like are acquired by practice, and we do not employ the way of logical demonstration in them. But medicine is acquired for the most part by the way of science, as was said. But were there another art, for instance agriculture, which investigates the nature of its subject – plants in this case – as a man investigates the human body; and were it to investigate their dispositions, then medicine would not exceed that [art] in its mode of knowing and then controversies cease....

The question arises how there can be theory in the arts. It can be said that a practitioner of an art (*artifex operatiuus*) is a theoretician insofar as he proves certain conclusions by means of logical demonstration. For example, when a carpenter concludes what the quantity of [timber in] a tree is by measuring its diameter, then he mixes geometry in his art; and when a farmer concludes that the middle of winter is not the time for sowing because the cold will corrupt the seminal heat, then he mixes in philosophy.

The question arises how there can be practice in philosophy. Dino [del Garbo] responds that natural philosophy is theory, but moral philosophy is practice. However, he says that theory and practice are different in medicine than in philosophy, because in medicine, theory is directed towards practice. But this is not so in the case of philosophy, because the theoretical is not directed towards the practical – natural philosophy is not directed towards moral philosophy....

The question arises whether the science of medicine is divided into knowledge (*scientia*) and application (*operationem*).... It should be considered that Avicenna intimates the proof of this conclusion, [namely that] both parts of medicine are "science," and he argues thus. The part of medicine by which its principles are known is true science because the principles of medicine are truly known by true demonstrations of natural philosophy and by the senses. And Avicenna understands this when he says that one [part of medicine] is for understanding the principles, as if he were saying that principles in this science are known and the part by which the *modus operandi* is known is true science because *modi operandi* are proven by these evident logical demonstrations. Therefore theory and practice are both true science.... And in this [medicine] differs from the mechanical arts like tailoring because [tailoring] teaches its *modus operandi* by practice alone. But [medicine] proves by logical demonstration....

"By 'theory' we mean ..." et cetera. Guglielmo of Brescia raises the question of how Avicenna can say that the theoretical part of medicine is for knowing the principles and not say this about practice, even though practice has its principles – for instance, that every cure is effected by what is contrary, and preservation [of health] is effected by what is similar. It is said that even though practice has its principles, nonetheless everything that is known in [those principles] is directed towards action. But what is known in theory is not directed in this way and therefore those are called principles that are, so to speak, prior to and removed from teachings about a *modus operandi*. Through theory it appears that the theoretical part [of medicine] is true science because it is truly demonstrative; for a physician proves by sufficient logical demonstration that there are three types of fever, as it appears in the first book of [Galen's] *On Distinguishing Fevers*, and that there are nine complexions, as Galen proves in the first book of *On Complexions*. None of this tells us the *modus operandi* for preserving [health] or effecting a cure....

"And by 'practice' we mean ..." et cetera.... Let us say that Avicenna imagines that the science of the *modus operandi* which is practice [is] written in a book or in the mind of the teacher – for example, repellents are suitable for the initial treatment of apostemes – and this is the division of [medicine called] "operation," that is, the part which provides a *modus operandi*. He imagines that this written science generates knowledge in our mind, and therefore he says that when we know it – namely, from a master or a book – it "helps us to acquire knowledge" – that is, it would then be knowledge within us. And this knowledge within us will be in a *modus operandi*, just as it was in the teacher or in the book. And this is what he says in the end. **Here systematic, rational instruction helps** you – because instruction whether oral or from a book creates knowledge within you – and **this knowledge proclaims** and so forth.... Otherwise we can say that practical knowledge, that is, knowledge of a *modus operandi*, will help in acquiring knowledge, because it spurs knowledge to go beyond itself. For one who hears that "the first agents to employ in apostemes" etc., immediately asks what an "aposteme" is, what "repelling" is, and so forth. And this (that is, this knowledge) spurs on to that, and so forth. Likewise it helps in acquiring knowledge, that is, a conception which is acquired from an habitual experimental condition. For men of knowledge who operate with the rules of the art are better at acquiring the experimental habit, which cannot be taught, as we said above.

Once [the character of the two divisions ... actually practice].... The question arises whether someone can be a perfect physician, perfectly instructed both orally and through reading, even though he never practices or has observed the practice that leads to perfection in him who is to practice. It seems that Avicenna would answer positively here. Galen in his commentary on the first aphorism [of Hippocrates] understands the opposite. In the writings of some of the Bologna doctors, we find that medical conceptions can be had by experience; therefore, no one can work well or be a good physician without reason (which would rectify experience) and without experience. In another way, [science] can be had through the instruction of books and by the voice of a teacher, and thus one can operate well and be a good doctor if one is instructed by reason alone, without experience. The answer is twofold. First, one who has the first act can move on to the second act; but one who has science to perfection has the first act, and therefore etc. Secondly, one who has a conception of the subject's means, its goal, and its usages can operate perfectly: but one who has the science of medicine through books has this. We say that he cannot be a perfect physician, even though he possesses all the written and oral science and knows all that can possibly be written down or heard. The reason is because from actual operation – that is, from seeing patients and from treating [them] – there is generated in the mind a certain conception which cannot be gotten from books or from oral instruction, and which cannot be taught, as Galen implies in *Therapeutic Method* book 12, when he speaks of the pain of colic. Moreover, to every proposition noted by the intellect in the act of operation, must be subsumed a particular proposition through an act of cognition, as we gather from Averroes's commentary on [Aristotle's] *On Sleep and Wakefulness*. But one who is practiced does this better, for practice adds something to the conception. What it adds neither impedes nor frustrates, and therefore it must help. Since the physician by this habitual condition of practice will operate better, he will therefore be imperfect without it. This is proved by numerous authorities, and first by Aristotle in the first book of the *Metaphysics*: those who are expert perform better. Alfarabi is of the same opinion in his book *On the Origin of the Sciences* in the chapter on civil science, where he says that the physician is not perfect except through two virtues (that is, two conceptions) of which one is mastery of the universal rules (*canonibus*) which he acquires from books on medicine, and the other is what is conveyed by frequent practice of medicine upon patients, and studying this through long experience and examination of the bodies of individuals. And through this, the physician can measure medicine and the treatment of people, or of a given body in a given disposition....

Be assured that the whole science of medicine is not put into practice perfectly by any individual save after much habituation and long experience. In sum, correct operation having its principles in the art, and following the way of demonstration, depends on a twofold habit, namely what is knowable and teachable, which is in the intellective mind and from experimental habit, that is, acquired through the exercise of the art upon particular cases. This habit is teachable, but [as something] to which one can become accustomed, as we said, and then the practitioner is made perfect.

44. IS MEDICINE A SCIENCE? (2): ARNAU OF VILANOVA ARGUES THAT MEDICINE TRANSCENDS THEORY

Arnau of Vilanova (ca 1240–1311) was born near Valencia in Spain, studied and taught medicine at Montpellier, and traveled widely. Arnau was a polymath, writing treatises on alchemy and astrology as well as medicine, translating texts from the Arabic, serving as a diplomat, and promoting schemes for educational and religious reform. Some of the latter got him into difficulties with his patrons, the kings of Aragon, as well as with the papacy.

A repetitio *is a student's transcription of a professor's lecture, as revised and approved for publication by the professor. This text is a* repetitio *of Arnau's lecture on Hippocrates's first aphorism, "Life is short and the Art is long; opportunity is elusive, experiment is dangerous, judgment is difficult. It is not enough for the physician to do what is necessary, but the patient and the attendants must do their part as well, and circumstances must be favorable." Arnau expounds mainstream doctrine on the three divisions of therapeutics and the regulation of the six *non-naturals, and adds four aspects of dietary or medicinal treatment: what one gives to the patient, in what strength, in what form, and in what order or sequence. This all sounds very logical and scholastic, but Arnau points out that logic has its limits when it comes to therapy. Even a well-considered plan of medical management has to cope with the uncertain and unexpected. Contingencies (*accidentia*) can sometimes be anticipated, but they often become apparent only after the fact. A physician has to know how to identify the factor that has derailed the treatment, so that he can correct it. Contingencies might seem irrelevant to "science" (at least as defined by Aristotle), but Arnau clearly believes that theory can give the physician some mastery over the unpredictable. He tries to convey these complex distinctions to his students through concrete case histories.*

Source: Arnau de Vilanova, trans. Michael R. McVaugh and Luís García Ballester, *Lecture on the Text "Life is Short" (Repetitio super canonem "Vita brevis"),* "Therapeutic Method in the Later Middle Ages: Arnau de Vilanova on Medical Contingency," *Caduceus* 11 (1995): 76–86. Latin.

... Now the physician's role regarding a course of treatment is like a sailor's, because both govern what is committed to them not by following necessary and permanent rules but by weighing contingent and variable factors. For the sailor has to alter the sails and other things as the winds change; the physician has to modify his tools and practices in accordance with the changes and variations in the illness as well as in the dispositions of the air and the other circumstances by which the body is affected. And thus because it is his responsibility to modify his procedures [when necessary], he must always keep in mind when instructing the attendants and patient that the aims of medical

practice will not automatically be reached at some definite time but will depend entirely on the knowledge or judgment of the person in charge, namely
the physician himself; and therefore he should tell them, you must follow
such-and-such a course of action until the evidence convinces me that it has
to be changed. Thus the physician will preserve his authority and will keep
the patient and the others from wondering or worrying when he changes his
approach – especially since he cannot avoid changing his approach if the art
demands it, whether as regards what he gives or its strength or its preparation
or the order in which he gives it.

[Adjustments Dictated by (1) Necessary Factors, Such as the Phases of the Illness]

The reason why an adjustment might have to be made in one of these four
areas is twofold: one is necessary and inevitable, the other is contingent. The
first has to do with the evolution of the illness, for every illness from which
someone recovers passes from onset (*principium*), through intensification (*aug-
mentum*), to *stasis (*status*), to recovery (*declinatio*). Thus a dietary regimen
will have to change in each of these four stages, as is fully plain in the first
part of the *Aphorisms* and in the *Regimen*, not just in one of these four but
in all of them. For someone who is given barley in onset should have only
almond milk in intensification; or it should be given thick and unstrained at
first, then strained. In stasis he should be given chickpea and barley water;
in recovery, first chickpea broth, then subtle and then grosser flesh little by
little until he can go back to a normal diet. Likewise a patient who is given
a strained, squeezed *tisane to drink during onset should be given it strained
but not squeezed in intensification; in stasis he should be given just sugared
water; in recovery weak wine at the beginning, the stronger little by little
until [he is] normal. In the same way it is necessary to alter the quantity of
food and drink in these stages, for in onset a patient may eat more copi-
ously, in intensification less, in stasis least, while in recovery the sequence is
changed so that the regimen begins with a small quantity and is gradually
increased up to the maximum, i.e. the normal, over as long a time as the first
three stages, as best the physician can judge (or, if it fails to equal it exactly,
is at least close). For these two phases of the illness are linearly equal either *in
se* or in their symptoms; as Galen proves in *On the Times of Illness* and Isaac
Judaeus [shows] in *On the Elements*, there is as long a period of time from the
final terminus of stasis till the end of recovery as there is from the beginning
of the illness to the end of stasis. And this calculation not only helps the
patient, it keeps the physician from confusion, because by this estimate the
physician can tell the patient, roughly, how long he will have to be obedient

to his commands, saying, "You will need at least so much time to recover completely; so obey me for that period and I will take care of your case." So too the physician will vary the quality of the food and drink [he prescribes] during these stages, for both should be physically hotter in onset and intensification than in stasis and recovery; and these stages likewise force him to alter the hour of meals, for in onset and recovery he ordinarily will recommend for this the [patient's] accustomed hour of mealtimes when healthy, as modified however by other circumstances, just as these stages required him to alter the regimen of food and drink.

The same thing is true of medicines, both as to the medicines themselves and as to their strength, and because teaching about practice is vague and useless unless it is brought down to particulars, let us give some brief examples of these things. First as to the medicines themselves. If someone with scabies in given a *syrup or *decoction of borage and fumitory during the onset, in stasis and recovery the fumitory must be changed to wormwood. For in the first stages the patient needs *digestion of the scorched *humor, while in the later stages [he needs] opening of the pores for its full *expulsion. If therefore in these [first] stages something is given that corrects the sharpness and dryness of the scorched humor, like borage, which also protects the heart and *spirits from its poison, and again if something is given that thins out the thickness [of the humor] and as it were scrapes it from the surface of the member and opens the pores of the body, like fumitory, this is obviously a sensible procedure – so long as nothing contraindicated occurs, like fear of abortion in women....

This is why the physician should be careful that his procedures do not prevent him from altering the strength of what he gives, increasing or decreasing it, whenever that should be necessary; errors frequently arise when this is forgotten. For it has happened that someone who is given the same vinegary medicine to drink all the way through to the end of stasis, without any diminution of its strength, finds once he has been freed from the *fever that he is constantly panting, with the tissues of his breast constricted.

There were once two physicians on the case of just such a patient, and once they had considered all the factors the elder said to the other: "I recommend that the vinegar be added to the syrup not now but each time that it is prepared, when the patient needs to drink it, and in this way we can keep taking into account the strength of the patient." It happened that the one who said this had to leave briefly. The one who remained took over the treatment but scorned to follow the advice of his colleague; but then, when the patient reached stasis, he began to suffer terribly from sciatica and gout. At this point the senior physician returned, and when he found the patient worse he asked about the regimen he had been following and discovered that he had been drinking a syrup of uniform strength and strong vinegariness. Then he asked the patient whether he had ever suffered other pains in those joints; he replied, "No, except once when I had to go barefoot in winter in a river for a long time, and after that my legs felt heavy but not very painful." And so the physician recognized that the evil of a cold *complexion had weakened those parts and sensitized them to the action of the vinegar. It should thus be plain how the [four] stages of illness force us to change the kinds and strengths of the medicines we prescribe; it should also be obvious that the same thing will be true of their quality, just as was explained in the case of food and drink. As for the time of their administration, [the four stages] affect it only slightly – unless the unexpected occurs, for if for example the patient should be attacked by vomiting or precordial pain at the moment when we had intended to administer a medicine, the time will have to be changed. But we will come back to the unexpected soon.

[Adjustments Dictated by (2) Contingent Factors, e.g. Unintended Side Effects of the Treatment Itself or Chance External Events]

Let us return to the second reason why a physician may need to alter his procedures, [namely] contingent rather than necessary factors. Again, the physician should know that they can require him to make changes to diet or medication in one of the four aforesaid ways. The contingencies that can arise (especially from external factors) are unforeseeable and innumerable, and more will be said about them below. But of all these factors, the physician must first of all keep in mind those that arise from his own treatment: for example, he may give a vinegary syrup to a patient with *ephemeral or *quotidian fever, and if he administers it for a long period he may hope – or better fear – that the liver will be chilled and the perfect digestion of blood be thereby impeded. So fear of this contingency over the course of time ought to induce him not only to decrease the strength of the vinegar but to give something else that will reinforce the liver, and this is why all the wisest [physicians] advise that in such a case the patient should be given *troches of eupatorium or the like every fourth and then every third [day]. Likewise it is plain per se how the contingencies that arise can force us to alter the strength or the quality of the medicine that we prescribe and even the moment when we administer it, and the same thing is true of the sequence in which we administer a series of medicines.

I give an example for students. It happened that a physician was treating a patient who had taken opium or henbane and was constipated by nature. So the physician sensibly commanded that at the beginning of the meal the patient should eat figs with nuts and at the end a dried pear; thus he would avoid constipation in two ways, one by starting with figs, because as Galen teaches they soften and cleanse the intestines, the other by taking a compressive *styptic like pears. The physician intended to counter [the patient's] flatulence with the nuts (which work more efficaciously taken with figs, because they are drawn to the intestines more speedily with something sweet).

After several days the patient was seized by a cough, which attacked him every day after a meal; believing that the amount of food he was eating was the cause, the physician ordered that it be cut back. When he saw that it did not stop, he prescribed things to soften the chest and lungs, and then finally because it did not stop he asked the advice of another physician whom he knew. His friend asked to visit the patient, and once he had studied all the facts and had learned what had been prescribed, he suggested that [his colleague] try roasting the nuts that he was giving his patient and administering figs with those nuts at the time he had been giving the pear [that is, at the end of the meal], and that [the patient] should begin [the meal] with a dried apple with sugar. This was done, and the cough ceased entirely in seven days. The physician came back to his friend to find out why the procedure had worked, and had it explained to him. Here, then, a contingency led to a change in what was prescribed (as regards the apple), in the sequence (as regards the figs and nuts [which were deferred to later in the meal]), and in quality (as regards the roasting of the nuts).

With regard to a program of medication – which is only for the sick, because medicines are prescribed for directly countering an illness – three things ought to be seen to: first, that the medicines be chosen properly; second, that they be prepared carefully; third, that they be administered appropriately. Concerning their suitability two things should be provided for. First, suitability as to effects: for example, if the patient needs [a medicine] hot and dry in the second *degree that the physician must select from the many with those qualities, melissa or mint or the like, he should always choose that medicine, whether *simple or compound, that will be of the greatest benefit to the patient and have the fewest harmful consequences. Secondly, suitability of that particular preparation, so that it be the strongest of its kind either absolutely or in relation to the illness for which it is prescribed: [for example] should figs (or ginger or dates) be given whole? Will this patient be better helped by figs from Persia or India or Damascus, or by Alexandrine or insular dates? There is great diversity found in things of the same kind, for example, plants that grow in the fields *versus* the same ones that grow in the mountains. As for the medicine itself, the physician should reflect on whether he can recognize it or not, and if he can he should ask to see it and judge it for himself. But if he is not acquainted with it, he should consider whether it has been described or depicted by the wise, and if so, when he has seen the plant, he should decide whether it corresponds to its description and [if so] choose it; while if it does not fit, he should not use it, but should choose instead something generally familiar and fitting the descriptions of the wise. For the students I give an example. You want to give eupatorium but you are unfamiliar with it and the apothecary brings you wild salvia. If you want to avoid deception, be sure you know how the wise describe eupatorium. In this way a certain physician discovered an error in his practice concerning the use of eupatorium and spica celtica and many other medicines. In the preparation [of a medicine] the physician must consider, in order, the cleansing, grinding, measurement, softening, and mixing [of its ingredients]. He should give instructions to his assistants, the apothecaries, about its mixing, telling them when [it is to be prepared], lest lacking his instructions they make it up later than they should. As for its proper administration, he should inform the attendants of the amount and the time and manner of its administration – that is, how big the dose should be, and in what hour it should be given, and how ([for example,] whether internally or externally, warm or cold, with fluids or without) – and with what [other treatment] ([for example] with a strong or light massage), and so on. And he should always command the patient to be obedient to the attendants in following his instructions at any hour. Thus we have seen in general from the aforesaid what the physician has to do himself, what he must know and what he must arrange and command; and we have also seen how he must encourage the patient to confidence in and compliance with both his physician and his attendants; and how the physician should instruct the attendants.

It remains to take up the fourth thing, namely to consider extrinsic contingencies and their sequence, and to clarify this we must first know why they are called extrinsic. One opinion is that they are called external or extrinsic contingencies because they fall beyond the rules of the art, as was said above. But taken strictly this would go against and contradict Hippocrates in his aphorism, since he says [there] that the physician must take into consideration – that is, consider and control – those things that are extrinsic; he therefore supposes that they fall under the practitioner's regulation, since he says they necessarily pertain to his consideration. This is why others want to say that they are extrinsic simply in the sense that they transcend nature and the force of the illness, as well as the common course and order of treatment. For the sound of bells, or the shouting of children and barking of dogs and rumble of carts, or the fire and wreck of a home, or flooding by rains and gusting of winds, or the rumor that something or someone beloved is lost, or the falling of a spider or scorpion into a jug, or such other things, when they befall a patient, do not do so as a result of his sickness or because of the natural powers of the things that must be used to treat him.

But there is still another problem: If such things are unforeseeable, how can the physician take them into account? The answer is that the physician can do so in three respects: he can consider them in themselves, or in their effects, or in their causes. In themselves they can be considered in either of two respects, one as regards the essence that they have when they act, the other as to their outcome, and they are uncertain in this latter respect because their outcome is not inevitable but contingent; in this manner they do not fall under the practitioner's consideration or reception, for he cannot know or control when and how they will act. But in the other three respects they do have some predictability, and to this extent they do fall under his consideration and regulation, though differently according to the differences in their predictability. For as to the first respect there is certainty to their existence; as to the second, of their possibility; as to the third, of their effectiveness.

In the first respect, therefore, he considers them as entities to be avoided. If a physician who enters the home of someone with *ophthalmia (or cardiac problems due to heat, or a cough) should find it full of smoke, he should recognize how bad this is for his patient and should command that he avoid it completely. If the patient suffers from headache, especially migraine [*galea*], the physician should react the same way, and if he notices barking dogs or shouting men or clashing cymbals outside the room, the patient ought [to be told] to avoid and shun them. When the physician observes such things, he can be certain that they exist, and so he can give orders concerning them. When he considers them as caused, then it is certain that they *can* exist, and then he can respond by anticipating and preventing them. Finally, when he recognizes signs in the patient that are unrelated to the force and nature of the illness or to the common nature of curative causes, he can be sure that these are signs of some unforeseen contingency, and therefore he should proceed to investigate and remove or correct it. It is in these last two ways of coping with the contingent that the physician's foresight and acumen will be most brilliantly displayed, and therefore any intelligent practitioner ought to work at them diligently. Here Hippocrates has bestowed a wonderful present upon us; indeed, the wise esteem it the best of all his gifts that he chose to exhort us to take external contingencies into account, since the need to deal with them is ordinarily less obvious than are the other things that he touched on. Therefore if we apprehend his purpose and recognize the import of his words, we will find his teachings here and elsewhere to be a deep well of wisdom; but we will not share his treasure if we simply take over his words unthinkingly.

Let us therefore see what fruit these two approaches will bear in guiding our practice of medicine, see what a precious pearl Hippocrates has wrapped up for us in the fabric of his eloquence. Remember that extrinsic contingencies can be considered in their causes or their effects, by anticipating their causes and observing their effects, so that the anticipated may be guarded against and the observed corrected. For example, the physician finds that his patient's home is situated at the foot of a bell tower; he can anticipate that the bells might cause a noise that would be unpleasant and harmful for someone suffering from headache. Likewise he anticipates that where there are many dogs there can be importunate and annoying barking. Likewise if he finds a north or south window in line with his patient's head, he knows that when those winds blow the patient's head will suffer unless his bed is moved or the window is tightly shut. Likewise if he sees that the bottle of syrup or decoction stands uncovered in some corner or window and he finds spiderwebs over it, he can anticipate that spiders may get into these vessels. If he finds that the patient's house is roofless and open, subject to the gusts of the winds, he can foresee that a patient with dysentery who lives in such a place may incur gripes or other lesions of the stomach when any light air blows. Likewise if he is treating cancers or *fistulas or swellings in the private parts and groin, and if these parts are exposed for any period of time, remaining so as long as the physician is at work cleansing or anointing or plastering, he can foresee that the patient may suffer problems with a chill in his hips or pains in the thigh or belly or other passions if he is not protected with hot air or warm cloths. If a patient suffers from hemorrhoids or has recently had a rupture of the lungs, so that it would do him harm to get upset and he must speak in a low tone, the physician can anticipate that the patient will have reason to shout or perhaps to become angry if he has an attendant who is deaf or careless or sleepy. And so we see how, by anticipating future contingencies through their causes, physicians can usefully give commands that will allow [the patient] to avoid harmful effects.

Now where a harmful effect appears in the patient that transcends the power of the illness and the common virtue of the curative causes, the physician can be certain that some unforeseen extrinsic contingency has intervened; he should therefore cast about, reflecting on all the things that he has used in his treatment, until he can identify the unforeseen contingency. But to be quick at this it will help to read through a table of the kinds and species of all medicinal healing agents that he can carry with him, if not in his heart then at least in a purse so that he can consult it more quickly. Once he has identified the contingency, he can correct the error. For example: a certain octogenarian physician, famous and experienced, wanted to use a steambath on account of his body's needs. He entered it one day and because he was old and weak in natural heat it did not seem to him that the air of the bath was hot enough; so he ordered lighted coals to be placed there, and a little afterwards one of his servants fainted and another, who himself was beginning to collapse, had to pull him out. Seeing his servant's condition, his master came out of the bath, and so that day he was unable to complete his treatment. The next day he wanted to go back in, but he did not want to bring with him the one who had fainted, and he called a young physician dear to him and asked him to consider and examine the lad's disposition, fearing from his collapse in the bath that some poisonous humor might be hidden in his viscera. Then the other servant who was there interposed, "Master, I think if I had stayed in a little longer the same thing would have happened to me, because I was already feeling my heart fail, and that's why I said I was afraid to go back." At this point the younger physician began to ask them whether they had entered the bath on a full stomach, and they said no. He asked if they had done anything just before, and they said no, except for this: he who had fainted said, "By my master's command, I heated the coals outside by blowing on them and then I entered the bath." Then the young physician replied: "The same thing will happen to you today if you bring live coals into the bath – for your master and lord right here well knows that man cannot live anywhere unless the air that is inhaled to temper [the heat of] the heart is colder or of weaker heat than the heart is. Because you young people, whose hearts abound in heat, were heating the air in the bath, you collapsed before your master did, but if he had stayed long he too would at last have been overcome." Then the old man, clapping his hand to his head, understood his mistake.

It happened to another physician in this town that for his body's needs he commanded the preparation of a *decoction of seaholly and licorice, on someone else's advice. A little after he took the decoction his bowels became upset, and he had pain and distress around the heart and vomited up the decoction and more; however, he did not attribute the event to the decoction but to other factors in his regimen. So the next day he again took a dose of the decoction and the same thing happened, still more severely. He was alarmed and astonished, and he reported this to the physician on whose advice he had begun to use the decoction, who replied that since such an effect was no part of the strength and nature of the decoction, some extrinsic contingency must have intervened, and that therefore he should check to see whether something had fallen into the container, and if not, that he should carefully investigate the vessels and strainers or other things that had been used to prepare the decoction. And in the end the patient discovered that the decoction had been strained through an unwashed colander that had been used the day before to strain a decoction of hellebore [*a powerful *purgative*].

It happened to another physician that every time he administered a decoction of *capilli veneris* [*maidenhair fern*] to a certain patient, the patient vomited excruciatingly; and finally after careful inquiry he found that the *capilli veneris* had been gathered in a large disused common cistern that still had a little water in the bottom. He went there to investigate and had himself shown the place where it was collected; and when he searched it carefully, he found the corpse of a toad at the bottom of the cistern, by which had been poisoned not only the moisture with which the plant had been nourished but the air around it....

Not many years ago it happened that a youth suffered a simple *flux; but despite the many antidotes he used to constrict his belly, they did him no good, and he developed an uncontrolled dysentery. He consulted a physician, who asked what medicines he had used and learned that they were the appropriate ones. Then he asked what food and drink the youth took, and when he learned that his patient was using water from a cistern for drinking and cooking, he asked whether the cistern were of stone or cement. The youth answered, stone, but that the stone had been found to have several cracks through which it lost water, so that it had been newly cemented throughout, though more thickly at the bottom. The physician suspected from this that the calcinated water had given his patient his dysentery, which was confirmed by the results; for once he gave up using that water, he immediately began to improve markedly....

If I were to tell you all that I myself have seen and heard, the day would not be long enough to describe the cases to you. Still, these will suffice to show why the physician must take extrinsic contingencies into account, how they help shape his practice, and how they fall under the precepts of his art.

45. IS MEDICINE A SCIENCE? (3): HENRI OF MONDEVILLE ON PROGRESS IN MEDICINE

Though Henri of Mondeville is surely one of the most vivid medical personalities of the Middle Ages, his life and career are surprisingly obscure. He was born in Normandy and apparently received his surgical education at Montpellier and Paris, perhaps under Lanfranc of Milan (doc. 58). He served as a military surgeon under Philip the Fair and Louis X, and taught anatomy and surgery at Montpellier in 1304 and at Paris beginning in 1312. He died sometime after 1316, before he could complete his vast textbook of surgery (Chirurgia). This work is notable for the way in which it applies academic styles of analysis to surgical decision-making. It also reveals Henri's colorful and combative personality and his concern to elevate surgery to the intellectual status of medicine (see doc. 59). For Henri, rational surgical knowledge can progress through cumulative experience, encompassing both ancient authorities and modern developments. Like all scholastic medical writers, he grounded his discourse upon the authority of the ancients, but he also believed that surgery — and medicine as well — was constantly advancing.

This sounds gratifyingly modern and progressive, but it is important to bear in mind that progress through experience and "invention" was a recognized part of scholastic medical tradition. Moreover, belief in progress and confidence in the ancient authorities were not mutually contradictory. This paradox was summed up in the famous image of the dwarfs on the shoulders of giants invoked in the passage below, which comes from the *antidotary that comprises book 5 of the Chirurgia. *Scholastic medicine saw pharmacy as a domain of medicine where knowledge was expected to develop and change, but the feisty Henri cannot resist using the opportunity to vaunt the advantage of the modern dwarfs.*

Source: trans. Faith Wallis from Henri de Mondeville, *Chirurgia* 5.1, ed. Julius Leopold Pagel, *Leben, Lehre und Leistungen des Heinrich von Mondeville* (Berlin: August Hirschwald, 1892), pp. 507–8. Latin.

There are seven reasons behind the composition of this antidotary. First: new surgical cases arise every day, and it is necessary to find new topical remedies to match them, because what occurs from something new needs a new prescription. Second: even if no new case emerges, nonetheless new modes of operation are discovered for ordinary old cases and these demand that one use new medications. Third: even supposing that no new case has arisen and no new topical remedy has been devised, it is possible that thanks to the experience of modern [practitioners], new virtues could be discovered for medications whose composition goes back to ancient times and it would be churlish to pass over these in silence. Thus recently, in our own day, it has been shown that contrary to the opinion of all the medical authors, all curable wounds are treated quickly and in the best and easiest manner with one single medicine, and that anointing [the wound] with a compound of marsh mallow is sufficient to destroy salty *phlegm and other similar ills. Fourth: because all the medications necessary for the art of surgery are not found in a single antidotary, but are dispersed among several, without being findable in all, it seems very useful to collect the topical remedies mentioned here and there and to compile a new antidotary to contain them all. Fifth: because there are many famous topical remedies which modern surgeons do not use any longer and which take up a lot of room in the antidotaries of the ancients, we should suppress them in the antidotaries of the moderns and not copy them any longer alongside our own [remedies]. There is nothing surprising about this, because Horace has already said, "Many which have fallen into disuse will be reborn, and what is strong is ruined by sudden chance." [Horace, *Ars poetica* 70 and Ovid, *Ex Ponto* 4.3.26.] Sixth, it is absurd, and almost heretical to believe that the glorious, sublime God should have given such mental aptitude (*ingenium*) to Galen that no one after him would ever be able to discover anything new. On the contrary: this would detract from God's own power. Does not God give to each of us, as to Galen, his own natural mental aptitude? Our mental aptitude would be rather poor if we always had to resort to what had already been discovered. Again, with respect to the ancients the moderns are like a dwarf on the shoulders of a giant, who sees everything that the giant sees and things beyond as well. That is why we are permitted to know things that were not known in Galen's time, and we need to write these things down. Seven: if something seems to hold true for a lesser case, it will also hold true for a greater one. Now, we see that in the case of the mechanical arts, for example in the arts of building, that if someone who excelled in the construction of churches and palaces in Galen's day were to be brought back to life today, he would not be worthy to serve under a modern builder. What is more, we see that ancient palaces and churches are demolished in order to be rebuilt in a better way. In a similar manner – indeed, all the more – the ancients can be corrected in the liberal sciences, and it is necessary to add and to write what is new.

46. THE SCHOLASTIC *QUAESTIO*: ARISTOTLE VS. GALEN ON THE GENERATION OF THE EMBRYO

One of the principal points on which Galen's medicine clashed with Aristotle's natural philosophy was the process of generation in higher animals. Unlike Aristotle, Galen knew of the existence of ovaries, which seemed to be homologues of the male testes. In conjunction with the presence of a semen-like moisture in the vagina during intercourse, the ovaries provided conclusive proof that the female produced a "seed" that played an essential and active role in conception, and accounted for children resembling their mothers as well as their fathers. Galen distinguished female seed from the menstrual blood that furnished the body of the embryo.

Aristotle, on the other hand, argued that sex difference would be pointless if men and women played the same role in conception. In his view, the male semen alone possessed the active power to bring about conception and to impart form to the fetus. Women contributed something totally different: matter. Matter was essential for conception, but as the passive recipient of form. This matter was menstrual blood; there was no female seed, and what looked like female "semen" was just a lubricating secretion.

The problem of the female seed was a classic topic for disputed questions in the medieval schools. Quaestiones disputatae *complemented lectures; they were, in effect, debates, conducted according to the rules of Aristotelian logic, about problems arising from an authoritative text. The point of reference was always what the authorities said, but the* quaestio *aimed nonetheless to prove or disprove a particular thesis. On the issue of the female seed, philosophers and theologians tended to favor Aristotle's position; physicians leaned toward the Galenic explanation.*

The Formation of the Fetus in the Uterus *is the work of the philosopher and theologian Giles of Rome (ca 1243–1316), a student of Thomas Aquinas and committed Aristotelian. While not explicitly a* quaestio disputata, *this treatise is in fact structured as one. Giles begins by laying out the argument he intends to refute, and then proceeds to demolish this position, point by point, while addressing objections that might arise from a hypothetical opponent. One of Giles's nicknames amongst the schoolmen was* doctor fundatissimus *– "the doctor who got to the very bottom of things" – a tribute to his thoroughness. His other nickname was, perhaps, a consequence of this:* doctor verbosus. *Even medieval readers, who had relatively long attention spans when it came to philosophic argument, found reading Giles something of an ordeal. In consequence, I have summarized his argument up to the point where he attacks the notion that female sperm can play any positive role in conception.*

Giles's medical counterpart was Jacopo da Forlì (ca 1350–1414), professor of medicine and philosophy at the university of Padua. His On the Generation of the Embryo *(De generatione embrionis) is a commentary on Avicenna's chapter on embryology (Canon book 3, fen 21, ch. 2) followed by a series of* quaestiones disputatae. *Jacopo homes in on the weakest point in Aristotle's model, namely that it cannot explain hereditary resemblance. His core argument is that male sperm must provide some matter as well as form; therefore the woman must contribute form as well as matter.*

a. The Aristotelian Position Defended: Giles of Rome on Conception

Summary of the argument thus far: in chapter 1, Giles analyzes Galen's seven arguments in favor of active *virtue or active power in the female semen. These are (1) the appetite of the uterus for male semen and its power to retain it proves that the uterus has active virtue, and if the uterus has this power, the female seed must as well; (2) women have testes – the ovaries – and therefore have seed; (3) a substance similar to semen is produced by the uterus and by female spermatic vessels, and this can be nothing other than semen; (4) women who abstain from intercourse for a long time can suffer from "suffocation of the womb" which is relieved by *evacuation (orgasm); suffocation is the result of thickening of the female seed, and so the seed must have active virtue; (5) women, like men, have seminal emissions (orgasms) in their dreams, and so must have semen; (6) women have spermatic vessels analogous to those of men; (7) unless the mother's seed has active virtue, the resemblance of a child to its mother cannot be explained. In chapters 2–5, Giles begins to demolish these arguments. Generation is the informing of matter, so it requires both form and matter. If both the man and the woman contributed both form and matter, nature would be reduplicating these functions unnecessarily. In chapter 6, Giles will argue that female sperm cannot play a role in

conception because a woman can conceive without emitting sperm, that is, without
orgasm. In chapter 7, he will explain what is the true function of female sperm.

Source: trans. Faith Wallis from *Tractatus aureus Egidii Romani de formatione corporis humani in*
utero ... (Paris: Ponset le Preux, 1515), fols. 13v–16r. Latin.

Chapter 6: That a Woman Can Be Impregnated without the Emission of
[her own] Sperm

In book 2 [c. 10] of his *Colliget*, Averroes proves by means of seven arguments that a woman can be impregnated without the emission of sperm [on
her part]. The first argument is taken from experience; the second is taken
from the attraction exerted by the uterus; the third is from what [the uterus]
spews forth; the fourth is from the necessity for the man; the fifth is from the
primacy of the heart; the sixth is from the nourishing of the members; the
seventh and final one is from the fact that female sperm is itself a waste product (*superfluitas*) The first reason is evident: indeed, it is a common experience
that someone who is not capable of violating a virgin can [still] impregnate
her; and this happens when sperm which is spilled outside the uterus is attracted by the heat of the uterus and impregnates the woman.

For it is a proven fact that a certain woman, uncorrupt in her flesh, conceived through the sperm of a man, as we ourselves have learned from those
worthy of belief, but before she could give way to desire for a man, she
submitted lest she be endangered with regard to the unborn fetus. Averroes
recounts the same thing concerning a certain trustworthy matron who was
his neighbor, and whose oath, as he says, he could rely on implicitly. She
swore upon her soul that she suddenly became pregnant in the hot water of a
[public] bath into which wicked men had ejaculated when they were bathing
there. Hence an emission of sperm on the part of the woman is not necessary,
but the sperm of the male suffices as the agent, and the menstruum [*menstrual
blood and matter*], attracted by the power of [the sperm] receives the sperm as
the agent, while [the menstruum] plays the role of matter.

The second reason is derived from the attraction exerted by the uterus.
Averroes says in the same place, citing the authority of Avicenna in what he
writes concerning sperm, that the uterus has the capacity to attract sperm by
its own proper virtue, which it has from its *specific form or total species.
Therefore the attraction of the sperm into the uterus is due not only to the
pleasure of sexual intercourse, but also to the proper virtue of the uterus
itself, which the woman possesses. If then the uterus attracts the sperm of the
man without emission of its own sperm, the conjunction of active and passive – that is, of male sperm and the menstruum – can be carried out by this
kind of attraction of sperm. For when the active is joined to the passive, the

former acts and the latter receives the action, as the Philosopher [Aristotle] says in *Metaphysics* 9. Since the effect can be produced through the action of the agent and the passivity of the passive [recipient], and since this [effect] can exist without the emission of female sperm, sperm of this kind will not be necessary. Emission of this type of sperm can contribute something suitable to or congruent with generation, but not something that is inevitable, so that generation could not take place otherwise.

The third argument (although Averroes puts in the last place) can be taken from the uterus's [action of] spewing out or ejaculation. For Averroes says that the woman's uterus spews out its own sperm in order to attract the sperm of the man into itself. If, then, the woman's sperm could have effected generation by itself and of necessity, the uterus would not spew it out. For just as at the time of impregnation it retains the sperm of the man which bestows form and the menstruum which assumes the role of matter, it would retain its own sperm if it were necessary for generation, and not spew it out in order to attract the sperm of the man. Therefore it could be argued in support of the contrary position that if the sperm of the woman contributes to generation, it does so as something which is necessary to attract the sperm of the male, and not in the first way (since it is posited that the uterus spews out its own [sperm] to attract the sperm of the man) nor in the second way (since this pertains to the uterus through its own virtue – it has a specific form which attracts the sperm of the man). Some experienced and eminent people say concerning this matter (and their statements are not to be utterly rejected) that when the orifice of the uterus senses its own sperm, it hastens to suck it up, and it sucks up the sperm of the male along with it. These people seem to imply that the female sperm is necessary in order that the uterus may be capable of sucking up the sperm of the male. But this necessity would not be absolute; rather, [it would be necessary only] with respect to a certain suitability or fittingness. For it is not that it could not take place any other way.... For as the Philosopher [Aristotle] claims in *On Animals* book 10 [*History of Animals* 10.5], when both sperms do not come together, impregnation does not take place. Hence he says that if the man emits his sperm quickly and a woman later on, this prevents impregnation. And Avicenna in *On Animals* book 10 says that impregnation happens when the two seeds come together at the same time, and he adds that when one is in advance and the other follows behind, impregnation does not take place. And he says that males who emit sperm later are more apt to generate, because the woman, being of a cold *complexion, emits sperm later. Therefore males who emit sperm later are more likely, all things being equal, to have their sperm join up with the sperm of the female; so unless something stands in the way, these men are more apt to generate. But all this should be understood in the sense of suitability, so that when it is said that two sperms must come together for generation to take place, it is because it is much easier and much more apposite that generation take place in this way, not that it is impossible that it could take place otherwise, or that such a coming together is necessary for generation. For those same people who say that the uterus sucks up its own sperm and the sperm of the man along with it, say that women, [speaking] on the subject of conception and sexual intercourse, claim that a woman is often impregnated without experiencing pleasure, and she also is impregnated when she does experience pleasure in intercourse. Though in woman the emission of sperm is attended by pleasure, a woman could be impregnated without emission of sperm. Indeed it is a proven fact that a woman who resists [coitus], or has no pleasure and who emits no sperm, can conceive.... For a woman can be impregnated without experiencing pleasure just as she can with pleasure, as some say, because impregnation can occur either way. Nonetheless, for it to happen with pleasure is more obvious and commonplace....

The fourth reason comes from the necessity for a man. For if a woman cannot conceive without emission of sperm, either this sperm brings about generation in itself, or if generation happened not to occur, it would be due to some circumstance. We propose to refute the idea that the woman's sperm contributes to generation in itself, since this sperm is something distinct from the menstruum and from the male sperm. If generation could in no wise take place without this sperm, it would seem to bring about generation by itself. But it does not do so as matter alone, because this matter is the menstruum, since blood is the ultimate food. The Philosopher says on many occasions in *On Animals* that blood is the matter of generation in blooded animals. So if the woman's sperm by itself could bring about generation, and if conception could not come to pass without such sperm, it would have some active force because it acts as an agent, and does not play the role of matter, and the male would be superfluous. As Averroes states in his *Colliget*: in order that the male not be superfluous, this [female] sperm is not completely necessary.

The fifth reason comes from the primacy of the heart, and this argument goes together with the fourth. For were this [female] sperm in itself disposed for generation, and were generation not possible without this sperm, then either it would bestow the form, and then the male would be superfluous, or it would take on the role of matter. But it is impossible for sperm of this kind to be the matter [of generation], because then all the members would be formed from it, and nothing would be formed from the menstruum, and no one makes that claim. This could happen in accordance with [the following] hypothesis, which Galen proposes: some members could be formed from the menstruum and others from this [female] sperm. But according to Averroes in book 2 of the *Colliget*, it should not be said that the sperm of the woman makes any members; regardless of how many members there are, they are one in their one principle, which is the heart. For the heart, as he says, is that which bestows potency upon all the members. Therefore we say that just as the sperm of the man comes from the heart, so the active generative virtue to make all the members is principally in [the sperm], although in this operation the testicles lend their aid. Just as the menstruum in the woman comes from the heart, so the nutritive virtue to make all the members is in it principally, although in this operation the liver lends its aid. Therefore the generative virtue is principally in the heart.... Therefore just as the sperm of the male has from the heart, as its principle, that from which all the members are made, and the menstruum of the woman has from the heart, as its principle, that from which all the members are made, we assign one thing which serves generation *per se* – namely the heart – to men and women alike. But just as there is in every human being, whether male or female, only one heart which is the principle of generation, so there is no single *humor there that serves generation. Since in women this [humor] is the menstruum, [the woman] does not eject sperm. We should say that in males there is one thing which makes everything, namely sperm, and in females there is another thing from which everything is made, namely the menstruum. Therefore female sperm is not suitable for generation, nor is it an agent, because it is not properly speaking sperm; nor is it like matter, because it is not properly the menstruum. And because it is not in itself suitable for generation, generation will be able to happen without this kind of sperm.

The sixth reason is taken from the nourishment of the members. For Averroes says in *Colliget* book 2 that what bestows nourishment must be what bestows matter. Therefore that which is the nutriment of the members will also be matter. And as Averroes himself says in the same place, it is impossible for members to be nourished by sperm, for blood would be more suitable for nutrition than sperm....

The final reason comes from the fact that female sperm is constituted like a waste product. Hence Averroes says in *Colliget* book 2 that female sperm is like a watery moisture, similar to the waste product urine. As he himself says there, the sperm of the woman is a certain waste product which is discharged because of pleasure, just as saliva is discharged from the mouth. And because generation can take place in the absence of something which is a waste produce like the waste product urine, it is appropriate that a woman can be impregnated without the emission of [her] sperm. And that is what we wished to declare.

b. The Galenic Response: Jacopo da Forlì

Source: trans. Faith Wallis from Jacopo da Forlì, *Expositio Jacobi super capitulum de generatione embrionis cum questionibus eiusdem* (Venice: Bonetus Locatellus, 1502), fols. 15r–v. Latin.

Question Four

Does the seed of the woman contribute actively to the generation of the fetus? It is argued that it does not, firstly because something cannot be at one and the same time the agent and the recipient of an action, with respect to the same thing, because then it would be at one and the same time in act and in potency with respect to the same thing, for it would be an agent insofar as it was in action, and the recipient of the action insofar as it was in potency, as we gather from [Aristotle's] *Metaphysics* 9.... Secondly, a material cause and an efficient cause can never coincide. Therefore something can never contribute both materially and efficiently to the same effect ... [as Aristotle says in] *Physics* 2. Since, therefore, the seed of the woman contributes materially to generation, it follows, etc. Thirdly, because it would then follow that the generation of a fetus could take place naturally within a woman without the help of a man ... because the active principle, together with sufficient material, is present in her.... Fourthly, the man's seed contributes to generation in a genuinely active way, and therefore the woman's seed contributes in a genuinely passive way ... because the woman's seed is not seen to contribute to generation in more ways than the man's seed: see [Aristotle's] *Generation of Animals* 1.

The opposite [opinion] is what Avicenna seems to uphold in this text, and also Galen in his book *On Semen*.

It should be noted that Aristotle and Galen are in conflict over this issue. Therefore I shall first discuss the Philosopher's [Aristotle's] position, and secondly, Galen's, which seems to me to be closer to the truth.

As for the first, this position advances the argument that the male sperm contains two different parts, namely a gross and corpulent [part] and a foamy [part].... The gross corpulent part does not contribute efficiently to generation, but is only a vehicle that carries the foamy part to the place of generation, and preserves it so that it does not easily dissipate and escape. In consequence, this [foamy] sperm alone is active in the generation of the fetus. It is like a craftsman, whose material is the menstrual blood. Therefore this position holds that the woman's sperm does not contribute necessarily to generation. For experience teaches that a woman can become pregnant without the emission of her sperm, because [she can become pregnant] without sexual pleasure, as [Averroes] says in *Colliget* 2. So if this sperm contributes to generation, it does so only as an extrinsic and accidental aid: firstly, so that the woman will have more pleasure in intercourse, and therefore the man's sperm will be more avidly attracted into the uterus; secondly, so that the mouth of the uterus may be moistened and lubricated so the sperm may more readily be precipitated into the uterus; thirdly, so that it may be rendered more subtle by the admixture of the man's sperm, so that it may open wider and so that [the sperm] may contact the menstruum more readily. From these are deduced the following conclusions: first, that the sperm of the man alone contributes efficiently to generation.... The second conclusion is that the man's sperm does not contribute materially to generation. The third conclusion is that the sperm of the woman contributes neither efficiently nor materially to generation. The fourth conclusion is that only the menstruum of woman is the material of generation.... The fifth conclusion follows: only the man contributes actively to generation, but the woman contributes passively.

As for the second, let us present as a first supposition that whatever things are essential to the species have the same active virtue, assuming neither [the male nor the female] is defective. This is obvious because whatever things are of this kind, are of the same grade of perfection, and this is very strongly argued from operation. Therefore, etc. The second supposition is that the resemblance of the fetus to its parents or to either of them, according to a particular disposition of a member (for example, face, color, a sickness, etc.), effectively depends on a particular *spirit detached from a particular member of the parent.... The third supposition is that any positive effect to which a positive agent corresponds, is produced [by that agent] in and of itself. The fourth supposition is that a natural agent, naturally inclined to produce a certain effect, but producing another [effect], does so accidentally. The fifth supposition is that sperm contributes to the generation of the fetus just as seed contributes to the generation of plants....

Then, as to the first conclusion, that the sperm of the man contributes materially to generation from its corporeal part, it is proven thus: the seeds of plants contribute materially to the generation of the shoot according to their corporeal part. The consequence follows from the fifth supposition. And experience shows this, for we see that beans will send forth a shoot without any external nutriment. The second conclusion: the sperm of the man insofar as the generative foam is included in it contributes in a genuinely active way to the generation of the fetus. All the authorities agree on this conclusion. The third conclusion: that the sperm of the woman insofar as it has a foamy part included in it, contributes efficiently to generation. This conclusion can be supported on many grounds. Firstly, a woman and a man, assuming neither are defective, and that each exists perfectly in its sex, are essentially of the same species; therefore, each of them contains active virtue and this follows from the first supposition. But in the man there is an active virtue which is productive of a fetus. Therefore, [in a woman there will be a like virtue], etc.

Secondly, if the opposite were the case it would follow that a woman could never generate a fetus which resembled her in the disposition of any member – for example, a scar, or something of the kind – and this is not borne out by experience. And the consequences follow, because a resemblance of this kind can only happen from a spirit detached from a particular member, according to the second supposition. But no spirit detached from a woman has the potency to create this resemblance through what is inimical, because no such thing can efficiently contribute to generation [*that is, a woman cannot pass on her traits through something which is not herself, namely the man*]. Therefore, etc. But perhaps in favor of this point it will be said that this resemblance happens because of a disposition of the menstruum. However, this answer is not valid, because it is not evident how menstrual blood can acquire a disposition so as to produce a member with a scar. Thirdly, it is argued on the same point as follows: it can happen that a fetus will resemble the mother and not resemble the father, just as a stallion, by mating with a she-ass, produces a mule, which resembles the ass more; a male dog and a female fox will produce an animal very similar to a fox in color and shape, and quite dissimilar to a dog. For frequently a father who is dark-complexioned and tall and hunched over will produce a son who is fair and short and upright like the mother. Therefore it is argued thus: such a resemblance of a fetus to its mother is a positive effect, and therefore it has a particular positive cause which in and of itself produces this effect. But this cause is not the father's sperm, since it would be naturally inclined to produce dispositions similar to the dispositions of the father. Therefore the cause is the sperm of the mother, and in consequence etc. The consequences follow from the third and fourth suppositions. How in such an assimilation there comes to pass such diversity that the fetus resembles the father in color and face, but the mother in sex (or vice versa) is set forth in [Avicenna's] text. The fourth conclusion: it follows that the sperm of the woman with respect to its corpulent part contributes materially to generation. This is proven in the same way as the argument was made for the male sperm. The fifth conclusion: although it is thus, nonetheless the sperm of the man contributes to generation more efficiently and the sperm of the woman more materially. This conclusion is sufficiently laid out in the text.

As for the principal arguments. To the first it is said by way of concession that something can be both agent and recipient of action, in action and in potency, with respect to the same thing, because of its different parts, just as the human body is at one and the same time something that moves through the soul, and something that is moved through the body. This is obvious to common sense, for it is quite impossible for something to be [both] totally active and totally passive. To the second, we can reply in the same vein, namely: something is never equally agent and equally matter with respect to the same thing. But nothing stops something from contributing both materially and efficiently to the same effect, and the authority of the Philosopher supports the first point. To the third it is said … that though there is active virtue in the woman's sperm, the virtue in it is not so totally active as to be sufficient to produce a fetus; it needs in addition the generative spirit included in the male semen. To the fourth it is said … that the position of the Philosopher should be taken according to the interpretation of Galen.

47. ACADEMIC DISSECTION AS "MATERIAL COMMENTARY" (1): MONDINO DE'LIUZZI

The groundwork for the introduction of dissection of a human cadaver (as distinct from that of an animal) to demonstrate Galenic anatomy was unwittingly laid down by Galen himself. Medieval readers were completely unaware that Galen never dissected humans; because he wrote so much about human anatomy, and recommended dissection so fervently, they assumed that he had. Even before human dissection was introduced in the northern Italian universities (doc. 42), some authors were assembling anatomy treatises that implied that human anatomy was based on human dissection. The anatomical treatise of Mondino de'Liuzzi (ca 1265–1326), professor of medicine at Bolonga, is based on knowledge of a human cadaver, acquired both through instructional dissections and through autopsies – though as the excerpt below indicates, animal dissection continued to play a role.

Mondino's approach was to combine the narrative of dissection with a Galenic analytical framework. By organizing his material according to the three *"venters" or principal body cavities (abdomen, chest, skull), he was able to fuse the visual evidence of dissection with an exposition of the Galenic physiology of the three organ systems: liver (*natural spirit), heart (*vital spirit), and brain (*animal spirit). In this way the dissection became a "material commentary" on the principal physiological texts of the "new Galen" curriculum, and notably On the Usefulness of the Parts. *Like his predecessors, Mondino wove a commentary on pathology into his description, but now the pathology was based on Galen's* On Affected Parts. *Thus he proposes to link the "anatomy of the dead" to the "anatomy of the living." Each organ is analyzed with respect to its position, connections, shape, parts, and function. In the case of the uterus, these analytic categories are used to explain why gynecological disorders affect so many parts of the body.*

Source: trans. Faith Wallis from *Anathomia Mundini* (Pavia: Antonius de Carcano, 19 December 1478), facsimile edition in Ernest Wickersheimer, *Anatomies de Mondino dei Luzzi et Guido de Vigevano* (Paris: Droz, 1926), pp. 7–8, 25–27; collated with the edition by Piero P. Giorgi and Gian Franco Pasini, *Anothomia di Mondino de'Liuzzi* (Bologna: Istituto per la Storia dell'Università di Bologna, 1992), pp. 96–110. Latin.

Galen, following the authority of Plato, says in the seventh book of his *Therapeutic Method*, "A work in any science or art is published for three reasons: first, to satisfy one's friends; secondly to give useful employment to one's faculties; and thirdly to compensate for the forgetfulness that comes with the lapse of time." Motivated by these [considerations], I have decided to compose a work for my students in medicine. Now in medicine a knowledge of the parts of the subject (that is, of the human body) and the location of those parts, form a division of the science, as Averroes says in the first book of his *Colliget* in the chapter on the definition of medicine. Therefore I propose to transmit, among other topics, some of that knowledge of the human body and of its parts that comes from anatomy. I shall not adopt an elevated style, but shall merely seek to convey such knowledge as manual practice requires.

Chapter 1

Having laid out the body of one that has died from beheading or hanging in the supine position, we must first gain an idea of the whole, and secondly, of the parts. For since all our knowledge begins from what is striking to us, and what is confusing is often more striking, and the whole is more confusing than the parts, let us begin by considering the whole. Concerning this whole, the first thing we ought to know is how man differs from the other animals. He differs in three ways, namely, in the form or position of his members, in his behavior and skills, and in certain parts. In form: because he is of upright stature and is so for four reasons. For the human body, compared to other animals, has matter which is very light, spiritous, and airy, and so able to rise upwards. Secondly, compared with other [animals] of the same size, man has more heat, and the property of heat is to rise upwards. Thirdly, man has a most perfect [intelligence], which he shares with the angels and intelligences that rule the universe, and thus he should be above his [body?] as he is above the universe. Fourthly, because of the end [for which he was made] his form and stature are erect, because his end is to understand, and this is what the senses are for, particularly the sense of sight, as is seen in the preface of [Aristotle's] *Metaphysics*. And therefore in man sight and the brain, and by consequence the head, should be positioned so as to receive the diverse impressions of the senses to the maximum degree. And because it can see many more things when it is raised up – which is why watchmen in cities are stationed in high places, as in towers and the like, as Galen says in the ninth part of his *On the Usefulness of Parts* – Avicenna in the beginning of book 3 of the *Canon* says that the human head had to be created on the top [of the body], not because of the brain or the ears or the mouth or the nostrils, but because of the eyes, for the reason stated. And so for all four reasons, man was given an upright stature. For this reason he is called *antropos* [*that is*, anthropos, *the Greek word for "human being," but here conflated with* tropos, *"turning"*] that is "with turned sole," and "microcosm," that is, the smaller world, because like the universe and the world, he has an upper and a lower part. This then is the first difference.

The second comes from behavior or art; because among animals he has the gentlest manners, for he is a political and civil animal. He lacks any natural art. He has no art implanted in him by nature, as do the spider, the bee, and their like. This is so that he can participate in every art, for had he any one art so implanted in him, he would have been deprived of every other, as Galen says in the fourth part of his *On the Usefulness of Parts*.

Thirdly, [man] differs also from other animals in his parts, for he lacks many parts with which animals are externally endowed by nature. He does not have the parts which nature has given them for defense, such as horns, beaks, and long claws. He is without these because he possesses the instrument of instruments, namely the hand, and with it he can manufacture any kind of weapon for his own defense, as Galen also says in the first part of *On the Usefulness of Parts*. For the same reason he does not have parts such as furry pelts, feathers, or scales, because he does not have much superfluous matter or earthy matter (from which these things are made). He also has no tail, for being upright in his gait, he rests by sitting down, and a tail would prevent this. So much for the anatomy of the whole.

The Anatomy of the Lower Venter

Although there are two kinds of parts, *similar and composite, I shall not make a separate anatomy of those that are similar [such as bones], for their anatomy is not fully visible in a body which has been cut up, but rather in one decomposed in streams of water. But in setting forth the anatomy of the organic members, I shall discuss the similar parts according to that which predominates in the organic member under discussion, for example flesh in the anatomy of the thigh, bones in the anatomy of the back and feet, and the anatomy of the *nerves in the anatomy of the brain and spinal cord. Concerning the *official [members], it should be known that in most of them, as far as anatomy of a dead body is concerned, there are six things to be observed, as the Alexandrian commentator says in his commentary on *On the Sects* [by Galen], namely what their position is, what their substance is, and consequently what their *complexion is, their size, number, shape, and connections [with other parts]. As for the anatomy of these [parts] made upon the living, two things should be considered which are also to some extent evident in the anatomy of the dead. The first is what is the use and operation [of the parts]; the second, what diseases can occur in them, and if there is an appropriate treatment, it will be shown.

The division and number of parts of the body is based on the fact that there are those that are called "external" or the "extremities," and those that are called "deep" or "intrinsic." Some of these are directly ordained for the preservation of the species, and some indirectly for the preservation of the individual. The first are the genital members, the second are the members that are contained in the venters. There are three venters in our body, the uppermost one that holds the animate members is the head; the lowest one that holds the natural members, and the middle that holds the *spiritual members. I shall first begin with the anatomy of the lowermost venter, because the organs there smell bad and therefore I shall begin with them so that they can be discarded first....

The Anatomy of the Uterus

To continue this discourse: if you make an anatomy on a woman, after the "spermatic" vessels [*Fallopian tubes*] you should observe the anatomy of the uterus just as you have done in the other members: first its position and the things to which it is attached; secondly its shape; thirdly its size; fourthly its substance; fifthly its parts; sixthly its purpose and injuries.

You will see its position, because it is situated in the hollow of the sacrum, and this hollow is surrounded by the joints of the [sacral vertebrae] and of the tail in the rear, and in front by the part called pubis or *femur*. It is positioned immediately between the rectum, which is, as it were, its keel, in the back, and the bladder in front. In particular as regards its neck, it is joined by this neck to the neck of the bladder, even though the concavity of the uterus lies above that of the bladder. [The uterus] is positioned exactly in the middle between the right and left [sides].

Next you may see the parts connected to the uterus, which are very many, since it has a connection with almost all the parts that lie above it: with the heart and liver through the median veins and arteries; with the brain by many nerves, and consequently, through both [veins and arteries] with the members which lie between, like the stomach, the diaphragm, kidneys and mesentery, and especially with the breasts, as already described, although it is also linked to them by means of other veins that have their origin in the chilic vein and arise from below the sternum, as will be stated below. It is also connected with the organs below it, such as the bladder by means of its neck, and with the colon. It is connected to the hips and to both joints by the sciatic [*nerves], which are thick strong [ligaments] that attach the uterus to the hips. Next to the uterus these ligaments are broad and thick, and next to the hips they are slender and issue forth like horns from the head of an animal. They are therefore called the "horns of the uterus."

The shape [of the uterus] is somewhat square, with a certain roundness, and it has a long neck below. This shape is [determined by] its confined location, and by its function or the necessity for which it was created, which will be explained later. It owes this shape to being divided into seven cells, as will be stated below.

Thirdly, you should examine its size. It is properly of middling size and is about the size of the bladder. But it varies because of other causes, since it grows larger or smaller because of pregnancy. For a woman who has borne children has a larger uterus than one who is barren. The second reason has to do with sexual intercourse, because a sexually experienced woman has a larger uterus than a virgin or than one who is continent. It is the same with lewd men, for use increases the size of an organ, according to Galen in *On Affected Parts*. The third reason is age, because a young woman has a larger [uterus] than a girl or an old woman. The fourth reason is *complexion or total constitution: this you can gather from the *Canon* of Avicenna, *fen* 2 in the third chapter. For these reasons, a woman I anatomized last year, that is, in the year of Christ 1315, in the month of January, had a womb twice as large as [the woman] that I anatomized in March of the same year. There may be yet another cause, which Avicenna puts forward, namely, that the first woman had just had her menstrual period, because at the time of menstruation the uterus becomes thicker and stouter. The uterus also shows variations in the amount it can generate, for the uterus of an animal that bears several young [at a time] is larger than that of one that bears only one. For that reason, the uterus of a sow that I anatomized in the year 1316 was a hundred times greater than I ever saw in a human female. This could also have been because the sow was pregnant and had thirteen piglets in her uterus, and in it I demonstrated the anatomy of the fetus and of pregnancy, which I shall relate to you.

Fourthly, you should look at the substance. The substance is sinewy and membranous, so that it can stretch to contain the fetus, and therefore it is of a cold and dry complexion. Also the substance is very thick, but it becomes thinner when it has to expand.

Fifthly, you should see the number of the parts [of the uterus], for it has external and internal parts. The external parts are first the sides on which are fastened the testicles [*that is, ovaries*] and the seminal vessels discussed above, and the horns and the neck, the end of which is the vulva. Note that the vulva is the length of a palm's breadth, just like the penis. It is capable of expanding in width and consequently it is a wrinkled membrane, having wrinkles like leeches so as to cause a tickling sensation when the penis is introduced. At the end of the upper or anterior part is the opening of the neck of the bladder, about two or three fingers' breadth from the vulva. At the end of the vulva are two membranes which may be raised or lowered over the orifice to prevent the entry of air and external matter into the neck of the womb or bladder, just as the membrane of the prepuce guards the penis. Therefore Avicenna [actually Haly Abbas, author of the Pantegni] calls them "the foreskin of the uterus" in the place cited above.

The inner parts you can see by cutting [the uterus] up the middle. Then you will see its "mouth" and cavity. The "mouth" is very nervous, made like the mouth of a new-born kitten or, to speak more properly, like the mouth of an old tench [a fish]. In virgins its surface is veiled with a thin veil, and when she is violated it is broken and therefore bleeds. The cavity contains seven cells, three on the right side and three on the left and one at the top or in the middle. These cells are nothing but cavities in the womb in which the semen can be coagulated with the menstrual matter, and be contained and connected to the orifices of the veins.

The purposes of the uterus are plain from this, for it is mainly for conception and secondarily for cleansing or *purging the whole body of superfluous, undigested blood. This applies to human beings only, because other animals do not suffer from the menstrual *flux, since in them superfluities are consumed in [the production of] hide, fur, claws, beaks and feathers and the like, which humans lack.

From this it is evident that the uterus must be subject to many diseases, and many members suffer in sympathy with it. It would take a long time to relate its diseases and particular accidents, their causes and treatments, and it would lie outside our purpose; but look it up in the appropriate places, such as [Avicenna's] Canon book 3, chapter 21, and in Serapion [Serapion the Elder, Yahya ibn Sarafyun, ninth c., or his homonym of the twelfth c.], Rhazes and our Johannes [Mesue].

These sympathetic diseases are as numerous as the organs to which [the uterus] is connected or locally attached. What these are has already been seen and stated, but there is one which you can learn about from anatomy. It is described by Galen in book 6 of On the Usefulness of Parts, namely: suffocation of the womb. This does not happen because the uterus is physically moved to the throat or the lungs, for this is impossible. But it comes about because when it is unable to expel the *vapors downward, it is moved by some cause, and contracted in the lower part, so that it expels them upward. Now if these vapors, by means of one of the attachments described above, should reach the stomach through the sympathies of the dorsal artery, they frequently cause hiccoughs or vomiting, and women say that they have their "uterus in their stomach." But if the vapors reach the lungs and hinder their action, or that of the diaphragm – namely, breathing – the women say that they have their "uterus in their throat," because the throat or trachea is in the first instance designed for breathing. But if the vapors reach the heart, which happens rarely, they suffer suffocation and fainting, and then the women say that their "uterus has reached the heart." But the fact of the matter is that this suffocation is from sympathy with the diaphragm, because of the attachment of the uterus to the diaphragm and loins. For nothing reaches these parts but the vapor. Now that you have seen how and by what means [vapors] could reach these [members], you can see how to treat them, and with what treatments, in the authorities. For the cure, look in the authorities. In these matters, anatomy mainly provides information about the places.

48. ACADEMIC DISSECTION AS "MATERIAL COMMENTARY" (2): ANATOMICAL ILLUSTRATION

Scientific illustration in the age of manuscripts presented enormous challenges because each image had to be copied by hand from another manuscript exemplar. Copying a scientific image demands some factual and analytical knowledge of the object being represented. The image might itself be a mental conception (for example, a geometric figure), or represent a viewpoint not accessible to everyday experience (for example, a map), or convey details that the scientific observer needs to notice, but that may be irrelevant, and hence "invisible," to others (for example, the number of petals in a flower). Consequently, even accurate and sophisticated images tended to degrade in quality as they passed from hand-made copy to hand-made copy. Nonetheless, many teachers and students of anatomy in the scholastic period found images to be a valuable adjunct to the experience of dissection: Henri of Mondeville used pictures (and even three-dimensional models) in the course of his lectures at Montpellier and Paris, and some in his audience made copies of them. A picture could help to fix information in the memory: the "Five Picture Series" illustrated below was created for that purpose. Alternatively, pictures could overcome some of the physical limitations of the dissection: this is the argument advanced by Guido of Vigevano. In the end, like dissection itself, these pictures were designed to be a vivid visual display of the basic teachings of Galenic anatomy.

a. The "Five Picture Series"

The "Five Picture Series" is an ensemble of diagrams illustrating the principal systems of the Galenic body. The album originated in the late antique medical schools of Alexandria as a teaching and study aid and it was widely copied in the Arab-Islamic world before coming to the West. In the twelfth-century German manuscript shown here, the five figures are spread across two facing pages. On the left-hand page, the two figures show (1) the arteries, with their origin in the heart, and (2) the veins, arising from the liver. At the top of the right-hand page are depicted (3) the bones (including the cranial sutures and teeth), and (4) the *nerves. At the bottom of the page is (5) the muscles. The squatting posture is standard in all copies and probably goes back to the Alexandrian original.

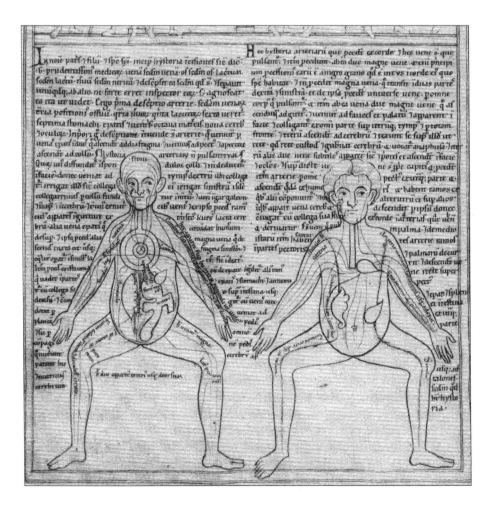

Source: MS Munich, Bayerische Staatsbibliothek CLM 13002 fols. 2v–3r, reproduced in Nancy Siraisi, *Medieval and Early Renaissance Medicine* (Chicago: University of Chicago Press, 1990), fig. 15, pp. 92–93.

b. The *Anatomy* of Guido of Vigevano

Guido of Vigevano was born in Lombardy around 1300. After a period of service with the emperor Henry VII, he joined the household of the queen of France, Jeanne of Burgundy. Royal treasury accounts indicate that he was in this post until at least 1349. He composed a number of works for the French royal house, including The King of France's Treasury *(Texaurus regis Francie), a combination of a regimen of health for a crusading army and an illustrated tract on military technology (1335). Guido's ten-part collection of medical works,* The Book of Notable Matters *(Liber notabilium), was dedicated to King Philip VII in 1345. It comprises Latin translations of a number of Galen's works, a regimen of health, and the* Anatomy for King Philip VII, *a set of anatomical drawings with captions and accompanying text.*

Guido's statement that the Church forbade dissection is, of course, not accurate and is belied by both his text and his illustrations, which explicitly show the anatomist opening each of the three *"venters" in turn. Indeed, Guido claims somewhat illogically that it was his extensive dissection experience and the Church's alleged prohibition that moved the king of France to commission the Anatomy. *Guido argues that pictures are superior in some respects to the actual experience. They offer views that would otherwise be impossible, and permit extended study without the time pressures imposed by putrefaction.*

Source: trans. Faith Wallis from Guido of Vigevano, *Anatomy for King Philip VII (Anatomia Philippi septimi)*, ed. Ernest Wickerheimer, *Anatomies de Mondino dei Luzzi et de Guido de Vigevano* (Paris: Droz, 1926), pp. 72–77, and plates from MS Chantilly, Musée Condé 569. Latin.

The Value of Anatomy and of Anatomical Images

This is the *Anatomy* for Philip VII, king of the French, depicted in images by Guido, physician to the aforementioned king.

Because it is prohibited by the Church to perform an anatomy upon a human body and because the art of medicine cannot be fully known unless one first knows about anatomy – as Galen says in book 1 of *On Affected Parts*, when he states that the condition of the anatomy of the members is no less useful than knowledge of what to do and how to help, since knowledge of anatomy conveys the characteristics and essence of each internal member – therefore I, the abovementioned Guido, in order that this book of noteworthy matters that I have extracted from the books of Galen may be more useful, will plainly and openly demonstrate the anatomy of the human body through illustrations, just as they are in the human body. [The anatomy] will appear in an evident fashion in the images below and rather better than it can be seen in the human body itself, because when we do an anatomy on a man, it is necessary to make haste because of the stench. Therefore doctors can only get an overall view of the inner organs, just as they lie there. Therefore, whoever wishes to see an anatomy well must see it many times, diligently, in detail, and one member after another. But since that cannot be done because the opportunities for obtaining a human body for an anatomy are rare and also because it is prohibited by the Church, I myself undertook to present an anatomy in pictures. And my qualifications to do so can be trusted, because I myself have done [anatomies] on the human body many, many times. And it should be known as an established fact that Avicenna, who wrote such a great book on anatomy, made mistakes in certain places and especially concerning the spleen, since he says [in *Canon* book 3, *fen* 15, tract 1, c. 2] that the spleen is elongated, whereas in fact it is just about completely round, with two or three nodules projecting below. And this is plainly apparent in a living man, because when the spleen is swollen in the belly, it is just about round when we palpate it. Whoever doubts this can make inquiries and ascertain the truth.

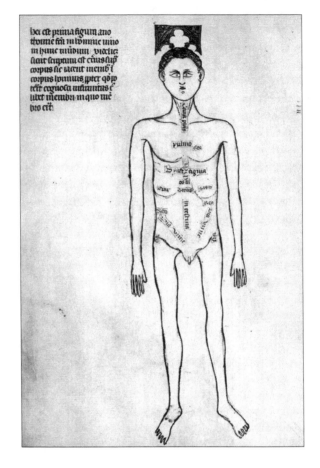

Figura 1: Surface of the Body and Location of Internal Organs
Anatomy depicted in the living man. The first image will be made such as to show a naked living man, and on the surface will be inscribed the name of every internal member that is in the body and its location.

This is the first image of the anatomy, showing a man alive in this world. Where the [internal] members of the body lie is as it is written on the surface of the body; this is so that a disease of any member can be recognized, and in what member it is.

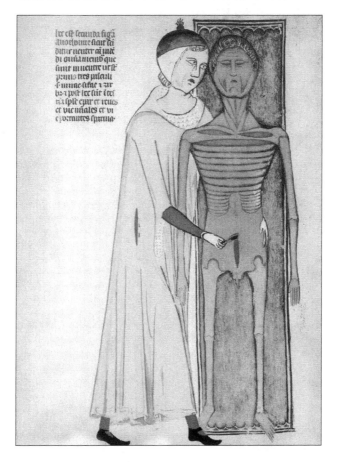

Figura 2: The Anatomist Opens the Abdomen

The second image of the anatomy. In the second image, the belly is opened
lengthwise, that is, from the bladder up to the entry to the stomach.

This is the second image of the anatomy. The belly is slit in order that all
the members which are in the belly may be seen. These are, first, the three
membranes – abdominal wall (*mirach*), peritoneum (*siphac*), and omentum
(*zirbus*) – and after them, there are the intestines, spleen, liver and kidneys,
the urinary vessels, and the vessels that carry the sperm....

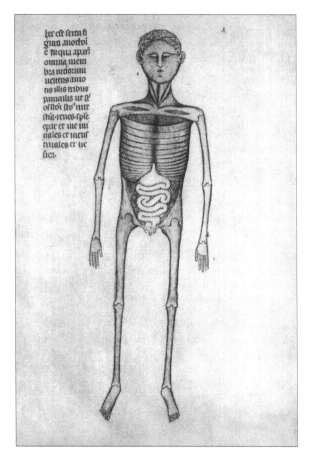

Figura 6: Abdominal Organs

The sixth image of the anatomy. In the sixth image, after the membrane called *zirbus* has been removed, all the internal members of the belly will appear in open view.

This is the sixth image of the anatomy, in which all the members in the interior of the belly appear after those three membranes have been removed. These are the entry to the stomach, the stomach, intestines, kidneys, spleen, liver, the urinal and menstrual vessels, and the bladder....

Figura 9: Esophagus and Digestive Tract

The ninth image of the anatomy. In the ninth image, since the *meri* or esophagus (which is the same thing) through which food and drink pass from the mouth to the entry of the stomach cannot be demonstrated, because it is covered by the trachea or pipe of the lungs (which is the same thing) as well as by

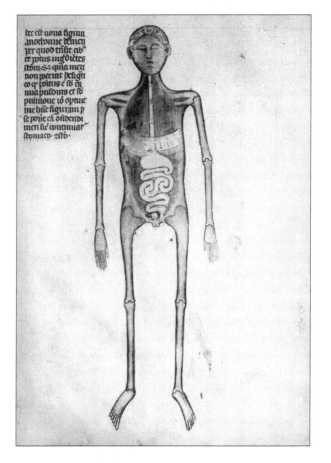

the lungs; and because the *meri* or esophagus is positioned on top of the spinal cord or vertebrae of the neck and shoulders, right down to the entrance of the stomach (which *meri* at the entrance to the stomach is called "mouth of the stomach"), I have made an effort to represent the *meri* alone in a single image. For it is highly necessary that this member, the *meri*, be actually demonstrated, because plasters are necessary for this *meri* and "mouth of the stomach," and it will be necessary to apply [the plaster] on the back, since the way to the *meri* is shorter from the back than from the front, given that the chest and lungs are on top of it.

This is the ninth image of the anatomy, showing the *meri* through which food and drink pass as they enter the stomach. But because the *meri* cannot be shown, since it is positioned under the pipe of the lungs and under the lungs, it was necessary for me to give it its own image for the sake of showing the *meri* as it is joined to the stomach.

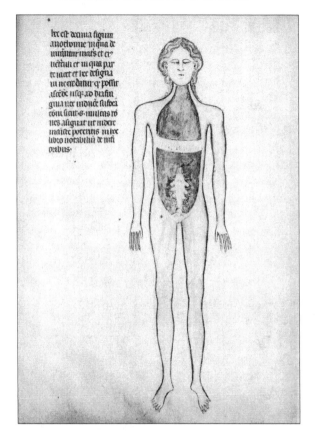

Figura 10: Uterus and Its Ligaments

The tenth image. The tenth image will be only for the sake of showing the anatomy of the uterus, because many, many physicians are wrong about the situation and condition of the uterus, since they say that it rises up all the way to the diaphragm and presses on the *spiritual members, and induces suffocation. This is false, as Galen says in his book *On Affected Parts*, for he says that the uterus does not rise up to the diaphragm, and not even to the stomach, since it has no ligaments above the navel. One should consult the book *On Affected Parts* and one will find plainly laid out Galen's refutation of those who understand nothing about the movement of the uterus.

This is the tenth figure of the anatomy in which is demonstrated the uterus and its *ventricles and in what region it lies. And I have depicted these things lest it be believed that [the uterus] can rise up all the way to the diaphragm and induce suffocation. Galen furnishes many arguments [against this] as you may plainly see in that book of noteworthy matters, *On Affected Parts....*

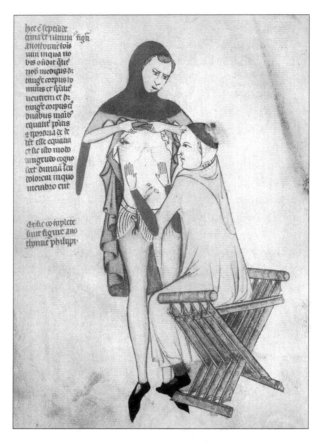

Figura 17: The Physician Palpates the Abdomen

The seventeenth image. In the seventeenth and final image, which completes the whole anatomy, when the patient senses some pain in his body, the physician must immediately know upon which member and in which member the pain is. Therefore, in this image the way of palpating the body is shown.

This is the seventeenth and last [image] of the anatomy of the living man, in which we show how the physician should palpate the body of a man, and particularly the belly. And he should palpate the body with both hands equally spaced, for the hypochondrium should be symmetrical. And in this way he will recognize in which member an induration or pain is located. And this completes the images of the *Anatomy for* [*King*] *Philip.*

49. SCHOLASTIC MEDICINE POPULARIZED: BARTHOLOMAEUS ANGLICUS ON DISEASES OF THE HEAD AND OF THE MIND

The Franciscan Bartholomaeus Anglicus (Bartholomew the Englishman) studied theology in Paris and lectured in the Order's studium *there before becoming lector or master of the* studium *in Magdeburg (Saxony) in 1231. His duties were to teach basic theology to novices, prepare the brighter ones for advanced studies in Paris, and perhaps also to teach secular students. He became the Order's minister provincial for Austria and then for Saxony, and died in office in 1272.*

On the Properties of Things (De proprietatibus rerum) was composed for Bartholomaeus's Magdeburg students and completed around 1245. This encyclopedia for preachers and students of Scripture enjoyed very wide circulation in the Middle Ages, including twelve printed editions before 1500. Its nineteen books cover the Creator, angels, and souls; human life (*humors and qualities in book 4; anatomy in book 5; life-cycle and estates of life in book 6; medicine in book 7); the heavens and time; the created world (organized around the four elements); and some miscellaneous themes such as the senses, number, etc.

Bartholomaeus's book is a compilatio, *not a philosophical work, and its underlying idea of nature as the "natures" or properties of individual creatures contrasts with the more abstract scholastic concepts of nature as law, blueprint, or principle of origin. Nonetheless,* On the Properties of Things *contains information that is completely consonant with the latest academic trends in medicine. For example, at the outset of book 7 on medicine, Bartholomaeus says that he will limit himself to discussing diseases mentioned in the Bible. Nonetheless, he treats his subject in the approved scholastic manner, quoting from the standard authorities and employing the conceptual framework of Galenism. He claims not to be concerned with the order in which he treats diseases, but in fact he adopts the standard head-to-toe order of therapeutic manuals. Bartholomaeus seems genuinely interested in disease and treatment, though he omits the pharmacological remedies found in his sources.*

So popular was Bartholomaeus's book that it was translated into several vernacular languages. The Middle English translation by the Dominican John Trevisa (1398) is itself a masterpiece of prose, and the French version by Jean Corbechon (1372), dedicated to King Charles V, survives in a number of exquisite illuminated manuscripts. The excerpts below are from the original Latin text. These are the opening chapters of book 7, which deal with diseases of the head, including mental disorders. Bartholomaeus draws on the standard models of psychology, which envisioned three cells or *ventricles in the brain, each responsible for a distinctive faculty: imagination (the capacity to form true mental images of phenomena in the world) was located in the front of the brain, reason in the middle, and memory in the back.

Bartholomaeus's account of mental illness is quoted by Gaspar Ofhuys in his account of the melancholic painter Hugo van der Goes (doc. 72).

Source: trans. Faith Wallis from *Bartholomaei Anglici De genuinis rerum coelestium, terrestrium et infer[n]arum proprietatibus* (Frankfurt: Wolfgang Richter, 1601), pp. 276–367. Latin.

Chapter 1. Headache and Its Causes and Signs

Now we must speak of the properties of these illnesses, that is, of their causes, effects, signs and remedies – not, indeed, of all of them, but only of those that are generally mentioned in Scripture. And so we need not concern ourselves with the order in which they are dealt with. First we will begin with afflictions of the head. Isaiah 1[:5]: "The whole head is sick," etc. As Constantine says [*Viaticum* 1.10], headache is called *cephalea*, and it comes about in two ways: either from the outside, as from a blow, or from dissolution by warm air, or constriction by cold air; or from within, and this either from a privy cause or from a remote cause – from a privy cause, which comes from nowhere other than the head, or from a remote cause such as the stomach. And if the pain is from a privy cause, it is either from a defect of a quality alone (particularly of heat or cold), or from a defect of the humors, such as blood, *phlegm, etc. If the pain is intermittent, and sometimes comes, sometimes goes, it is a sign that it is from the stomach. Hence Galen [says, in *On Compounding Medicines according to Place* 2.1, cited in *Viaticum* 1.10]: If there is pain in the head, and it comes from no identifiable external cause, then sharp humors are oppressing the stomach. If it is without intermission, it is from the humors. If it is from the blood, the head will suffer from heat, with heaviness in the forehead (because the anterior part of the head is the seat of blood), the eyes will be red, and the veins of the face full. If it is from *choleric fumes, heat will be felt in the nostrils, dryness in the tongue; there will be wakefulness and thirst, the pain will be greater on the right side than on the left, because that is where the seat of choler is. The face and eyes will be yellow and there will be a bitter taste in the mouth. If it is from *melancholy, the pain will be more intense on the left side, and accompanied by cold, wakefulness, and heaviness. The face will be livid, like the color of earth. The eyes are hollow and inflamed, and there is an acid taste in the mouth. If it comes from phlegm, a heavy pain results, there is running from the nose and the mouth, sometimes with coughing and gasping for breath and groaning. The face is pallid and somewhat swollen; there is inflammation of the eyes, an insipid taste in the mouth, and the pain is greater in the back of the head, for that is the seat of phlegm. Hence Galen in his book of instructions [says that] one should know that the head is divided into four parts. For blood dominates in the forehead, choler on the right, melancholy on the left, and phlegm in the occiput. Headache occurs in these and many other ways, such as from the pungency of strong wine, whose fumes pierce the membranes surrounding the brain, and produce a severe headache. Here ends what Constantine says.

Chapter 2. Medicine and Remedies for Pain and Affliction of the Head

The head suffers from a certain internal pain which the physicians (as Constantine says) call migraine [*Viaticum* 1.11], and according to Constantine, it is very severe. It feels as if there is hammering and pounding in the head. Sound or talking is unbearable, as is light or glare. This pain arises from hot, choleric fumes, together with *windiness. And so one feels piercing, burning and ringing [*Viaticum* 1.12]. The head may also be afflicted externally on the skin with pustules and scabies, with a discharge of *sanies like honey, and so this type of scabies is called "honeycomb" (*favus*) by Constantine [*Viaticum* 1.17]. For these pustules have small holes from which the sanies comes out. This *favus* arises from viscous humor which breaks out or ulcerates on the surface of the skin. In children, the head is afflicted by a similar condition which Constantine calls "scale," and which we call "grub" [*tinea, that is, ringworm*] because like a grub it eats away the surface of the scalp, and clings to it inseparably. This affliction generates a terrible itching and when it is scratched, scales fall away. This affliction often happens to young children because of the abundant moisture and softness of their skin and the fact that they eat more abundantly. As Constantine says, we cut back on their food and, when the underlying humor has diminished, apply ointment. Constantine says that the best remedy for nursing children is to open a vein behind the ears and withdraw blood, and then anoint the sore place with the extracted [blood] while it is hot; when it penetrates, it breaks up and consumes the [morbid] matter [*Viaticum* 1.18]. And because these scales often cling to the roots of the hairs, it is not easy to cure them unless it is uprooted from the head. If this affliction becomes entrenched, it can scarcely be healed any further, for when the "grub" is healed, it always leaves some vestige behind on the head. Again, the head is afflicted externally by loss of beauty when the hair falls out or it goes bald…. In its hair, the head suffers that flaking and blemish that doctors call "bran" [*that is, dandruff*]. For sometimes scales like bran arise around the roots of the hairs on the head. This happens either because of a defect of the brain or from a defect of the fumes that exit from the head and nurture the hairs. But this filthy condition is to be diligently cleansed by purifying cleaning agents and by medicines, just as lice and nits and almost undetectable worms are to be removed from the region of the head by appropriate medications. According to Constantine, the abovementioned afflictions of the head can be quickly taken care of. If the pain arises from a defect in a humor – for example, a surfeit of blood or another humor – we withdraw blood from the cephalic vein, and we *purge the body with suitable and appropriate medicines; especially if the [morbid] matter is in the stomach, we induce vomiting and bring it out with a suitable medication [*Viaticum* 1.10, 11]. When the body has been purged, we pour lukewarm water over the head, hands, and feet in order to open the pores and let the fumes evaporate easily. If the back part [of the head] hurts, we open the broad vein in the forehead and withdraw blood [Platearius, *Practica* 2.6], and this helps, as Constantine says; or else we *scarify the shins, and so the humors and fumes and *spirits which are the cause of the pain are drawn down from the head to the lower parts [*Viaticum* 1.10]. If the front part [of the head] hurts, we induce a nosebleed. And if the humor is hot and choleric, we resort to cold medications. We anoint the temples, nostrils and pulsating veins with rose water, together with the milk of a woman who is nursing a male child, and we induce sleep. If the [morbid] matter is cold and viscous, and digested matter is resting at the mouth of the stomach, we administer a Patriarchal *Emetic Filtrate to provoke vomiting; thus let us draw it out from the bottom of the stomach with a suitable medicine, and we use warm *fomentations and ointments, and prescribe a moderately warm diet, and thus we heal contraries with contraries. But if there is headache with defect of a humor through excess of any quality, then the patient does not need purging, but rather *alterative remedies. So for morbid qualities, we supply contrary qualities. If the pain comes from repletion from too much food and drink, as often happens when one is drunk, the best remedy is to drink a very large quantity of warm water, and then after a short interval to induce vomiting. If you wish to use stronger medications, consult the *Viaticum* of Constantine. This much suffices for the purposes of a wise man.

Chapter 3. Catarrh and Flux of the Head

Judith 8[:3]: "A burning heat came upon the head of Manasseh, and he died," etc. The reason why Manasseh's death came on suddenly was an immoderate *flux of *rheum from the head to the internal parts from the intensity of the heat and of its warmth, which dissolves the humors of the head, as Bernard [*possibly Bernard of Provence, a late 12th c. author*] observes. The doctors call a flux of this kind *"catarrh" and it happens in the head for many reasons. Sometimes the heat of the air dissolves fluid humors. Sometimes cold air constricts the brain and expels its liquid parts. Sometimes an abundance of humors, dissolved by internal heat, flows out incontinently; or it is compressed and pressed out by the cold. Sometimes it is lubricated by humidity; sometimes it dissolves due to the liquid and flowing nature of the humors; and sometimes from weakness of the retentive faculty. These are the signs of a flux coming from a great abundance of humors: the body appears plethoric and replete, the face is somewhat puffy, the eyes protrude, there is an abundance of superfluities coming from the mouth and nostrils, and the body is heavy. These are the signs of dissolving heat: a red color in the face, with redness of the veins, particularly in the eyes; hot tears flow, which sting the eyes; the skin is hot and the heat is felt deep within. Constricting cold is recognized by these signs: the color of the face is pallid, there are cold tears, and the cold is felt deep within. If it comes about from liquidity of the humors, it is recognized by the quantity of superfluities from the mouth and nostrils, and these are fluid, and distil without congealing. If superfluity is the cause, it is cured by removal of the superfluity (especially if the flux tends towards the respiratory organs), and through constricting the fluid humor [Platearius, *Practica* 2.3]. If the flux is especially cold and moist, hot and dry remedies will do well to counteract it, and to constrict and consume the humors, such as laudanum, frankincense, storax, and *castoreum. If it is a hot flux, it should be constricted by a cold fomentation, by a *decoction of roses in rain-water, and by applying these roses to the openings of the nostrils. It should be noted that as long as the flux of the catarrh is violent, no ointment or fomentation should be applied, because this will make for a greater dissolution, as Constantine says. Nor should water be poured upon the head, save perhaps rose water, or water of willow in cases where the cause is heat.

Chapter 4. Frenzy: Its Causes, Signs and Remedies

Deuteronomy 28[:28]: "[The Lord] will smite you with madness and insanity and stupor," etc. [The Bible] calls frenzy "madness." It is described thus by Constantine [*Viaticum* 1.16]. Frenzy, he says, is a hot *aposteme in one of the membranes of the brain, and it is the consequence of sleeplessness and raving. The word "frenzy" is derived from *frenes*, that is, the membranes that surround the brain. It comes about in two ways. [First], from red *bile which is made light by its innate heat and by the heat of a *fever, and then stirred into a rage and carried upward by the veins, *nerves, and arteries; this is collected into an aposteme, and causes true frenzy. Alternately, it is caused by fumes ascending from the body to the brain, and perturbing it, and this is "parafrenzy," that is, not true frenzy. A person suffering from frenzy has dreadful symptoms, namely, great thirst, a dry, blackened and roughened tongue, great torment and anguish, fainting because of deficiency of spirits, and the transformation of natural heat into unnatural heat. If the cause is blood, [the patient] becomes red; if it is choler, yellow. This affliction befalls hot and dry people in the summertime, and all these things are related to choler. But parafrenzy is generated from adhesions of other members, for example, from an aposteme in the stomach or uterus. When these members are restored to their original state, the brain also returns [to normal] and the parafrenzy is cured. But when the aposteme is in the substance of the brain, then the frenzy is very bad indeed and extremely distressing, and hence very dangerous. The signs of frenzy are: discolored urine, great insanity with fever, continuous wakefulness, roving and distended eyes, flailing of the hands, shaking of the head, grinding and chattering of the teeth. [Patients] always want to get out of bed. Sometimes they sing, sometimes laugh, sometimes cry. They freely bite and scratch their caregivers and doctors. Rarely are they silent, and they shout a lot. These people are very dangerously ill, and yet they know not that they are ill. Help must be given quickly, lest these people perish; this should be both in the form of diet and of medication. The diet should be very light, namely, breadcrumbs washed several times in water. The medication is that the sick man's head should first be shaved and washed with lukewarm vinegar. He should be held or bound in a dark place. He should not be presented with a variety of faces or images lest his insanity be irritated. His attendants shall keep silent, and not reply to his foolish speech. At the beginning of the treatment, about an egg-shell full of blood shall be let from the vein in the forehead. Before all else, and in the beginning, if strength and age permit, he shall be bled from the cephalic vein. Let *digestion be procured and choler extinguished by medication. Above all, bring on sleep with ointments and fomentations. His shaven head should be plastered often with the lung of a pig or a sheep. Temples and forehead should be anointed with juice of lettuce and poppy. If following this treatment the insanity persists for three days with insomnia and discoloration of the urine, there is no hope of recovery; but if the urine takes on a good color and the bad signs diminish, one may hope.

Chapter 6. Of Insanity [*amentia*]

Amentia and insanity are the same thing. And Platearius [*Practica* 2.5] says that madness is an *infection of the anterior cell of the head with loss of the imaginative faculty, just as melancholy is an infection of the middle cell with loss of reason. As Constantine says in his book *On Melancholy*, melancholy (he says) is a suspicion that overmasters the soul and that induces fear and sadness. These afflictions are distinguished according to the different kinds

CHAPTER SEVEN

THEORY AND PRACTICE IN SCHOLASTIC MEDICINE

The Galenic triad of "body," "signs," and "causes" were the conceptual pillars of a medical curriculum designed to encompass both theory and practice. This chapter presents documents that illustrate how doctors and surgeons strove to re-orient their ideas of practice in the light of medical theory. Essentially, this involved endowing existing elements of practice, such as diagnosis and therapeutic intervention, with a theoretical rationale. For example, pulse and urine remained the principal clues to detecting and identifying disease, but they were now integrated into the physiology of the natural and *vital spirits (docs. 50–51). Early medieval texts on diseases are largely concerned with description and cure; by contrast, scholastic treatises, like the ones on epilepsy in doc. 52, focus on the logical links between cause, symptom, and treatment. Alongside the traditional forms of pharmaceutical literature such as antidotaries and catalogues of ma-teria medica, the scholastic doctor now had to compose arguments about how drugs worked (doc. 55). In the case of surgery, the stakes were particularly high. For both ideological and political reasons, the public rift between physicians who used their brains and surgeons who used their hands became more emphatic in the late Middle Ages.

There were significant regional differences here. In Italy, all graduate physicians were considered to be competent as surgeons, but the reverse was not true. Surgery was taught in universities, but most surgeons felt they did not need a surgery degree. The distinction between physicians and surgeons was supposed to be absolute in Paris, but in fact it was never as clear-cut or as acrimonious as it is often made out to be. Nonethe-less, authors of surgical texts felt obliged to address the question of surgery's status as a scientia (docs. 58–60). They were grappling with two interrelated problems: how surgery related to medicine (for example, in the gray zone of "surgical diseases" – see doc. 62), and the degree to which surgery could be subjected to the types of analysis characteristic of scholasticism.

50. SIGNS AND DIAGNOSIS (1): GILLES OF CORBEIL ON URINES

In scholastic Galenism, urine is what the body discards when it *digests food to make blood; it is therefore an index of how well the *natural spirit is faring. Pulse, the pulsation of the heart and arteries, is likewise a "read-out" of the working of the vital spirit. The most widely copied school text of uroscopy was On Urines *by Gilles of Corbeil. Gilles was born around 1140, studied at Salerno, and returned to Paris sometime between ca 1180 and 1194. There he taught medicine until his death around 1214. His major medical works were two poems,* On Urines *and* On Pulses. *Though based on the two parallel texts in the* Articella, *Theophilus's* On Urines *and Philaretus's* On Pulses, *Gilles's texts were considered much superior. The 1270–74 statutes of the Paris Medical Faculty listed both as "optional" reading (doc. 40b), and they were the subject of numerous commentaries. Like the* Epitome on Pulses *(doc. 51), Gilles's urine treatise provided a mnemonic schematization for judging the condition of urine. Color was the major sign, combined with texture. Each "tone" of urine was decoded. Though causal explanations were missing, Gilles linked diagnostic signs to a theoretical model of disease.*

Source: trans. Michael R. McVaugh in *Sourcebook in Medieval Science*, ed. Edward Grant (Cambridge, MA: Harvard University Press, 1974), pp. 748–50 (n. 100.1). Latin.

Part 1

Urine may be so called because it is unified in the kidneys (*fit in renibus una*) or from the Greek *urith*, which means demonstration, or else because it corrodes, dries and burns (*urit*) whatever it touches. As a clear humor separates from serous milk, so the fluid urine leaves the bulk of the blood. Urine is the serum of blood, the subtle residue of the *humors, which are created by the directive force ruling the second *digestion, formed by the filtration of aliment, when the pure part is separated from the impure.

The physician who wishes to be considered an expert judge of urine must consider with care the following things: what sort, what [it is], what is in it, how much, how often, where, when; age, nature, sex, exercise, anger, diet, anxiety, hunger, movement, baths, food, ointment, drink. But the first four, which are particularly important, form the best basis of judgment. Health or illness, strength or debility, deficiency, excess, or balance, are determined with certainty by examination in this way.

Urine can be of twenty colors, which you can learn from the descriptions below....

A large quantity of urine, darkened throughout by a black cloudiness, and muddied with sediment, if produced on a *critical day [of an illness] and accompanied by poor hearing and insomnia, portends a *flux of blood from the nose; depending on whether the other signs are ominous or favorable, the patient will die or recover....

If the urine is livid, the lividity is partial or total. If total, it means the mortification of a member or of its humors. Livid near the surface, it suggests various things: a mild form of *hemitriteus fever; falling sickness; ascites; *synochal fever; the rupture of a vein; *catarrh; *strangury; an ailment of the womb; a flux; a defect of the lungs; pain in the joints; consumptive *phthisis; the extinction of [natural] heat. These are the causes of lividity – interpret them according to [other] symptoms.

A very limited quantity of urine, passed with difficulty, livid and oily, foreshadows death; livid, passed frequently but in scanty quantity, points to strangury; lividity coupled with minute, distinct particles consistently indicates respiratory trouble; a grainy lividity foretells affliction of the joints and rheumatism. If the womb presses upon the spine or diaphragm, it gives the surface of the urine a livid tinge.

Thin urine, white in color, is a sign of spleen, *dropsy, intoxication, nephritis, delirium, diabetes, rheumatism, black *bile, epilepsy, dizziness, chill of the liver, or (with a bilious fever) death; in the old it is a sign of debility or childishness; in those suffering in the neck or shoulders, of lipothymia [fainting]; in women, it is a sign of a number of complaints of the womb; and it also signifies hemorrhoids and condylomata [a callous lump or knob on the skin]....

If the urine is wine-colored, it means danger to health when it accompanies a continued fever; it is less to be feared if there is no fever. [It can be produced when] a caustic humor inflames the kidneys and liver; or when the renal vein ruptures; or when, its vessel broken, the menstrual blood passes from a woman's body. Dancing, overmuch coitus, running, and immoderate exercise produce the same signs in a healthy body. Blue-black urine follows this pattern too.

Urine tinged green indicates jaundice, spasm, severe fever, and finally death.

Part 2

The color of urine often misleads the physician in his assessment of it; but there is an exact law, a definite rule for judgment, to be found in its contents. Hippocrates, an author knowledgeable about nature, deferred other considerations and drew the seeds of his true doctrine from these things. Now we will enumerate, in order, the things contained [in urine] and will explain the significance of each.

[The possible contents are] the circle; bubbles; grit; cloudiness; spume; pus; grease; *chyme; blood; sand; hair; bran; lumps; scales; specks; sperm; ash; sediment; and rising *vapor.

If there is a thick, watery circle in the urine, the posterior part [of the head] is afflicted with *phlegm. Purplish and thick, the front of the head is afflicted with blood; pale and thin, the left side is afflicted with black bile. If the circle is reddish and thin, fiery *choler rages on the right side of the head. A leaden color means that the root of the senses is attacked, and that the affliction is passing on to the branches. If it turns from livid to red, the natural state of the brain is improving, and strength restored. If it takes on a greenish color, in fever, the bilious humor is bringing on delirium. If it is tremulous, the spinal members are affected; if black, it means either mortification or *adustion, depending on whether it was previously been greenish or livid.

Swollen, airy, persistent bubbles [rising to the top] indicate crudeness of the humors causing the illness; also prolongation of the illness, with nephritis, headache, *rugitum* [*rumbling of the guts*], vomiting, and diarrhea....

Color, consistency, duration, form, and place are the determining characteristics of urinary sediment. The color should be white, the consistency continuous, the form conical, the place the bottom of the vessel, and the duration marked. If the sediment is all these – white, continuous, lasting, conical – digestion will be good, *virtue strong, and natural action will flourish with a triple activity: it whitens, it cleanses, and it condenses, concentrates, and unites. [This shows that] the natural heat is dissipating *ventosity and absorbing vapor; that the natural force is absorbing what is beneficial and resisting what is not; that nature's actions are not interrupted or stopped. The sure indication of health derives from these signs. Let the fever have a favorable *crisis, and the illness will be of short duration....

51. SIGNS AND DIAGNOSIS (2): *EPITOME ON PULSES*

Galen wrote many treatises on pulse and promised his readers that he would one day produce a comprehensive overview. He never did, but the anonymous thirteenth-century Summa pulsuum *(Epitome on Pulses) set out to fill that gap in a format suitable to scholastic medical instruction. Pulse is the sensible manifestation of the heart, just as urine is the sensible manifestation of the liver (two of the three "principal organs" of the Galenic system). It should be borne in mind that according to Galenic physiology, the function of the pulse is to cool the heat of the body, to impel *spirit through the arteries to the members, and eventually to discharge waste *vapors via exhalation. The different rhythms of the pulse were decoded to reveal the body's condition, both psychological and somatic. But pulse was also a prognostic sign, particularly when an element of* *quantification was thrown in: it is instructive to compare this to the quantification of pharmacy illustrated in doc. 55.*

The legend alluded to in the first paragraph relates that St Basil of Caesarea (330– 379), hearing that the Jewish physician had foretold his death after taking his pulse, prayed to God to delay his death a short while in order to demonstrate that the divine will override the laws of nature. Basil's prayer was granted and the Jew was converted. It is somewhat ironic that Archbishop Alfanus (Constantine the African's patron) was allegedly more impressed by the Jew than by the saint! In the chapter on differentiating pulses, only the first "consideration" is included in this translation. The second discusses the significance of the condition of the artery (hard or soft, full or empty, hot or cold). The third defines systole and diastole as the contraction and dilation of the vessel and explains the significance of systoles of various lengths. The fourth discusses the meaning of pulses that are growing stronger or weaker. The final consideration examines specific irregular pulses.

Source: trans. Michael R. McVaugh in *Sourcebook in Medieval Science*, ed. Edward Grant (Cambridge, MA: Harvard University Press, 1974), pp. 745–48 (n. 99) Latin.

Of all the indications of the internal disposition of the body, two are most reliable, the pulse and the urine. Now there are two principal members in the structure of the body, which sustain or transform the substance of the whole: these are the heart and the liver. According to Galen, all the *powers of the body are founded on these two members; they are alike in composition, and cause the whole body to be uniformly disposed. The heart and the liver fill the same places in the microcosm as the sun and moon do in the greater world. Just as innate heat passes from the sun through the air as a gift to all living things upon the earth, so too heat progresses from the heart, its source, via the *vital spirit; it consumes wastes and is propagated in many ways in generously supplying the [body] from the middle to the extreme [parts]. And the liver is analogous to the moon: for just as the moon communicates moisture to the regions next it, and as the full moon is adorned in fullest roundness when the sun casts its own rays upon it, just so the liver generates *humors and bestows a suitable humor on every member, while the strengthened substance of the members is sustained with the aid of the heart. Should the sun not regard the moon, the moon would suffer an eclipse, and the substance of the air be wholly darkened. Likewise, when the aid of the heart is lacking, and with it the members' nutriment, the relation of the distant parts to their neighbors is destroyed, weak associations are broken, and the marvelous union of the soul with the body is undone in many ways.

The urine, then, indicates the state of the liver and proclaims any hindrances to the internal members, as well as proclaims their functions. The pulse, on the other hand, reveals the condition of the heart and the general tenor of life, and by elucidating the passions of the soul, manifests the mind's secrets. Since, therefore, the life of the body and nutrition of the members is most excellent, a knowledge of the pulses far outweighs an understanding of urine. For this reason we have written this our epitome on pulses, fully and clearly compiled from Galen's great work on pulses, his epitome on the same, and the *Summa pulsuum* [*Epitome on Pulses*] of Archbishop Alfanus [of Salerno], skilled in both Greek and Latin. Archbishop Alfanus studiously pursued a knowledge of the pulses, led on by envy of the Jew who (as is told in the legend of St Basil) accurately foretold the saint's moment of death from a knowledge of his pulse.

The Definition of the Pulse

The pulse is the motion of the heart and arteries in diastole and systole so as to cool the natural heat and to expel vaporous waste. It is a motion of the heart, and from the heart to the arteries; but it is not a reversible motion, since it is not a motion of quality or alteration, nor is it an essential or general motion. It is thus a local motion, either direct or circular, and since it is not circular, it is direct. It is not simple but compounded of diastole and systole, of motion upwards and downwards. Its function is to cool the innate heat and to expel the vaporous waste, so that the spirit may be purified and tempered; this allows the establishment of bodily harmony, namely the conjunction and union of several distant parts. For since the soul (*anima*) is incorporeal and distant from the body, it could in no way inhere in bodily substance did not the spirit (*spiritus*), like an incorporeal body, serve as a middle term, to bring together distant substances and associate them harmoniously. Although the soul is simple in nature and neither inheres in the greater members to a greater degree nor in the lesser members to a lesser, it resides principally in the brain and heart, which it moves by its essence. But the agents of the soul differ naturally in competence. The heart is hollow, formed like a smith's bellows, containing heat, spirit, and humor. When the heat *resolves the blood into spirit and vapors, the spirit is taken up into the concavity of the heart, so that the substance of the heart is enlarged; a contraction follows, due to heaviness and the exhalation of spirit. The soul thus moves the pulse, like an artificer; and in the same way, with the artificer absent, his instruments are stilled.

The Different Kinds of Pulses

The varieties of pulses are differentiated by the physician in a number of ways, in particular according to five considerations: (1) motion of the arteries;

(2) condition of the artery; (3) duration of diastole and systole; (4) strengthening or weakening of pulsation; (5) regularity or irregularity of the beat. Ten varieties of pulse derive from these five considerations.

From the first consideration several varieties are derived. They are based on the quantity of arterial motion, of necessity either great, little, or in-between. These quantities can be classified as long, short, and intermediate; broad, narrow, and intermediate; obvious, hidden, and intermediate. A long pulse is that which can be felt over a space of four fingers or more; a short pulse does not occur over a full four fingers; an intermediate one is neither greater nor less. A broad pulse is felt over a width of four fingers or more; a narrow one occurs as if in a taut cord; an intermediate one does not surpass either limit. An obvious pulse is manifest to the touch; a hidden pulse escapes the sense of touch; and an intermediate pulse is felt to a moderate extent.

A long pulse indicates a plenitude of spirits filling the artery lengthwise: a short pulse, a deficiency of spirits. A long pulse signifies hotness; a short one, coldness; an intermediate one, temperateness. A broad pulse indicates moistness; a narrow one, dryness; an intermediate one, temperancy between the two. An open pulse indicates strong *virtue and a healthy organ; a hidden pulse, weak virtue and an unhealthy organ; and an intermediate pulse, the mean between the two. A long, broad, open pulse is called great; a short, narrow, hidden pulse is called small; and an in-between pulse is created of the means between these. A pulse can be long either naturally or unnaturally: naturally long means a lavish nature; unnaturally long means abundance and intensity of heat. A naturally short pulse indicates weakness and inadequacy for great undertakings; an unnaturally short one indicates weakness of heat and of the heart. A broad pulse and abundancy of moistness can occur either naturally or unnaturally: if naturally, it indicates a pliant nature and weakness in action; if unnaturally, it indicates dissolution of the humors and members. A naturally narrow pulse indicates constancy; an unnaturally narrow one aridity of the members and material solidity. An open pulse, natural or unnatural, indicates prodigality, effusiveness, and officiousness; also strength of heat and ease of arterial dilation. An unnaturally open pulse reveals a plenitude of vapors and excess heat, as in the drunk or feverish. A hidden pulse can also be either natural or unnatural; natural, it indicates taciturnity, secretiveness, and scanty heat or vapor; unnatural, it indicates a weakness of natural heat and the natural virtues. A long pulse can be either long and broad or long and narrow; similarly a short pulse can be either short and broad or short and narrow. Long indicates hotness, broad moistness; therefore long and broad shows that it results from a hot and moist humor, namely blood. Long and narrow indicates hotness and dryness and thus derives from a hot and dry humor, namely choler. Short and broad indicates the frigidity of earth and moistness and is thus derived from cold and moist [humor], namely phelgm. Short and narrow indicates coldness and dryness and derives from a cold, dry humor, namely *melancholy. An unnaturally long and broad pulse thus indicates the excessive domination, qualitatively or quantitatively, of blood. In quantitative excess, the contraction of the pulse to expel waste vapors from the heart is greater than its dilation to attract cold air to the heart; in qualitative excess, however, the dilation of the pulse to attract the frigid air is greater than its contraction to emit the vapors. Thus, when blood is in excess qualitatively and quantitatively, the pulse is unnaturally long and broad. When it produces *fever, the pulse is hot and biting; when it does not, the pulse is neither distempered in hotness nor biting. [A long, narrow pulse indicates] excess of choler, quantitative or qualitative. If the excess is quantitative, the pulse is not biting and contraction is greater than dilation; if it exceeds qualitatively, the pulse is biting and dilation is greater than constriction. A short, broad pulse indicates excess of *phlegm, either qualitatively or quantitatively. If qualitatively, the pulse is biting and dilation is greater than contraction. If quantitatively, the pulse is not biting and contraction is greater than dilation. A short, narrow pulse, which indicates melancholy, indicates qualitative excess when it is biting and dilation is greater; if it is not biting but slow, and the contraction is greater, it indicates quantitative excess.

A second variety of pulse derived from the first consideration, namely the motion of the artery, is taken from its quickness, slowness, or intermediate speed. A rapid pulse is a dilation that ends more rapidly than it begins; a slow one is a dilation that ends more slowly than it begins; and an intermediate one is midway between the two in rapidity. A naturally rapid pulse indicates capacity for resolution and sharpness of dissolving heat, as in a person with quick breathing or quick speech. An unnaturally rapid pulse indicates overabundance, while a naturally rapid pulse shows the man to be quick in all the works he undertakes.

A third variety of pulse is taken from its strength or weakness. A naturally strong, great, rapid pulse indicates a strong man; a weak pulse indicates failure of strength....

On Foretelling Life and Death by the Pulse

The hour of death can be foretold by the failing pulse on a *critical day, and the hour of convalescence determined by a rising one. Suppose, for example, that the patient has a failing pulse; whether he will die or not from this sickness is determined thus. You must reckon from the first failure of his pulse to the second, [finding] the time of day when it happens and the number of beats between the two – say you find thirty beats between the first and second failures at the third hour of the day. But since it is improper for you to stay there in continual calculation, come back the next day at the same hour and count the beats of his pulse again. The first day you counted thirty beats between one failure of the pulse and the next; if now the failure comes on the fifteenth beat, so that you have fifteen strong beats where before you had thirty, it is a sign that when the same number of hours have passed once more, having lost [a further] fifteen beats, the patient will die at that moment.

You should treat a rising pulse in the same way. Suppose someone has a faint pulse, almost failing; you should reckon from the first slightly stronger pulse to the second, determining both the time of day and the number of beats between the two strong pulses. Suppose between the first and second slightly stronger pulses you find thirty beats to occur, so that the thirtieth beat is stronger than the other beats – this at the third hour of the day; and suppose the next day at the same hour you count his pulse again. The first day you found thirty beats between the first and second stronger pulses; now on the fifteenth beat you find a stronger one, so that the patient has picked up fifteen beats in those twenty-four hours. This is a sign that in the next twenty-four hours the patient will not lose but will gain another fifteen beats, and that at that moment the *crisis will pass and the patient be relieved and improved.

If you cannot return to the patient at the same hour when you first counted his pulse, and must come back earlier, or later, then, taking his pulse, determine precisely the number of beats, and the number of hours that have passed, and carefully calculate according to the above procedure, taking into account the large or small time difference; you will then be able to make marvelous predictions.

52. CAUSES: THE CASE OF EPILEPSY

In The Sacred Disease, *Hippocrates argued that epilepsy was not divine possession, but a purely natural disorder caused by excessive *phlegm blocking the channels to the brain. Though* The Sacred Disease *was not available to western medieval readers, its explanation of epilepsy filtered through ancient and Arabic sources to shape the scholastic view of this disease. Perhaps because it was so dramatic and frightening, epilepsy became something of a showcase for discussing rational theories of disease causation or *etiology. Arnau of Vilanova (see doc. 44) takes full advantage of the occasion to lay out the physiological origins of epilepsy and to elaborate a differential diagnosis. Bernard of Gordon (fl. 1283–1308) follows a different path. Though trained in the same Montpellier medical tradition as Arnau and, like him, a professor, Bernard is less systematic in his thinking and seems more attuned to clinical realities – what the patient experiences* *and what the doctor sees. Bernard was apparently the first medical writer to distinguish* petit mal *from* grand mal *epilepsy.*

a. Arnau of Vilanova, *Breviary of the Practice of Medicine* (*Breviarium practicae medicinae*), Chapter 22

Source: trans. Edna P. von Storch and Theo. J.C. von Storch, "Arnold of Villanova on Epilepsy," *Annals of Medical History*, n.s. 10 (1918): 252–54. Latin.

... I hold that epilepsy is an *occlusion of the chief *ventricles of the brain with loss of sensation and motion; or epilepsy is a non-continuous spasm of the whole body. This disease takes its rise from different causes, such as superfluous foods and drinks, or poisons, the bites of mad dogs or reptiles, from poisoned, corrupt, and pestiferous air. When the pores are constricted, and superfluities are retained, and natural heat is lessened, there follows a filling up of the chief ventricles of the brain. And these are the three causes which principally induce epilepsy.

Epilepsy is of two kinds, one true, the other false. True epilepsy comes from phlegm; false epilepsy comes from *melancholy mixed with phlegm. Likewise there are three species of epilepsy according to the threefold diversity of places in which the cause itself is contained. The first species is properly called epilepsy. It comes from a defect of the brain, or from matter existing in the brain and not coming from outside. Of this type, the infallible sign is that victims suddenly fall, emit a great foam, and do not speak. They have a heaviness in the head and there are not present the same signs as in other types. There is a second type called *analepsy. This comes from matter existing in the stomach, not in the cavity of the stomach itself – as some have maintained, and erroneously – but in the veins, arteries, and *nerves of the stomach, through the midst of which the matter, boiling over, is snatched up to the brain. In this type, when the patient falls, he feels in the beginning of his attack a certain biting and gnawing in the stomach, a ringing in the ears, and this is because the fumes which then ascend from the stomach to the brain occlude the ventricles of the brain itself. Sometimes this type is accompanied by vomiting at the onset of the attack. There is a third type, called catalepsy, which comes from matter contained in the extremities, such as the hands, feet, etc. Such victims, at the onset of the attack, feel in their extremities a forcible carrying away, as if by ants, from the matter ascending upward. They are saved by constricting the extremities, as Galen tells about a certain writer who felt in his foot the matter of this disease ascending to his brain. Galen had him bind his tibia and thus prevented the matter from rising any higher. If the matter of this disease is contained in the intestines, during the attack such patients void the feces. If it comes from some defect in the womb, or the semen too long retained and turned into poison, they void, during the attack, the menses, or semen, or urine. Whichever *humor be the cause, it is recognized by the following symptoms. If blood be the cause, there will be a sanguinary disposition in the body, with flushed countenance and swelling of the veins. When age, preceding diet, hot or wet climate, time of the year all coincide in heat and moisture, they are clearer symptoms. When phlegm is the cause, it is recognized by a phlegmatic disposition of the body, by superfluities abounding in the mouth and nose, tastelessness in the mouth and heaviness in the head; when there is pallor on the surface of the body, and diet, climate, age and season of the year coincide with it, they make us more certain. When melancholy is the cause, it is recognized by a melancholic disposition of the body, by the roundness and surface of the body, which is of an ashen color. Likewise age, climate, season of the year, and similar details indicate the same thing. From choler this disease does not come. Note also, that when it does come from blood or phlegm, it is more manifest, and the patient falls at the full moon. But when it comes from melancholy, the patient falls at the new moon. Note, too, that when this disease occurs between infancy and puberty in males, or infancy and the first menstruation in females, it can be cured; after that, only rarely and with the greatest difficulty will it be cured.

b. Bernard of Gordon, *Lily of Medicine (Lilium medicinae)*, Part 2, Chapter 25

Source: trans. Adrian P. English in William G. Lennox, "Bernard de Gordon on Epilepsy (trans. by Adrian P. English)," *Annals of Medical History*, 3rd ser., 3 (1941): 373–74. Latin.

Epilepsy is a disease of the brain, removing sensation, motion and erection from the whole body, accompanied by a very serious disturbance of movement, because of an occlusion made in the non-principal ventricles of the brain.

The cause of this disease is a humor or coarse *windiness occluding the non-principal ventricles of the brain, impeding the passage of breath to the members, and therefore [the patient] is driven to fall suddenly to the ground. He feels absolutely nothing, nor can he in any way stand erect, but necessarily falls, unless the epilepsy be very mild, as will be seen. The movement of the feet and hands is agitated, disordered, and so is the breathing. Therefore, because of the disturbance in the breathing, there is always foam in the mouth. If the principal ventricles of the brain were to be occluded, it would be *apoplexy, because the matter is the same in both cases and it is in the same part of the body, save that in apoplexy the great and principal ventricles are occluded, but in epilepsy the small ones. Therefore the paroxysm of epilepsy is short, and not of itself fatal; but a paroxysm of apoplexy is continuous until death, which comes in a short time. If it happens that the paroxysm passes off within four days, the patient will be freed, but will lapse into paralysis.

Since, then, the matter of epilepsy is in the non-principal ventricles of the brain, and is situated near the heads of the nerves, the matter is grounded in the nerve, and the nerve is distended sidewise and curtailed lengthwise. And so epilepsy is a spasm, or accompanied by a spasm filling the whole body. The nerves are shortened, and drawn toward their source, so that, as Avicenna says, they can the better expel what is injuring them. Yet sometimes the matter is so subtle that a spasm is not greatly in evidence. Such an occlusion comes from phlegm, and this very often. Next, it comes from melancholy, then from blood, although rarely from blood alone. It comes less from *choler than from any other humor, for it comes from coarse windiness and *vapors and *resolved humors, but always the matter is poisonous, fetid, and disgusting.

Helping causes are the South Wind and the North Wind when it follows upon a South Wind; and everything which quickly and suddenly heats the head, such as a long stay in the sun, or bath, or close to the fire; or else excessive coldness, or abundance of food and drink, drunkenness, abundance of smoky foods, such as garlic, onions, and the like, and in all cases a poor regimen, since this disease comes only from a poor regimen and bad diet, as Galen writes on the aphorism [of Hippocrates beginning] "Epilecticorum uero iuuenibus" [Aphorisms 2.35 "In curing epilepsy in the young ..."]. This disease, which is so disgusting, comes only from a disordered diet, and particularly in those who had a head weak from birth, because in these cases only a slight disorder is sufficient, but in others it must be severe.

Epilepsy, then, comes from either a secret cause or from some antecedent and remote cause. This is said because it sometimes comes from the brain, sometimes from other parts, since the evil, poisonous fumes sometimes ascend from the chest to the head, occluding the ventricles, and so induce a paroxysm of epilepsy. Sometimes it comes from the stomach, sometimes from the liver, the spleen, the kidneys, the intestines, the bladder, the feet, hands or thumb.

Epilepsy sometimes observes periods, sometimes not, so that it sometimes follows the motion of the sun, and comes once from year to year. Sometimes it follows the motion of the moon, so that it sometimes occurs in the first quarter, which is very moist, and the second, which is much more moist, if not actually, at least apparently, and according to rarefaction. Sometimes it occurs in the days after a full moon and then a colder matter is indicated. Sometimes two or three or even more cycles pass. Sometimes it comes from defects in the womb and the corruption of semen and menstrual blood. This may, perhaps, not be corrigible by the cure. Sometimes it comes from the uterus. Sometimes the paroxysm is very long and violent, sometimes short. I have often seen it so short that the patient had only to lean against a wall or the like, rub his face, and it ceased. Sometimes he did not need a support, but there came to him a dizziness in the head, and blindness in the eyes, and he himself, sensing it, recited the Hail Mary, and before he had finished it, the paroxysm had passed off, and he spat once, and the whole thing passed off, and it used to come often during the day. There are some who after a paroxysm remember absolutely nothing about the attack, nor their affliction, and there are some who remember and are ashamed. Some defile themselves during a paroxysm, some vomit, some defecate, some suffer a pollution [*emission of semen*]. All of these things occur according to the diversity of the matter in quantity, quality, and site in the particular patient. Sometimes epilepsy comes because of worms. Sometimes it is a composite disease, because it is joined with *syncope, as in widows and chaste men, since the vapor of the corrupted semen, being turned into poison, goes to the heart and induces syncope, passing thence to the head and inducing epilepsy. It comes also from a horrible sight, such as the sight of lightning, or of a great sound, as of thunder, or a loud bell or the like. It comes also on account of those things which by their very nature induce epilepsy. There are many things of this kind, such as: if a boar be excoriated, and immediately a naked man dons the skin, he will become epileptic: also, if the man be *suffumigated with the horns. The same is true of galbanum, myrrh, and garlic. Epilepsy often comes to children either because of some disorder in their nurse, or when the children drink wine, and become drunk; and sometimes epilepsy comes on account of poisonous reptiles.

53. SCHOLASTIC THERAPEUTICS (I): RHAZES, *BOOK FOR ALMANSOR*

Abû Bakr Muhammad b. Zakariyyâ' al-Râzî (d. 925), known in the West as Rhazes, was the most prolific and formative medical author of the Arab-Islamic world. Like Avicenna, he thought of himself as a philosopher as well as a physician and tacitly modeled himself on Galen, even though he criticized many of Galen's tenets. For his patron al-Mansur, governor of Rayy (near modern Tehran), Rhazes wrote a comprehensive treatise on therapeutics. It was translated into Latin by Gerard of Cremona in the late twelfth century as the Book for Almansor. *By the fourteenth century, book 9 of this treatise – a head-to-toe survey of diseases – had a firmly established place in the medical curriculum. The excerpt from the chapter on weakness of the stomach translated here is accompanied by the commentary of Syllanus de Nigris of Pavia. Syllanus was enrolled in the College of Physicians in Milan on 23 March 1458, but otherwise he seems to be a rather obscure medical figure, and this is his only traced work. The commentary can hardly be described as profound or brilliant, but its very banality makes it a good illustration of how therapeutics could be subjected to scholastic methods.*

Source: trans. Faith Wallis from Rhazes, *Almansoris liber nonum cum expositione Sillani* (Venice: Bonetus Locatellus, 1490), fols. 46r–47v. Latin.

When weakness of the stomach occurs with little thirst, with the food passing out of the stomach slowly, and with acid belching, and when all these symptoms are minor and not long-standing, the stomach should be treated with *troches of roses; the patient should take in the morning one and one-half times the weight of a gold coin, together with one ounce of a *decoction of seeds [*that is, plants and spices*]. Now the decoction of seeds is [prepared like] this. Take Nabatean sermountain and cow-parsley; boil it in 100 drams [of water] until the water turns red. Afterwards, give it as a drink together with the troches of roses, as we said above. Troches of roses are [prepared like] this: take 3 drams of powdered red roses and 1 dram each of aloes wood, spikenard, mastic, cassia wood, camel's hay, cinnamon and wormwood; moisten with old wine and form into troches. Let [the patient] be nourished with things that are easy to *digest and which produce little in the way of *humors or superfluities, and which are seasoned with aromatics and spices.... Let him take vigorous exercise before his meal and drink less water than usual, and after the meal let him sleep a good deal, and he should drink a small amount of pure, old wine. And let him reduce his total intake of food.

Syllanus de Nigris's Commentary

[The author] *determines concerning weakness of the stomach, and [the determination] is divided into three. First he sets out the treatment when [the condition] arises from cold; secondly, [when it arises] from heat; thirdly from dryness.... The first is divided into two: first, he sets out the treatment when the weakness of the stomach is recent, and secondly, when it is long-standing.... [Of these], the first is [divided] into two. First he sets forth the treatment with troches of roses and the decoctions of seeds; secondly he sets forth a description of the decoction of seeds and the troches.... Concerning the first, it is said that weakness of the stomach occurs with little thirst, delayed passage of food through the stomach and acid belching. From these signs it should be inferred that the weakness comes from cold. The reason is evident. Secondly he says that where the aforementioned signs are minor and not long-standing, the stomach should be treated by giving troches of roses in a *potion, one and one-half the weight of a gold coin every day in the morning with one ounce of the decoction of seeds. The reason is because these things are hot and *styptic. Troches of aloes wood are effective for the same condition. Troches of capers are effective for the same condition, and also troches of *diarodon* [*a compound remedy based on roses*].... He sets out the description of the decoction of seeds and of the troches of roses; first he sets out the first, and secondly the second.... Concerning the first he says what the decoction of seeds is. Take Nabatean sermountain and cow-parsley and boil it in a *mina* [of water] until the water turns red and give some of this with the troches. Then he sets out the description of the troches of roses, which is: take 3 drams of [powdered] red roses and 1 dram each of aloes wood, spikenard, mastic, cassia wood, camel's hay, cinnamon, and wormwood; moisten with old wine and form into troches. For the same: if one ounce of distilled spirits (*aqua vitae*) can be given in the drink each time.... He sets out the dietary treatment, saying that the patient should be nourished with things that are quickly digested. The reason is because the digestion is weakened. Secondly: he says that those things with which he is nourished should produce little in the way of superfluities. Thirdly: he says that these things should be seasoned with aromatic spices. These are galingale and other spices that open the stomach, like pepper and ginger, cloves, cow-parsley, and the like. Fourthly: he says that before dining he ought to take much vigorous exercise. The reason is that that it refreshes and warms the stomach. Fifthly: he says that he should drink less water than usual. The reason is because [water] chills and relaxes the stomach. Sixthly: he says that after dining he should sleep a good deal. The reason is because it helps with the consumption [of the food], strengthening digestion and restoring heat. Seventh: he says that he should drink pure, old wine, because it warms the stomach. Eighth: he says that he should take less food than usual. The reason is that the *vital power is insufficient to digest a great quantity of food. Note that suitable foods are the flesh of rams, kids, of chickens, of flying and walking birds, of hen-pheasants, pigeons, quails and the like, roasted rather than boiled, and seasoned with spices, [as well as] soft-boiled eggs, and foods of this kind.

54. SCHOLASTIC THERAPEUTICS (2): JOHN OF GADDESDEN ON SMALLPOX

John of Gaddesden (ca 1280–1361) received his medical education at Oxford and also trained in theology. He was a distinguished medical writer in his day: in the Canterbury Tales, *Chaucer's Physician was said to be well versed in "Bernard and*

Gatesden and Gilbertyn" – that is, Bernard of Gordon (see docs. 52b and 55), John of Gaddesden, and Gilbert the Englishman (see doc. 69a). The title of John's treatise on therapeutics, The Rose of Medicine (Rosa medicinae), *was probably suggested by Bernard of Gordon's* Lily of Medicine (Lilium medicinae). *John claims that he chose the title because the rose has five petals, and his book was divided into five parts; moreover, just as the rose excels all other flowers, so his book is superior to all other treatises on medicine.*

Instead of the conventional head-to-toe order, John organized his material into three books on "common diseases" and two on "particular diseases." Within the individual chapters, however, John follows the usual template of a practica: *the definition of the disease is followed by its causes, symptoms ("signs"), prognosis, and cures.*

Smallpox is an exceptionally virulent disease; unless vaccinated, almost all who are exposed to it contract it. The pathogen travels in the powder or dust of dried pustules and can survive for a long time on clothing, furniture, etc. Hence the argument that it was either congenital or environmental made sense to pre-modern observers; indeed, John never mentions that smallpox is communicable. The appearance of the pustules coincides with a drop in the *fever – *a fact that reinforced the perception of the body successfully expelling morbid* *humors *from its interior to the surface. Humoral theory also allowed medieval physicians to explain the variable symptoms of smallpox.*

John's use of "color therapy" reflects an ancient belief that enveloping or surrounding the patient with the color red could speed recovery from smallpox and inhibit scarring. It is found even in ancient Chinese medicine and was still the subject of experimentation at the turn of the twentieth century. John had a personal interest in this treatment because he attended one of the sons of King Edward I when he fell ill with smallpox, and apparently he cured him by this method.

Source: trans. Faith Wallis from [John of Gaddesden], *Rosa anglica* (Pavia: [Leonardus Gerla, 2nd press, for] Joannes Antonius Biretta, 24 Jan. 1492), book 2, c. 4, fols. 50r–51v. Latin.

On Smallpox

Smallpox (*variole*) are so called from the multifarious manner (*varie*) in which they lie upon the skin, because they take hold of diverse parts of the skin by forming *apostemes and by *infecting with corrupt blood, and in this respect they differ from *morbilli* [*probably chicken-pox*] and *punctilli* [*probably measles*]. *Morbilli* are small apostemes on the skin generated by red *bile, and they are diminutive apostemes because they take up less space due to the sharpness of *choleric matter. For in true smallpox there are choleric matter and very small pustules. But *punctilli* are bloody infections that resemble flea-bites, except that they persist. And there are two kinds of *punctilli*: large and small. I have spoken already about the small kind. But the large ones are infections which are extensive, red, and not easily seen, on the shins of people who are poor and *consumptive, and who regularly sit close to the fire with their shoes off; in English they are called "measles." Smallpox is defined as small apostemes or pustules appearing on the skin, mostly red in color, sometimes extending deeply into the flesh, and infecting the whole body. It arises from the corruption of menstrual blood, and runs in a course of dangerous crises. It is generally preceded by a short *putrid fever, that is, a continuous [fever originating] in the blood. This is also the case with *morbilli*, except that they are smaller and [arise] from choler.

Cause. According to Haly [*'Alî ibn Ridwân, ca 998–1061*] in his commentary on part 2 of Galen's *Art of Medicine* [the passage beginning] "Unnatural swellings ...", these diseases come about because in a person in whom there is residual menstrual blood or corrupt blood which is in a state of ebullition, nature expels all the superfluity of a bloody fever or a continuous choleric fever to the surface of the body. Smallpox and *morbilli* are generated from these things, because they come about from menstrual blood. Averroes says in his chapter on *morbilli* that no one can avoid incurring smallpox. And these are his very words: Because every member has an expulsive *virtue which commands the other, this is the cause of smallpox and *morbilli*. And for this reason, no one can escape from these two [diseases], because they arise from bad material which is embedded in the nutriment of the embryo, that is, in the menstrual blood. Therefore, a *sanguineous continuous fever often arises. And these [diseases] are generated accidentally if conception takes place during the menstrual period, and in that case such a person can only rarely escape leprosy or a terrible illness. Likewise [these diseases] are generated from foods and from humors that are easily thrown into a state of ebullition, such as animal blood and broth; and in a similar manner from watery foods, when something hot is consumed directly afterwards – for example if one takes wine on top of milk or ginger on top of fruit and garlic and onions on top of fish, because this causes ebullition – and [also from] sexual relations with a menstruating woman and eating the flesh of cattle or drinking a lot of wine or new ale, as well as neglecting bloodletting. And it sometimes happens that a person can get smallpox twice, when the [morbific] matter is not completely expelled the first time. [It also happens] when a person eats figs frequently, because this expels matter to the surface. Likewise a pestilence of the air can generate [these diseases]. And therefore a hot and humid *complexion is more susceptible than a dry one, and the time of infancy and childhood and sometimes adolescence more than youth or old age, because in old age it does not occur except in [periods of] great heat, or in a region which is hot and humid. But as Isaac [Judaeus] says in his *On Fevers* 5, it never affects those who are extremely old. As for the season of the year, these [diseases] happen more in spring than in winter, and more in autumn, particularly towards the end when preceded by a hot, dry summer; likewise in a season when the south wind is blowing more than at any other time, and remaining under a hot sun makes the blood ebullient and helps to generate this disease. And there are four types of smallpox: sanguine, which are [characterized] by broad red [apostemes]; choleric, which have [apostemes] that are red, pointed, stabbing and not very broad; *phelgmatic, which have broad, white ones; and *melancholic, which have black or purplish or livid or green according to the state of the melancholy, whether its material is natural or more or less *adust. Here it should be further noted that smallpox does not strike a fetus in the maternal womb, because in [the fetus] the heat is dampened and so there is no ebullition; secondly, because the natural virtue is intense, in order to shape the members; and thirdly because the *emunctories are wanting; fourthly, because the heat of the womb preserves the menstrual blood so that it does not become ebullient or corrupt. Again, one should note that it is not necessary for everyone to incur smallpox, although Isaac in *On Fevers* 5 says that this is so. But it should be understood this way. People will be susceptible to this [disease] because of menstrual blood remaining in the fetus after birth, unless it is expelled in the urine and stool or sweat or through bloodletting. A man will incur [smallpox] in reality, or he will be susceptible of leprosy more than others, unless the conception take place in a woman who is cleansed (that it, healthy) after her menstrual *flux, and unless the father is healthy and follows a good regimen, and the fetus have a good complexion, and unless the person lives in a moderate fashion, not gluttonous and ill-regulated. This, however, is rare, because as [Hippocrates] says in *Prognosis* 2, people do not exert themselves except to eat. Again it should be noted that there are two kinds of smallpox: [smallpox] in the strict sense, and [smallpox] in the loose sense. [Smallpox] in the strict sense arises from menstrual blood that becomes ebullient within, and this particularly happens in children. [Smallpox] in the loose sense arises from corrupted food that has been attracted from the interior of the body to the surface by strong external heat, and this can happen at any age, and they can itch. And therefore Avicenna says in book 4 of the *Canon* that sometimes a person can have smallpox twice, once in the strict sense and the second time in the loose sense. So much for this.

Signs. If the smallpox arise from the blood, then [the pustules] will be pointed at the top and broad at the base. They will quickly *ripen and be converted into *sanies. They are healthy, because their matter is blood, and blood is the friend of nature and amenable to *digestion. And if [the patient] is of a hot and moist complexion and the season is spring and the [wind] southerly and all these [circumstances] come together, then it is certain that [the smallpox] comes from the blood. If they are choleric, then [the pustules] are pink tinged with yellow, small, round and their tops are pointed. They produce a stabbing pain like a pin, because of the sharpness of their matter. In reality, they are *morbilli,* and if the *concocted [matter] appears in the urine on a *critical day with diminution of the pain and fever, and if the pox appear, and then moisture emerges from them, then it is a good sign. If they are phlegmatic, then they are white and broad and soft and difficult to digest. The matter which is prepared or putrefied under the skin generates a great itching, if the phlegm is salty. And when they begin to itch, they break open and emit stained [?] and putrid matter. If the urine is unconcocted, they presage death. Melancholic ones are livid to start with and then virid, that is, blackish. There is no moisture in them; they are large and hard, like big warts. Hence they are the worst, and they have no quality which is capable of being brought to maturation. Therefore they dry out and crack open, and this produces fainting and loss of strength, and when these [signs] appear, one can prognosticate death. In a blood-based fever, the signs which precede smallpox are headache and backache, because of the great quantity of corrupt blood spreading through the vein on the back. In smallpox [there is] redness and swelling of the face, turbulence of the eyes and tears; but in *morbilli* there are more tears, and less back pain, because the [pustules] are generated from the vehemence of the evil nature of a small amount of corrupt blood. But in this case there is great swelling and distress. Heaviness of the head also precedes smallpox; pain and stabbing precede smallpox, because it affects all the members of *similar parts, seen and unseen, so that it causes itching in the lining of the lungs and the throat and sneezing in the nostrils, sharp pain in the chest, and hoarseness of voice. Continuity [of the flesh] is broken because of the exiting [of the morbific matter], as if thorns or needles had pierced it. Sleep is anxious and the sputum thick … the patient seems to see lights. And when [the pustules] begin to appear, they are like pinheads, or grains of millet, or like the head of an ant. Then they start to multiply and grow larger; then they form a crust and produce sanies; and then they dry out and fall off. Avicenna says that sometimes they emerge in double form, with one inside the other, and these are very bad. And the sign of the magnitude of the [morbific] matter is its viscosity; therefore [the pustules] are fatal in those whose *powers are weakened. And then when they [are doubled] like this, there is pain deep down in the pustule and likewise on the surface, and after they fall off another remains, and so on.

Prognosis. We can prognosticate that the white [pustules] are better when they are few in number and large in size and emerge easily with little distress and a slight fever. The fever diminishes when they appear, and its course will resemble that of tertian or quartan [fever.] If they are large and white and numerous, close together without merging together, they are less bad. But if they are white, small, hard, close, and come out with difficulty because the matter is gross, then they are bad and will cause frequent distress before they can ripen. But if the smallpox emerge in a variable fashion, so that sometimes [the pustules] appear and sometimes they are hidden, and particularly if they are purplish, with debility of strength, these are fatal. But if strength is not debilitated, there is hope for a good outcome. And therefore if they are inclining towards blackness, and if they are large, they are fatal in most cases....

Cure. There are many things to be done to cure this disease. First, one should *evacuate [the patient] with bloodletting and an *emetic which is slightly cooling or constricting, not one which attracts or dissolves. Secondly, one should *alter [the patient] within by means of acidic substances, provided that constriction of the chest does not impede this, or else with cold and strengthening digestive remedies – *styptics, so to speak. Thirdly, one should give [the patient] those things that help readily to expel [the pustules]. Fourthly, one should protect the eyes, chest, nostrils, and bowels from [the pustules] with *repellent [remedies], because of the noble nature of these organs. And the repellents should work to drive the poisonous matter from the interior [of the body] to the exterior. Fifthly, [the patient] should be dried out with infusions; this cannot be done before ripening is complete. Sixthly, on the day after [the pustules] erupt, dry, clean, and consolidate [them]. And if they do not erupt on their own, they should be opened with a golden needle. Seventh, one should eliminate all scars of the smallpox, and cure them, and fill them in. As to the first [treatment]: know that if the body is *plethoric or if blood dominates, and if the vital power is strong and the age of life and other circumstances are in agreement, one should let blood at the outset from the common median vein and then from the tip of the nose, particularly in children, because this kind of bloodletting preserves the upper parts from the evil nature of the smallpox and it is easy for infants....

As to the third: ... take red scarlet [cloth] or another type of red fabric, and wrap the smallpox patient up completely in it, as I did with the son of the most noble king of England when he was sick with this disease, and I made everything that was around his bed to be red; and this is a good cure. In consequence, I cured him without any vestiges of the smallpox. However, one should take care not to anoint the region of the smallpox after [the pustules] emerge, because this will block the pores. [The patient] should not be exposed to cold air unless the [surrounding] air is very hot. In that case the air should be tempered with willow leaves and by sprinkling water and roses and camphor about the house, and with water combined with camphor. Likewise the limbs of the patient should be bound, or he should wear gloves all the time, lest he scratch himself; and he should not touch himself, because that will make an ugly pit in the skin. Then take juice of fennel and of parsley, and when this is lukewarm, soak linen cloths in it and wrap up the whole body. For this will draw the [morbific] matter to the surface and partially consume it. Or make a decoction of senna or parsley in water with lentils and dried figs, and then soak a linen sheet in it, and squeeze out the juice, and wrap up the patient. After this – but not at the beginning [of the disease] – anoint [the patient], not with oil, but with the blood of an animal which is of a warm nature, such as a chicken, pigeon, or sheep, and afterwards let him be wrapped up in the aforementioned sheet. Do this often, but take care lest the dressings be roughly pulled off, particularly with children....

55. SCHOLASTIC PHARMACOLOGY: BERNARD OF GORDON

Bernard of Gordon's (see doc. 52b) On the Preservation of Human Life *grew out of his lectures to medical students, but its four component sections (on bloodletting, urines, pulse, and regimen) often circulated as independent treatises. Bernard's remarks on mathematical pharmacy are from the section on urines.*

*The impulse to quantify the action of drugs is rooted in Arabic Galenism's doctrine of grades or *degrees of intensity: *simples were classed as hot, cold, wet or dry on an ascending scale of one to four. Quantification received additional endorsement in Galen's* Art of Medicine, *where Galen remarked that if a part of the body were ten times hotter than normal and seven times drier, one would have to apply a remedy ten times colder and seven times wetter. Bernard's exercise in applying principles of quantification reflects the exceptional attention to the issue of degrees at Montpellier: it was a problem where natural philosophy, mathematics, and medicine intersected.*

*The context of Bernard's comments is a discussion of illness due to excess *phlegm, *where indigestion and fatigue are the presenting symptoms. Bernard offers a classic two-phase therapy: diet and pharmacy. His approach to compound drugs, however, departs from convention. Bernard not only analyzes the ingredients according to their "primary" and "secondary" qualities, but calibrates these to the "prime dose," or lowest effective* quantity. *Each degree is then assigned a mathematical weight expressed as a ratio of the quality to its opposite:*

> *hot in 1st degree* = *hot/cold ratio of 2:1*
> *2nd degree* = *4:1*
> *3rd degree* = *8:1*
> *4th degree* = *16:1*

Ingredients are then selected according to their qualities and weighed out in proportion to their degree-weight. To calculate the final "complexion" of the compound, multiply the number of prime doses used by the degree-weight.

But it is unlikely that doctors really constructed their prescriptions using this elaborate method. The second excerpt below is taken from the section of Bernard's famous manual of practice, the Lily of Medicine, *on indigestion. Bernard ascribes *digestion to a multitude of potential causes, including excess phlegm, which is the condition for which Bernard devised his model recipe in* On the Preservation of Human Life. *Notice that the recipe for the *syrup in the* Lily *uses the same ingredients, more or less, as the recipe in* Preservation; *however, that is where the similarity stops.*

a. Pharmacy in Theory:
On the Preservation of Human Life

Source: trans. Michael R. McVaugh, "Quantified Medical Theory and Practice at Fourteenth Century Montpellier," *Bulletin of the History of Medicine* 43 (1969): 409–13. Latin.

Chapter 8. Concerning Urine of Pale Color, Tending to Thickness in Substance, and Concerning the Cure of Phlegmatic Matter

A color tending to paleness, with substance tending to thickness, indicates the dominance of natural phlegm without *fever. The paleness of the urine is due to indigestion, the indigestion due to coldness; and the thickness is due to moistness mixed substantially with wateriness. Such a color tends towards milky or greyish or yellowish-green or yellowish, depending on the different degrees of indigestion, the different mixtures, and the various types of phlegm; by itself, however, it indicates nothing but abundance of phlegm. It is possible that there may be fever, but this cannot be discerned from the urine. The symptoms that commonly accompany indigestion and abundance of phlegm are heaviness of the stomach, little thirst, nausea and little appetite, loathing [for food?], heavy sleep with dreams of water, heaviness of the eyes and head, lassitude, indolence, a slow and feeble pulse, and poor memory and slow understanding (since according to Galen, part three of *De interioribus* [*On Affected Parts*], coldness in the first *degree and moistness in the second accompany mental confusion, so that such minds are weak and easily changed).

Abstinence is most suitable for the cure of such cases, for they carry food and drink with them: according to Galen, phlegm is changed into blood in time of need. Let them thus avoid all things moist and watery, all fruits, all oils, all fish, broths, egg-yolk, and bones. Wakefulness, exercise, dry and fried things are good for them. The [phlegmatic] matter is digested with those things that heat and dry, and with those things bearing on the stomach, since it is the part of the patient [involved]; we must therefore bear in mind the *dyscrasia and the part of the patient. Let them also avoid completely, from the very beginning, those things that are very hot, lest the matter heat up and so decay.

First of all, therefore, hyssop is prescribed, since it heats and dries in the third degree. The phlegm in the body is colder than it is, so that hyssop is suitable with respect to the primary qualities, since it renders subtle, while phlegm is gross, viscous, and *ventose; it is suitable with regard to the secondary qualities, and it is also suitable with regard to the tertiary qualities, since it evacuates the crude humors. Thus, because it has many profitable effects and none harmful, we make hyssop the base; and since according to Mesue we can use a great quantity of such things, of hyssop take one-half pound. Secondly, mint is prescribed, for according to Avicenna it is hot and dry in the second degree, and it has the property of strengthening the stomach and preventing decay; it soothes phlegmatic nausea, strengthens the appetite, and renders subtle. It is thus marvellously suitable. But since (according to Avicenna) it has excess moistness, reduce its quantity, and use four ounces. Thirdly, absinth [*the herb* Artemesia absinthium, *or wormwood*] is prescribed, which is hot in the first degree and dry in the second. It has many varieties, but the whitish one is not suitable in this case, since many of its virtues are remitted. Absinth *stypticifies, opens, and softens; by virtue of its stypticity it fortifies, but it opens and softens by virtue of its bitterness, and thus that which is not bitter is not suitable here. The stypticity of this variety is helpful, but many of its other properties due to its earthiness are not, especially when it is mixed with earthy substances, so that its quantity should be reduced; and since it is made abominable by its bitterness, we reduce it further and use three ounces. Fourthly calamint is prescribed, hot and dry in the third degree; and because it does not fortify and is of scant virtue, we reduce its quantity in comparison to the base, and use two ounces. Then aromatic seeds may be added, hot and dry, such as the seeds of fennel and anise; they are exceedingly *aperative and *subtiliative in relation to the material in the stomach, so we reduce their quantity and use one ounce of each. Because all these medicines are hot, we weaken them with roses. Use one ounce of roses to weaken them; and since [roses] strengthen and are aromatic, add another ounce, which makes two. If it is summer, this medicine is made up with loaf sugar; if winter, with honey, thus:

```
hyssop – one-half pound
common mint – four ounces
green-leaved absinth – three ounces
calamint – two ounces
anise
fennel – one ounce each
red roses – two ounces
```

loaf sugar – one pound
and make up a syrup.

This can also be made into an *electuary, or a condiment, an oil, a plaster, or a *decoction, with a little honey in an elixir if the patient is poor; and if he is naturally weak, remove the absinth and replace it with lemon rind, for lemon rind is hot in the first degree and dry in the third; and the odor of lemon, according to Avicenna, rectifies the *corruption and pestilence in the air. Thus in the composition of a medicine we must consider the errant matter, the dyscrasia, and the part of the patient involved.

Because the intensity of the medicine must be increased according to the degree of the dyscrasia, we must therefore know in what degree and fraction of a degree the medicine's intensity lies; if not precisely, at least approximately near the truth. For this we must turn to my book *On Degrees*, where the nature of this gradation is perfectly explained. But in order to make an approximation it is necessary to reduce the medicine to prime doses, and to set the qualities of one kind in one column and the others in another column; then compare them by the twofold method according to the rules given in the book *On Degrees*.

Let us say, for example, that the prime dose of hyssop in the fifth climate [*geographic zone of latitude*] is three ounces; then, since there is one-half pound of hyssop in this recipe, it contains two prime doses. From the first prime dose it has eight hot parts and one cold, and from the second the same; we have therefore 16 hot parts predominant, and two [parts] cold. In the second place came mint: let us suppose that four ounces is its prime dose, so that upon first being administered it can heat to the second degree. It will provide therefore four hot parts and one cold. We join these with the first, and in the column of hot there are 20 parts, while in the column of cold there are only three. In the third place came absinth: let us suppose that its prime dose is three ounces. It will have two parts hot and one cold, and if we join these with the others, there will be 22 parts hot and four cold. In the fourth place came calamint: supposing that two ounces is its prime dose, we have eight parts hot and one cold; adding, we get 30 parts hot and five cold. Fifth came the seeds: supposing that the dose of each is an ounce, there will be two prime doses. Thus from fennel, which is hot in the second degree, we get four parts of hot and one of cold; but since anise is in the third degree, supposing that one ounce is its prime dose, this gives us eight parts of hot and one of cold. If we now add, we have 42 parts hot and seven cold. Sixth were the roses, and supposing that their prime dose is one ounce, there being two ounces used, they will provide four parts of cold and two of hot; add, and there will be 44 parts of hot and 11 of cold. Now suppose that this medicine is compounded with sugar, let us say one pound of it; sugar being in the first degree of hotness, suppose its prime dose to be four ounces, and there will then be three prime doses; we get from the first dose two parts hot and one cold, from the second the same, and from the third likewise, and thus we will have six parts hot and three cold. Add, and there are 50 parts hot and 14 cold. (Although, according to Galen, *De simplici medicina* [*On simple medicine*] book 1, water is cold, we do not include it; for according to Galen's *Regimen* it is a constituent of foods and medicine, and so, being a constitutive material, is hot when in hot things and cold in cold. We therefore disregard it here.)

[Bernard's formula looks like this:

6 oz. hyssop	*3° H*	*16 : 2*
4 oz. mint	*2° H*	*4 : 1*
3 oz. absinth	*1° H*	*2 : 1*
2 oz. calamint	*3° H*	*8 : 1*
1 oz. fennel	*2° H*	*4 : 1*
1 oz. anise	*3° H*	*8 : 1*
2 oz. red roses	*1° C*	*2 : 4*
1 lb. sugar	*1° H*	*6 : 3*

50 : 14]

That we may see the degree resulting from the twofold method, let us see what ratio the dominant qualities have to the dominated. It appears that they are more than double, for then there would be only 28 parts hot – if it were so, it would be hot precisely in the first degree. Nor are they quadruple; then there would be 56, and it would be precisely in the second degree. Therefore, since they are more than double and less than quadruple, the medicine is hot between the first degree and the full second degree.... The gradation is quite rough, but it suffices for novices, since the doctrine is exactly and precisely communicated in the book *On Degrees.*

Let it be understood that the prime dose should be reduced for the inhabitants of the fourth climate, and increased for inhabitants of the sixth and seventh. I do not claim that these are the precise doses, but rather approximations of a sort; nor do I claim that the syrup is gradated to absolute perfection, only approximately. And it is to be understood that if the syrup is made with honey, the hotness is greater. It should also be understood that as has been said concerning the gradation of the active qualities, so too the gradation of the passive qualities proceeds by the double and by the half. And it should be further understood that in what follows I do not intend to assign a degree to each medicine, since that would be onerous for me and tedious for you. Rather, what I have said is to be taken as an example in accordance with the method of my book, since the theory of gradation is not enough by itself.

b. Pharmacy in Practice: The *Lily of Medicine*

Source: trans. Faith Wallis from Bernard of Gordon, [*Lilium medicinae*] (Venice: Bonetus Locatellus, 1498), *Particula* 5, c. 3. Latin.

On Indigestion of the Stomach Due to External Causes, and Internal Ones, Which Are: *Apostemes, Wounds, Pain, Debility, Excessive Sensation, and Some *Humoral Disorders

It should be understood that these things are very close to one another; it is virtually impossible to have one without another and the cures are all but identical. The stomach's [power of] *digestion is sometimes removed, sometimes diminished, sometimes corrupted. And these take place according to *intention and *remission, and the quality of the causes....

Cure

... But if the indigestion is due to cold humoral disorder, then it should be cured first. Let the patient take garlic and strong wine in small quantity, and keep the exterior members warm. And place leeches on the stomach, and take anise, sermountain, *ameos* [*possibly cow parsley or wild angelica*], cicely, spikenard, and aloes wood, and take a *potion seasoned with nutmeg, *diatrion pipereon* [*a compound medicine based on pepper*], and ginger.

And if the coldness is joined to dryness, reduce intake of hot and evaporative [foods]; and take milk, and barley-water with honey, and wine with water, and take this medicine:

Recipe: mastic and spikenard, boiled in oil, and applied to the stomach. Or soften wax in oil, mix with a small amount of naval pitch, and use as a plaster on the stomach.

And if the coldness is joined to wetness, eat boiled foods, and wine from the Black Sea, and take pepper and cinnamon, and use this syrup:

Recipe: 3 oz. each of hyssop, absinth, and calamint; 1 oz. each of anise, fennel, *ameos*, cicely, spikenard, *squinanti*, and aromatic cane; 1 pound of honey and roses. Make into a syrup. And with these ingredients one can make an oil, or an ointment, or [mix with] wax, and anoint the stomach with oil of balsam.

And if phlegm or *melancholy dominates in the stomach, let it be *purged, as stated above [in the section on] stomach pain.

And it should be known that if a little boy or girl is placed on the stomach, the digestive virtue is greatly strengthened. However, provided they do not sweat, a puppy or at very least a hand should be held on top of the stomach for a long time.

56. A PRIMER ON BLOODLETTING (1): LANFRANC OF MILAN'S SCHOLASTIC PHLEBOTOMY

*Galenic physiology posited that the body was constantly manufacturing blood from food. This blood was stored in the veins and taken up as needed by the various organs of the body. If the body produced more blood than it consumed, a medically dangerous state of *plethora might ensue, leading to *corrupt *humors and *fevers. Hence bloodletting was regularly practiced as a prophylactic measure. During illness, bloodletting could serve as an extreme *evacuation measure if diet or drugs failed to expel the morbific matter. It could also be deployed to shift morbific matter from one part of the body to another in order to facilitate its evacuation, or to steer it away from one of the principal organs.*

Lanfranc of Milan was one of the pioneering proponents of the new "rational surgery" in thirteenth-century Italy (see doc. 58). Around 1290, Lanfranc left his practice in Milan, possibly for political reasons, and emigrated to France, first to Lyons and then around 1295 to Paris. There he taught a course in surgery at the Faculty of Medicine. The following discussion of bloodletting is from Lanfranc's Great Surgery *(Chirurgia magna), completed in 1296.*

Source: trans. Michael R. McVaugh from Lanfranc of Milan, *Magna chirurgia*, tract 3, doctrine 3, c. 16, in *Sourcebook in Medieval Science*, ed. Edward Grant (Cambridge, MA: Harvard University Press, 1974), pp. 799–802. Latin.

*Phlebotomy is an artificial diminution of the blood contained in the veins. You know that although, because of our pride, the office of phlebotomy is today left to barbers, it was once the work of physicians, particularly when surgeons carried it out. Oh Lord, why is there such a distinction made today between the physician and the surgeon? Perhaps because physicians abandoned manual operation to laymen? Or because, as some say, they disdain to work with their hands? Or, as I believe, because they do not understand the method of operation which is necessary? This false distinction is so entrenched, because of surgery's earlier disuse, that some people believe that it is impossible for one man to have a mastery of both. Let everyone know, therefore, that a man who is wholly ignorant of surgery cannot be a good physician. Moreover, a surgeon who is ignorant of medicine ought to be held as nothing – rather, it is necessary for him to know every aspect of medicine well.

We use phlebotomy, generally, for three things: to preserve health, to protect it from possible sickness, and to remove an existing illness in one of the first two ways (which seem the same, but are different). Phlebotomy is called elective, since we can choose the time and hour, climate, or disposition of the patient, considering many particulars and waiting for the ideal time and moment. Although we consider many particulars when need be, nevertheless sometimes, omitting other particulars, we insist on nothing except the strength of [the patient's] forces. Actually, necessity may sometimes compel us to bleed him when his forces are weak, but then we do in three or four successive operations what could be done with stronger [patients] in one. We employ phlebotomy with those who eat considerable meat and drink good wine, and whose faculties (*virtutes*) produce considerable blood, even though it be healthy blood, and who take little exercise; particularly the young and certain old people who are used to it. This method of treatment is allied to the conservation of health. Secondly, we bleed those who suffer with a *sanguine pain in the joints, or a constant fever (*synocha*), or *quinsy, or pleurisy, or an intermittent pain. All these things can be avoided by treatment before the normal time of onset of the sickness, and this method is called preventative. Thirdly when a man suffers from a strong pain in the head without fever, from quinsy, pleurisy, pneumonia, hot *apostemes of the internal members, or any other illness that derives from an overabundance of blood, phlebotomy is performed to remove the incipient or established illness, and this method of treatment is called curative. The necessity for bleeding is common to these three general treatments; still, it is much better for a man to be governed by a regimen including adequate exercise and temperate food and drink, and better to live moderately and abstemiously when he feels himself replete, than to live in such fashion that he comes to require phlebotomy. I would say that this is equally true of laxative medicine.

Let me now propose three universal headings for phlebotomy, under which I will arrange my teaching on the subject. First will be what sort of man the bloodletter should be, and how he should carry out his office; second, who those people are who require phlebotomy; and third, which those veins are on which bloodletting should be carried out and how each vein should be opened.

A bloodletter should be a young man, neither a boy nor old; he should have steady hands and be wholly strong of body; he should have good and subtle sight, and should be able to recognize the veins, and to differentiate them from *nerves and arteries; and he should know the different places in which the veins that are to be bled may be opened, and should know how to avoid all danger in those places where the veins come near the nerves and arteries. He should also possess several lancets (*phlebotomos*) of steel, bright and clean, of different shapes, some of which should be fine and some somewhat bigger, some short and some longer, so that when it is necessary to open a large vein and make a large incision he may use a larger lancet, and the smaller one in the contrary case. He should hold the lancet with the thumb and index finger of his right hand and boldly palp the vein beforehand to find the best place for bleeding; and then, with these two fingers, insert the lancet in whatever vein he wishes.

As to the second topic, you should know that children should not be bled before puberty, save in urgent necessity – for example, if you saw someone suffocating from too much blood, as evidenced by shortness of breath, by the fullness of the jugular veins in his neck, by the redness of his whole face, or its fullness and humors, and by the bearing of his body. In such a case, before you bleed him, speak to his parents and friends as follows: "Do not say that I advised you that he should be bled, because I am not saying this; but I will say that phlebotomy is necessary in order for him to live. If he is bled and should die, it will not be because of the phlebotomy; but if he is cured, it can only be by bleeding; and if he were my son, I would have him bled, seeing no other way. Still, you choose whatever you or others think best." You should speak thus in all uncertain cases where something dangerous is to be done. Likewise old men should not be bled, particularly the more decrepit – although this rule is sometimes contravened, since there are certain old people whose forces (*virtutes*) are stronger than those of some young people. And those recovering from illnesses should not be bled, particularly when they have had a good, full *crisis; nor should pregnant women, particularly in the first three and last three months, even though they may be accustomed to being bled regularly, before and after the life [*that is, quickening?*] of the embryo, without it harming them. Youths whose color is white and pale, and whose beard is scanty and thin, and who have tiny veins, difficult to find, are not suited to bleeding; nor are those whose bodies contain crude and *melancholic humors, and who have little good blood, for that little blood should be guarded like a treasure. In this respect the French do much harm, since they bleed themselves when they are filled with gross, cold, corrupt humors; they see the *putrid, corrupt blood [drawn off] and think they have done very well to remove such blood. The barber will say, "See how much you needed that bloodletting; it will be necessary to draw some more soon"; but a man who goes to the barber all the time will be destroyed by [blood] letting. It is thus better for him to conserve his blood and to evacuate the corrupt humors by other means. Phlebotomy is also not proper for those who have the first stages of *cataract, nor indeed is any diminution of blood, especially with *cupping-glasses. But phlebotomy is proper in all the cases named above, for if a man eats much meat and drinks much wine, other things being in accord, he is not safe. Sanguine illnesses may be generated in him, or perhaps he may drop dead suddenly. But if he is bled, his health can be preserved longer. Likewise, he who habitually suffers from a sanguine rheumatism will no longer have pain if he is adequately bled before the time of its onset, unless you do something else harmful. This is true of all illnesses that are due to too much blood. In the case of one who suffers from a constant fever, phlebotomy is so necessary that to bleed him until he faints, before the fourth day, will either remove the fever or will so far reduce the matter that the remainder will not putrefy; but if he is not phlebotomized, the blood sometimes boils up into his chest because of the heat and collects there in such great quantity, given the size of the place, that the patient suffocates. Sometimes a vein bursts in the chest or in the lung, and if its flow is not restrained, the patient will die – unless his natural strength moderates the flow, as sometimes happens.... Generally, therefore, it is useful in all sanguine illnesses, which can never or rarely be cured without it.

Third, while the veins which branch from the ramose vein, which comes from the curve of the liver [*portal vein and vena cava*], continue to branch many times over, and although many people have extensively described their possible incisions, in the interests of brevity I will discuss here only the opening of those veins that are in use. There are three particular sites in either arm which are customarily bled. First, the cephalic vein, which is bled in two places, near and slightly above the bend of the elbow. You must bind the arm above the site and compress it slightly until the vein appears, and you should cut it broadly (*large*) since its narrow (*stricta*) incision can create numerous apostemes. You must beware lest you touch the muscle, which lies very near. This vein is also bled between the thumb and index finger, at and a little above their conjunction. It is bled for hot ailments of the head, and of the neck and the members from the breastbone up, generally. The basilic vein is bled in the lower part of the arm, where it too lies near the bend of the elbow; it is right over a large artery, or quite close to it, so that you must pay the greatest attention lest you touch it. It is also bled between the little and ring finger of either hand. Its bleeding is good for all ailments from the breastbone down and is also valuable in pursuing a preventive regimen against ailments of the head. The median vein is formed from the basilic and the above-mentioned cephalic veins and likewise opens in the lower arm near the elbow; you must be careful not to touch one of the two nerves between which it lies. Bleeding it is useful when you mean to evacuate the body, and therefore assists against ailments of the heart and of all the pectoral members, once these ailments are well-established – for before they establish themselves it is more useful to bleed from the basilic vein. [It is also good] against incipient ailments of the head, those which have not yet become established, since after their establishment bleeding is better from the cephalic vein, as has been said. Bleeding from the vein of the thumb is good for head ailments; so is bleeding from the cephalic vein, from which the vein of the thumb arises, but bleeding from the thumb weakens the patient less, and no mistake can arise from its bleeding.... I had as a patient a woman who had an almost unbearable pain in the head, whom I bled from the hand and also purged, to no avail; there was still more material in the front of the head, and the vein [in the forehead] was more prominent than usual, so that I ordered that it be opened, and she was soon well. When you want to bleed from this vein, constrict the neck, and cut the vein lengthwise. Sometimes this vein is also cut at its highest point; this is good for hardened ulcers of the head, for instance *saphati*, and for sanguine tinea, particularly if the head is bathed with the blood drawn off.

The veins in both temples may be bled for headache and eye ailments. I once treated a young man who was suffering from [a] persistent hot headache, repeatedly purged and bled him, and although he found some relief he continued to be troubled with the same thing. Then I cut the vessel (*arteriam*) on the afflicted side, cauterized it (lest it consolidate further), and thereafter his cure was lasting. Likewise, it is good for facial sores and headache to bleed from the veins in back of the ears. Incision of the veins of the tongue is good for quinsy, apostemes of the tongue or throat (when preceded by a bleeding from the cephalic vein), for acute *rheum of the eyes, prurigo, nasal sores, and dizziness, whenever these things are of a sanguine origin. Sometimes the jugular veins in the neck are bled when suffocation from excessive blood is feared, and sometimes too in cases of leprosy. The veins in the lower lip are bled for hot sores in the mouth, and for apostemes and hot ills of the gums. In the feet, three veins in each foot are frequently bled: one under the curve of the knee, bled for illnesses of the womb and to bring on menstruation – this vein strongly evacuates the entire body; another is between the heel and the ankle, on the inner side (called the saphenous vein), which is bled for diseases of the womb in women, and for apostemes of the testicles in men – always preceded by bleeding of the basilic vein on the opposite side; and on the outside lies the sciatic vein, which is similarly bled between the heel and the ankle, on the outside, for sciatica – this will cure it, as I have said.

Note that when you mean to bleed a second time at the same place, as sometimes happens (namely when you need to remove a great deal of blood but dare not do it all at once), then make the wound very broad, so that it will not consolidate; [and when you wish to bleed again,] bind the limb and rub the wound to make the place bleed again. Likewise, should you want to use phlebotomy to draw matter to the opposite side, when you have drawn off one third of the blood you wish to remove, put your finger over the wound so that no blood be lost, and make the patient spit; then let the blood flow again. Do this three or four times, for in this way the blood is better diverted to the opposite side and the patient's strength better conserved. Again, note that if the patient usually faints when he is bled, let the bleeding be done with him lying down; it is also good for him to eat beforehand a mouthful of dry bread in pomegranate wine. All veins should be opened along the length of the limb, although some men hold the opposite, except that if the veins of the foot are so fine that blood will not flow through a longitudinal incision, they should be cut laterally. When the veins of the head running from the neck are to be bled, as required above, the neck should be constricted until they stand out, and held tight until the desired quantity of blood is available. When the veins of the arm are to be bled, the arm should be ligatured four fingers above the place to be bled; but it should not be bound so tightly (as is done by some) that all feeling be lost to the arm. If you wish to bleed the veins of the hands or the feet, they should be put in hot water to warm for an hour, and constricted above the wrist or ankle; continue to keep the hand in hot water until you have withdrawn as much blood as you wish.

57. A PRIMER ON BLOODLETTING (2): THE "SIGN MAN": AN ASTROLOGICAL GUIDE TO *PHLEBOTOMY

This image is taken from a small folding almanac designed to be suspended from a doctor's belt. These almanacs contain medical information such as summaries of the diagnostic meanings of different colors of urine, alongside calendrical, astronomical, and astrological materials. The latter were chosen for their medical pertinence. Documents in chapter 8 explain in some detail the role of astrology in medical theory and practice; this "sign man," however, applies medical astrology to bloodletting. The underlying idea is that blood in the body, like the tides in the ocean, is controlled by the moon. As the moon makes its monthly circuit through the twelve constellations of the zodiac, it will cause blood in a specific part of the body to increase. For example, when the moon is in Aries, blood augments in the head; when it moves on into Taurus, blood increases in the throat, and so on through to Pisces, when blood swells in the feet. A physician should locate the moon in the zodiac before prescribing bloodletting, because it might be dangerous to perform this procedure from a part of the body where blood was thus augmented. The image shows the constellation figures in relation to the affected body parts; the surrounding text is translated below. Elsewhere in the almanac, there are tables showing the phases of the moon and its location in the zodiac.

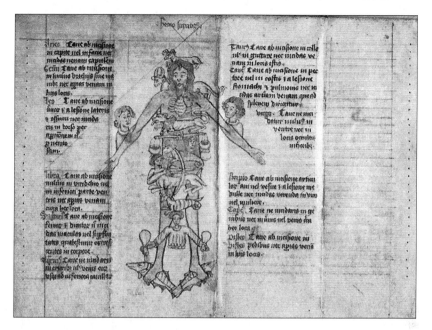

Source: Illustration from London, Wellcome Library MS 40 (folding almanac, late fifteenth c.). Surrounding text trans. Faith Wallis. Latin.

Aries: Beware of incision in the head or in the face, nor should you make an incision in the great vein of the head.

Taurus: Beware of incision in the neck or in the throat, nor should you make an incision in a vein in these places.

Gemini: Beware of incision in the person's arms or hands, nor should you open a vein in these places.

Cancer: Beware of incision in the chest or in the ribs, and of injury to the stomach or lungs; nor should you make an incision in the arterial vein, which leads to the spleen.

Leo: Beware of incision in the sinews and of injury to the sides and the bones; nor should you make an incision in the back either through an opening or by means of a *cupping glass.

Virgo: Beware of incision that makes a wound in the belly or in the internal organs.

Libra: Beware of incision that makes a wound in the navel or in the lower part of the belly; nor should you open a vein in the vicinity of these places.

Scorpio: Beware of incision in the joints, the anus or the bladder, and of injury to the marrow; nor should you make an incision in the private parts of man or woman.

Sagittarius: Beware of incision in the thighs and fingers, nor should you incise blemishes or any superfluities whatsoever that flow from the body.

Capricorn: Beware lest you make an incision on the knees or in the sinews or veins in the vicinity of this area.

Aquarius: Beware lest you make an incision in the legs or in their veins, down to the lower part of the ankles.

Pisces: Beware of incision in the feet, nor should you open a vein in these places.

58. IS SURGERY A SCIENCE? (1): LANFRANC OF MILAN DEFENDS THE INTELLECTUAL DIGNITY OF SURGERY

*Medieval Galenism set out three avenues of therapy: regimen, pharmacy, and surgery. Regimen or hygiene was grounded in the theory that health consisted of a balanced *complexion maintained through adjustment of the *non-naturals; pharmacy likewise could be justified and explained in terms of elemental properties and mathematical *degrees. But it was much more difficult to argue that surgery was a "science" in the sense that Avicenna or Aristotle understood the term (see doc. 43). The key issue was that surgery was carried out with the hands and with instruments, and not with ideas, words, and books. Hence practitioners of surgery were (at least in some medieval settings) distinguished from physicians on a social and legal plane; in many universities, especially north of the Alps, surgery was marginalized.*

But some surgeons held that their branch of medical practice was indeed a body of rational knowledge grounded in philosophical theory. This document and the two that follow illustrate different ways of claiming a scientific pedigree for surgery. Lanfranc of Milan (see doc. 56) argued that theory makes for better surgery. Indeed, his Great Surgery defended surgery as a science precisely because it requires knowledge (scientia) of medical theory. In a sense, Lanfranc absorbed surgery into medicine. He also adopted academic styles of discourse and argument, particularly in his lavish citation of medical authorities – Hippocrates and Galen, but also the Arabic writers Isaac Judaeus, Avicenna, Haly Abbas (author of the Pantegni*), Serapion, and Mesue. The greatest medical authorities are thus appropriated for surgery.*

Source: trans. Faith Wallis from *Chirurgia magna* 1.1.2, in *Ars chirurgica Guidonis Cauliaci* ... (Venice: Giunta, 1546), fol. 208rb. Latin.

That a surgeon must possess direct (*sensualiter*) knowledge of the *complexions of the body and its parts, and of medicines, is demonstrated in this way through a concrete case (*experimentum*). Suppose that two men of identical age are wounded at the same moment and in the same location – say, pierced through the middle of the arm by a sword or a similar blade. However, one of them is of a hot and humid complexion and the other is cold and dry. The practice and prevailing view of laymen concludes that both can be treated in the same way, but the science of complexion, which is confirmed rationally by the practice of surgery, teaches us that both cannot be cured in one and the same way. On the contrary: in the case of the first man – the one who is of a hot complexion – we will be apprehensive lest he fall into a *fever and lest a hot *aposteme overtake the [wounded] member. For Galen says, "Members which have a hot aposteme act like a wellspring to fever and like a furnace to the body." For this complexion is more susceptible than all the others to fever, as Galen, Isaac [Judaeus], and Avicenna attest.

So, what should be done? One should consider whether a large amount of blood is flowing from the wound. If so, that is a good thing. If not, we will have the patient bled from the opposite arm or from the foot on the same side, if his vital *powers and his age can bear it; or we will apply *cupping glasses to his thighs, if his vital powers are weak, and we will make him have a bowel movement once a day (if he does not do so naturally) by means of a suppository or an enema. And we will bring the parts of the wound together with a suture, if this is required, or else with compresses and a ligature alone, if a suture is not required; and we will do other things about the wound, which will be discussed below in its proper place. But we will apply to the wound a defensive medicine made of *Armenian bole, oil of roses, and a small amount of vinegar, so that the medicine can penetrate to the bottom of the wound, lest the *humor descend to the wounded area. And we will forbid him to consume wine, meat, milk, eggs, fish, and foods that generate a large quantity of blood. He will be content to sup on porridge of oats or barley with almonds and generally keep to a light and restricted diet until the aposteme is no longer dangerous. And if we know that he should be defended from aposteme and fever, it is the science of complexion that teaches us that he should be swiftly cured or released.

But the other [patient] should not be bled, nor should cupping glasses be applied, because in people like this, blood should be guarded like treasure. They should not be denied meat or wine, because the stomach and digestive powers are weak and cannot generate the matter required for the wound. We should not be afraid that he will fall into a fever, because his complexion is not suited to fever. Besides, we find that the identical medicine, prepared in the identical fashion, will have a manifestly different effect when it is applied to different bodily complexions. For if Roman vitriol (which in French is called "cuperosa") is applied to wounds on dry bodies, it helps in generating flesh. But it not only does not help moist [bodies], it corrodes them. Now the action of vitriol is constant, although different effects result because of differences in the bodies to which it is applied, just as the sun's action is diverse, not because of the sun, but because of diversities in the body on which it acts. For vitriol is extremely desiccative and in dry bodies *consimilar members put up a strong resistance to its force; for this reason it can only dry out the superfluities of the wound which it finds, and when they are dried out, flesh generates naturally. In moist bodies, however, because the debility of their members cannot resist the force of the vitriol, they suffer under it and are converted into fluid; hence *corruption in the wound is increased by the vitriol.

What was just said about the different complexions of the body, was said by Galen with respect to the different complexions of the members. If two wounds are equal in *sanies, but one is in a dry member and another in a moist member, the [wound] in the dry [member] requires a drier medicine. And if there are wounds in two members of similar complexion, but one has a lot of pus and the other little, the one which has a lot of pus requires a drier medicine. John Damascene [Mesue, *Aphorism* 106]: "Medications and dressings ought to be of the same quality as the members to which they are applied." And Galen: "A natural entity should be preserved with things that are similar to it; but what is contrary to nature should be ex-pelled with things contrary to it." Therefore if the surgeon does not know about natural complexions, how can he vary the medications according to the different complexions of members and bodies, particularly if he does not know about the complexions of medicines and their degrees? For the surgeon should know about the generation of the humors, which are the third of the *naturals, and he should know about the science and cause of apostemes.... He should know about the differences between members and their use and functions, so that he knows which members exert great action within the body and which are of great sensitivity and will not tolerate strong medicine. It is necessary that he understand the powers, so that he will recognize when the action of any particular virtue is diminished, and so come to the aid of the member that ministers to this damaged operation. And if he possesses knowledge, the notion of powers, operations, and *spirits will not be hidden from him. All the above are naturals, and this constitutes the first branch of theoretical medicine.

In the same way, it is necessary that he have knowledge of the *non-natural things so that he may know how to choose air which is suitable for a patient who is wounded or suffering from an aposteme. For wounds do not dry out in moist, misty air, and so wounded patients must move from an atmosphere like this to one that is bright and fragrant. In winter they must be defended from cold, because nothing damages wounded sinews and bones like cold; in summer, however, the necessity to temper the air is not as great. [The surgeon] must also know how to regulate diet.... Again, it is also necessary that he govern motion and rest in the patient in accordance with what is suitable, for if the patient is wounded in the head or has a punctured sinew, he must rest; he should keep quiet, and have a soft, level bed, lest the limb suffer any discomfort. But if there are old wounds on the arms, and they are painless, it would be good for the patient to walk about with his arm in a sling. And if he is wounded in the legs and feet, it would be good for him to lie down and exercise himself with his hands. Likewise, the surgeon should temper the patient's sleep, in so far as he is able. For excessive sleep generates superfluities, debilitates the powers, and chills and slackens the whole body. Excessive wakefulness dissipates and consumes the spirits, stirs up the humors in the wounds, brings on unnatural dryness, and causes pain. Again, it is incumbent upon him to *evacuate repletion and gratify hunger so that he can restore the patient to a *temperate state, for otherwise the wound will never be closed. And he must temper the passions of the mind in the patient, for because of anger, much spirit is poured out, and for this reason it often happens that the limb becomes inflamed. But fear and sorrow and lack of confidence concerning his health draws the [patient's] spirit into the interior [of the body], and hence the powers are debilitated and unable to generate the matter required to repair the wound. These are the six non-natural things, the second branch of theoretical medicine.

[The surgeon] must know about the third branch, [namely] what a wound is, an ulcer, cancer, aposteme, and so forth, so that he may know upon what, for the sake of what, and to what purpose he should apply his exertions. For all these [conditions] are different, and in accordance with these differences, they require different treatments. For example, he should know the cause of the condition, for wounds inflicted by a sword are cured otherwise than wounds made by the impact of a rock or by a fall. And wounds from the bite of a dog can turn out to be rabid, as will be discussed later on. [The surgeon] must know the incidental circumstances surrounding the wound, so that he may know whether the wound cannot be cured unless these incidental circumstances be first removed, as will be discussed in the chapter on this subject. These three – the disease, the cause, and the incidental circumstances – with the abovementioned six [non-naturals] and seven [naturals] make up the whole of theoretical medicine. Also the surgeon ought not to lack familiarity with the two instruments of practice which come before the surgery itself, for he must regulate the diet in different ways.... It is even more necessary that he know how to administer a *potion when this is expedient. Galen [says]: "[*Purgative] drugs and vomiting are of great assistance to those who have very serious and *putrid wounds. For when the body is purged of bad humors, the diseased matter is shifted from the location of the wound, and the wound consolidates more quickly." So he who considers all the parts of medicine will clearly discover that it is necessary for a surgeon, along with the other gifts which nature bestows (as explained in the preface [of this work]), to learn about medicine in its entirety.

59. IS SURGERY A SCIENCE? (2): HENRI OF MONDEVILLE DEFENDS THE SCIENTIFIC CREDENTIALS OF SURGERY

Henri of Mondeville and his textbook of surgery have been introduced in connection with his views on progress in medicine (doc. 45). He probably received his academic training in Paris under Lanfranc of Milan, and, like his master, he was concerned to elevate surgery's intellectual prestige. To achieve this end, he had to convince Parisian academic doctors that operative surgery was a rational and scientific pursuit, and he had to convince craft surgeons that learning medical theory would enhance their success as practitioners. His hopes for integrating surgical education into the medical faculty were dashed in 1311, when King Philip IV elected to regulate surgery as a licensed craft, supervised by sworn master surgeons.

In this extract, Henri displays his scholastic virtuosity by tackling the controversial issue of the proper treatment of "simple" wounds, such as straightforward cuts without complications. Should they be left open to heal by what a modern surgeon would call "secondary intention" (from the bottom up, by the filling of the wound with granulation tissue), or closed over to heal by "primary intention"? Should the surgeon provoke the formation of pus, or impede it? Henri argues for the minority view promoted by Teodorico Borgognoni (doc. 62), defending his position not merely from his own experience, but from physiological and pathological theory.

Source: trans. Michael R. McVaugh from the French version of the *Chirurgia* edited by E. Nicaise, *Chirurgie de Maître Henri de Mondeville* (Paris, 1893), in *Sourcebook in Medieval Science*, ed. Edward Grant (Cambridge, MA: Harvard University Press, 1974), pp. 803–6 (no. 115.2). French.

Tract II, *Notula* 21

It is extremely risky for a little-known surgeon to treat any case other than as his colleagues generally do, for example to treat wounds as Theodoric [Borgognoni] instructs in the first part of his *Great Surgery* ... [*that is, by closing the wound, applying a dry dressing, and leaving it to heal*]. Master Jean Pitart [surgeon to Philip IV of France] and I, who were the first to bring this method into France and first to use it in the treatment of wounds at Paris and on a number of military campaigns, did so against the will and advice of everyone, in particular the physicians. We had to endure scorn and contemptuous words from laymen, and menaces and threats from our colleagues, the surgeons. From some laymen and from physicians, every day and at each new treatment, we suffered such violent attacks that, nearly exhausted by so much opposition, we were about to give the treatment up, and would have given it up entirely, God knows. But the most serene prince Charles, count of Valois [the brother of Philip IV], came to our aid, as did several others who had previously seen us in the camps curing wounds by this method. Moreover, we were sustained by the truth, for which man should sooner accept death than yield to error. Is not God the Truth, and was he not willing to suffer death for it? Yet if we had not been strong of faith, royal physicians upheld by the king, of some little literacy, we would surely have had to abandon this treatment....

Tract II, Doctrine I, Chapter 3

Throughout this book, we have been supposing that every simple wound can be cured without producing a notable quantity of pus, on condition that it be treated according to our own doctrine, that of Theodoric, without deviation. We must now see if this is possible.

It may be said that this is not possible, since in every member that is nourished, whether it be large or small, healthy or unhealthy, the third *digestion takes place; and in every digestion wastes are produced, especially within wounded members, and these wastes compose the matter of pus. The weakened [natural] heat is the agent of this transformation; and when an agent and the object on which it acts are both present, it is impossible that its action should not take place; and it is thus impossible that pus should not be engendered in a wound. The fact is proved on the authority of all the authors in medicine and surgery, and by all the practitioners. The contrary is shown by Theodoric throughout his *Great Surgery* and we ourselves can also attest it from experience.

It must be concluded that every wound treated thus can be cured without producing a notable quantity of pus. This can be proven in two ways, by experience and by reasoning: by experience, since we see that it often happens thus; by reasoning, because where the cause is lacking, the effect will be lacking too – and in every simple wound treated by our method we can avoid all the causes of the formation of pus, therefore, and so on. The major [premise, namely, that where the cause is lacking, the effect will be lacking too] is proved on the authority of the Philosopher [Aristotle]; the minor results from the fact that according to experience and to authorities, there are just five causes of the formation of pus in wounds (although Haly gives only three: excess of nourishment, unhealthy quality, and application of unhealthy medicine). The first cause is the alteration caused in the wound by the air; we can avoid this by rapidly closing the wound and maintaining this closure. The second cause is a too violent *flux of *humors toward the wound. We avoid this by an *evacuation, which will divert the humors, by raising the injured member, by an artfully made bandage, by *fomentations of hot wine and application of wine to the wound, all things that dissolve a part of those humors that have already reached the member and that repel those that would have come to it; this is because they strengthen the member and expel the humors by constriction, as the press squeezes juice from the grapes. The third cause is the weakness of the injured member, which receives wastes from other parts; we can avoid this by a suitable bandage and by employing wine and other *temperate remedies, internally and externally, in moderate quantity – that is, sufficiently to sustain the organic force; these medicines strengthen the natural *complexion of the member by their aromaticity. The fourth cause is an excess of nourishment taken, or its unhealthy quality, or both; we avoid this by a light regimen, scanty, easy to digest, and one that forms good dry blood, not burnt. The fifth cause is the application of a suppurative medicine; but the wine and bandages which we use do not have this effect, rather they dry and dissolve; thus, and so on. If any other cause of this sort is given by authorities under another name, I believe that it will be reducible to one of these [that] I have just given.

It follows that the minor [premise] is proven and that in every simple wound we can avoid the causes of the formation of pus; moreover, from this results the primary conclusion that it is possible to cure every wound, as a wound, without creating a significant quantity of pus, when treated in this manner. As for the reasoning that maintains the contrary, it should be said that it concludes correctly that pus is formed in every wound where wastes are produced in sufficient quantity to engender a great deal of pus, but this reasoning does not prove that pus is formed in considerable quantity in those wounds where scant wastes are produced. To the authorities it must be replied that their conclusions are valid for those wounds for which one prescribes a cold, humid, suppurative regimen, or the like.

Moreover, once proven and agreed that it is possible to cure all wounds thus treated without producing pus there in significant quantity, we can ask, which of the two treatments is the more healthy, that in which the formation of pus is produced or provoked, or that in which this formation is avoided completely or as much as possible? It may be argued that the treatment in which the formation of pus takes place or is provoked is preferable to that in which it is completely avoided, since the treatment by which we free nature from wastes appears preferable to that which does not have this result – that is the case here, therefore, and so forth. The major premise is evident; the minor premise is proven by the fact that nature discharges herself by suppuration; therefore, and so on. It is also supported by Galen, commenting on the *Aphorisms* [of Hippocrates], Part V: "In serious wounds the hard is bad, the soft is good;" therefore, and so on.

The contrary is supported by Avicenna's authority, Book I [of the *Canon*], fen 4, chapter 29 – "On treatment by *solution of continuity, and of the kinds of ulcers" – where he says that one should set himself three goals in the treatment of the fleshy members, of which the third is to prevent suppuration as much as possible; therefore, and so on. This can also be supported by the authority of Galen, who says the same thing (in Book IV of the *Megategni*, chapter 4): dessicative medicines are suitable for all wounds, from first to last, save only those which involve a contusion, that is to say, an old contusion. And dessicatives do not engender suppuration; therefore suppuration must not be provoked in wounds, and so on. Moreover, in the *Tegni* (treatise on causes, chapter 34 ...), explaining the treatment of *apostemes, Galen says that after having first *purged the body, it is necessary to try to repel [wastes]; then, if that is impossible, to dissolve them; and finally, if that does not succeed, he says that it is necessary to *ripen and provoke the suppuration. It is clear that Galen is trying first to cure by the best method of treatment; therefore, and so on.

It must be concluded that the treatment in which no pus is formed, in which one avoids it as much as possible, is better, surer, and more healthy than that in which it is produced or is provoked. The reason for this is as follows: the treatment which least troubles the patient or the surgeon; in which there is no loss of substance; in which the least *spirit and vital heat is lost, and by which the least external cold penetrates (both are in fact contrary to the principles of life); which involves neither hot aposteme nor *fever; by which the lips of the wound can be more exactly joined – that treatment is preferable to one which does just the contrary. But this is the case here; therefore, and so forth. The major [premise] is self-evident; the minor can be proved by going over each of the parts of the argument; therefore, and so on. Besides, it is useless to do with more [what can be done with less], and so on; thus, it is in vain that we provoke suppuration in wounds, because according to the opinion of Galen and Avicenna, the dessicatives are appropriate for all wounds from first to last, therefore, and so forth.

To the first argument, which says that nature is relieved by suppuration, we should rather answer that to provoke suppuration is to injure nature, on the authority of Hippocrates (aphorism of part II on the formation of pus). It is however true that once pus is formed, its expulsion is a relief, and true that it is necessary that it then be expelled; but it would be better if it were never engendered nor expelled, for wounds heal more easily before suppuration than after. Likewise, as there are more people who know how to induce suppuration than how to dry it up, it can happen that suppuration thus provoked cannot be stopped. Then the surgeons announce that St. Eloi's sickness has *infected the wound, or something of this sort, so that the people will not criticize them – indeed, they withdraw with honor and no longer concern themselves with the treatment – when neither the patient nor even the saint to whom they ascribe it ever suffered from the disease.

As for Galen's statement, "The hard is bad, etc.," it should be said that Galen meant it not for simple wounds, but for complicated wounds, involving apostemes, contused and of long standing, whose development is so advanced that they cannot be cleared up by [the normal] evacuation, repercussion [*that is, diverting*] and *solution, without provoking suppuration. From the moment a wound develops complications, the sooner it becomes soft and fluid, the better it will be; and the longer it remains hardened, the worse it will be. Some, misunderstanding this opinion of Galen's and applying it to simple wounds, have harmed many people by provoking suppuration in them. Perhaps this statement has been more harmful than useful, since a statement misunderstood leads to error – but all this was contrary to Galen's own intentions.

60. IS SURGERY A SCIENCE? (3): GUY OF CHAULIAC'S HISTORY OF SURGERY

Educated at Toulouse and Montpellier, Guy of Chauliac (d. ca 1368) also studied surgery and anatomy in Bologna. He practiced in Paris and Lyons but spent much of his career in Avignon as surgeon to popes Clement VI (1342–52), Innocent VI (1352–62), and Urban V (1362–70). He composed an enormously successful textbook of surgery, the Inventarium *or* Great Surgery *(Chirurgia magna), around 1363. It was subsequently translated into many vernacular languages.*

Compared with the other surgeons who spoke on the subject of the status of their discipline, Guy was not particularly concerned with defending surgery's rationality or with policing the frontiers to keep out barbers and empirics. The fact that he had a medical degree may have contributed to this sense of security. He seems to have learned surgery in the context of his medical studies, though he certainly differed from most physicians in choosing to write for surgeons. Perhaps as well, his comfortable status as a cleric with a benefice placed him above the fray of inter-professional rivalry. On the other hand, Guy had a strong sense of the importance of historical change in establishing surgery's distinctive identity, though his picture of progress toward academic respectability was not borne out by contemporary trends.

Source: trans. James Bruce Ross in *The Portable Medieval Reader*, ed. Mary Martin McLaughlin (New York: Viking, 1949), pp. 640–49. Latin.

The workers in this art, from whom I have had knowledge and theory, and from whom you will find observations and maxims in this work, in order that you may know which has spoken better than the other, should be arranged in a certain order.

The first of all was Hippocrates who (as one reads in the *Introduction to Medicine*) surpassed all the others, and first among the Greeks led medicine to perfect enlightenment. For according to Macrobius and Isidore, in the fourth book of the *Etymologies* (and as is also related in the prologue to the *Continens* [of Rhazes]), medicine had been silent for the space of five hundred years before Hippocrates, since the time of Apollo and Asclepius, who were its first discoverers. He lived ninety-five years, and wrote many books on surgery, as it appears from the fourth [book] of the *Therapeutics* and many other passages of Galen. But I believe that on account of the good arrangement of the books of Galen the books of Hippocrates and many others have been neglected.

Galen followed him, and what Hippocrates sowed, as a good laborer he cultivated and increased. He wrote many books, indeed, in which he included much about surgery, and especially the *Book on Tumors Contrary to Nature*, written in summary; and the first six books [of] *On Therapeutics*, containing wounds and ulcers, and the last two concerning boils and other maladies which require manual operation....

After Galen we find Paul [of Aegina, seventh c.] who (as Rhazes attests in his *Continens*, and Haly Abbas in the first book of his *Royal Disposition* [*an alternative title for the Pantegni*]) did many things in surgery; however, I have found only the sixth book of his *Surgery*.

Going on we find Rhazes, Albucasis [d. ca 1013], and Alcaran....

Haly Abbas was a great master and besides what he sowed in the books on the *Royal Disposition*, he arranged on surgery the ninth part of his *Second Sermon*.

Avicenna, illustrious prince, followed him, and in very good order (as in other things) treated surgery in his fourth book.

And we find that up to him all were both physicians and surgeons, but since then, either through refinement or because of too great occupation with cures, surgery was separated and left in the hands of mechanics. Of these the first were Roger [Frugard], Roland [of Parma], and the Four Masters, who wrote separate books on surgery, and put in them much that was empirical. Then we find Jamerius [fl. ca 1230–52] who did some rude surgery in which he included a lot of nonsense; however, in many things he followed Roger. Later, we find Bruno [of Longobucco, fl. ca 1252], who, prudently enough, made a summary of the findings of Galen and Avicenna, and of the operations of Albucasis; however, he did not have all the translation of the books of Galen, and entirely omitted anatomy. Immediately after him came Theodoric [Borgognoni], who gathering up all that Bruno said, with some fables of Hugh of Lucca [d. ca 1252–8], his master, made a book out of them.

William of Saliceto [ca 1210–ca 1280] was a man of worth who composed two compendia, one on medicine and the other on surgery; and in my opinion, what he treated he did very well. Lanfranc [of Milan] also wrote a book in which he put scarcely anything but what he took from William; however, he changed the arrangement.

At that time Master Arnau of Vilanova was flourishing in both skills, and wrote many fine works. Henri of Mondeville began in Paris a very notable treatise in which he tried to make a marriage between Theodoric and Lanfranc, but being prevented by death he did not finish the treatise.

In this present time, in Calabria, Master Nicholas of Reggio [d. 1350], very expert in Greek and Latin, has translated at the order of King Robert [of Sicily] many books of Galen and has sent them to us at court; they seem to be of finer and more perfect style than those that have been translated from the Arabic....

In my time there have been many operating surgeons, at Toulouse, Master Nicholas Catalan; at Montpellier, Master Bonet, son of Lanfranc; at Bologna, Masters Peregrin and Mercadant; at Paris, Master Peter of Argentière; at Lyons (where I have practiced for a long time), Peter of Bonant; at Avignon, Master Peter of Arles and my companion, Jean of Parma.

And I, Guy of Chauliac, surgeon and master in medicine, from the borders of Auvergne, diocese of Mende, doctor and personal chaplain to our lord the pope, I have seen many operations and many of the writings of the masters mentioned, principally of Galen; for as many books of his as are found in the two translations, I have seen and studied with as much diligence as possible, and for a long time I have operated in many places. And at present I am in Avignon, in the year of our Lord 1363, the first year of the pontificate of Urban V. In which year, from the teachings of the above named, and from my experiences, with the aid of my companions, I have compiled this work, as God has willed.

The sects that were current in my time among the workers in this art ... were five.

The first was of Roger, Roland, and the Four Masters, who, indiscriminately for all wounds and boils, produced healing or suppuration with their poultices and cataplasms; relying for this on the fifth [part of Hippocrates's] *Aphorisms*, "The loose are good, and the hard are bad." [*Aphorisms* 5.67]

The second was of Bruno and Theodoric who indiscriminately dried up all wounds with wine alone, relying for this on the fourth [book of Galen's] *Therapeutics* [*that is, Therapeutic Method*], "The dry comes closer to the healthy, and the wet to the unhealthy."

The third sect was of William of Saliceto and of Lanfranc who, wishing to hold the middle ground between the above, cared for or dressed all wounds with unguents and sweet salves, relying for this on the fourth [book] of the *Therapeutics*, that there is only one way to healing, namely, that which is done safely and painlessly.

The fourth sect is composed of all the men at arms or Teutonic knights and others following war; who treat all wounds with conjurations and liquors, oil, wool, and cabbage leaves, relying on this, that God has put his efficacy in words, in herbs, and in stones.

The fifth sect is composed of women and many ignorant ones who entrust the sick with all maladies only to the saints, relying on this: "The Lord has given it to me as it has pleased him; the Lord will take it from me when it shall please him; blessed be the name of the Lord, Amen." [Job 1.21] ...

The conditions required of a surgeon are four: the first is that he be educated; the second that he be skilled; the third, that he be ingenious; the fourth, that he be well behaved. It is then required in the first place that a surgeon be educated, not only in the principles of surgery, but also of medicine, both in theory and practice.

In theory he must know things *natural, *non-natural, and unnatural. And first, he must understand natural things, principally anatomy, for without it nothing can be done in surgery, as will appear below. He must also understand *temperament, for according to the diversity of the nature of bodies it is necessary to diversify the medicament.... He must also know the things that are not natural, such as air, meat, drink, etc., for these are the causes of sickness and health. He must also know the things which are contrary to nature, that is sickness, for from this rightly comes the curative purpose. Let him not be ignorant in any way of the cause; for if he cures without the knowledge of that, the cure will not be by his abilities but by chance. Let him not forget or scorn accidents; for sometimes they override their cause, and deceive or divert, and pervert the whole cure....

In practice, he must know how to put in order the way of living and the medicaments; for without this surgery, which is the third instrument of medicine [*that is, the third avenue of therapy, following regimen and drugs*], is not perfect. Of which Galen speaks in the *Introduction*: as pharmacy has need of regimen and surgery, so surgery has need of regimen and pharmacy.

Thus it appears that the surgeon working in his art should know the principles of medicine. And with this, it is very fitting that he know something of the other arts. That is what Galen says in the first [book] of his *Therapeutics* ... that if the doctors have nothing to do with geometry, or astronomy, or dialectics, or any other good discipline, soon the leather workers, carpenters, smiths and others, leaving their own occupations, will run to medicine and make themselves into doctors....

61. A SURGICAL SAMPLER (1): GUY OF CHAULIAC ON THE TREATMENT OF WOUNDS

Wound treatment is one of the most ancient and widely practiced forms of surgery, but that did not prevent scholastic surgeons from reframing the process in the light of new styles of medical thinking. First, Galen's categorization of "break in continuity" (solutio continuitatis) as a distinct category of illness, elaborated in book 4 of Avicenna's Canon, widened the category of wounds to include any injury where the skin is broken (for example, ulcers). Second, wound treatment was rationalized by emphasizing general principles and by imposing step-by-step order on the narrative of the treatment procedure. Rationalizing also meant citing authorities, justifying treatments by invoking medical theory, and incorporating anatomical details. Guy of Chauliac's discussion of abdominal wounds exhibits all these traits. It also exudes confidence in the ability of rational surgical management to cope with dire situations, as when the belly has been perforated and the intestines protrude or are injured. Roger Frugard (doc. 38) was very pessimistic about penetrating abdominal wounds, but Guy presents himself as one who is in command of an array of well-attested techniques for replacing the guts within the body cavity and suturing the wound.

Source: trans. Faith Wallis from Guy of Chauliac, *Inventarium sive Chirurgia Magna*, ed. Michael R. McVaugh (Leiden: Brill, 1997), vol. 1, pp. 200–204, and ill. p. 203. Latin.

Treatise 3: On Wounds. Doctrine 2: Wounds in Compound Organs. Chapter 6: Concerning Wounds in the Belly and Its Parts

As there are two parts in the belly, namely that which is contained and that which contains (as was explained in the Anatomy [in the first Treatise of the *Inventarium*]), so also wounds sometimes occur in the containing part and sometimes in the contents. Thus, wounds of the belly are sometimes external and do not penetrate to the inner parts, and sometimes they do penetrate to the inner parts. Of those that penetrate to the inner parts, some are of such a nature that nothing of the interior members protrudes; but sometimes the omentum protrudes, or the intestines, or something else. Wounds in the contained parts are sometimes in the omentum, sometimes in the intestines, sometimes in the stomach, and so forth. These are the distinctions on which indications and treatments are based.

The **causes** of these wounds are the same as those of other [wounds]: sword, lance, arrow, and anything capable of cutting and perforating.

Signs and indications. A sign that a wound in the belly does not penetrate is obtained by visual inspection, by [exploration with] a probe, and by the fact that nothing comes out of it. But a sign that it does penetrate is obtained when the probe enters deeply and when the omentum, intestine, or some other member comes out of it. A sign that the omentum has protruded and has been altered is when its substance, fatty and full of veins, is visible, and when it appears livid and dark. A sign that the intestines are wounded is the issue of feces from [the wound]. The sign indicating whether it is the large or small intestine is deduced from the location, for the small intestine is above the navel and the large intestine below. A sign that the stomach is wounded is that *chyle issues from it and that [the wound] is located in the front. A sign that the liver is wounded is the issue of blood and [the wound] is located on the right side. A sign that it is the spleen is the issue of feculent matter and [the wound] is located on the left side. A sign that it is the kidneys is the issue of watery blood, and also the site. In *Therapeutic Method* book 6, Galen expresses the view that wounds and sutures are more dangerous and difficult when they are in the middle of the belly than when they are on the flanks, because the [middle] parts contract more due to their muscles and the intestines can more easily protrude. It is also judged that unless one comes quickly to their aid and reintroduces them, the intestines will swell up and inflate because of the coldness of the air, and then it will be difficult to reintroduce them. Hippocrates in the sixth part of the *Aphorisms* also concludes that unless one counteracts the protrusion of the epiploon or omentum or *zirbus* quickly, it will very rapidly be *altered and corrupted. For this reason, physicians cut off what is exposed and altered. According to

Galen's commentary [on the *Aphorisms*], while this is not always the case, it is for the most part the case. In *Therapeutic Method* book 6, Galen also expresses the view that the large intestine can readily heal, but the small intestine heals with difficulty, and the jejunum not at all, because of the multitude and magnitude of the vessels and the thinness and sinewy character of the tunic. Also, this intestine receives bile in its undiluted form and is closer to the liver than the other [organs]. Moreover, one may venture to treat the lower parts of the stomach because they are fleshy and also because medications can remain in that location; but in the orifice of the stomach, [medication] touches the afflicted parts only in passing, and its sensitive nature repels treatment....

Treatment. There is nothing distinctive about the treatment of wounds of the belly which do not penetrate, apart from the ligature.... Their treatment is the same as that of flesh wounds: with a suture if they need it, and with other things that help the production of flesh. Penetrating wounds where no internal part protrudes or is wounded are treated in the same way, except that they have their own particular suture.

Suture of the belly. This suture takes different forms according to different circumstances. Some, such as Galen, prescribe that [the belly] be sutured so that the peritoneum is joined to the abdominal wall, because being in itself without flesh (since it is bloodless and sinewy), it cannot readily be consolidated, and because of the laxity of the abdominal wall a rupture may follow. The first stitch is made by inserting the point of the needle through one lip [of the wound] so that it does not touch the peritoneum; then by piercing the other lip from the inside, it penetrates all [layers] including the peritoneum, and it is knotted on the outside. In the next stitch, the needle, entering through the lip, pierces everything, including peritoneum and abdominal wall; re-entering through the other lip, it avoids the peritoneum and only pierces the abdominal wall, and it is knotted on the outside. Let the other stitches be made in this way until the whole [wound] is adequately sutured.

Galen relates another method, which Albucasis [*Abû al-Qâsim al-Zahrâwî*, fl. ca 1000] adopts. It is the general method, and it is easier, but not safer, and it is to suture all four margins of the two lips together with a single stitch and a knot. As many stitches are made as are necessary.

Albucasis describes a third method. One pierces [the lips] with needles, as he says, and then leaving the needles in place, one winds a thread over their tops as women do in [lacing up] sleeves....

The fourth method is Lanfranc's and Henri [of Mondeville] adopts it. A threaded needle is stuck in on the outside of one lip and pierces the whole peritoneum and abdominal wall; then coming out through the other lip from the inside, it again pierces the peritoneum and abdominal wall. Then, at a distance of one's little finger from the first stitch, make a second stitch with the same needle and thread, without cutting or knotting it, in this way: insert the needle in the lip that was last perforated from the outside towards the inside, then insert it in the other lip from the inside towards the outside, always including both the peritoneum and the abdominal wall. Near the needle, you will find the end of the thread, which you initially left outside. Tie the two ends of the thread together, making a single knot on the side for every two stitches, because in this way the thread will never pass on top of the lips of the wound, but will only appear on the sides. When the suture is finished, apply other remedies, and bandage up....

In a penetrating wound of the belly in which the inner organs are wounded and do not protrude, if the belly wound is large enough (and if it is not large enough, it can be enlarged with an appropriate instrument, to be described below), let [the internal parts] be carefully pulled out. If they need to be sutured and if this can be done successfully – as for example the fundus of the stomach or the large intestine – let them be sutured with a furrier's stitch and not with ants' heads, as some practitioners say (for so Albucasis testifies), because it is both disagreeable and ineffective, as the facts show. Some, such as Roger [of Parma], Jamerius, and Teodorico, insert a tube made of elder wood into the intestine so that the feces do not corrupt the suture; but others, as Gugliemo [of Saliceto] relates, put in a section of the intestine of some animal, or according to the Four Masters, a piece of a trachea. This does not seem reasonable to me, because nature, bent on expelling foreign bodies, expels and removes it from the suture, and so the purpose for which these things were applied is frustrated. In my view, it is better, after the intestine has been sutured as stated above and cleaned of all filth, to apply externally a powder which will preserve the suture, and that [the organs] be reinserted into the belly according to the method which will be described.

If the omentum has protruded and is blackened and corrupted, let the blackened parts be tied up with a loop, and let the part outside the loop in the lower end of the sewing of the belly be cut away, leaving the heads of the loop and of the thread which sutures the said intestines outside, so that suppurating matter may drain out of the wound. When the omentum has been sutured or ligatured, it should be reinserted into the belly as stated, and let the wound in the belly be immediately sutured as stated. Under no circumstances should it be opened until the internal organs are healed, as Jamerius and Roger prescribe, and Lanfranc follows them on this point. This is because nothing is more harmful to internal members and to natural heat than contact with air which has not been altered by [the body's] nature. Because of this [patients] fall victim to that pernicious occurrence, pain and griping of the intestines, and this causes them to fall into spasms and consequently die.

And along with this, the open wound, which was of necessity large because of the operation, continually predisposes the guts to extrude, which is harmful and dangerous in the extreme.

Things of this nature are provided from the outside; but on the inside, let there be administered what Avicenna says – centaury and *terra sigillata – and the things that are mentioned in connection with wounds of internal organs of the chest, because they will also be suitable for these [wounds]; and in Galen's *On Simple Drugs* 6, horse-tail is highly recommended by some for wounds of the intestines and bladder. And Galen in *Therapeutic Method* 6 prescribes *clysters of sharp, black, tepid wine, especially in a case where the perforation is right down to the inner cavity.

At least for the first seven days, let the diet be light and such that it does not produce stool or superfluities that cause putrefaction, but rather, those that consolidate…. If [the patient's] strength is weak, one can give chicken broth [simmered] to the point where the cooked parts dissolve; and if some tragacanth and gum arabic can be added in, which will not make it taste sharper, this would be best. And Guglielmo praises effusively water from the *decoction of incense and mastic.

In a penetrating belly wound in which the intestines or some other part protrude, wounded or not, sutured or bandaged, Galen and Avicenna identify four tasks: the first is to restore what is protruding to its proper place; the second, to suture the wound; the third, to apply drugs; and consequently the fourth is to ensure that no internal part suffers swelling or pain.

The first [task] is accomplished if the wound is large enough that [the protruding part] can be introduced with the hands, using a gentle pressure; or [the patient] can be shaken by elevating the hands and feet, and in this way [the organs] are re-introduced, according to Roger. If they cannot be replaced in this way, because they are swollen or because the wound is small, is it not then necessary (says Galen) to do one of two things: either *evacuate the *windiness, or make the wound larger? But I think that the first [option] is better, if it can be carried out successfully. How will it be carried out successfully? By removing the cause of the windiness. And what is this? The coldness of the surrounding air; and so healing is carried out by heating. One must therefore steep a soft sponge in hot water and warm the guts with it. In the meantime, let some sharp warm wine be prepared, because this warms much more than water does, and strengthens the guts. Some, indeed, like Roger and Teodorico, split suckling pigs or other animals down the middle and apply them to the guts as warm as they can, and they repeat this until the guts are warmed and deflated and go back to their place. Haly Abbas prescribes that the patient be suspended by his extremities over a bath and shaken, or that the guts be anointed with oil of violets (or with warm pig grease, as Jamerius says), and in this way the guts will go back to their place.

But if, after you have done all this, the guts remain swollen, Galen and the others prescribe that one cut open the belly wound enough to allow what is protruding to be replaced. Suitable (according to [Galen]) for such incisions are what are called double-headed syringotomes, namely those which are curved and rounded back and at the end – not pointed – the shape of which Albucasis describes thus:

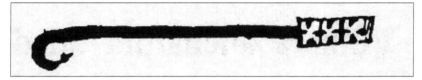

A suitable position for the patient is on his back, but with the wounded part elevated; the point of both is to avoid any harm to the protruding part from the other internal organs.

The second task is accomplished when a competent assistant brings the whole gash together by pressing from outside with his hands, and then opens it little by little while the entire wound is sutured by the physician in an assured manner. How the suture of the belly is made has been described above.

The third task is accomplished, according to Galen, with the drugs called sanguinolentive [*promoting the flow of blood*] and which, as we have shown in previous [sections of this book], consolidate wounds in other parts. These are, namely, the powder that conserves sutures, and *stupes with wine, and plasters, and other remedies that generate flesh. A bandage on the outside is in this case more necessary than the bandage which we said ought to be worn in the case of the chest.

The fourth part of the treatment does not differ greatly from that used in other cases. However, one ought to measure out soft wool in proportion to warm oil, to infuse everything in the vicinity, and to cover the area between the swelling and the armpits. But it is better to introduce something into the intestines with a clyster for such a purpose. Concerning the treatment of abdominal *dropsy by incision, Avicenna in *Canon* book 3 says that it may transpire that pain and perforation follow the incision, and then it is necessary to administer an effusion of oil of dill and camomile to the perforation, and to place upon the spot where the incision was made a plaster made from fenugreek and linseed and the seed of marsh mallow and the like. But some, such as Henri [of Mondeville], in order to eliminate such unbearable perforative griping, boil salt with wine, and add bran until it thickens, and place it in a sack which they apply to all the painful parts, as hot as possible, and a bandage is put over it. And when it has cooled down, it is changed for another of the same kind, and this is repeated until the pain and griping subside. There is no need to attend much to any matter which might remain in the cavity of the belly, because it cannot be of any great quantity, since these parts are not heavily supplied with blood. And as Guglielmo says, nature resolves it or else dispatches it to the inguinal region, and there let it be treated as is customary for other swellings in this area....

62. A SURGICAL SAMPLER (2): TEODORICO BORGOGNONI AND THE NEW SURGICAL DISEASES

As they devoured the Arabic treatises on surgery, notably book 4 of Avicenna's Canon *and the* Surgery *of Albucasis, western practitioners discovered a hitherto unknown domain of "surgical diseases." These were pathological conditions that originated within the body as a result of *humoral imbalance but that manifested themselves outside the body or in an accessible body cavity. They were traditionally treated as medical problems to be confronted with drugs or regimen, but the Arabs taught that they could also be treated surgically. Kidney and bladder stones were a case in point. The Arabic texts, while elaborating the conventional non-surgical therapies, such as diet and baths, also described invasive operations by which bladder calculi could be removed. In the life and work of one surgeon, Teodorico Borgognoni (1205–98), we can see the impact of these enlarged possibilities. Teodorico learned surgery from his father Ugo (Hugo) of Lucca, the town surgeon of Bologna. Though he joined the Dominican Order and later became a bishop, Teodorico continued to practice surgery and composed a textbook on the subject. Its first edition, completed in the mid-1240s, did not mention operations for the stone; but after reading Bruno Longobucco's* Great Surgery *of 1252, Teodorico completely revised his book to reflect its Arab-inspired teachings. The passage reproduced below is from the third and final recension.*

By expanding surgery into the interior of the body, Teodorico and his fellow surgeons were colonizing terrain that hitherto had belonged only to doctors. This is especially evident in the case of urinary stones, which start in the kidneys (where they can only be treated medically), before descending to the bladder, where they may be treated surgically. Ironically, given the delicacy and danger of many of these new operations, the learned surgeons actually expressed a preference for treating their patients by non-surgical methods as far as possible. Yet even as the surgeons boldly exploited this blurring of boundaries, the physicians prepared to fight back. In France, for instance, they lobbied for more rigorous regulations to separate medicine and surgery and ensure the latter's subordinate status. And if surgeons displayed a laudable reluctance to actually operate for bladder stones, there were plenty of empirics – ancestors of the professional lithotomists of the early modern period – who were ready to cut for the stone. Surgical diseases thus proved to be something of a professional snare for the ambitious, literate surgeon.

Source: trans. Eldridge Campbell and James Colton, Teodorico Borgognoni, *The Surgery of Theodoric ca. AD 1267*, book 3, ch. 44(New York: Appleton-Century-Crofts, 1960), vol. 2, pp. 119–32. Latin.

Stones in the Bladder and Kidneys

Sometimes a stone is generated in the bladder, sometimes in the kidneys; and just as the authorities say, in youth a stone is generally generated in the kidneys, while in children it is in the bladder, the mouth of which is narrow, prohibiting the material from which the stone is made from escaping. But although it is no part of our intention in this book to discuss the cause and cure of the stone that gathers in the kidneys (inasmuch as it is never cured by benefit of surgery), yet on account of the close relationship which it has in its medicinal cure with the stone in the bladder, we shall write somewhat briefly in this chapter about its cure. We shall speak first, nevertheless, about the stone in the bladder to which surgical operation applies.

I say therefore that according to the opinion of the authorities the cause from which a stone arises in the bladder is a thick and viscous humor. And the indications by which it is manifested are many. For among these there is the fact that the urine issues from the bladder white and thin with sandy excrement, and with difficulty and severe pain in the pubic region; and a boy holds his [penis] with his hands and rubs it and works with it and often the [penis] is erect and the anus protrudes; and in drawing the hand over the bladder it feels hard.

Now the appearance of the stones is various. For some are small, some large, some smooth, some rough, some long, some round, and some branching.

The issuance of a smooth and round stone is, of course, easy. But of one which is rough and branching, the issuance is more difficult; wherefore it is necessary for you to bring about its fragmentation.

Likewise, as Rhazes says, one type is that which is broken up by medication, another is not so broken up; and therefore it is necessary to test it for some time with medications before an incision is made.

And we shall speak first of stones in the kidneys and bladder and how they ought to be treated with medications. Next we shall speak of how a stone in the bladder for which medications are not effective ought to be treated by surgery.

And when a stone has gathered in the kidneys, the signs of it are pain of the spine and of the spinal muscles; and deep in the area around the kidneys the patient feels pain and heaviness and sluggishness (especially around the head of the rectum), and sluggishness of the legs and thighs externally, and prickling of the toes.

But the signs of a stone in the bladder are a frequently aggravated pain in the pubic regions and strangulation of the urine and sometimes [suffering in the iliac region] and colic.

But whether it arises in the kidneys or in the bladder, if it has arisen from a hot cause and not a chronic one, the signs are these: a sharp and pungent pain, and with urine of excessive sharpness there follows *strangury; and straining produces red or reddish urine (sometimes with drops of blood), and sand which is red or reddish, or green, or black.

If it arises from a cold cause, coldness is felt deep inside, and in the area of the collection, heaviness. The urine is sometimes thin, sometimes thick and turbid; the sand is black or white or ashen.

But if the stone has been formed from both causes, the urine appears fatty, discolored, noticeably livid, always with scaly and *sanious sediment, sometimes with bloody sediment.

Likewise it sometimes occurs in youth, sometimes in old age, sometimes in childhood.

In youth more frequently it occurs in the kidneys because the humors grow stony there from the heat and dryness of the kidneys. But in childhood it more frequently occurs in the bladder, because then viscous humors are generated that grow stony by reason of the narrow neck of the bladder.

But if it occurs in the kidneys and the stone has become hardened, it can scarcely if ever be cured.

If the stone is in the bladder and has grown old there for whatever reason and at whatever age, it can scarcely if ever be cured except by surgery.

But if the stone has not grown old, in the case of one originating from a hot cause, the matter may be *digested by administering *diaprunum morning and evening; after the use of this *electuary you may follow with hot *oxysaccharum. An inunction ought to be made also on the outside with the fat of rabbits or hares, and with butter in the case of one originating from a cold cause. In the case of one originating from a hot cause, with oil of violet over the place where the stone is, for the purpose of digesting the matter.

Medications

The digested matter may be *purged with an electuary of rose juice; on the third day employ a bath with a *decoction of French mercury [*the herb Mercurialis annua*], wormwood and the leaves of willow and grape leaves, of tormentilla, lesser plantain, acedula; and to the patient as he emerges from the bath offer *trochees of madder with a decoction of hart's tongue; on the following day exercise *phlebotomy from a crural vein, if the stone is in the bladder or from an exterior cause. If the stone is in the kidneys, then offer medications that break up the stone.

An excellent powder for breaking up the stone: take the head, feet, and whole skin of a hare, and burn them together in an earthenware pot, and pulverize them; afterwards add some salvia and millefolium, and give it to the patient with his food, or with hot wine in which saxifrage has been cooked; and put it with the aforementioned powder to strengthen the kidneys and bladder, so that they will not be injured by the great strength of the powder....

Against inability to urinate, Galen in his book on the cure of diseases, mentions a medication that breaks up the stone and expels it little by little until the bladder is cleansed and the urine issues forth clear and pure. In this a very great mystery is considered to exist, especially since it completely cures this disease, so that the stone is not generated thereafter, and it is: take the seeds of sweet cucumber, and likewise the seed of ferula [*asafoetida], the seed of olixatrum, and of myrrh, six pennyweight of each; of purple xilocassia, and of cinnamon, four pennyweight of each, and pulverize them, and put them together with clarified honey, and let the patient take a quantity as much as a lupine [bean]. But as for one who is about to compound this medication, in order to keep it sacrosanct, let him not grind up these ingredients in anything except a wooden mortar with a wooden pestle, not allow anything iron about it or around it or anywhere about, for in this chiefly consists its mysterious power....

And you should know, my friend, that Alexander [of Tralles] says that for those in whose kidneys stones are generated the bath is the most useful thing, for it is able not only to alleviate pain but also to effect a cure. When the nephritic person has washed himself, the painful areas should be anointed with camomile oil and massaged for a long time. Indeed this ought to be done not merely once a day but a second or third time and he ought to bathe often too....

If the pain persists and the stones cannot be broken up, stronger medicines must be summoned up. Take therefore the blood of a he-goat, mix it in a mortar with fermented meal, and after grinding them make a poultice and apply it. The aforesaid poultice acts upon the pores and stones in the kidneys and bladder in marvellous fashion....

Use of the Catheter

Likewise if he cannot be cured thus, prepare a bath up to his umbilicus with a decoction of mallows, and althea [*marsh mallows*], and [cow-parsnip root]. And when he emerges from the bath anoint him in the region of the bladder with butter, and introduce one ounce of *petroleum oil through a catheter if his body seems to be *choleric or attenuated. And let the catheter be of silver; and let it be done for as much as four days. And on the fifth day let him be put again in the bath, and then insert a catheter of silver, or gold, or brass, through the neck of the bladder until it touches the stone; and then let the stone be strongly pushed with the catheter; and if it can be done, let the stone be brought down from the neck of the bladder as far as the base; and there it can stay for forty years without any annoyance....

As for diet, vegetables ought to be given: endive, lettuce, mallows, beets, and orach, and those things that cool and moisten. But [cabbage] and calamint, rocket root, [parsley root], garlic, and onion, should be avoided as unsuitable. Of the light foods, there are domestic hens, pheasant, pullets, partridges, blackbirds, and fig peckers.

Surgery

But when the patient has been treated for a month very carefully with all the means of medicine, and his urine is not provoked and sand does not issue with it, then you must assume that the stone is completely solidified and it is not susceptible to being broken up. At that time, therefore, you must have recourse to surgery. But you should not presume, nevertheless, that you may extract a stone from a man who is advanced in age, nor if the stone is excessively large, since as Albucasis says, there is danger lest some part of the bladder be cut and the patient die, or he may suffer the continuous passage of urine because the area does not ever heal up. It has already been determined by the wise ancients that the cure of the stone by the knife is easy in children up to the age of fourteen years, and difficult in the old, since as Haly Abbas says, their bodies are dry, on which account their wounds have difficulty scarring over. But in youths the treatment is of medium difficulty and the cure of one whose stone is large is easier, and that of one whose stone is small is just the opposite. Now this fact is evident since a large stone, because of its heaviness, tends to locate at the base where it is more quickly found and can more easily be drawn to a place suitable for incision, and there an incision may be made more safely.

For those who are not able to be incised because of some one of the aforesaid reasons, we have already told how they are to be helped, namely, that the patient should be bathed in water in which there are soothing herbs cooked up, such as mallows, violet, pond lily, [marsh mallow], [cow-parsnip root], and the like, so that the urinary passage may be enlarged. Then a catheter without syringe (smeared with oil or butter as has been said) may be introduced with ease into the penis, and by pushing and thrusting the stone may be removed from the neck of the bladder and you may push it to the base of the bladder.

However, some proceed otherwise. For they introduce a finger into the anus and with this they draw down the neck of the bladder, and thus little by little they move the stone back and push it to the base of the bladder, and there, as has been said, it can remain for forty years without bother to anyone.

Incision

However, when you wish to extract a stone you should first see that the patient is cleaned out completely with a *clyster, which draws out all the feces from the intestines so that it does not prevent you from finding the stone when you are looking for it. Or you may let the patient fast for two days so that he eats very little, and then instruct the patient that he should jump many times from a high place to a low place so as to move the stone and bring it down from the upper portion of the bladder to the neck. Then prepare a plank in a place where there is plenty of light. Let one man sit at the end of this and hold the patient in front of him, but let his thighs be bound with long bandages to his neck so that the whole bladder is sloping downward; or let the man who is holding him take hold of his legs (especially if it is a small child), elevate them high, and not let go of them until the operation is completed. Then smear the finger of your left hand with oil and introduce it into the anus of the patient, and with your other hand press the bladder above the pubic bone downwards; and seek for the stone until it rests under your finger; and bring it down little by little to the neck of the bladder. Then press upon it with your finger and push it downward toward the place in which you wish to make an incision; and instruct the assistant to stretch the testicles and penis upwards with his hand; and with his other hand let him pull back the skin which is under the testicles away from the area in which the incision is to be made. Then make the incision over that stone between the anus and the testicles, but not in the middle, but rather towards the left side of the buttocks, so that the incision may be big enough lengthwise and limited internally to the size that the stone requires to emerge. Then introduce an instrument with a curved end and draw the stone out with it. And very often the stone will emerge into the incision by the compression of the finger which is in the anus without any difficulty and without the introduction of the aforesaid instrument. But if there is more than one stone, then Albucasis advises that you press down first the large one towards the mouth of the bladder and then make your incision over it and extract it; after this moreover push down the small one. You will do the same if there are more than two. But when you have completed your operation, then place pads soaked in rose oil and cold water or in white of egg to calm the hot abscess. Then bring together the two thighs of the patient if it is a child, and bind them properly with bandages, so that the medication over the wound can be kept in its proper place. If a hot abscess should supervene, however, poultice the spot with a decoction of mallows, mallow paste and the like, so that the heat of the urine may be lessened and the passage enlarged through which, if any superfluity remains, it is possible for the stone to emerge freely with the urine.

However, the wound posterior to the narrow neck of the bladder, if it has been brought together with a suture, may then be cared for like other wounds until it is healed. And you should know that very often it happens that blood congeals in the bladder and an [*aposteme] occurs there, and a stoppage of the urine follows. And the sign of this is the passage of blood with the urine. On this account, if the wound is large you ought to extract this blood with your finger. And if the wound is narrow, evacuate it with an instrument. For if that blood is not extracted, it will provide putrefaction and *corruption in the bladder. Then the wound should be washed with vinegar and water, or with hot wine.

Now you should be solicitous about [what] I am telling you; and both when you are making inquiries about the treatment for the stone and when you are trying to find the stone, you should first prepare for yourself the necessary things, such as instruments and the medications which remove blood. Then search for it and when you have found it do not let it go in the hope of finding it again on the other side, but rather make your incision right there and extract it; for very often the searching is more painful to the patient than the incision. And you should have with you many kinds of instruments that extract a stone; and they should differ from one another in size and the length of the curve at their extremities; and there should be available whatever one of these is most convenient at the necessary time.

As a matter of fact it sometimes happens that when the stone is small it ascends to the passage of the penis and a stoppage of urine follows from this. Then hasten its treatment according to what I tell you, and this is: that you should bind the penis with one thread below the stone so that it may not return to the bladder and you may bind it again with another thread above the stone; then cut over the stone into the penis between the two bindings and extract it. And after having loosened the bindings cleanse the wound of blood, and no bandage is necessary over it, because when the thread is released after the extraction of the stone, the skin returns to its proper place and covers the wound. Therefore it is necessary in applying the ligature of thread to stretch the skin upward, so that when it returns it will cover the wound and healing will take place more easily.

63. A SURGICAL SAMPLER (3): OPHTHALMIC SURGERY

*One consequence of the learned surgeons' promotion of the possibilities of their science was to raise the public's expectations of surgical efficacy. Complex operations, however, such as the ones described by Guy of Chauliac and Teodorico, required not only technical knowledge but consistent practice. Eye operations such as couching for *cataract were also risky and needed both trained assistants and specialized equipment. This is one of the many reasons why, ironically, learned surgeons left these more spectacular interventions to empirics and specialists who did only one procedure, but practiced it continuously. These men were certainly not unskilled, and many, like the thirteenth-century Italian Benvenutus Grassus, were also literate. Though little is known about the career of Grassus, his book was highly prized and translated into a number of vernacular languages.*

*Cataract was defined as both a physical obstruction and an accumulation of ocular *humor, so it could be treated either surgically or medically. Most of the major surgical authors of the thirteenth century were familiar with the couching operation described below, and Benvenutus Grassus's account of the technique may owe something to reading their works. Nonetheless, he adds details that could only have come from his extensive practice. He also takes the opportunity to vaunt his own "patented" remedies, notably his special *purgative called "Jerusalem pills."*

Source: trans. Casey A. Wood, Benvenutus Grassus, *De oculis eorumque egritudinibus et curis* (Stanford, CA: Stanford University Press, 1929), pp. 31–36. Latin.

Chapter 4. On Cataract

We must now consider diseases of the eye and their causes, the first of these being cataract. I tell you that there are seven kinds of cataract, four of them curable and three incurable.

First of all let us talk about the curable varieties, and distinguish well-defined sorts from the doubtful.

The first of the curable cataracts looks like the purest white chalk. The second is bluish-white and is due to errors of diet causing excretions from the stomach. These are carried to the brain, thence to the eye, where they cause the disease. The third kind is also bluish-white and is caused by severe headache, such as migraine, by excessive cold, too much worry, wailing and weeping, and similar troubles. The fourth variety of curable cataract is of a yellowish cast and arises from excessive drinking and eating, from the pain and complications of childbirth, and from the *melancholic humor.

Chapter 5. Of the Treatment of Cataract

Having spoken of the characteristics and causes of curable cataracts, let us consider their cure. In the first place, they cannot be entirely cured until they are complete [*ripe] and properly formed. The proof that this stage is reached is the patient's inability to see clearly the sun by day or the light of a candle at night. Some ignorant physicians attempt to remove the cataract by *purgation, powders, and *collyriums. They fail because the disease cannot be controlled by such remedies; the trouble lies within the coats of the eye, especially the albugineous, and is the result of a disintegration of that humor so that a coagulated watery substance is poured out between the light and the crystalline humor. On this account both the Saracens and the Arabs call this form of cataract *linzaret*, that is, fluid that has petrified in the eye. The doctors of the Salerno School give it a Latin name, *catharacta*, because the foul fluid has fallen down between the tunics and the light of the eye. It cannot, therefore, be cured by medicaments that do not reach the inside of the eye, but only by the most approved and tried practice of our art.

Chapter 6. The Operation for Cataract

A proper cure begins with a purgative, using my Jerusalem pills, compounded only by me. The formula of these is spurge, half an ounce, hepatic aloes, five ounces, to be ground with sugar of roses. After purgation, at the third hour, the patient should be placed astraddle a bench, as if on horseback. Now be seated on the same bench face to face with the patient, who will keep one eye closed. So begins the operation in the name of our Savior Jesus Christ.

With one hand raise the upper lid, and with the other hold a silver needle and direct it toward the outer lacrimal region. Then perforate the eye coats, pushing and turning the instrument around with your fingers until you touch the diseased matter, which the Saracens and Arabs call *linzaret* (but which we call cataract), with the point of the needle and dislodge it from its position in front of the pupil. Then push it well below, holding it there until you have said four *pater nosters* [*the Lord's Prayer*]. Then carefully and slowly turn the needle back to its first position in front of the eye. If the cataract follows the instrument and shows itself in front, you must again depress it, pushing it this time as much as possible toward the ear. Then withdraw the needle in the same manner as it was inserted. And note well that having entered the instrument you must not withdraw it until you are convinced that you have depressed the cataract in the manner just described.

After the operation the patient's eye must be closed, and he should be kept in bed on his back in a shady part of the house. He must not be moved nor allowed to look at a light for eight days, during which period the eye operated on must be dressed with white of egg twice a day and twice during the night. His diet should be soft, fresh eggs with bread. If the patient is young, let him drink water; if old, he may drink a little wine well diluted with water. Many [physicians] allow such patients the meat of chicken, but I prohibit it as being too heavy. That sort of diet causes a rush of blood to the eyes and interferes with natural healing. Finally, after eight or nine days, let the patient make the sign of the Cross and leave his bed. He may now bathe in cold water and so accustom himself to that practice.

Such is the procedure with all curable cataracts, whether they be chalk-white, bluish, blue, or yellowish. Pay no attention to any kind of treatment except that given in our book....

The needle should be made of gold or silver. I am opposed to the use of steel, which has at least three disadvantages: first, it is much harder than silver and on that account injures every part it touches; and remember that the cataract is also hard, and in operating the point of a steel needle might break off and remain in the eye. In that case the whole eye might be destroyed by the pain that results; for severe pain may bring on cold abscess and an obstinate and continuous flow of tears unfavorable to the cure of the cataract. A steel instrument is also very heavy, and the patient experiences more pain in its use because of its weight and hardness than if it were made of gold or silver, that are less harmful on account of their purity and softness. Take note, also, that a gold instrument especially clarifies objects with which it comes in contact because of its inherent power over cold and dampness....

64. A SURGICAL SAMPLER (4):
SURGICAL ANESTHESIA?

One of the most delicate problems encountered in studying pre-modern surgical texts (and medical texts, for that matter) is that not every procedure described or recorded was actually implemented in practice. Sometimes the author will describe an operation but advise that it not be attempted. In the case of the "soporific sponge," often taken uncritically to be a widely used form of general anesthesia, the authors may be trying to articulate the possibilities of surgery rather than describing an actual practice.

Recipes for anesthetics in the form of a sponge soaked in narcotic substances or in the form of a drink are not uncommon in medieval medical texts. The soporific sponge described by Teodorico Borgognoni (see doc. 62) closely resembles the one in the *Antidotarium Nicolai (doc. 36b) and can even be found in ninth-century manuscripts. Nonetheless, it may be a "literary recipe." Teodorico claimed to have learned it from his father Hugo, but there is no intimation that he ever used it himself. The recipe does not appear in all recensions of his Surgery, and it is absent from the writings of other major thirteenth-century surgeons. Only Guy of Chauliac mentions the sponge, but as something he encountered in Theodoric, not as something he used himself.

Source: trans. Eldridge Campbell and James Colton, Teodorico Borgognoni, *The Surgery of Theodoric ca AD 1267*, book 4, ch. 8 (New York: Appleton-Century-Crofts, 1960), vol. 2, pp. 212–13. Latin.

The composition of a savor to be made by surgeons, according to Master Hugo, is as follows: take of opium and the juice of unripe mulberry [*blackberry*], hyoscamus [*henbane*], the juice of spurge flax, the juice of leaves of mandragora [*mandrake*], juice of ivy, juice of climbing ivy, of lettuce seed, and of the seed of the lapathum which has hard, round berries, and of the shrub hemlock, one ounce each. Mix these all together in a brazen vessel, and then put into it a new sponge. Boil all together out under the sun during the dog days, until all is consumed and cooked down into the sponge. As often as there is need, you may put this sponge into hot water for an hour, and apply it to the nostrils until the subject for operation falls asleep. Then the surgery may be performed and when it is completed, in order to wake him up, soak another sponge in vinegar and pass it frequently under his nostrils.

Likewise the juice of the roots of hay may be put under the nostrils, and the patient will soon be roused.

CHAPTER EIGHT

CONTESTED FRONTIERS OF SCHOLASTIC MEDICINE: MEDICAL ASTROLOGY AND MEDICAL ALCHEMY

*Its association with natural philosophy or *physica committed university medicine to an ongoing engagement with the scientific disciplines of the arts curriculum. Astronomy was the most important of these: its subject matter was uniquely noble – the cosmos itself – and it had exceptional explanatory power, because in the Aristotelian geocentric universe, the movements of the stars and planets generated the changes experienced on earth. Celestial movements were mathematical and predictable, but could predicting the movements of the heavens help doctors to foresee the outcome of disease or plan therapeutic strategies? Medicine was certainly tempted to adopt astronomy/astrology as an auxiliary science, and yet the response was far from unanimous. As we have already seen in relation to the Bologna curriculum (doc. 42), astronomy and astrology formed a very significant part of medical education in Italian universities; in northern universities, on the other hand, its presence was somewhat marginal. Moreover, there were many different types or levels of medical astrology in the Middle Ages, ranging from a generic astrological meteorology that linked the seasons to the *humors, through more focused applications such as the "sign man" for bloodletting (doc. 57), to full-dress medical horoscopes. Finally, there was a lively academic debate about the practical limits of astrological prediction, as well as its moral implications. Not all doctors thought astrology was valuable, or even licit.*

Medicine's involvement in alchemy had a rather more tangled genesis, with roots in both natural philosophy and the world of pharmacy (see, for example, the chapter on ceruse in the Antidotarium Nicolai, *doc. 36b). Learned alchemists claimed that their art had a fully scientific basis: the alchemist in his laboratory was simply replicating nature's own processes of change and transformation, but in a controlled and accelerated manner. Like alchemy, pharmacy combined and processed substances, sometimes using heat, or even distillation. Both alchemy and pharmacy manipulated substances in order to extract, purify, and intensify their natural properties The attraction of alchemy was particularly strong in those corners of medieval pharmacy that used mineral substances, notably in surgical ointments, *styptics, oils, and so on. The potent effect of distilled alcohol fascinated surgeons and doctors alike. In some circles, there was also a strong interest in the use of gold as a medicinal substance, because its chemical stability seemed to indicate exceptional preservative powers. But alchemy's association with craft work, its occasional esoteric pretensions, and its unsavory reputation as a bag of tricks for counterfeiters, made some doctors cautious and skeptical.*

65. PANACEA OR PROBLEM? (1): THE CASE FOR MEDICAL ASTROLOGY

The Summary on Crises and Critical Days *(Aggregationes de crisi et creticis diebus) was written in second half of the thirteenth century by an unknown author, identified in some of the earliest manuscripts as "Master B." It built on and supplemented two treatises used in the "new Galen" curriculum (see doc. 41),* On Crises *and* On Critical Days*. A "*crisis*" is a sudden alteration in the course of a disease: it could lead to recovery, or to death. A "*critical day" is when a crisis occurs or can be expected to occur. Ever since Hippocrates, western doctors had assumed that crises followed a predictable temporal rhythm. This rhythm could be a simple count of days, beginning from the onset of the disease, or it could be determined by macrocosmic factors, for example, the phase of the moon. The* Summary *takes this to a new level of sophistication, using mathematical astrology derived from Arabic sources. This was "cutting edge" science.*

The treatise is in four chapters. Chapter 1 defines "crisis" and distinguishes various types of crisis. Chapter 2 discusses critical days. Chapter 3 is about clinical signs, particularly those connected with crisis. Finally, chapter 4 dispenses rules and advice for making a medical prognosis. The extract below is from the section of chapter 2 where the author explains how critical days are determined by the heavenly bodies. His explanation rests on the core scientific idea underpinning learned astrology, namely the concept of "celestial influence." The heavens move, while the stationary earth is the passive recipient of the changes that their motion sets in train. The planets also radiate particular qualities that vary with their position vis-à-vis one another. Both ideas of "influence" would later be invoked to explain the universality of the Black Death (see docs. 84–85). Acute diseases were particularly sensitive to the influence of the moon's monthly cycle of visible phases. During this cycle, the moon not only moves through the twelve signs of the zodiac but also changes its angular relationship to the sun (its "aspect"). It is "in square" when it is positioned at 90 degrees from the sun along the zodiacal circle, "in trine" when it is separated by 120 degrees, and "in sextile" when separated by 30 degrees. In technical astrology, these "aspects" signify positive or negative relationships between the planets.

Source: trans. Faith Wallis from *Aggregationes de crisi et creticis diebus*, c. 2, ed. Cornelius O'Boyle, *Medieval Prognosis and Astrology* (Cambridge: Wellcome Unit for the History of Medicine, 1991), pp. 64–72. Latin.

Although the superior bodies exert an influence on those below and although we receive some of the power of all the stars, and notably of the planets, nonetheless two planets have a stronger influence: the sun and the moon. The sun does this on its own, and has no need of either the moon or the other stars in its main operations. The moon on the other hand has need of the sun in all it does. The influence of the sun on the things that lie beneath it is evident, in that it creates the four seasons. For as Galen says in *On Critical Days* 3, none of the other planets can stand in its way as it climbs up to the Tropic of Cancer and makes summer (at which time it is directly over our heads), when it drops down to the winter tropic and makes winter, and when its path is tempered [between the two tropics] and it makes the temperate seasons of spring and fall. Its influence is seen in the generation of animals and plants and in the way animals are aroused to sexual intercourse. This is evident, because when [the sun] is in the first degree of Aries [in mid-March] and starts to climb up [towards the Tropic of Cancer] everything flourishes, grows and multiplies, and animals are aroused to sexual intercourse. Hence the Philosopher [Aristotle] says in *On Generation and Corruption* 2, "The position of the sun beneath the ecliptic is the cause of generation and corruption in things." It is also visible in the ripening and swelling of fruit. The influence of the moon is also seen in the things which are beneath it and is particularly evident in wet things, so that it is seen in the flow and ebb of the sea, and in the regular flow of menstruation, and in the growth and diminution of brains and bone marrow, for bones are found to be full of marrow at the full moon. It is also seen in changes in the atmosphere, for often before and after [the moon's] conjunction with the sun, there is a change in the atmosphere. This is because when the upper extremity of the [crescent] moon is clearly tilted after its [initial] appearance, it signifies the blowing of the north wind and clear weather. If it is lying flat, it signifies that the south wind will blow. This happens in most cases.

More than the others, these two planets make a strong impression upon, and produce change in, the things that are beneath them. Therefore, since all motion and change in lower things comes from these two and since a crisis is a motion or sudden change, therefore a crisis must be caused by the motion and influence of these two planets. And because what causes a crisis in disease is vital power, and vital power is moved, strengthened, or weakened in different ways and under different influences, therefore crisis and motion in diseases are caused by the motion of these two planets. And because some diseases are chronic and some acute, chronic diseases are determined by the movement of the sun and acute [diseases] by the movement of the moon. This has a twofold cause: first, because matter which is cold and gross needs a stronger motive force, while warm and subtle [matter needs] a weaker one; secondly, matter which is slow in motion needs a slow motive force and that which is swift in motion needs a swift one. Hence the Philosopher says in *On Generation [and Corruption]*, "Those things which act and those things which receive action must be proportional."

So first, let us examine how the motion and influence of the moon determines acute diseases, and secondly, how chronic diseases are determined by the motion and influence of the sun.

Concerning the first, there are three things that should be noted. The first concerns why there is a diversity of critical days running according to periodic intervals, in accordance with the motion of the moon....

About the first point, it should be noted that the influence of the moon is twofold. One is common, and that is to make things warm, to make things cold, and to moisten things. [The moon] does not have this influence of itself, but receives it from the sun. Hence Galen says in *On Crises* 3, "Whatever the moon does, it does because of the light it receives from the sun, because its light is not visible except when it is separated from [*not in conjunction with*] the sun." Hence all the changes produced by the moon come only from the degree of its longitudinal distance from the sun; and it exerts its influence in different ways according to the different shapes which it receives. It has its proper influence and this is both fortunate and unfortunate. The moon has this double influence upon a crisis. Hence Constantine [the African] in *The Theoretical* [*Part of the Pantegni*] book 10 says: "Nature is the thing that is most similar to the moon, for just as the moon receives its light from the sun and is assimilated to it, so nature is assimilated to the moon, and fits together with it."

First, let us demonstrate how [the moon acts] according to its common influence. One should know that (as Constantine says in book 10) the moon receives from the sun eight shapes, and these are prominent and evident. The first is when it is distant from the sun by 45 degrees and it is called a "razor-edge" moon. It takes this shape on the fourth day [of the lunar month], and then it is said to be "approaching sextile." The second is when it is 90 degrees from the sun and is half full, and then it is said to be "in square." The third is when it is 130 degrees distant from the sun and it is called "gibbous"; then it is said to be "above trine," and it takes this shape when it is eleven days old. The fourth is when it is opposite the sun, and separated from it by 180 degrees. Then it is said to be *bederem* [*Arabic for "full moon"*] or full, and it is said to be "at the diameter," and this takes place on the fourteenth day. The moon receives these four shapes in its rise towards the east [when waxing]. Likewise, it receives four other shapes in its descent [when waning]: the first on the seventeenth day, the second on the twentieth, the third on the twenty-fourth, and the fourth on the twenty-seventh. On the seventeenth it is gibbous, and "above trine." And on the twentieth it is quadrate, and "in square." And on the twenty-fourth it is said to be "above sextile," and on the twenty-seventh it is "at conjunction." So since as it runs its course through its orbit from quarter to quarter it receives these shapes, in which it exerts a stronger influence, therefore the days which run from quarter to quarter are more powerful in a crisis. And because it exerts a stronger influence when it is at the diameter than when it is in square, therefore the fourteenth day is more strong than the seventh and the twentieth, inasmuch as it derives from a superior root. And because [the moon] exerts a stronger influence when it is in square than when it is in sextile or trine, therefore the seventh and twentieth days are more powerful in a crisis than the fourth, ninth, eleventh, and seventeenth. For this reason, those days in which the moon is at the diameter or in square or in conjunction are critical, namely the seventh, fourteenth, twentieth, and twenty-seventh; the others are indicative [of a crisis], namely the fourth, eleventh, seventeenth, and twenty-fourth.

Thus it is apparent how the moon, possessing common power, is the cause of diversity, possessing its proper power. To know this, one should pay heed to the rule set forth by Galen in *On Critical Days* 3, and the astrologers confirm this. And this extremely important rule is the basis of prognostication and the method by which astronomers make prognostications about things. And it is: that the moon alters the things that it alters with a stronger alteration, for good or ill, at intervals of seven days, and it is weaker at the mid-point of these seven-day [periods]. And along with this, one ought to take into account the starting point of the thing that is undergoing change, and the [zodiac] sign, and the degree in which the moon is then situated. For example, let us suppose that a woman conceives or gives birth, or that a certain action is starting to take place, and the moon is in Taurus. The greatest change in that thing will then take place when the moon, passing through the circle of the [zodiac] signs, will be in Leo, or in Scorpio, or in Aquarius, because when it is in Leo it is in square [with respect to Taurus], and when it is in Scorpio it will be at the diameter. And when it is in Leo, the first period of seven days will be completed, and the second seven when it is in Scorpio, the third seven when it is in Aquarius, and fourth seven when it returns to Taurus. This is because the moon traverses the circle of the [zodiac] signs in about 27 and one-third days (that is, eight hours) more or less. And since [the moon] finishes up the whole circle in that number, then it finishes up the quarter in seven days and a bit over. And from this it is evident that the section of the moon that cuts the quarter circle does not happen in seven whole days.... Therefore the moon exerts stronger impressions as it cuts the circle from one seven to the next seven, and weaker ones in the mid-points of the sevens, be it for good or ill. Because when the moon is in square or at the diameter and emits a fortunate influence, then there is a great change in the situation for the good; and if it emits an unfortunate influence, then there will be a marked change in the situation for the bad. And when the moon is in the middle of the quadrant and it emits a fortunate influence, then there will be a modest change for the good, and the opposite, if it [emits] the opposite.

Should you ask how one knows whether the moon is emitting a fortunate or an unfortunate influence, I reply that to know this one must (as we said before) diligently ponder the starting-point of the situation in which the change occurs, and take into consideration the sign and degree in which the moon is found, and whether there is a "fortunate [star]" in that sign – that is, a benevolent star which emits good fortune, like Jupiter, Mercury, or Venus, or an "unfortunate star" emitting misfortune, like Mars or Saturn. Let us suppose that a man is born and a fortunate star is in Aries and an unfortunate one in Taurus; then when the moon is in Aries, or in one of the two signs in square with it, or in the sign opposite Aries, the moon will emit good fortune, and the man's disposition will be a good disposition on those days. And when the moon passes through Taurus or in one of the two signs in square with it or the sign opposite Taurus, then it emits misfortune and then the disposition of that man will be a bad disposition on those days, all his life long, and he will be better prepared for things to go badly. And just as this is true in health, so it is the case in sickness. Suppose that a certain acute disease befalls a man when the moon is in Aries, or in square with it in Cancer, or opposite it in Libra, or in [square in] Capricorn; then these diseases will be safer and it is more likely that he can escape them. And if the illness begins when the moon is passing through Taurus or is in Leo or Scorpio or Aquarius, then the illness will be worse for that man and more likely to lead to death, seeing that it is from a higher root. Galen says all this in *On Critical Days* 3, but obscurely....

It is obvious, then, from what has just been said, that the moon exerts a stronger influence for good or ill at the sevens and weaker at the mid-point of the sevens. For this reason, the days that fall on the sevens (like the seventh and the fourteenth) produce stronger crises and the days falling in the middle of the sevens (like the fourth, eleventh and seventeenth) produce weaker ones.... And if you ask how I would know if the starting-point of a disease is good or bad, I reply (following Galen) that when a disease begins when the moon is in a sign in which there is a fortunate [star], or in another which is in square or opposite it, then the starting-point of the illness is a good starting-point for that man who has the illness. And if the disease begins when the moon is in a sign in which there is an unfortunate [star], or in one of the two [signs] which are in square with it, or opposite it, then the starting-point of the illness is called a bad starting-point. Suppose then that for a certain man, an illness starts today; consider, then, whether the starting-point of the illness is a good starting-point, and if it is, when the moon will arrive at the mid-point of the quarter – that is, on the fourth day. Then there will be a modest change in the disease for the better. If his *powers are very strong and the [morbid] matter is small in quantity and very obedient [to treatment], there will then be a complete termination for the good. But if he is not fully powerful and if the matter is not fully obedient, then if nature is strengthened, good will come about on the seventh day. The obvious signs of *digestion [of the morbid matter] will appear – for example, urine with red sediment or [urine that is] white in the upper part. And if it is a *choleric disease in which little or no sediment appears, then a change of color will be visible. Later, when the moon is in square on the seventh day, the disease will undergo a marked change for the better. Then, if the vital powers are strong and establish dominance over the matter of the disease, and the matter is completely digested, then the crisis will be complete. But if not, some of the material at least will be *evacuated, and the patient will be somewhat relieved, and then the crisis will occur on the fourteenth day. This varies with the variety of [morbid] matter and adaptability of individuals to cold and heat.

From this it is plain that the physician, when making a prognostication of death or life, should consider the proper influence of the moon and compare it to the strength of the vital power and of the illness and then it will be easy to prognosticate. Some astronomers in prognostication only take into account the influence of the superior bodies. But doctors in prognostication compare the strength of the vital power and of the illness. And judgment made from comparing the vital power and the illness with respect to power [will reveal] with greater certainty which of these will prevail. For if the vital power is strong and the [morbid] matter obedient, even though the moon emits an unfortunate influence, the crisis will be good, albeit incomplete, or perhaps the crisis will be delayed. And if the disease completely prevails, I say that although the influence of the moon is good, it will end badly, although perhaps the bad [end] will be delayed....

66. PANACEA OR PROBLEM? (2): JACQUES DESPARS'S RESERVATIONS ABOUT MEDICAL ASTROLOGY

Jacques Despars (ca. 1380–1458) was a regent master in the Faculty of Medicine of Paris from 1411 to 1419. From 1420 onwards he lived alternately in Cambrai and Tournai, whence he was frequently summoned to serve the dukes of Burgundy. His commentary on books 1, 2 and 4 (fen 1) of Avicenna's Canon, *composed between 1432 and 1453, was deeply influential. Though Despars was a scholastic doctor through and through, his commentary includes a remarkable amount of information about the author's own clinical experience.*

Despars expresses his skepticism about astrology in his commentary on Canon 1,

fen 4, ch. 20, where Avicenna discusses the timing of bloodletting. He surveys the different styles and levels of medical astrology, each of which requires a reference manual.
Any ordinary calendar would show the Egyptian Days, that is, the two days in each
calendar month that are supposed to be of evil omen for any human undertaking.
But for full-dress Ptolemaic planetary astrology, which based predictions on planetary
"aspects," one would need an almanac showing the zodiacal position of each planet
every day. A more modest almanac would show the moon's zodiacal position, plus
conjunctions (when the moon and sun are in the same sign and degree) and oppositions
(when they are at opposite points of the zodiac). A really pared-down almanac would
contain only the most essential information for bloodletting, namely, the sign of the
zodiac in which the moon would be found (doc. 57).

Source: trans. Faith Wallis from Jacques Despars, commentary on Avicenna, *Canon* Book 1, *fen* 4,
ch. 20, in Avicenna, *Canon* (Lyon: Johannes Trechsel, 24 Dec. 1498), fols. aaa 1r–2v.

Avicenna's Text

Know, furthermore, that there are two times for bloodletting, namely the
time of choice and the time of necessity. The time of choice is during daylight
hours, and after digestion is completed and superfluities have been evacuated.
The time of necessity is whenever it must be done and when one ought not
to delay, and when one should pay no heed to contrary indications.

Despars's Commentary

*Despars discusses the distinction between the two times for bloodletting. He then turns
to criteria for selecting a time for bloodletting.*

First, be aware of the fact that the only real time of choice for bloodletting is
in the spring. According to Averroes in *Colliget* book 7, chapter 3, the suitable
time for bloodletting is spring. Summer is contraindicated for bloodletting
because of the weakening of the vital power in that season and the slack-
ness of the *spirits. Of course, you should do it if the nature of the disease
demands, but in small quantity. Winter is contraindicated for bloodletting
because the blood is congealed and thick in that season. Autumn just after the
end of summer, which is warm and dry in *temperament, is not suitable because of its dryness, because of the perturbation of the winds, because of the
weakening of the vital operations, and because of the preceding hot weather.
Not that bloodletting should be totally banned when the nature of the disease
demands it, but the quantity should be reduced. That is what [Averroes] says.
    Secondly, be aware of the fact that some people, in choosing the time for

bloodletting, insist on diligent attention to the state of the heavens. And of these, some are particularly attentive to the quarters of the moon, because [the moon] exerts power over the moist parts of the body and because it is the planet closest to us. And among these, some decree that bloodletting should take place in [the moon's] first quarter, because it is warm and humid and this corresponds to blood, while others [do it] in the middle of the third quarter because then the *humors are neither constricted nor too abundant. Others follow this [mnemonic] verse: "Old folk need an old moon, young folk need a new." Others assiduously avoid the two Egyptian Days that are inscribed in each month of the calendar. Others do not consider all this to be sufficient, but decree that the moon should be in a propitious sign [of the zodiac] and that it should not be in a malefic aspect with other planets, nor others with it. And so they equip themselves with a large almanac for each year, by means of which they can readily know on any given day what sign each planet is in, and what the aspects are. Others are content with a mid-sized almanac that indicates when the moon enters each [zodiac] sign, the conjunctions and oppositions of sun and moon, the preferred days for bloodletting and the preferred days and nights for taking *purgative medicines. Others are content with a small almanac that just indicates when the moon enters each sign.

But Galen our master and model (*patronus*), Rhazes, Avenzoar, the Prince [Avicenna], and Averroes pay little heed to all this. This is because the heavens are the most remote cause of human dispositions and it is enough for the doctor to understand their more immediate causes. It is also because the judgments of astrology are for the most part uncertain, unstable, ambiguous, and often deceptive for those who make them and those who trust them, due to the diversity of intermediate causes and circumstances and of countless different things that often impede and check the influence of the heavens. But because it pleases princes and nobles (and even common folk) to put their trust in these judgments, even though they are often deceived by them, we concede that on account of their rank one should pay heed to these things in choosing a time for bloodletting. But I advise doctors that they not avoid necessary bloodletting because of the disposition of the heavens, nor defer it for very long. Indeed, if when the sun and moon are in conjunction or opposition, there should come to you a person with a stroke or *quinsy, suffering from a *plethora or with a great amount of blood, severely bruised by a fall or blow, or if a high *fever or an *apostemic lassitude is on the very point of spontaneously being transformed into corruption of the blood, then perform bloodletting on the spot.

67. ROGER BACON: ALCHEMY AND THE MEDICAL PAYOFF OF "EXPERIMENTAL SCIENCE"

Roger Bacon was born in England about 1219 and studied at the University of Paris, where around 1237 he delivered some of the earliest recorded lectures on Aristotle's scientific treatises. He underwent an intellectual conversion experience when he read The Secret of Secrets, *an Arabic work that claimed to be a letter of advice from Aristotle to Alexander the Great. The* Secret of Secrets *implied that knowledge acquired through experience and experiment, rather than through logical analysis, held the greatest hope for bettering the lot of mankind. Bacon decided to return to Oxford to pursue this "experimental science." He joined the Franciscans in 1257, but a few years later was accused of holding suspect ideas and was transferred to Paris. Between 1266 and 1268 he wrote, at the request of Pope Clement IV, a number of manifestos in which he outlined his proposals for a new approach to integrating science and theology, and appealed for research funds. Clement IV died in 1268, and Bacon returned to Oxford, where he continued to write philosophical and theological works. For some reason not entirely clear, Bacon may have been placed under arrest by his Order in 1277. He died in 1292.*

Bacon's "experimental science" encompasses all the ambiguous meanings of the Latin word experimentum: *"experience," "trial," "test," "experiment," "something proven by experience but rationally inexplicable" (see doc. 81). In Bacon's view, experimental science was the way for medicine to make progress, notably in finding remedies against old age. In his treatise* The Errors of the Doctors, *Bacon hurls the usual accusations against physicians (for instance, that they were pretentious, argumentative, and hide-bound), but spends most of his energy arguing that medicine would only discover effective cures by investing in the study of alchemy. Alchemy, as a technology for extracting and separating metal from ore, could be harnessed to isolate and purify the active power in plants and other* materia medica, *leaving the useless or harmful parts behind. In the passage below, we pick up the thread of his argument at the point where he proposes that medical education shift its priorities radically and embrace the new sciences of power.*

a. Medicine and "Experimental Science": The *Opus maius*

Source: trans. Robert Belle Burke, *The Opus maius of Roger Bacon* (Philadelphia: University of Pennsylvania Press, 1928), vol. 2, pp. 583–87, 617–19, 626–27. Latin.

Having laid down fundamental principles of the wisdom of the Latins so far as they are found in language, mathematics, and optics, I now wish to unfold the principles of experimental science, since without experience nothing can be sufficiently known. For there are two modes of acquiring knowledge, namely, by reasoning and experience. Reasoning draws a conclusion and makes us grant the conclusion, but does not make the conclusion certain, nor does it remove doubt so that the mind may rest on the intuition of truth unless the mind discovers it by the path of experience; since many have the arguments relating to what can be known, but because they lack experience they neglect the arguments, and neither avoid what is harmful nor follow what is good. For if a man who has never seen fire should prove by adequate reasoning that fire burns and injures things and destroys them, his mind would not be satisfied thereby, nor would he avoid fire, until he placed his hand or some combustible substance in the fire, so that he might prove by experience that which reasoning taught. But when he has had actual experience of combustion his mind is made certain and rests in the full light of truth. Therefore reasoning does not suffice, but experience does....

He therefore who wishes to rejoice without doubt in regard to the truths underlying phenomena must know how to devote himself to experiment. For authors write many statements, and people believe them through reasoning which they formulate without experience. Their reasoning is wholly false. For it is generally believed that the diamond cannot be broken except by goat's blood, and philosophers and theologians misuse this idea. But fracture by means of blood of this kind has never been verified, although the effort has been made; and without that blood it can be broken easily. For I have seen this with my own eyes, and this is necessary, because gems cannot be carved except by fragments of this stone. Similarly it is generally believed that the *castoreum employed by physicians [is] the testicles of the male [beaver (Latin: *castor*)]. But this is not true, because the beaver has these [castoreum glands] under its breast, and both the male and female produce testicles of this kind. Besides these [castoreum glands], the male beaver has its testicles in their natural place; and therefore what is subjoined is a dreadful lie, namely that when the hunters pursue the beaver, he himself knowing what they are seeking cuts out with his teeth these glands. Moreover, it is generally believed that hot water freezes more quickly than cold in vessels, and the argument advanced in support of this is that contrary is excited by contrary, just like enemies meeting each other. But it is certain that cold water freezes more quickly for any one who makes the experiment. People attribute this to Aristotle in the second book of the *Meteorology*; but he certainly does not make this statement, [although] he does make one like it, by which they have been deceived, namely that if cold water and hot water are poured on a cold place, as upon ice, the hot water freezes more quickly, and this is true. But if hot water and cold are placed in two vessels, the cold will freeze more quickly. Therefore all things must be verified by experience.

But experience is of two kinds; one is gained through our external senses, and in this way we gain our experience of those things that are in the heavens by instruments made for this purpose, and of those things here below by means attested by our vision. Things that do not belong in our part of the world we know through other scientists who have had experience of them. As, for example, Aristotle on the authority of Alexander sent two thousand men through different parts of the world to gain experimental knowledge of all things that are on the surface of the earth, as Pliny bears witness in his *Natural History*. This experience is both human and philosophical, as far as man can act in accordance with the grace given him; but this experience does not suffice him, because it does not give full attestation in regard to things corporeal owing to its difficulty, and does not touch at all on things spiritual. It is necessary, therefore, that the intellect of man should be otherwise aided, and for this reason the holy patriarchs and prophets, who first gave sciences to the world, received illumination within and were not dependent on sense alone. The same is true of many believers since the time of Christ. For the grace of faith illuminates greatly, as also do divine inspirations, not only in things spiritual, but in things corporeal and in the sciences of philosophy; as Ptolemy states in the *Centiloquium*, namely that there are two roads by which we arrive at the knowledge of facts, one through the experience of philosophy, the other through divine inspiration, which is far the better way, as he says....

Therefore since all the divisions of speculative philosophy proceed by arguments, which are either based on a point from authority or on the other points of argumentation except this division which I am now examining, we find necessary the science that is called experimental. I wish to explain it, as it is useful not only to philosophy, but to the knowledge of God, and for the direction of the whole world....

Another example can be given in the field of medicine in regard to the prolongation of human life, for which the medical art has nothing to offer except the *regimen of health. But a far longer extension of life is possible....

Therefore in regard to this we must strive, that the wonderful and ineffable utility and splendor of experimental science may appear and a pathway may be opened to the greatest secret of secrets, which Aristotle has hidden in his book on the regimen of life [i.e., *Secret of Secrets*]. For although the regimen of health should be observed in food and drink, in sleep and in wakefulness, in motion and in rest, in *evacuation and retention, in the nature of the air and in the passions of the mind, so that these matters should be properly cared for from infancy, no one wishes to take thought in regard to them, not even physicians, since we see that scarcely one physician in a thousand will give this matter even slight attention. Very rarely does it happen that any one pays sufficient heed to the rules of health. No one does so in his youth, but sometimes one in three thousand thinks of these matters when he is old and approaching death, for at that time he fears for himself and thinks of his health. But he cannot then apply a remedy because of his weakened *powers and senses and his lack of experience. Therefore fathers are weakened and beget weak sons with a liability to premature death. Then by neglect of the rules of health the sons weaken themselves, and thus the son's son has a doubly weakened constitution, and in his turn weakens himself by a disregard of these rules. Thus a weakened constitution passes from father to sons, until a final shortening of life has been reached, as is the case in these days....

Since I have shown that the cause of a shortening of life of this kind is accidental, and therefore that a remedy is possible, I now return to this example which I have decided to give in the field of medicine, in which the power of medical arts fails. But the experimental art supplies the defect of medicine in this particular ...

But the medical art does not furnish remedies against this corruption that comes from lack of control and failure in regimen, just as all physicians expert in their art know, although medical authors confess that remedies are possible, but they do not teach them. For these remedies have always been hidden not only from physicians, but from the whole rank and file of scientists, and have been revealed only to the most noted....

Bacon argues that the "elixir" to retard old age would be a compound in which the four elements are perfectly in balance.

If the elements should be prepared and purified in some mixture, so that there would be no action of one element on another, but so that they would be reduced to pure simplicity, the wisest have judged that they would have the most perfect medicine. For in this way the elements would be equal. Averroes, moreover, asserts in opposition to [Galen] in the tenth book of the *Metaphysics* that if a mixture was made with an equality of the miscibles, the elements would not act or be acted on, nor would they be corrupted. Aristotle also maintains this view in the fifth book of the *Metaphysics*, where he has stated definitely that no corruption occurs when the active potencies are equal; and this is an assured fact.

For this condition will exist in our bodies after the resurrection. For an equality of elements in those bodies excludes corruption for ever. For this equality is the ultimate end of the natural matter in mixed bodies, because it is the noblest state, and therefore in it the appetite of matter would cease, and would desire nothing beyond.... Scientists, therefore, have striven to reduce the elements in some form of food or drink to an equality or nearly so, and have taught the means to this end. But owing to the difficulty of this very great experiment, and because few take an interest in experiments, since the labor involved is complicated and the expense very great, and because men pay no heed to the secrets of nature and the possibilities of art, it happens that very few have labored on this very great secret of science, and still fewer have reached a laudable end....

b. In Alchemy Lies the Salvation of Medicine: Bacon's *On the Errors of the Doctors*

Source: trans. Mary Catherine Welborn, "The Errors of the Doctors According to Friar Roger Bacon of the Minor Order," *Isis* 18 (1932): 31–33. Latin.

15. The fifth deficiency [in physicians] is that they are ignorant of alchemy and agriculture; while on the contrary it is quite evident that practically all *simple drugs are discussed in these two subjects. There are a great many difficulties that arise on account of the lack of knowledge of alchemy, because when the art of medicine teaches the use of the virtues of drugs without the substance, and it is necessary to do this in an infinite number of cases on account of the whole mass of poisonous earthy material, no distinction between them can be made except by means of alchemy which alone gives the method of extracting each virtue from any substance whatsoever; because it is necessary in working with drugs that there be resolutions and dissolutions [*that is, extraction*] of one thing from another which cannot be made without the aid of alchemy which gives the method of resolving any one substance from any other.

16. There are numerous examples of this: for instance, from the kinds of rhubarb used for *purging *phlegm the *virtue alone should be taken and not the whole substance, of which fact practically the whole world of doctors is ignorant; although it is a most beneficial thing and especially good for the human body, and among all medicines it alone strengthens the natural heat and invigorates the body, just as is shown by Aristotle in the [*Secret of Secrets*], and I too have observed this in my own body. For every other drug weakens either a little or a great deal as everyone knows, and this alone strengthens. There is practically an infinite number of other similar examples [of drugs] from which the virtue should be extracted in order that they may be taken easily and without danger, as is shown in books dealing with drugs. But not only should the useful virtue be separated from the substance, but also the poisonous virtue from the useful substance, as for example in viper's flesh, in the head of the dragon, and in many others, it is necessary not only to extract the poisonous virtue but also other useless things, and not only this but it is also necessary to make a variety of resolutions of bodies from other bodies, as in the extraction of elements of various kinds, and various kinds of water,

and many other things, and whether those substances from which they are extracted are altogether useless, or poisonous, or indifferent, or useful for many other purposes. For thus by means of alchemy is extracted the *blessed oil from bricks, rose water from roses, *et cetera* which can and should be much improved by alchemical methods rather than by the untutored. Again many drugs should be sublimated, just as Avicenna and others have clearly told us.

17. In addition to these and similar ways in which alchemy is useful in medical practice, the application of its methods is always valuable in medical theory and highly necessary, since it explains inclusively the entire development of things from their elements through the simple humors and then composite ones even up to the parts of animals and plants and men, as has already been touched upon; medicine does not explain this development but constantly sends the doctors to alchemy, as is shown by Avicenna in many places, and by other authors of medical works. Whence this alone of the sciences, that is alchemy, dares to explain what are the first four elements, then the second four, and a third four, up to twelve, from which man and the whole lower world are made. Whence there are twelve corporeal substances that have within themselves the power to determine the species of things and exist in the world *per se*, and the natural philosopher deals with only four of these elements. However the doctor, although he touches upon these things, does not explain them but sends the medical students to alchemy....

68. BISTICIUS: A FLORENTINE GOLDSMITH AND MEDICAL ALCHEMIST

Bisticius (d. ca 1487) is a shadowy figure, though he is mentioned in several fifteenth-century Italian sources. Some contemporaries characterized him as an illiterate silver-smith who gained a reputation as an alchemical healer. On the other hand, there is documentary evidence that Bisticius bequeathed books to the library of the monastery of San Marco in Florence. Some of these books survive; a note in one of them gives Bisticius's full name as "Master [the title of a learned man] Lorenzo son of Master Jacopo Filippe de Bisticcio" and states that he was a famous professor of medicine. A manuscript of alchemical and medical treatises written out by one Bartholomaeus Marcellus, and now in Venice (San Marco lat. VI 282), says that Bartholomaeus copied many alchemical works from books owned by Bisticius. It adds that because Bisticius was a goldsmith and knew about sublimations, he "became a marvelous doctor, beyond the most famous physicians of this age, so that he seemed no empiric but the supreme monarch of medicine, and was so courted by all the nobles, lords and princes of Italy, as if he had been the oracle of Apollo and with immense gain for himself, and there seemed to be in him the soul and reason of most holy Hippocrates of yore" (as cited by Thorndike [see source note below], p. 42). This same manuscript contains some of Bisticius's own recipes, supposedly written in his own hand.

Source: trans. Lynn Thorndike, *Science and Thought in the Fifteenth Century* (New York and London: Haffner, 1967), pp. 266–67.

The first medicine, oft tested by me, Bisticius, is against *tertian and *quartan fever. So in the name of Jesus Christ collect on three days three leaves of salvia or, if you wish, all three at once on one day, with the greatest devotion and faith repeating a paternoster [*the Lord's Prayer*], Ave Maria [*"Hail, Mary ..."*], creed, and Salve Regina [*the hymn to the Virgin "Hail, Queen ..."*], and after collecting these three leaves write on the first thus: "The Father is peace"; on the second, " + The Son is the life"; on the third, " + The Holy Spirit is the cure and health." But I have tried, too, writing all these on all three leaves, and at the same time those other words that follow and are similarly efficacious, namely, " + Christ was born, + Christ died, + Christ rose again," and these are written in the same way on leaves of salvia and are eaten on three days on a fasting stomach, one on each day.

Recipe for a balsam oft tested in many and the greatest emergencies. Take a pound of turpentine; of frankincense, two ounces; of aloes, lemon, one ounce; of mastix, gariofle [*cloves*], galange, cinnamon, nux, must, cubebs, one ounce each; of gum elemni [*resin from an unidentified plant*], called apretitreos, six ounces; of ardent water [*distilled alcohol*] four times distilled, one pound. Grind all of them that can be ground, and mix together, and put in an alembic and seal it so no vapor can get out and place it in a furnace for the purpose, namely a distillery, and distill it with a slow fire. The first water [*that is, the first product of distillation*] will be clear as spring water, the next will begin to show color and to thicken and it will float on the other water and they won't mix. But the third water will be still denser and thick like honey. It may fitly be called the balsam of water and will appear thick in its distillation, and in every test its *virtue is as the virtue of balsam. But note that in case you wish to make an unguent, you should use in place of *aqua vitae* [*distilled alcohol*] laurel unguent and put the mixture in a well sealed bottle in a dunghill for eight days, and 'twill be good for colds, no matter how windy and watery they may be. Observe that the first water burns like *aqua ardens* [*distilled alcohol*]. The second coagulates milk, and if you put one tepid drop of the said water in a saucer of tepid milk, it immediately coagulates the milk.... The first water that is drawn off is called water of balsam. The second is called ivory of balsam. The third is called artificial [*manufactured*] balsam. The first is good, the second better, the third best. The first burns itself without burning a cloth, but leaves it dry. The second is combustible and burns a cloth too. The third is stronger by a hundredfold, and the more it is worked over and redistilled, the stronger it will be to a hundredfold. Therefore during distillation it burns wood and anything which is put in it....

To break any stone in the human bladder and eject it: the most approved experiment for those who cannot urinate because of stone. Take a hare that hasn't been skinned and put it in a clean pot and cover the pot. Then put it in a furnace till it is well burnt and becomes a black powder, and give a little of it to the patient with an egg and he will be cured and there's no doubt of it. Be sure you put the hare in alive with all his intestines in the aforesaid pot. And if you wish to prepare the patient, follow this procedure. Cook rock parsley with oil, then wring out the oil and place the parsley before and behind the patient; then after a bit give him some of the aforesaid powdered hare and he will be cured right away, and let this be done until he is cured.

To cure films in the eyes of beasts, grind glass thoroughly and sift it well with a sieve and put it in the beasts' eyes and within five days they will be cured. For the same: burn well human excrement and put it in the eyes of beasts which have leucoma, using a tube, and they will be cured.

PART III.

MEDICINE AND SOCIETY (1100–1500)

Part II of this book explored medicine's metamorphosis into a learned profession from the inside, so to speak – that is, through the voices of people who taught medicine or composed texts for the use of doctors. This final section switches to a wide-angled lens, presenting documents that reveal how healers and patients interacted within an increasingly complex and articulate society. One might expect that scholastic medicine, with its heavy investment in scientific definitions and logical explanations, would clarify what disease was and what the experience of illness meant. The texts presented in chapter 9 show that clarity was not easy to achieve. Diagnosis was the exegesis of symptoms, and the meanings elicited were symbolic as well as clinical. Moreover, formally educated physicians were not the only people in the shifting social landscape of late medieval Europe who claimed to discern these meanings and to bring help to the suffering (chapter 10). From the university-trained doctor's point of view, the case was clear: practice without theory, the hallmark of the ancient Empiricist school, now became the stigma of the "empiric" who presumed to treat without benefit of formal learning. As doctors organized professional guilds and colleges in imitation of university faculties, they geared up to lobby Church and Crown to make *physica the one true, licit medicine. Their success, however, was mitigated: "empirics" could advance arguments of their own, and the persistence of older, less sharply defined models of medicina *provided room for informal avenues of healing.*

Learned doctors fought back by claiming that their medical practice was especially secure and effective. In chapter 11, we shadow these physicians as they seek to back up that claim in practice, encountering patients at the bedside, advising them by letter, and above all, offering what only an academic doctor could offer: a scientific explanation for an unprecedented medical catastrophe, the Black Death. Peering over the doctor's shoulder was an increasingly obtrusive body of ecclesiastical regulations and secular laws designed to ensure that the doctor acted in accordance with the precepts of the Christian faith and for the public good (chapter 12). But the ambition of the Church after the eleventh-century Gregorian Reform to fashion Europe into a fully Christian society also stimulated more visible and corporate expressions of the core Christian value of charity. Medicine and charity intersected and overlapped in the medieval hospital (chapter 13).

To realize its project of reforming society, the Church embarked upon a campaign of educating Christians of all ranks to internalize the demands of the Gospel. Its principal tactic was the ritual of moral diagnosis and therapy called confession; its goal was to Christianize all aspects of lay life, from the battlefield to the bedroom, from the marketplace to the palace. This great religious enterprise had a medical cognate: the cultivation of health in daily life (chapter 14). Like preachers and confessors, doctors laid down regimens for the good life, and in so doing they helped to shape the European concept of self-regulation and self-fashioning. But rules have a way of provoking resistance. The final chapter of this book listens to medieval voices that lampoon or lash out at the intellectual and moral failings of doctors. If some of these texts speak with the accents of late medieval anti-clerical protest, this only confirms medicine's position as Christianity's secular shadow.

CHAPTER NINE

WHAT IS DISEASE? WHAT IS ILLNESS? DOCTORS' DILEMMAS AND THE MEANING OF SUFFERING

In the middle of the seventeenth century, the English physician Thomas Sydenham (1624–89) proposed that diseases should be studied as if they were plants, that is, as distinct species with consistent characteristics and uniform life-histories. This proposal was an important milestone on the path to the modern conception of disease specificity. The road would eventually lead through pathological anatomy, which showed how diseases leave distinctive lesions on particular parts of the body, to the germ theory, which exposed some diseases as the actions of living organisms that invade the body. By the mid-nineteenth century, medicine accepted that diseases always behaved in more or less the same way, regardless of who had them.

Few learned doctors prior to Sydenham's day would have entertained such a view of disease. There were, to be sure, named diseases with distinctive patterns of symptoms (John of Gaddesden's description of smallpox is a good example: doc. 54) and it was important to distinguish these symptom patterns (for instance, the differentiation of pleurisy and pneumonia in the Liber tertius: *doc. 6). The true nature of a disease, however, resided in its cause, and that cause was not an entity with a separate existence in the natural world. Setting aside trauma or malformation, disease was primarily an event – some disruption in the state of the body's* *humors *and* *spirits. *Exposed to the* **"non-natural"* *influences of the environment or behavior, humors and spirits could augment or diminish, accumulate in different locations and move to other locations, become overheated and scorched, exude fumes, generate winds, putrefy, and be tainted or poisoned. Every* morbus *or named disease was the consequence of such a disequilibrium or change. The doctor's business was to go to the root of the problem and bring the body back into its right humoral mix, its* *temperament. *Symptoms such as* *fever *or swelling needed to be brought under control, but these were essentially tactical moves; the grand strategy was to* *evacuate *corrupt *humors from the body and help the individual's nature to return to equilibrium.*

In this chapter, we shall examine how this dynamic and individualistic model shaped medieval approaches to three difficult diseases: leprosy, cancer, and mental illness. Medical anthropologists point to the distinction between the disease *that the doctor names and knows, and the* illness *that the patient experiences. In the medieval context, what a disease was and what an illness meant were rather closer together than they are in the modern world. Not far below the surface of the medical descriptions of leprosy and cancer lurk savage beasts: leprosy threatens to transform human faces into those of lions*

337

or human flesh into the scales of a serpent; cancer is a voracious animal devouring the breast from within. Mental illness as well was both a natural affliction and a sign of spiritual distress. Hence when people turned to the renowned visionary and medical writer Hildegard of Bingen (doc. 73), they were seeking both prophecy and prognosis.

69. INTERPRETING SYMPTOMS:
THE DIFFICULT CASE OF LEPROSY

Historians at one time treated leprosy as the quintessential medieval disease. It was presumed to be everywhere, and at almost epidemic levels. Medieval people were portrayed as obsessively afraid of leprosy, which they considered highly contagious. It was assumed that leper hospitals were designed to isolate and confine lepers and that lepers themselves were cut off from society, even to the point of being ritually declared dead. However, in recent years, thanks to innovative research by François-Olivier Touati in France, Luke Demaitre in the United States, and Carole Rawcliffe in England, this sensationalist and distorted picture is being dismantled. That being said, leprosy was a disease that lay at the intersection of complex cultural and religious responses and it could entail significant and sometimes negative social consequences for individual sufferers. Ironically, hostile attitudes toward lepers seem to have intensified from the fourteenth century onwards, when the disease itself was in sharp decline and its identity was becoming more and more medicalized.

For scholastic medicine, leprosy posed particular problems of adapting Galenic theory to the pressing realities of practice. Doctors were trained to think of disease as a fluid event taking place in the body of an individual with a distinctive *temperament. In the case of leprosy, though, they had to confront the fact that patients and their communities just wanted to know whether this specific disease was present or not. Doctors began de facto treating leprosy as an entity separable from the individual patient. Once detected, leprosy was presumed incurable, though medical authors proposed a number of palliative treatments.

The two texts presented here deal with the difficulties of diagnosing leprosy. Leprosy causes thickening, degeneration, and destruction of the normal cell structure of the skin, nerves, mucosa, and lymphatic glands. But the resulting symptoms can vary considerably: skin nodules and sores, impaired breathing and hoarseness, loss of eyebrows, and the loss of sensitivity along nerve trunks. Gilbert the Englishman (fl. ca 1250) recognized most of these symptoms correctly, but he also struggled with the fact that many of them could be signs of other diseases. Gilbert nonetheless remained loyal to the idea that the cause of leprosy was humoral imbalance; indeed, the humoral model furnished a plausible explanation of why leprosy symptoms varied so widely.

In the clinical manual ascribed to Jordanus de Turre (fl. 1310–35) the symptoms were reduced to essentials, with practical, step-by-step advice for testing. Jordanus gestured toward Galenic diagnosis by excreta and pulse, but he was really concerned with the more pertinent changes in mucosa, skin, and nerve sensitivity. However, he took pains to present the reason (in Galenic terms) why a given sign was diagnostic. Aware of the patient's desire to conceal his condition and avoid a diagnosis of leprosy, Jordanus advised the doctor to examine the interior nasal mucosa (a sign inaccessible to the patient himself), and described an ingenious way of testing whether the patient had lost sensitivity, even if the patient were trying to hide this fact.

a. Gilbert the Englishman: The Symptoms of Leprosy

Source: trans. Michael R. McVaugh from Gilbert the Englishman, *Compendium medicine*, in *Sourcebook in Medieval Science*, ed. Edward Grant (Cambridge, MA: Harvard University Press, 1974), pp. 752–54 (no. 101.1). Latin.

The General Symptoms of Leprosy

It is important to recognize the disease of leprosy, together with its antecedent and conjoint causes, from its proper symptoms; first in general, then after analysis according to its species, for a clearer understanding.

One symptom is a permanent loss of sensation, coming from within, particularly of the last digits of both the hands and feet, namely the smallest digit and the one next to it; and of the muscle, from the little finger to the elbow or even the shoulder, and from the toe to the knee and sometimes above. A coldness in these places named above is another sign.... This coldness sometimes occurs without any clear external cause and is in some cases permanent. Should there be an external cause of cold, these places are easily chilled; from such causes there may be produced a brief numbness and prickling in the forehead, palate, tongue, eyelids, and brows – first as if from ants, then as if from needles, and finally as if from large spines. Prickling is an equivocal symptom, though, and may mean leprosy or paralysis. Leprosy is in the muscles and flesh and the external parts; paralysis is in the nerves and is accompanied by debility of the nerves. Lucidity of the skin is also a symptom, seen because the natural folds of the skin are not present; it is instead stretched into a similitude to very thin polished leather. There is consumption of the muscles, leaving empty space, but this is equivocal and may also indicate a wasting disease. Similarly, distortion of the joints of the foot and hands, and of the mouth and nose [is a symptom]; this is preceded by a tickling sensation, as if some living thing were fluttering about within the body, the thorax, the arms, or the lips. A motion can be felt there which is even apparent to the sight; it sometimes affects the eye and distorts it. This is a very sure symptom. There will be fetidity of the breath, the sweat, and the skin, although this indication can be erroneous. The site [of the disease] will lose its hair, and the hair that grows back will be very fine, so fine that it cannot be seen unless looked at against the sun. Sometimes none grows back at all. When the eyebrows and lashes lose their hair, it is the worst of all signs. Hoarseness and obstruction of the nostrils are also general signs, [assuming they do not derive] from any other cause. When the affected parts are washed, water will run off the skin, just as if it had been oiled; this is a very bad sign; so too if the place is rubbed briskly and the water disappears. The corners of the eyes grow round and brilliant. The skin rises into little pimples, like those that appear on the skin of a plucked goose, even if there has been no touch or chilliness to cause this. The blood drawn off in *phlebotomy is greasy and contains sand.... Tumors accompany the loss of hair from the eyebrows. Lepers search for sexual pleasure more than usual and more than they should; they are ardent in the act, yet find themselves weaker than usual. Their skin is tormented by a persistent itching; they suffer inordinately now from heat and now from cold. They do not often come down with fever nor suffer with a *quartan fever. When they do, it comes on them only once or twice; or if it comes on more often, it indicates the *resolution and cure of the leprous matter.... They will suddenly feel a coldness, as if cold water were passing between their skin and their flesh or over their skin; it sometimes seems to them as though drops of rain were striking them on the face or on some other part of the body. They become enraged more easily than usual. Their blood, washed, is lumpy and has a fetid odor. Their eyes become distorted, rimmed with red, striking horror into those who see them. Grains will be found under their tongues, as in leprous swine. Also, if blood is rubbed in the palm of the hand and squeaks or is too greasy, or if the blood passing into clear still water remains on the surface, it is a sign of leprosy.... If urine poured over blood mixes easily with it, it is a bad sign. If vinegar poured over blood bubbles and does not mix with it, as it would mix with something dry, it is a sign of corruption; so is fetidity of the blood. The urine of lepers is thin of substance, sometimes containing hairs and sand.

The Symptoms Proper to Each Kind of Leprosy

Now that we have described the symptoms [of leprosy] is general, we will discuss them in relation to their antecedent causes, namely the four humors. The leprosy cause by *adust *melancholic blood, or blood *infected with adust melancholy, is called *elephantia* [*"elephant disease"*]; that caused by adust *choleric blood, or choler scorching and infecting blood, is called *leonina* [*"lion disease"*]; that caused by adust *phlegmatic blood, or blood infected with adust phlegm, is called *tyria* [*"serpent disease"*]; and that caused by blood adust and corrupt in its own right, or corrupted by something external, is called *allopicia* [*"fox disease"*]. These varieties are rarely found uncombined; indeed, we frequently find two or three or four forms occurring together. The combination is to be interpreted according to the symptoms of the individual varieties and a compound medicine administered according to the combination of symptoms.

b. Jordanus de Turre: Diagnostic Protocol for Leprosy

Source: trans. Michael R. McVaugh in *Sourcebook in Medieval Science*, ed. Edward Grant (Cambridge, MA: Harvard University Press, 1974), pp. 754–55 (no. 101.2). Latin.

Lepers can be recognized by five signs: by the urine, by the pulse, by the blood, by the voice, and by the different members. Whoever wants to determine whether someone has leprosy should first make him sing. If his voice is harsh, it may be a sign of leprosy, but if it is clear, it is a good sign. (Proceed as follows: take a tablet and write the good signs on one side and the bad signs on the other, and you will not become confused.)

It is also possible to judge by the urine, and this in four ways. First, the urine of lepers must be white with a certain transparency. Moreover, it must be clear and thin. As for the contents, they will be clotted and should look like flour or ground bran. Finally, if the urinal is shaken, it should make a sound; the reason is that while with fevered patients there would be no noise, because of the oiliness removed from the body, with lepers there will be, thanks to the earthiness and dryness of the matters contained in it.

It is also possible to recognize lepers by the pulse, which should be weak. Avicenna gives the reason for this, that it has little force because of the artery, which is almost entirely dried up.

Similarly, they can be recognized by the blood. You should bleed the patient from a vein in any part of the body so that the blood is collected in a clean vessel; leave it until a residue is formed, which should be put into a linen cloth and shaken in fresh water; squeeze it gently until the water is no longer appreciably tinted. Then take what is left in the cloth after the squeezing, and if you see brilliant white corpuscles there, looking like millet or panicum, it is a sign of leprosy. Or put a large lump of salt in the liquid extracted from the blood; if it melts or dissolves, this is a good sign, but if not, if it remains whole, it is a sign of leprosy. The reason for this is that in leprous blood there is no good warm moistness able to dissolve it, only a thick earthiness by which it cannot be dissolved. Or pour strong vinegar onto the blood; if the vinegar foams, it is a sign of leprosy, just as when you pour it on the ground it foams, because of its dryness. Finally, you can pour urine onto the blood; if it sinks and mixes, it is a sign of leprosy, and if not, not. The reason for using urine and not some other liquid is that urine is a very subtle, penetrating substance and also has a greater suitability for use with blood, being its filtrate.

It is also possible to recognize lepers by examining the different members. First, because lepers have thin, fine hairs, so that they thicken at the roots; moreover, their hairs are pale and grey. This is due to the fact that the material from which the hairs are formed is lacking and cannot be exhaled through the pores, because the pores are [almost] closed. It is advisable to examine the hairs in sunlight, to see if they are thin and straight, like pigs' bristles.

They are also recognized by the skin of the head, which is lumpy, so that one area is higher than the next; and by the lack of hair on the eyebrows, since lepers have no hair there, particularly at the corners; their brows have a curvature, seeming almost round and spherical. They are recognized, too, by the roundness of the eyeballs, which seem to be starting from their sockets, so that a leper's face is horrible to see; its natural expression being distorted, it is a terrible sight. These are the most obvious signs.

But it can also be recognized by a wound in the nostrils, which can be examined in the following manner. Cut a small wooden wand and fork it like tongs and introduce it into the nose, expanding it; then examine the interior with a lighted candle. If you see within an ulceration or excoriation in the deepest part of the nose, it is a sign of leprosy itself; this is a sign which is known not to all but to the wise only. Or it can be recognized by the bridge of the nose, where there should be a depression like a thread stretched lengthwise along it; for the cartilage which joins the two parts is eaten away, leaving a furrow.

They can also be recognized by the veins around the eyes and by the veins of the chest, which are very red, since the arteries and veins are bleached out by desiccation, while the blood is red, so that their red color is seen; for contraries stand out when juxtaposed. Or they can be recognized by the tongue. Draw out the tongue, using a cloth, and if you can see white corpuscles at its root, like grains of millet, it is a sure sign of leprosy.

Having done all these things, you must examine the patient completely naked, to see whether his skin is darkened and to see if its surface feels rough with a certain smoothness at the same time; if so, it is a sign of leprosy. Then sprinkle cold water on the shoulders; if it is not retained, it is a sign of leprosy. The reason is that the oiliness of the skin is weakened by the excess heat beneath the skin and water will not stay on this oiliness; and so it is a sign.

Or make the patient cover his eyes so that he cannot see and say, "Look out, I'm going to prick you!" and do not prick him. Then say, "I pricked you on the foot"; and if he agrees, it is a sign of leprosy. Likewise, prick him with a needle, from the little finger and the flesh next to it up to the arm. The reason for doing it in these fingers rather than others is that they are the weakest and therefore the ones which are first lost to the natural state.

These are the universal signs of leprosy, which are not dependent on any of its forms. But any of the latter can be known, [for example] whether it is leonine, by using the signs listed above with those given by Avicenna in

Book 1, *fen* 2, of the *Canon*.... If you find signs of blood, you are dealing with the variety called "alopecia," for there their hair falls and they seem flayed like a fox, whence the name. If you find signs of phlegm, it is the variety called "tyria," whose name comes from the serpent "tyro." If you find signs of choler, it is the leonine variety, which gets its name because the face [of the patient] looks like that of a lion. But if symptoms of melancholy are found, it is the variety called "elephantia," in which the skin seems flayed away.

70. METAPHOR AND MALIGNANCY – THE DIFFICULT CASE OF CANCER (1): JEAN OF TOURNEMIRE DIAGNOSES HIS DAUGHTER'S BREAST CANCER AND RECEIVES DIVINE MEDICAL AID

*"Cancer" in medieval medicine was a term that covered gangrene (*cancera*), lupus, *erysipelas, penetrating abscesses, canker sores, shingles, and "St Anthony's fire," as well as what a modern person would recognize as cancer. Nonetheless, from the medieval perspective it was something quite precise. Morbid swellings (*apostemes) that were hard, spread quickly, sent out dark branches like the legs of a crab, and eventually produced ulcers that corroded the flesh were typically "cancer." The defining factor was the cause, namely *melancholy that had been *corrupted or *adust (scorched) and had thickened and hardened within the body. Some cancers were also understood to begin with a latent or hidden phase (*cancer absconditus or occultus*), but the latter term could also apply to any cancer that was embedded in *nerves and blood vessels, particularly cancer of the breast. Cancer was an especially malign and insidious disease. Like the animal for which it was named, it moved in an unpredictable fashion, burrowing into the flesh, grasping and gnawing its prey with dreadful tenacity. Its sibling disease, lupus, was named for the ravenous wolf, because it seemed to chew off the flesh. Cancer was always "wild" and "evil," and the prognosis was always bad.*

Jean of Tournemire (fl. 1380) was a graduate of Montpellier; he went on to teach there, wrote a number of conventional scholastic medical works, and eventually became physician to the Avignon popes. In 1387, he diagnosed his own eighteen-year-old daughter Marguerite with breast cancer. She was healed through the relics of St Peter of Luxembourg, the boy-bishop of Metz, who died that very year at the age of eighteen at the papal court, attended by Jean of Tournemire himself. Jean told the story of Marguerite's miraculous healing to a commission examining evidence for the canonization of Peter. The commissioners were particularly concerned that Jean explain his initial diagnosis. His criteria echo those found in the major scholastic treatises: a hard tumor, which begins as a small swelling like a hazelnut and then grows in an alarming manner.

Cancer was thought to be stimulated by being touched – hence treating Marguerite by rubbing her cancer with the relic of St Peter was doubly miraculous.

Source: trans. Faith Wallis from *Acta Sanctorum* Julii Tomus Primus (Paris: Victor Palme, 1867), pp. 525–27. Some corrections to the text have been introduced following the readings of Ernest Wickersheimer, "Les guérisons miraculeuses du Cardinal Pierre de Luxembourg (1387–1390)," *2e Congrès international d'histoire de la médecine, Paris 1921* (Évreux: Herissey, 1922), pp. 371–89. Latin.

Witness 45 was questioned concerning article 182 of the said articles, which begins thus: "*Item*, that Marguerite, daughter of master Jean of Tournemire, physician of our lord the pope, residing the city of Montpellier," etc. [Jean of Tournemire] said that he knew this much about the contents of the article, namely, that in the year of the Lord 1387, and at the beginning of the month of September last, he (the witness), physician to our lord the pope, and on active service, wished to visit his home in Montpellier. And when he arrived there, he discovered that his daughter Marguerite, wife of Pierre Saisse, eighteen years of age, was stricken in her left breast with a hard tumor and with pain. When he asked her how this had come about, she said in reply (her mother being present) that it had started as a nodule like a hazel-nut, hard to the touch, and painful when touched. Eventually this nodule and induration expanded over a great part of the breast. [Jean] saw that she was pregnant, and said that doubtless it was because of the unborn infant. But her mother replied, "How can that be, when it is not in the other breast?" The witness gave her what relief he could, saying that it was a cancerous disease, a hidden cancer (*cancer absconditus*), which is a mortal illness. Indeed, when it breaks out onto the surface of the breast and it starts to ulcerate, [patients] die within a year or a year and a half, from the flesh being gnawed away, for gradually the breast is completely gnawed away. Nor did he ever see anyone suffering from such a disease who was alive after a year and a half or two years at the most. For although this gnawing away can be remitted by a physician applying ointments, he did not see anyone surviving beyond two years, but rather, they died. This violent gnawing is ferociously gruesome in its advance, and although some women are robust they usually do not survive the second year. Rather, the breast is, so to speak, gnawed away within this time. This disease is called *noli me tangere* by some, because the more it is handled, the worse it gets, unless it be with an ointment selected by an excellent physician.

Seeing this, [Jean of Tournemire] was deeply perturbed. He said to his daughter's mother, and to [Marguerite] herself, "Do not do anything apart from avoiding certain things, namely, salted meats, cheese, legumes, fruits with hard flesh, chestnuts, pears. And show devotion to the most glorious cardinal, Lord Peter of Luxembourg, and permit the said daughter to visit his image in the church of Notre Dame des Tables with your offerings; and show devotion to him twice a day in the morning and the evening, calling upon him and upon his aid on naked bended knees." His daughter said to him that they should send her a piece of the robe [rauba] of the said lord cardinal with which she could touch her breast. [Jean of Tournemire] took his leave of them in tears, and returned to the service of our lord the pope at court. The next day, he went to the tomb of the said lord cardinal to bow down in reverence before the lord cardinal. In tears, he made his trouble known to [the saint], beseeching him to display the power and might which he possesses together with the holy Godhead. A few days later he went to the lord bishop-elect, and now bishop of Coutances, beseeching him to give him a little of the robe of the said lord cardinal. [The bishop] replied that he did not have [the robe], but only the linen garments in which the cardinal died. And he opened his coffer, and gave [Jean de Tournemire] a small piece of one of the linen garments. And he showed him a knotted cord [that is, a belt], all bloodied, with certain knots; and when he saw this, the witness asked him to give him a little piece of this cord, and he replied that he did not dare to do so, save at the pope's command. Nonetheless, as a special grace, [the bishop] gave him a thread of the fringe of this cord, shaped like a needle.

[Jean de Tournemire] received this with all the humility of which he was capable, and wrapped it in fine linen. From messengers he learned that the breast had broken open, and was beginning to be painful. For as is the nature of this cancer, ulceration had set in. When he heard this, he ordered his wife to take the piece of cloth, together with the thread tied up in the fine linen, and to rub the breast morning and evening with the said cloth, especially the hard cancer, and to insert the thread into the opening of the ulceration. When the feast of All Saints arrived [1 November], the witness was notified that his daughter was doing poorly, because she had miscarried. He was upset, and having received leave from the pope, and having heard Mass on the feast of All Saints, he departed from the present city [of Avignon] and rode eleven leagues, notwithstanding that the days were short. On the following day he arrived at his home around the fourth hour and found his daughter Marguerite very weak. Despite her weakness, he wished to see the cancerous breast and he discovered that the induration was oozing laudable pus, not fetid [pus], and this is contrary to the nature of cancer. And he discovered that the breast was not ulcerated from the eruption, which was also against the nature of cancer. When he saw and considered these things, he judged that it was the doing of God and the said glorious lord cardinal that in such a short time the cancerous induration was oozing laudable, not fetid pus, and there was no ulceration of the eruption. And he judged that this was not done by nature but by God, at the intercession of the glorious lord cardinal. He swore on his conscience that he had practiced for forty years and had never seen anyone suffering from a similar disease cured. Indeed, despite the application of remedies, [a patient] will die within a year or a year and a half, or within two years at the longest, with the expulsion of very fetid pus and ulceration of the breast. For within this time the breast is ulcerated, devoured, and [women] die from this devouring and from the intolerable stench. For this reason, due to the fact that there was no ulceration of the flesh, according to the nature of ulcerative cancer, and that there was no fetid and horrible pus, which is also natural in such a case, and the fact that she was cured in five weeks with the application of simple remedies and the avoidance of the diet mentioned above, he judged this to be a particular gift of God and to have come from God at the intercession of the said lord cardinal.

[Jean of Tournemire] was asked how he knew that this was the cancerous disease or aposteme called "cancer." He said that he judged from the way in which it became manifest that this aposteme was a hidden cancer, on two points: first, it started from a small induration like a hazelnut; secondly, it was not painful unless the spot was touched. These are two conditions that are proper to [this disease]; they are not found in other apostemes which are *phlegmatic, *sanguine, or *choleric, but are specific to melancholic apostemes, generated from adust melancholic matter. Such an aposteme is called a "hidden cancer" by doctors. This hidden cancer is not mortal, nor will [patients] die, unless it erupts as an ulcer. For this reason Hippocrates said, "It is better and safer not to treat a hidden cancer than to treat it; good regimen is sufficient" (*Aphorisms* 6.38). Hippocrates's reasoning was that by treating a cancerous aposteme of this kind with *resolvent ointments, one hastens its eruption [on the surface of the body], and when this eruption takes place, which is corrosive because of the nature of the adust material, this hastens death.

For a cancer, after it is ulcerated, is a completely incurable ailment, especially in the breast and in any place where it cannot be completely rooted out with a razor (for in a place where it can be completely rooted out with a razor, it is curable). Indeed, Rhazes says in his *Continens* that he had tried in his day to cure an ulcerated cancer of the breast, and had advised that the entire breast should be removed with the razor. Faced with the pain, the woman was in danger of death, but because she would die in a short time, they wanted to try to treat her, with the consent of her friends. And because some heads of the cancer had invaded the other breast and they were not uprooted with the razor, the cancer remained in the other breast, which shortly thereafter began to ulcerate, and thus she died within a year. Asked if he believed that his daughter had been cured by the prayers of the said lord cardinal, [Jean of Tournemire] replied in the affirmative, on the grounds that (as he said) the disease was incurable in the breast.

Asked what he had done with the thread, he said that twice each day, mother and daughter would place it on the eruption of the cancer. And he said that Marguerite would say to him, her father, that when the thread was applied, she felt great relief. Asked how long she remained with an erupted cancer before she was healed, he said that she was totally cured in five weeks; no other medication was applied save the linen cloth upon the said breast, and the thread within the eruption. Asked if he had made a vow, he replied that he had, in these (or similar) words: "Glorious cardinal, if you have power before God, cure my daughter." He offered these words with great contrition and tears and promised to carry a pair of breasts made of wax to his shrine. Asked why he had acquired such a devotion [to St Peter of Luxembourg], he replied that he had formed this devotion both from the miracles that were said to have been performed after his death in response to his prayers, and from his way of life when he was alive. Although [Peter] was stricken with a raging and tormenting disease, he bore his *consumption most patiently and was never moved to anger or despair – on the contrary, he frequently smiled in the midst of his afflictions. Asked how he knew this, [Jean of Tournemire] replied that he had frequently attended [Peter of Luxembourg] in his terminal illness and had seen the little cord which he was said to wear, knotted and bloodied, when he was alive. Asked if anyone else had been present when he had made the vow, he replied that there was not.

71. METAPHOR AND MALIGNANCY – THE DIFFICULT CASE OF CANCER (2): GUILLAUME BOUCHER TREATS A PARISIAN LADY WITH BREAST CANCER

Eye-witness reports of what medieval doctors actually did at the bedside are rare. Moreover, most such reports are also first-person accounts: autobiographical anecdotes inserted into the textbooks of practical medicine or into collections of tried-and-true remedies called experimenta *(see doc. 81). However, the document presented here furnishes a third-person account by an informed observer of what the practice of early fifteenth-century Parisian physicians was actually like. The text is identified in its sole surviving manuscript as* The Secrets and Consultations of Drs. Guillaume Boucher and Pierre d'Ausson *(Secreta et consilia Carnificis et Danszon). It was composed by an anonymous German doctor doing post-graduate studies in Paris. During this period of study, the German master had the privilege of accompanying the eminent Parisian doctors Guillaume Boucher (d. 1410) and Pierre d'Ausson (d. 1409), who were royal physicians and professors in the Faculty of Medicine. The title gives a somewhat misleading impression of the contents, for while it contains "secrets" or* experimenta, *and therapeutic advice or* consilia *(see docs. 82–83), the text can more accurately be described as a collection of case records. It is a rich lode of information about clinical encounters (see doc. 80).*

The German master's style suggests that this is a relatively "unprocessed" personal record, not a text worked up for publication. Also remarkable is the detached perspective of the author. His aim (as his brief preface indicates) was simply to record what he saw these doctors do, in the event that the experience might eventually prove useful in his own practice. He was not himself an actor in these encounters, and he seems to have had no vested interest other than to learn something. As a result, he records ambivalent outcomes and even failures as well as successes in a matter-of-fact way. The literary lens of our German master also takes a wide-angle shot of the principal practitioners, their associates, the other health-care professionals (surgeons, apothecaries, and so forth), and, of course, the patients.

In the case of the Parisian lady with breast cancer, the therapy seems to have been palliative from the outset, though the doctors felt that there was at least something they could do to extend the woman's life and reduce her suffering. The use of crayfish is interesting, as the term "cancer" means crab. So is the use of precious metals and precious stones: gold never tarnishes, and was used as a sovereign preservative of life in medieval tonics and antidotes, while precious stones could diffuse their power through internal remedies, by external application, and perhaps also through the eyes.

Source: trans. Faith Wallis from Ernest Wickersheimer, "Les secrets et les conseils de maître Guillaume Boucher et de ses confrères. Contribution à l'histoire de la médecine à Paris vers 1400," *Bulletin de la société française d'histoire de la médecine* 8 (1909): 89–91. Latin.

Concerning ulcerated cancer of the breast, for a bourgeoise, whose breast cancer was ulcerated and had spread over almost her entire chest, and this was because she did not put her trust in a learned physician, but rather in an itinerant healer who had opened [the cancer], just as if it were any other *aposteme, against the teaching of the doctors.

Boucher's regimen. Before all else, let her trust in the sacraments and receive them, because death, when it comes [in cases like this, comes] suddenly; so let her receive [the sacraments] as one who is about to die. Therefore let his woman continually take these two herbs, namely carnation and tormentil, in her *decoctions, and she should always eat them with her food.

As for local remedies, the place and the interior of the cavity should be washed through and through with water of black morels and water of coriander, purslane, lettuce, rose, houseleek, and sangreen or of willow leaves (a mixture of some or all of the above), with the cleansing and purifying of the *putrid matter with these herbs. Then twice or three times a day, apply a chicken or hen, or the lung of a freshly killed pig or sheep. And the chicken or hen should be cut open straight down the back, and it should be fresh, with its blood fresh, and also with its intestines. Let it be applied gently to the spot, so that she does not feel any pain. And under the body of the chicken or hen, thus applied, place the following green herbs, chopped, and the whole thing should remain applied for one hour. Take a sufficient quantity each of herb robert, scarlet pimpernel, winter cherry, *herba tunica*, tormentil, mullein, firwort, mouse-ear hawkweed, and knotgrass. And then from these herbs which have been under the chicken, make a vapor inhalation which will contain the power of these herbs; the sore place and all the ulcerated members will be soothed by reason of its natural heat. Then afterwards let it be taken as a decoction; or else place threads of clean, white, old linen clothes pulled apart from one another so that they may return to their pristine nature, into the ointment that follows all at once, so as to receive the power of the ointment. And then, when this [decoction] has been cooked, or with these [threads] dissolved and steeped together in the ointment that follows, let them be applied on top of the ulcerated, broken and abraded areas, and into the deep cavities of the area, and onto the regenerated spots (*renovacionibus*). Do this often: that is, four or five times a day, and even at night, or more often.

Here follows the ointment. Take pure tutty [*zinc oxide*] with half an ounce of rose water and water of black morels, three drams each of litharge [*lead oxide*], washed gold, and rinsed ceruse [*lead carbonate*], one ounce each of juice of black morel, juice of clover, and juice of figwort root, half a quart of oil of roses, two and one-half drams of camphor. Mix it up, and make a liquid ointment, working it vigorously in a lead mortar with a lead pestle, and mixing it for a long time, so that it receives some of the power of the lead. This ointment is very effective among all prudent things, insofar as they might come to the attention of human beings.

Also let her make *purgatives from crayfish taken from good waters, boiled and dressed with herbs. Likewise she should eat crayfish (that is, river crabs), small and large, for it is a wonderful food and particularly good for this woman. Likewise, let cabbage with clean barley be prepared with the said crabs. Let her take what follows below for ten or fifteen days with her meals, a piece about the size of one or two florins in the morning, or of two florins in the morning or at dawn, in case her belly is constipated, with goat's milk or whey – a goblet of one or the other – more or less frequently, as her stomach can tolerate it, for I believe that according to the authorities on ulcerated cancers and those that are not ulcerated, it is good for the belly always to be kept fairly loose. Take one ounce of Cremona dodder, one half dram of flowers of sweet william, one and one-half dram of bugloss flowers. Make a coarsely-ground powder.

Then to sooth the members and revive the spirit, let her take once or twice each week, or more often, two drams of the *electuary which follows, without drinking afterwards. Rather, she should go to sleep immediately if she can.

Take one dram each of dyed silk and safflower seed, half a dram each of the bone from the heart of a deer and "Byzantine purple," one scruple each of shaved ivory, ash [of ivory?], and chips of jacinths, emeralds, and sapphires, half a scruple each of filings of gold and silver, and two drams each of the seeds of melon, gourd, cucumber, and watermelon. Mix them and pulverize them, and grind them up with sugar dissolved in bugloss water, and with the juice of very fragrant pears. Make an electuary in lozenges of two drams, up to three quarts or one pound, and keep in a dry place.

It would also do her good if she kept near her, and continually wore about her, the following precious stones: emeralds, sapphires, and rubies.

Here ends Boucher's regimen, prescribed for an ulcerated cancer.

72. THE ENIGMA OF MENTAL ILLNESS

The Flemish painter Hugo van der Goes of Ghent (1433/40–82) entered the Red Cloister of the reformist Congregation of Windesheim near Brussels in 1475 as a conversus. *A* conversus *ranked above a laybrother (*donatus*), and slightly below a choir-monk.* Conversi *lacked the learning to participate in the* opus Dei, *but they often worked as craftsmen. Prior Thomas became head of the Red Cloister in 1475, the same year that Hugo entered. He was described as a pious and good-natured man and a talented calligrapher.*

Hugo may have had an intimation of his unstable mental condition at the time he entered the Red Cloister. He had just finished the Portinari Altarpiece, *a commission from the head of the Medici Bank in Bruges, Tommaso Portinari, for the church of Sant' Egido at the hospital of Santa Maria Nuova in Florence. The painting is now in the Uffizi Gallery. Its central subject is the birth of Christ, but the painter compels the viewer to focus on the prominent foreground still life. The species of flowers represented, their number and color, are all commentaries on the religious significance of Christ's birth, life, and death. Violets, for instance, represent humility, and the three* *red carnations (also called "nail flowers") recall by their name both the Incarnation and the nails of the cross. The grapes on the albarello or drug jar and the sheaf of wheat allude to the wine and bread of the Mass, the "spiritual medicine" of the ailing soul. The albarello that normally held medicinal herbs now holds the floral emblems of Christ's Passion: lilies and irises. Thus, the Mass, the redemptive suffering of Christ, and the healing vocation of the hospital converge in the image. But it is the black columbines in the glass that point directly to Hugo's illness. The word for columbine in Flemish is akeleyen, and in French, ancoiles or anacolie. This puns with the second half of the word melancholia, and the first part – melan – is the Greek word for "black" (*melancholy is "black *choler" or black *bile). Columbines were conventionally the attribute of the Holy Spirit, but Hugo's choice of the color black and the nexus of symbols of suffering and healing in which he situated these striking flowers suggest that he was introducing a private prayer for healing into his masterpiece.*

Some thirty years after Hugo's death, Gaspar Ofhuys, a brother of the Red Cloister, set down a circumstantial account of the painter's distressing mental illness. Clues to Ofhuys's motives may be found in the text itself. When he begins to speculate about the natural or divine cause of Hugo's affliction, the narrative subtly shifts into a sermon. We might infer, then, that the sad story of Hugo van der Goes had become a kind of exemplum *in the collective memory of the Red Cloister – raw material for homilies or meditations on worldly pride and expiatory suffering. The account ends by pointing to the location of Hugo's grave in the forecourt, a daily visual reminder of the frightening spectacle of insanity and its moral messages. Gaspar Ofhuys presents various theories about the cause of Hugo's condition (compare these to Bartholomaeus Anglicus's account in doc. 49). In the end, he declares himself agnostic on the subject.*

a. Gaspar Ofhuys's Account of Hugo van der Goes's Mental Illness

Source: trans. Faith Wallis from the edition by W.A. McCloy, "The Ofhuys Chronicle of Hugo van der Goes," PhD thesis, State University of Iowa, 1958, pp. 10–15. Latin.

In the year of the Lord 1482, Brother Hugo the *conversus*, who made his profession in this house, died. He was so celebrated as a painter that people said that there was no one at that time who was his equal on our side of the Alps. He and I – the present writer – were novices together. Prior Thomas himself allowed [Hugo], while he was being received into the order and undergoing his noviciate, to retain many of the enjoyments appropriate to worldly people, thinking that this was for the better, seeing that he enjoyed esteem amongst worldly people. These things inclined him more to the pomp of this world than to the path of penance and humility. This displeased some people, who said, "Novices should not be exalted, but humbled." And because he excelled in painting pictures, he was visited by nobles and others, and even by the most illustrious Archduke Maximilian [in 1478]. They were eager to see the works which he had painted. Because these guests came on account of [Hugo], Father Thomas allowed him to go upstairs to the guest chamber and enjoy a meal with them.

A few years – perhaps five or six – after his profession, this *conversus* brother set out for Cologne, if I recall correctly, along with his half-brother Nicholas, who was professed here and who was a *donatus*, as well as Peter, canon regular of Marienthron (but dwelling then at the Jericho Monastery in Brussels), and others. As I learned from the account of his brother Nicholas, the oblate, it was then that our brother Hugo the *conversus* incurred a strange disease of his cognitive faculties (*fantasialem morbum*). Because of this, he kept repeating that he was damned and condemned to eternal damnation; and because of this, he even tried to do himself bodily harm and to kill himself – [and would have done so] had he not been forcibly restrained with the help of bystanders. Because of this strange infirmity, the end of that journey was filled with considerable sadness. Looking for help, they arrived at Brussels and without delay summoned Father Thomas to come there. When he had looked everything over and listened to everything, he suspected that [Hugo] was afflicted with the same disease that had tormented King Saul. Then recalling how Saul felt more cheerful when David played his harp, he permitted not only much melody to be played before brother Hugo, but also the performance of other entertainments. It was his intention that these should expel the mental fantasies. But throughout all this, brother Hugo did not improve; rather, he declared that he was a son of perdition, uttering strange things. Thus stricken, he entered this house.

The ministrations and assistance of the choir brothers, who displayed charity and compassion day and night, shall be remembered by God to eternity and beyond. Although all this was in plain view, many people, even people of rank, spread different stories. Again, different people held different views as to what the disease of this *conversus* was. Some said it was a kind of great frenzy. Others claimed he was possessed by a demon. Now there were some indications of both these afflictions, but nonetheless I always heard that never once in the whole course of his illness did he want to injure anyone except himself. That is not what one hears about the frenzied or the possessed; and so I believe that God alone knows what is was.

Consequently we can speak of the infirmity of this our *conversus* artist in two ways. First, one can say that it was natural – some species of frenzy. For according to the *[non?]-naturals, several species of this disease are generated – "sometimes from melancholic foods, sometimes from drinking strong wine which scorches the *humors and turns them to ashes, sometimes from the passions of the soul like anxiety, sadness, excessive application and fear, sometimes from the malignancy of a *corrupt humor which dominates in the body of a person predisposed to a disease of this kind." [*Ofhuys is quoting here from Bartholomaeus Anglicus, On the Properties of Things 7.6*] As for the passions of the soul, I know for a fact that this brother *conversus* was gravely burdened by them. For he was exceedingly anxious about how he would carry out the works he was supposed to paint. At the time, people said that he would hardly be able to finish them in nine years. He gave a great deal of time to studying in a Flemish book. I fear that his natural tendencies were undoubtedly aggravated by drinking wine on account of his guests. Over time, therefore, the matter for his great infirmity could have been generated from these things.

Secondly, we can discuss this infirmity by positing that it came upon him from God's most tender-hearted providence, who (as it says in 2 Peter 3) "deals patiently for our sake, not willing that any should perish, but that all should be brought around to penance." For this brother *conversus* was highly exalted in our order because of his special skill and enjoyed greater fame than if he had remained a layman, and since he was a human being like other human beings, his heart was lifted up by the honors shown to him, and the various visits and greetings. For this reason, the Lord, not wishing him to perish, mercifully sent him this humiliating infirmity, by which he was greatly humiliated indeed. The brother himself realized this, and as soon as he had convalesced, he humbled himself greatly, voluntarily leaving our refectory and humbly taking his meals with the lay-folk. I have taken the trouble to recount this here because, in my view, God permitted all these things not only to punish the sin or to reproach and correct the sinner, but also so that we might learn something.

Let us take it that this infirmity happened from a natural cause. This teaches us to repress the passions of the soul, and not to allow ourselves to be dominated by them, for otherwise we can be irreparably harmed in our natural constitutions. It was said at the time that this brother, who was a famous painter, had been damaged in a certain vein in the region of the brain by excessive imaginings, fantasies, and anxieties. They say that there is in the region of the brain a very small, slender vein that nourishes the power of imagination and *fantasy. Therefore when imaginations and fantasies abound in us, this little vein becomes agitated, and if it is sufficiently agitated and harmed, it ruptures, and the person falls into a frenzy or insanity. Let us set a limit, then, to our fantasies and imaginations, our conjectures, and other pointless and useless cogitations, lest we fall into so great and irremediable a peril. For we are human beings: could not what happened to this *conversus* because of fantasies and imaginations also happen to us?

Let us suppose that this misfortune came not from a natural cause, but from the infallible providence of God, who furnishes the means of repentance and return for the elect and predestined if they fall into error. What, my brothers, shall we say to this? It is better to be afflicted for a space of time than to suffer torment for eternity. Hence the condemned man, buried in hell, prayed: "I beseech you, father Abraham, that you send Lazarus to my father's house, for I have five brothers, lest they also come to this place of torments (Luke 16:27–28)." It is as if he said: I know that they live in a way worthy of damnation, and unless they do penance and are afflicted in the world for their sins, they will incur these torments. Are you afraid to be afflicted here [on earth]? Eternal affliction is much more greatly to be feared. So if you are afraid of God's temporal affliction, you should be that much more afraid of infernal affliction. And since no one is ashamed of sin who lacks an appreciation of justice, then sinner, correct yourself! If you are proud, humble yourself mightily before God and his vicar, your priest; because unless you mend your ways (because you are elect, and one of the predestined), God himself – who resists the proud, not wishing you to perish, and whom you cannot resist – will humiliate you that you may be an example to others.

Is our Lord not placated by humility and appeased by penance? Therefore, humble your soul before his face, mend your evil ways, resolve in sincerity to live well and in a disciplined fashion, turn away from evil and do good, and you will obtain his mercy; you will temper temporal affliction and escape eternal punishment.

[Hugo] was buried in our forecourt (*atrio*) under the open sky.

b. The *Portinari Altarpiece* and the Detail of the Flowers

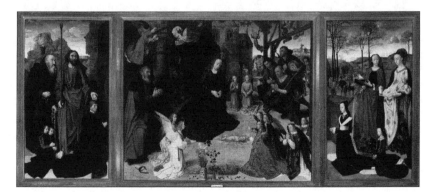

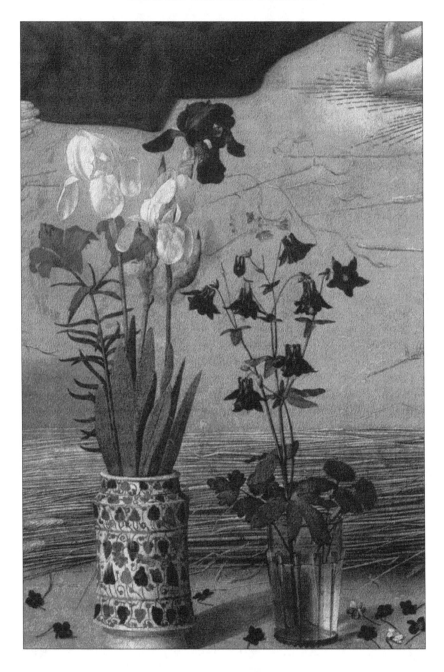

73. PROPHECY AND HEALING: THE MEANING OF ILLNESS ACCORDING TO HILDEGARD OF BINGEN

The Benedictine abbess Hildegard of Bingen (1098–1179) was a most original and striking individual. She was famous in her day as a visionary, but also known for her vigorous preaching and her skill in healing. Prophecy and healing were conjoint vocations for Hildegard: indeed, the main manuscript of her Causes and Cures *closes with the colophon "Here ends the prophecies of St Hildegard."* Causes and Cures *is not easy to characterize. It fuses together a cosmography, an account of the effects of the Fall interwoven with reflections on the nature of physical and psychological illness, and an extended discussion of conception. The text is loosely knit – it may, in fact, have been assembled from fragmentary writings after the abbess's death – but it is typically Hildegardian in its attention to the theme of Adam's fall and the grandeur and misery of the human body and spirit, prey to both demons and *humors.*

Hildegard also maintained a lively correspondence with people who sought her spiritual and medical advice. In the first of the two letters reproduced below, she seeks to explain the relationship between demonic torment or possession and the afflictions of body and mind that result from humoral imbalance. In the second letter, Hildegard offers advice to a priest suffering from nightmares. Her diagnosis is a typical mixture of humoral physiology and Christian moral theology; her cure includes one of the most widely used of Christian "charms" against illness, namely the recitation of the opening word of St John's gospel. Hildegard's ideas about sin and physical or mental illness are not expressed in terms of straightforward causal relationships.

a. Hildegard's *Causes and Cures*

Source: trans. Faith Wallis from Hildegard of Bingen, *Causae et Curae*, ed. Laurence Moulinier (Berlin: Akademie-Verlag, 2003), pp. 183–84. Latin.

But there are certain people called *"sanguine" in whose blood black *bile often arises, which makes their blood black and which dries up the water within them, so that because of this, they are often gravely wearied both when they are awake and when they are asleep. For when Adam knew what was good and by eating the apple did what was evil, black bile rose up within him in reaction to this change. Without the suggestion of the devil, [black bile] is not present in humans, either when they are awake or when they are asleep, because the sorrow and despair which Adam experienced in his transgression arise out of black bile. When Adam disobeyed the divine command, black bile at that very moment coagulated in his blood just as brightness vanishes when a lamp is extinguished and the glowing, smoking wick is left stinking. And so it was with Adam, because when the brightness within him was extinguished, black bile coagulated in his blood, from which sorrow and despair arose within him. For at Adam's fall, the devil scorched the melancholy within him, and in this way [the devil] sometimes makes a person subject to doubt and lack of faith. But because the form of the human person is limited so that it cannot rise excessively above itself, therefore, he loves God and is sad and thus in his sadness he often despairs that God is watching over him. And because the human person is formed in God's image, he cannot cease to fear God....

But when evil *fevers are in the human person and when evil humors begin to overflow in him, he is assailed by heaviness of body and tedium of mind, and the soul, naturally sensing this, as if affected by tedium, yields to the body, and raises up and extends the body and its veins somewhat, just as it does when it must depart from the body.

As well, evil humors sometimes make smoke, which rises up to the brain and so *infects it that people become stupid, forgetful, and insensate.

The pain which is called hiccough is generated from cold in the stomach. This cold wraps around the liver and stretches around the lungs so that even the vital *powers of the heart are moved, just as a person will shake from the cold and his teeth will chatter. And so a person will have a hiccough with a vocalization.

Often black bile will rise up in a person and a foggy smoke will spread within him, which constricts his veins and blood and flesh for a long time, until it has ceased to spread through his body. But it often transpires that bile abounds to excess in the human being so that it also spreads through the whole body. And so the human being suffers as it were stinging nails in his flesh until such time as the superfluity of bile subsides.

Before Adam transgressed the divine command, what is now bile in the human body shone like a crystal within him, and he experienced a taste for good deeds. And what is now black bile in the human body was as radiant as the dawn in [Adam] and he possessed in himself knowledge and the perfection of good deeds. But when Adam transgressed, the radiance of innocence was darkened in him and his eyes, which before this had seen heavenly things, were snuffed out, and bile changed to bitterness in him and black bile into the blackness of impiety, and he was utterly changed into another form. And so his soul contracted sorrow and immediately looked to make excuses by getting angry. For anger arises from sorrow, whence human beings as well have contracted sorrow and anger from the first parent, as well as other harmful things.

b. Hildegard Advises the Afflicted

Source: trans. Joseph Baird and Radd K. Ehrmann, *The Letters of Hildegard of Bingen*, 3 vols. (New York and Oxford: Oxford University Press, 1998–2004), Letters 287 (pp. 83–84) and 293 (p. 93). Latin.

Letter 287, to a Priest (?), ca 1173–79

In a true vision I saw the following regarding the matters you ask about and regarding that insidious devil who ensnares many by his devious machinations. For because of their sins the devil is near people at the very beginning of their deception, and he looks them over from head to toe to see whether they will give in to him or renounce him. If they yield, he runs to them, but if they reject him, he flees from them. Then, he scrutinizes the former, like a potter examining his fragile vessels, to see how they can please him, and because he was close at hand when they first began to sin, he never leaves them, for he says that they were born to do his work. Therefore, because of an imbalance of blood or black *bile or *phlegm, pestilential diseases afflict certain people.

Those who have an excess of blood are suddenly struck with horror and readily give way to anger, and so they often cry out and shriek insanely, because of the attack of devilish machinations. Therefore, they think they hear people talking to them although there is no one there. And so they do not speak out against God totally, but, in fact, sometimes speak of him lovingly, and sigh to him. But if, by God's permission, a malignant spirit takes possession of someone's body, that person does not speak of God with faith but sometimes, because of the devil's spells, speaks of him deceitfully. Many with a surfeit of blood, however, think that they are possessed even when they are not, for if they were possessed, they could be quickly liberated, because sometimes the devil is expelled by exorcisms and prayers and fasts [Matt. 17:20]. These people with an excess of blood sometimes weep and mourn and sigh, but those who are possessed are always hard-hearted and cruel and do not willingly follow other people's advice, but, rather, do whatever they wish.

Those who have an excess of bile are not insane, but they are assailed by many wicked thoughts in denial of God, and they think of this state of mind as a great affliction and even as a sickness unto death. Thus they put the devil to flight. People think, however, that they are possessed although they are not. If they persevere under this heavy affliction, they become martyrs.

Those who abound in phlegm are always weighed down with sickness of body, and yet they still have a good will. The devil rejoices in all their bodily sufferings, because they are in great pain. Still, he can do them no further harm, save insofar as God permits it, because all these things happen by God's judgment.

God sometimes permits all these afflictions to come upon a person because [the person] fully acquiesces in the devil's intrigues, and, refusing to rely on God's help, turns wholly to the devil. Therefore, for the reasons enumerated here, we must hasten to God in our prayers, wherever a person has been overwhelmed in such a manner.

Letter 293, to a Priest (ca 1173–79)

O servant of God, you who are an ornament in Christ's service, do not fear the heaviness that rises in you on account of your terrifying dreams, for these are caused by bloody *humors in conjunction with melancholia. Your sleep is troubled, but your dreams very often are not true, because the ancient deceiver (although he does not harm your physical senses) troubles you by these deceptive dreams. It is by the dispensation of God that you are chastened by such an affliction, so that through this fear all your carnal thoughts will be sharply restrained.

Every single night, place your hand on your heart, and, with sincere devotion, read the gospel "In the beginning was the Word" [John 1:1], and afterward say these words: "Lord God almighty, who in your full goodness breathed the breath of life into me, I beseech you through the holy garment of the gentle humanity of your Son (which he put on on my account) that you not suffer me to be torn apart by the bitterness of this great distress any longer, but through the love of your only begotten Son and your great mercy free me from this tribulation, and defend me from all the snares of the spirits of the air."

May the Holy Spirit make you a tabernacle of sanctification so that in the joys of supreme bliss you may live always with God.

CHAPTER TEN

WHO CAN HELP? PHYSICIANS, "EMPIRICS," AND THE SPECTRUM OF PRACTITIONERS

The emergence of an institutionalized academic form of medical education had consequences that went well beyond the shaping of medical knowledge: it created the European medical profession as a visible occupational caste. The form of the university itself, a self-governing guild of masters, served as the model for city guilds and colleges of medical practitioners. Just as the university had won the right from ecclesiastical and civil authorities to police admission to the teaching profession, so the medical guilds sought to gain the collective right to examine all who wished to call themselves physicians and practice in a given jurisdiction. Academic solidarity was the template for professional solidarity.

Not every city had a medical guild, and even where guilds existed, their form and ⁺powers varied widely. In Paris, for example, the university's medical faculty doubled as the city's guild. Its standards for qualification were, understandably, explicitly academic, and it had high ambitions to bring all medical activity in the city under its supervision. Elsewhere, a university degree was not always required by the guild, but they all administered some formal test of medical learning along broadly scholastic lines to candidates. Like all guilds, physicians' guilds aimed to protect the value of their product; that product was "medicine" as defined in the universities. This definition drew a line between the trained physician and all other purveyors of medical care. Even in places where there were no guilds, the model of the learned physician tacitly defined expectations about qualified medical practice. Indeed, people who could not or did not attend universities could still be recognized as physicians if they presented themselves and their practice as congruent with this model. This was the situation of many Jewish doctors, for example (doc. 77), who trained through family-based apprenticeships.

Medieval physicians, unlike their modern counterparts, did not want to monopolize health care; instead, they lobbied rulers and courts to be recognized as the highest rung of a hierarchy of practitioners. Below the physician, in roughly descending order, were learned surgeons; craft-trained surgeons; barber-surgeons, who combined bloodletting with the removal of "superfluities" from the skin and head; itinerant specialists such as dentists and oculists; empirics; midwives; clergy who dispensed charitable advice and help; and, finally, ordinary family and neighbors. All ranks on this ladder could administer some kind of drug therapy, and some possessed the skill and training to perform surgery. But only the educated physician could pronounce a diagnosis, because only he understood the hidden causes of disease. A corollary of this was that only the learned physician could prescribe treatment, though others might carry it out. Learned physicians were in consequence especially sensitive to the activities of empirics such as

Jean Domrémi (doc. 76), who claimed to diagnose by urine inspection, or Jacoba Felicie (doc. 75), who prescribed food and drink – "regimen" in other words – for her patients. These people were the target of lawsuits, not because they cared for the sick, but because their style of practice implied an understanding of disease that was the monopoly of the academic doctor.

The efforts of urban governments, large and small, to persuade a learned physician to settle in town and serve the populace indicate that most ordinary people were willing to take the learned doctors at their own valuation. But even in towns that were well supplied with doctors, patients took a pragmatic approach in their everyday quest for healing. Cure-contracts, for instance, show that they were ready to trust their health to a wide range of practitioners, but on a strictly business basis.

74. SHOULD CLERGY AND MONKS PRACTICE MEDICINE?

Schools and universities were nominally clerical organizations; many medieval medical practitioners held clerical status at some level and received ecclesiastical benefices. The emergence of a visible learned profession of medicine, however, raised the question of whether a cleric could belong to the "estate" of the physicians. The debate was exacerbated by the fact that in the nascent money economy of the twelfth century, medicine was a profitable line of work. Medicine was beginning to look like a secular occupation for laymen, and in the aftermath of the eleventh-century reform movement, the Church was particularly sensitive to reinforcing the distinction between clergy and laity.

The documents translated below reveal how the Church reacted to the new social context of being a doctor. Once a suitable and praiseworthy activity for a bishop or monk, medicine now involved specialized study in distant schools and seemed inevitably tainted with social and economic ambition. The decree of the second Lateran Council of 1139 repeats verbatim decrees promulgated in two regional French synods (Clermont in 1130 and Reims in 1131), which suggests that the rules were actually difficult to enforce. Indeed, there is evidence that some cash-strapped monasteries were sending monks away for medical training and then hiring them out as physicians. The canon enacted by Pope Alexander III at the Council of Tours in 1163 found a place in many decretal collections and even in the cartulary of the University of Paris. However, it is important not to exaggerate the effect of such prohibitions. For the most part, they targeted monks and cloistered regular canons, not the secular clergy, and official dispensations were always possible. Was surgery a particular problem, given its inevitable association with shedding blood and the risk of death of the patient? Innocent III's response to one monk-priest's inquiry in 1212, later included in Gregory IX's Decretals, *suggests that the latter might have been a serious issue, but only for those in major orders such as priests. Even then, there was considerable latitude in practice, as the career of the Dominican friar, bishop, and surgeon Teodorico Borgognoni illustrates (see doc. 62).*

a. The Decree of the Second Lateran Council of 1139

Source: trans. R.J. Schroeder, *Disciplinary Decrees of the General Councils* (St Louis: Herder, 1957), p. 201. Original text in *Conciliorum oecumenicorum decreta*, ed. J. Alberigo et al., 3rd ed. (Bologna: Istituto per le Scienze Religiose, 1973), p. 198. Latin.

Monks and Canons Regular Are Not to Study Jurisprudence and Medicine for the Sake of Temporal Gain

An evil and detestable custom, we understand, has grown up in the form that monks and canons regular, after having received the habit and made profession, despite the rule of the holy masters Benedict and Augustine, study jurisprudence and medicine for the sake of temporal gain. Instead of devoting themselves to psalmody and hymns, they are led by the impulses of avarice to make themselves defenders of causes and, confiding in the support of a splendid voice, confuse by the variety of their statements what is just and unjust, right and wrong. The imperial constitutions, however, testify that it is absurd and disgraceful for clerics to seek to become experts in forensic disputations. We decree, therefore, in virtue of our Apostolic authority, that offenders of this kind be severely punished. Moreover, the care of souls being neglected and the purposes of their order being set aside, they promise health in return for detestable money and thus make themselves physicians of human bodies. Since an impure eye is the messenger of an impure heart, those things about which good people blush to speak, religion ought not to treat. Therefore, that the monastic order as well as the order of canons may be pleasing to God and be conserved inviolate in their holy purposes, we forbid in virtue of our Apostolic authority that this be done in the future. Bishops, abbots, and priors consenting to such outrageous practices and not correcting it, shall be deprived of their honors and cut off from the Church.

b. Canon 8 of Pope Alexander III Enacted at the Council of Tours, 1163

Source: trans. Darrel W. Amundsen, "Medieval Canon Law on Medical and Surgical Practice by the Clergy," *Medicine, Society, and Faith in the Ancient and Medieval Worlds* (Baltimore: The Johns Hopkins University Press, 1996), p. 230. Originally published in *Bulletin of the History of Medicine* 52 (1978): 22–44. Latin.

The ancient enemy's hatred does not strive with much effort to ruin the weak members of the Church, but he sends his hand against her more desirable members and attempts to trip up the elect, for the Scripture says, "The elect are his food." Therefore he thinks that he has caused the fall of many when he has drawn away a more precious member of the Church by his cunning. And, of course, it is then that, by his usual habit, he entices away from their cloisters certain regulars for the study of law and for pondering medical concoctions under the pretext of aiding the bodies of their ill brothers and performing ecclesiastical affairs more proficiently. On this account, so that, by the pursuit of knowledge, spiritual men be not entangled again in the affairs of this world and be not lacking in things of the soul, believing themselves thereby to provide for others in external matters, we decree with the consent of the present council, that no one at all is permitted to depart for the purpose of studying medicine or secular law after having taken the vow and profession of religion in any religious place. If he does depart and does not return to his cloister within the space of two months, let him be avoided by all as if excommunicate, and in no case, if he dares to present a defense, should he be heard. When he has returned, however, let him always be the last of the brothers in the choir, in the chapter, at table, and in the rest, and let him lose hope of every advancement, unless, perhaps, by the pity of the Apostolic See.

c. Rescript *Tua nos* of Innocent III (1212)

Source: trans. Darrel W. Amundsen, "Medieval Canon Law on Medical and Surgical Practice by the Clergy," *Medicine, Society, and Faith in the Ancient and Medieval Worlds* (Baltimore: The Johns Hopkins University Press, 1996), p. 236. Originally published in *Bulletin of the History of Medicine* 52 (1978): 22–44. The italicized passages are in the original version, transmitted through the *Compilatio quarta* 5.6.3 of the *Quinque compilationes antiquae*, ed. E. Friedberg (1882; reprinted Graz: Akademische Druck- und Verlagsanstalt, 1956); they are omitted in Gregory IX, *Decretales* 5.12.19, ed. E. Friedberg, *Corpus iuris canonici*, 2 vols. (1879; reprinted Graz: Akademische Druck- und Verlagsanstalt, 1959). Latin.

Your brotherhood said that we should be consulted. You asked *to be advised by the Apostolic See* what must be decided concerning a certain monk who, believing that he could cure a certain woman of a tumor of the throat, acting as a surgeon, opened the tumor with a knife. When the tumor had healed somewhat, he ordered the woman not to expose herself to the wind at all lest the wind, stealing into the incision in her throat, bring about her death. But the woman, defying his order, rashly exposed herself to the wind while gathering crops, and thus much blood flowed out through the incision in her throat, and the woman died. *She, nevertheless, confessed that she was responsible because she had exposed herself to the wind.* The question is whether this monk, since he is also a priest, may lawfully exercise the priestly office. We therefore reply to your brotherhood that, although the monk himself was very much at fault for usurping an alien function which very little suited him, nevertheless, if he did it from piety and not from cupidity, and was expert in the exercise of surgery and was zealous to employ every diligence which he ought to have done, he must not be condemned for that which happened through the fault of the woman against his advice. Then, with no penance being required, he may be permitted to celebrate divine service. Otherwise, the fulfilling of the sacerdotal office must be strictly forbidden him.

75. THE FACULTY OF MEDICINE OF PARIS *VS.* JACOBA FELICIE

This is the account of a trial held in 1322. The plaintiff was the Faculty of Medicine of Paris, acting as the guild of the city by virtue of a royal privilege granted some fifty years earlier (see doc. 76); the defendant was a female healer accused of illicit practice, named Jacoba or Jacqueline Felicie. The minutes of the trial are a treasury of information about the practice of medicine in the fourteenth century. Jacoba was technically an empiric, since she had no formal educational accreditation. But she seems to have conducted her practice in a manner that was very close – perhaps too close – to that of learned doctors. She also had a rather distinguished clientele: empirics were by no means only the doctors of the poor. Ultimately the arguments on both sides appear to revolve around Jacoba's gender (although the accusations and the testimony, curiously, do not). In the end, Jacoba lost her case.

Source: trans. James Bruce Ross in *The Portable Medieval Reader*, ed. Mary Martin McLaughlin (New York: Viking, 1949), pp. 635–40. Latin.

Witnesses were brought before us ... in the inquisition made at the instance of the masters in medicine at Paris against Jacoba Felicie and others practicing the art of medicine and surgery in Paris and the suburbs without the knowledge and authority of the said masters, to the end that they be punished, and that this practice be forbidden them....

The dean and the regent masters of the Faculty of Medicine at Paris intend to prove against the accused, Mistress Jacoba Felicie, (1) that the said Jacoba visited, in Paris and in the suburbs, many sick persons afflicted with grave illnesses, inspecting their urine both in common and individually, and touching, feeling, and holding their pulses, body, and limbs. Also (2) that after this inspection of urine and this touching, she said and has said to those sick persons: "I shall make you well, God willing, if you have faith in me," making an agreement concerning the cure with them, and receiving money for it. Also (3) that after the agreement had been made between the said defendant and the sick persons or their friends, concerning curing them of their internal illness, or from a wound or ulcer appearing on the outside of the bodies of the said sick persons, the said defendant visited and visits the sick persons very often, inspecting their urine carefully and continually, after the manner of physicians and doctors, and feeling their pulse, and their body, and touching and holding their limbs. Also (4) that after these actions, she gave and gives to the sick persons syrups to drink, comforting, laxative, digestive, both liquid and nonliquid, and aromatic, and other drinks, which they take and drink and have drunk very often in the presence of the said defendant, she prescribing and giving them. Also (5) that she exercised and exercises, in the aforesaid matters, this function of practicing medicine in Paris and in the suburbs, that she has practiced and practices from day to day although she has not been approved in any official *studium* at Paris or elsewhere....

Jean Faber, living near the Tower in Paris ... when he was asked if he knew the parties, said that he knew some of the masters by sight, others not, but that he knew the said Jacoba, because she has done well by him, as he said. Asked what he knows of those matters contained in the articles, he replied that he was suffering from a certain sickness in his head and ears at a time of great heat, that is, before the feast of the nativity of St John [24 June], and that the said Jacoba had visited him, and had shown such great care for him that he was cured from his illness by the potations which she gave him, and by the aid of God. When he was asked what *potions she had given to him, he answered that Jacoba had administered potions to him, of which the first was green, and the second and third more or less colorless, but how they were made he did not know. Asked if the said Jacoba has been wont to visit the sick, he said that she has, as he has heard many say. When he was asked if he had made a contract with her about curing him, he said that he had not. After he had been made well he paid her as he wished....

The lord Odo de Cormessiaco, a brother of the hospital of Paris, a witness, when he was asked what he knew of the matters contained in the articles, etc., answered this by law on his oath, that is, that when, around the feast of the nativity of St John, he had been seized by a severe illness, to such an extent that his own limbs could not support him, Master John de Turre had visited him, and many other masters in medicine, Masters Martin and Herman and many others. And he had himself taken to the house of the said Jacoba, and was there for a while, and then afterwards this Jacoba visited him both at the baths and in the aforesaid hospital. And Master Jean, who lives with this said Jacoba, gave him a *purgative, and they prepared many baths and bandages for him, and anointed him very often. The said Jacoba and Jean worked over him with such great care that he was completely restored to health. They also gave him herbs, that is, camomile leaves, melitot, and very many others, which he did not recall. Also, on the advice of the said Jacoba, the said Jean made a certain charcoal fire of the length and breadth of the witness, and upon this fire he placed many herbs and afterwards he had him lie down on these herbs, and lie there until this made him sweat exceedingly. Afterwards they wrapped him in linen cloth and put him in his own bed, and cared for him with such diligence that by means of God's help and the said care, he was cured. When he was asked if Jacoba had made a contract with him concerning visiting and healing him, he said she had not. He paid as he wished when he got well, and he believed better than otherwise....

Jeanne, wife of Denis called Bilbaut, living in the Rue de la Ferronnerie in Paris … answered on oath that around the feast of St Christopher [25 July], just passed, she had been seized with a *fever, and very many physicians had visited her in the said illness, that is, a certain brother de Cordelis, Master Herman, Manfred, and very many others. And she was so weighed down by the said illness that on a certain Tuesday around the said feast, she was not able to speak, and the said physicians gave her up for dead. And so it would have been, if the said Jacoba had not come at her request. When she had come, she inspected her urine and felt her pulse, and afterwards gave her a certain clear liquid to drink, and gave her also a syrup, so that she would go to the toilet. And Jacoba so labored over her that by the grace of God she was cured of the said illness.…

These are the arguments which Jacoba said and set forth in her trial.…

The said Jacoba said that if the statute, decree, admonition, prohibition, and excommunication which the said dean and masters are trying to use against her, Jacoba, had ever been made, this had been only once, on account of and against ignorant women and inexperienced fools, who, untrained in the medical art and totally ignorant of its precepts, usurped the office of practicing it. From their number the said Jacoba is excepted, being expert in the art of medicine and instructed in the precepts of said art. For these reasons, the statute, decree, admonition, prohibition, and excommunication aforesaid are not binding and cannot be binding on her, since when the cause ceases, the effect ceases.…

Also the said statute and decree, etc., had been made on account of and against ignorant women and foolish usurpers who were then exercising the office of practice in Paris, and who are either dead or so ancient and decrepit that they are not able to exercise the said office, as it appears from the tenor of the said statute and decree, etc., which were made a hundred and two years ago, at which time Jacoba was not, nor was she for sixty years afterwards, in the nature of things; indeed, she is young, thirty or thereabouts, as it appears from her aspect.…

Also it is better and more becoming that a woman clever and expert in the art should visit a sick woman, and should see and look into the secrets of nature and her private parts, than a man, to whom it is not permitted to see and investigate the aforesaid, nor to feel the hands, breasts, belly and feet, etc., of women. Indeed, a man ought to avoid and shun the secrets of women and their intimate associations as much as he can. And a woman would allow herself to die before she would reveal the secrets of her illness to a man, because of the virtue of the female sex and because of the shame that she would endure by revealing them. And from these causes many women and also men have perished in their illnesses, not wishing to have doctors, lest they see their secret parts.…

Also, supposing without prejudice that it is bad that a woman should visit, care for, and investigate, as has been said, it is, however, less bad that a woman wise, discreet, and expert in the aforesaid matters has done and does these things, since the sick persons of both sexes, who have not dared to reveal the aforesaid secrets to a man, would not have wished to die. Thus it is that the laws say that lesser evils should be permitted, so that greater ones may be avoided. For this reason, since the said Jacoba is expert in the art of medicine, it is, therefore, better that she should be permitted to make visits, in order to exercise the office of practice, than that the sick should die, especially since she has cured and healed all those....

Also, it has been ascertained and proved, that some sick persons of both sexes, seized by many severe illnesses and enduring the care of very many expert masters in the art of medicine, have not been able to recover at all from their illnesses, although the masters applied as much care and diligence to these as they were able. And the said Jacoba, called afterwards, has cured these sick persons in a short time, by an art which is suitable for accomplishing this.

76. THE FACULTY OF MEDICINE OF PARIS *VS.* JEAN DOMRÉMI

Jean Domrémi was another successful empiric, or informally trained medical practitioner. He worked in Paris during the troubled early decades of the fifteenth century, when France was invaded by the English and civil war broke out between the Duke of Burgundy and his supporters and those loyal to the Valois dynasty. On the eve of Joan of Arc's campaign, Domrémi went to court to appeal an attempt by the Faculty of Medicine to prosecute him for illicit medical practice.

The right of the Faculty of Medicine to control the conditions of medical practice in the city of Paris was enshrined in the statutes of 1270–71. These statutes empowered the Faculty to punish offenders through the Church courts – the university being technically under the authority of the bishop of Paris – where the penalty would be excommunication. A royal edict of 1352, however, transferred cases of illicit practice, at least in principle, to the secular courts. When the Faculty hauled Domrémi before the bishop's court and threatened him with excommunication, he appealed to the royal justice system. This document chronicles the hearings held before the Parlement, the highest royal court. It is written in French, interspersed with numerous Latin phrases and citations, and is at once ponderously legalistic and briskly stenographic. Though peppered with court-room jargon, it catches the tone and inflections of the participants in a vivid way.

The chaotic conditions in Paris might explain how this enterprising empiric managed to defy for so long the attempts by the Faculty of Medicine to get him to desist, but this does not detract from the fact that Domrémi was very resourceful. He seems to have been particularly adept at absorbing the discourse, techniques, and social postures associated with scholastic medical practice. The record of his appeal trial brings into sharp focus some of the key questions surrounding the attempts by guilds and colleges to control medical practice, such as the definition of competence, the role of literacy, and the meaning of techniques such as urine inspection. We do not know the outcome of the appeal, though there is evidence that Domrémi was still active in Paris a decade later.

Source: trans. Faith Wallis, in Geneviève Dumas and Faith Wallis, "Theory and Practice in the Trial of Jean Domrémi," *Journal of the History of Medicine and Allied Sciences* 54 (1999): 55–87. The original text is in *Cartularium Universitatis Parisiensis*, ed. Henri Denifle and Emile Chatelain (Paris: Delalaine, 1891–97), vol. 4, pp. 425–28. Middle French.

Tuesday, 23 November 1423

Between Master Jean Domrémi, physician and surgeon on the one hand, and the dean and masters of medicine of the University of Paris, and the said university, on the other. Domrémi protests that he does not wish to offend anyone, nor to detract from the privileges of the said university. And he says that he has practiced for 43 years in Paris and during that time he has lived among, has had converse with, and has been in the company of the most notable physicians and surgeons of this kingdom, and he names several of these. And he says that because he cured Sire Guillaume de Sens, president of the Grands Jours [*royal assizes*] of Troyes, he [Guillaume] advised him to come to Paris, and he came, and since then has practiced, and has been summoned for graduation with the late Master Guibert de Celsoy and other notable physicians and surgeons who listened readily to his opinions. And he brought about very fine cures, but in spite of this and suddenly, because he cured a woman of this city who was pregnant, whom he names, the physicians became annoyed, because they had attended her for a long time and could see no other remedy except to open up the woman to save the infant; and yet Domrémi has cured her and she is in good health and her child is alive. Furthermore, he says that the late king [Charles VI, d. 1422] retained him as a surgeon, and made him inspector general of surgeons in this kingdom. And notwithstanding, his opponents have denied him learning, forbidden him to practice, and forbidden herbalists or apothecaries to furnish him with herbs or drugs for his practice, and have sought without cause to excommunicate him, and through the provost of Paris have enacted certain particular prohibitions against him. He lists as well the writs and prohibitions made against him. He also recounts the legal proceedings brought against him in the Church court and other vexations. He recounts, moreover, the contents this matter, there are papal and episcopal statutes and ordinances which are maintained and applied, even in the time of the late Bishop Stephen of Paris, and a while ago when the [Latin] patriarch of Constantinople administered the diocese of Paris. Likewise King Charles, king of France and Navarre, and King John, and Charles V made similar ordinances and prohibitions touching the practice of the art of medicine, and these have been observed, and when anyone wanted to do the contrary, he was corrected and punished by justice. In particular, Jean Thion and Guillaume de Beauval were prohibited from practicing medicine because they were ignorant, and nothing but cobblers. Likewise others, whom they name, were forbidden by this court. And the said dean and Faculty and the said University, as far back as anyone can remember, possess [the right] to prevent anyone from practicing against their statutes and ordinances, and possess [the right] to act against them and impede them, and to punish them or cause them to be punished by justice according to the said ordinances and statutes. They say, furthermore, that because recently they caused the said statutes and ordinances to be published by the bishop's court, the said Domrémi, who held that this prohibition included him, brought proceedings against them in the bishop's court, which ordained that Domrémi should be examined, but Domrémi did not put in an appearance and was declared in contempt of court. They recount the trial and the content of the royal letters obtained by them, addressed to the provost of Paris, ordering him to publish their prohibitions, statutes, and ordinances in general terms, and which were published in general terms as stated. But Domrémi was not content, and turned to the king, and obtained letters to launch his suit, and other letters [permitting him] to present his case before my lords the presidents [of the Parlement] during the vacation. And in the course of this hearing, [Domrémi] said that he was a sworn [member] of the science and art [*that is, guild*] of surgery. However, the surgeons brought proceedings against him, and Domrémi answered that he was not a surgeon, but that he was a physician. And notwithstanding that he styles himself a physician, he does not understand either French or Latin, nor knows how to read, and therefore he cannot be a physician, because this is not a science that one can known by hearsay, and one is not a physician by art, or by nature, or by revelation. And if he says that he knows [medicine] from experience, experience is never certain unless it proceeds from science. Hence the masters say *qui vult artem aliquam exercere racione et experimentorum* [*sic*] *uti debet* [*he who wishes to practice any art should make use of reason and experience*]; otherwise *experimentum est fallax et nebulosum* [*experience is misleading and obscure; quoting Hippocrates, Aphorisms 1.1*]. And there is too great a danger *in re publica* [*for the public*] in allowing such folk to practice who have no art, reason or science behind their experience. And no matter what Domrémi says, he has only if he was involved in surgery, it would have been secretly and on diseases on the surface of the body, and he would never be involved in medicine except covertly and would fail if he were involved in medicine without approbation, and there would be abuses and attacks on the statutes and ordinances. And he did not comport himself like a physician in his dress and was accustomed to wear a short gown, like a peddler of *theriac. And he has never lived in Paris, and he came to Paris in the year 1418 after the entry of the Burgundians, and he was armed and very menacing, and he kept company with armed men, and threatened Master Jean Avantage, now physician to the duke of Burgundy. And now he wears a long robe, and if he knew about drugs and herbs, he would [still] not be a physician, and no apothecary or herbalist should be a physician; it would be perilous and inconvenient, and anyhow, he does not know anything about either subject, and if he has at his lodging waters and herbs, [the waters] stink and frogs sing in them in the summertime. And he has ointments which he uses for any and every illness and which have no efficacy or benefit, unless it is *a casu et fortuna* [*by chance and luck*]. And suppose he does know something about medicine and surgery – which he does not? Ought this to be a pretext for breaking and overturning all the statutes and ordinances and all the laws? Certainly not, *quia de hiis que raro accidunt non est fienda lex* [*because law ought not to be based on exceptional occurrences*]. Hence it would be better if Domrémi went to some village, or to Châlons or Troyes, if they will have him, where he can earn his living if he knows something – which he does not. Furthermore, they recount certain abuses and exploits of the said Domrémi concerning the wife of Aguillon, procurator of the Châtelet, and the wife of Ymbert des Champs, of whom mention is made in a civil suit, who say that by the incompetence of the said Domrémi the wife of the said des Champs *pepit abortivum* [*had a miscarriage*] due to an overdose of *scammony. Likewise the wife of the hatter Jean de Chambly, who lives opposite the Palace, *pepit abortivum* as above, through the incompetence of the said Domrémi. Also they recount that a cooper whom Domrémi bled against all the rules of medicine from the foot into water *uisa egritudine* [*when the disease manifested itself*], died on the following day. Moreover they tell of a draper whom Domrémi attended and for whom he prepared a prescription, for which he demanded only one gold écu, even though the ingredients cost more than four gold écus. They told of Marion Lyonne, whom he over-treated so much that she died, [and] about the master du Saint-Esprit [*probably a title: master of the Order of the Holy Spirit*] who died of the incision which [Domrémi] made and rid the world of his body, and of many others of which [Domrémi] does not boast; and he only boasts of those who escape from the peril of being in his hands. And concerning what Domrémi says about his cure of the pregnant woman, that great hatred was conceived against him, one cannot provide a good rational explanation and which are frequently and everywhere experienced in medicine. And suppose that Domrémi cannot speak Latin: that does not signify that he is not a physician or a clerk, for Aristotle could not speak any Latin, because the sciences have been translated into all languages. Domrémi also has Galen, Hippocrates, Avicenna and the other doctors in French. According to the Philosopher *cecus a natura potest a<c>quirire scientiam [a blind man can acquire knowledge from nature]*. And suppose that Domrémi cannot read: he has his son with him who is a good clerk and a good apothecary, who lived for a long time with the late Jenson Derpy, and knows how to read [to] Domrémi. And moreover *Omerus fuit cecus [Homer was blind]* and a very great clerk. Domrémi adds that he has cured many whom the said physicians of Paris had abandoned, especially the said pregnant woman whom the said physicians wanted to open up in order to kill mother and child. Domrémi delivered her from an *aposteme and cured her, and she was not *in statu crisis [in a state of crisis]* at the time, but that time had passed, and a week, indeed three weeks, had gone by. And Domrémi did not cure her *a casu [by chance]*, because he has done many other cures. Likewise, concerning the wife of the late master Philippe Vilate, who was in pain and who was judged to be pregnant by the physicians of Paris; and shortly thereafter Domrémi was called in, who judged by her urine that she was not pregnant, and judged that she had a swelling in her body, and declared the causes, which were found to be true, just as Domrémi told. The physicians of Paris were greatly amazed at this and among them in particular Master Guillaume Boucher, who had been of the opinion that the said Madame Vilate was pregnant. He wanted to know who this Domrémi was, who was summoned to the lodging next door to Vilate's; and he [Boucher] stationed himself in a room near where Domrémi was, where he interrogated him on the subject of three or four urine samples which he brought to him, of which [Domrémi] made good and accurate judgment according to the statement of the said Boucher, who considers him a man of great expertise and who would willingly have given him his daughter in marriage had he been in a position to marry. He recounts as well many cures and experiences: concerning the wife of the merchant Marestot de Audry, who was attended by Master Jean Le Lievre and other physicians for a case of *carbuncles and epidemic sickness, and who was cured by Domrémi; who also cured Master Pierre Godet of a serious disease which the physicians did not know how to cure. Likewise Martin de Neauville, whom the physicians did not know how to cure, and they said that he could not possibly have gout and nevertheless Domrémi cured him. Master Laurent Lamy was also cured by him, and the armorer of the count of Nevers Jean de Savoie and his wife, and many others whom he named. He produced manifest cures for which he only demanded a small fee and he was content with a franc or an écu, whereas the physicians were wont to demand 50 or 60 écus, and from the receiver of Paris, whom Domrémi cured, they had more than 200 écus. And it is well known for 30 or 40 leagues around Paris that Domrémi is a man of expertise and practices in Paris and he cured Colart Godait, bailiff of Beauvais. And the physicians knew and know that he practices and has practiced for a long time. And those who accuse and pursue him learned from him and kept company with him for a long time to learn his judgment on medicine and urines and practice, for instance masters Jean Warin, Jean Colin, Cotereau, and the dean of the Faculty. And it is not at all true that he uses one ointment for all diseases; he has more medications in his house than in any house in Paris. And if Domrémi used scammony, he used it moderately and knows its virtue well; but there are many of the aforesaid physicians who use it any way they want and do not understand it, and not long ago none other than Master Bernard Nivart sent a prescription to an apothecary who refused to make it up for him, because he had put in enough scammony to kill an ox. The accusations that he has used it heedlessly are not true and he has caused no harm to man or woman with scammony or any other medicine he has prescribed. And he never gave any medicine to Marion Lyonne or to others [concerning whom] they wish to charge him, but they were attended by Tanquart and by Blanchchape; to try to charge Domrémi is nothing but idle jesting. He also says that Pierre Hemon was being treated by Master Henri Doigny, was abandoned, and was cured by Domrémi, as was the late Master Jacques Philippe, royal notary. And if he attended some who did not come to convalescence, *non est medico semper relevetur ut eger* [*a patient is not always relieved by a physician*], as his opponents themselves admit. And furthermore Domrémi proposes that several sick patients be visited first by the physicians and then by Domrémi, and that inquiry be made into the causes of the diseases and the judgments of urines, and it will be found by the report of the said patients that Domrémi will judge just as well and accurately as the said physicians, and that he is sufficiently competent and expert, as much as they are, who have conceived this envy and hatred against him....

Wednesday, 14 December

In the case between the masters and dean of the Faculty of Medicine on the one hand, and Jean Domrémi. Continuing his plea, Master Jean Domrémi says that he is not, nor has he ever been a weaver. Also that those who have frequently profited from the experience of simple folk ought not to reject [that experience], just as Arnau of Vilanova tells of a cardinal who was cured through the experience of a very simple man. And it is true that Domrémi has considerable expertise and cured Master Jean de Martroy, a physician, who was gravely ill and who could find no remedy, and whom Domrémy cured. And Domrémi should not be charged with what is written in the *Codex* [of Justinian, under the title] *de professoribus et medicis* [*concerning professors and physicians*] because this refers to physicians ordained to teach in school, and there are no ordinances against him, and they do not include people of expertise. Also, they would be abolished *per contrarium usum* [*because custom opposes it*]; there have been many, and still are more than a hundred in Paris who have practiced and are practicing, men and women, who are not graduates; there was Master Salmon who understood Greek and did not understand any Latin, and others who have practiced like La Calabre [*a female empiric*], who cured diseases physicians did not know how to deal with. And there are decrees for La Gousse and others, who have been allowed to practice notwithstanding the opposition of the physicians. And it does not pertain to the bishop's court to decide on this matter, which is secular *et de layco* [*and concerns a layman*], and it has acted against the public welfare, and the judge appointed by the emperor [*that is, the king*] to be aware of these things should be aware of this. And he says that proceedings were launched against Domrémi *ad excommunicacionem* ["to excommunicate him"] without [due legal] warning by defaming him by libelous statements and defamatory words, and although the commission was given in general terms, nevertheless it was applied particularly against Domrémi, and the commission was indeed specifically [against him], contrary to judicial procedure, and because of this Domrémi requested that the episcopal court attend to this matter, but they did not wish to grant him counsel, and the episcopal court did see to this, but without allowing a proper avenue of justice. And for this reason he obtained royal letters from the king to be received in opposition and so he will be received as plaintiff and that he will not be deprived of his estate or his practice, and that he was approved, admitted and accepted by the former masters, and the new ones want to chase him out even though he is very expert and has a good practice, and they launched against him the said opprobrium, threats, and insults and called him a deceiver and charlatan, and made him look like a liar before the episcopal court in his own hearing. And so he will be received as plaintiff, and his letters will be ratified, and during the trial he will enjoy [his rights] because it is in the public interest, and Domrémi is defendant and opposing party, and he will not be deprived. He concludes as above....

Wednesday, 4 January 1424

In the case between the masters of the Faculty of Medicine and the university on the one hand, and Jean Domrémi on the other. The masters say that if Domrémi has traveled, he has had ample opportunity to study. And although experience counts for much, it profits and does more for people who have science *quia ars reddit facilem* [*because art makes things easy*] and one cannot have good judgment if one does not have science. And Galen says that no one should undertake medicine unless he is a philosopher and a graduate, and has the principles of the science. And if one says that Apollo, Galen, and Hippocrates discovered medicine by experience, one ought not to compare Domrémi to them, who were great clerks and great philosophers, *doctissimi viri* [*very learned men*]. But Domrémi does not know how to read French or Latin, and it would be very dangerous to depend upon such people, for the greatest clerks and those who have studied and study every day find judgments in medicine difficult enough, and for this reason were the laws and statutes of the university made. And Domrémi has only one book on surgery which he gives to a child who does not know how to read, and one could not learn anything from it save how to cure a minor wound *ad extra* [*on the surface of the body*]. And if anyone convalesced when [Domrémi] was in attendance, perhaps it was because they were not really very sick, and nature would have done the job, or he could have cured them *sorte et non arte* [*by chance and not by skill*]. And if he enjoys fame among simple and ignorant people, that in no way proves his competence *quia vulgus peritum ab imperito nescit discernere secundum dictum Ypocratis* [*because, as Hippocrates says, ordinary people do not know how to distinguish between a competent and an incompetent (physician)*]. Also Domrémi does not boast of the many who died or got worse when he was in attendance. And it would be very dangerous to allow anyone [to practice] without approbation and without examination, because then the studies and the statutes of the university would be for nothing. And in other professions where the danger is not so great, it is plain that no one is admitted as a master unless he has been first examined, approved, and sworn in, and no barber, tailor, or cobbler would be admitted otherwise, or [anyone in] any other craft, where neither the danger nor the effort is as great as in medicine. And despite what is said, the ordinances have always been maintained and observed, and neither Salmon nor La Calabre nor the others practiced medicine, and had they involved themselves in medicine, it would have been covertly, or a long time ago when the population of Paris was large [*that is, prior to the Black Death*] and many things were done which went unnoticed, and if La Calabre and others were involved in attending pregnant women, this would be women's business according to the law *de ventre incipiendo* [*on opening the womb*], and they did not involve themselves primarily in medicine, and prohibitions were issued by court decree against those who did. Therefore Domrémi will not be received as opposing the ordinances, statutes, and decrees cited above. Thus it is concluded, as above. And the court will be back after the recess because both parties are founded in their rights....

a. A Jewish Doctor Is Accused of Abortion and Malpractice

17 November 1298

Against Isaac the Jew, surgeon [*sic*].

In the name of the Lord, amen. In the year of his incarnation 1298, on 17 November, an inquiry was made on the part of the court of the Hospital of Manosque concerning what had come to the hearing of the court with loud insinuation: that Isaac the Jew, son of Resplanda and son-in-law of Joseph of Alesto, Jew of Manosque, calling himself a physician, practicing and comporting himself as a physician in the city and valley of Manosque, visited and prepared a poisonous medication for Uga, daughter of the late Peire of Die, who was pregnant. He made her drink the aforementioned poisonous medication, so that the infant in the belly of the said Astruga died and was still-born, and [he did this] so that the said Astruga should not be defamed because of the aforementioned pregnancy, such that from the aforesaid *po- tion or poisonous medication the aforementioned infant was still-born. Since these [deeds] would constitute a bad example and are worthy of correction, the aforementioned court therefore proceeds to launch an inquiry against the aforementioned Isaac and all and sundry who might be found guilty in the aforementioned affair....

In the same year on 18 November, Master Guilhem Rocencus of Manosque, witness, was sworn in and summoned [to testify] on the first point, which was first carefully read out before him. He said that he knew nothing except that Master Bertrand, then archpriest of Manosque, and brother Arnaud the prior, asked him on Palm Sunday if he knew that the said Huga was pregnant. The said Guilhem said to them that he did not know whether she was pregnant or not. And they told him that she was, indeed, pregnant and that the said woman was at that time a widow and ill, and that she had died of her illness in the inn that now belongs to Raimon Desderii, in which the said Huga was staying. Asked if he had seen Master Isaac, the Jew and doctor, enter on a certain day into the house where the said Huga was staying, he said yes, at some time. Asked about the second point he said that he had heard it said that it was so, namely from the aforementioned Lord Bertrand and the abovementioned prior and some other people....

On the same day Guilhem Pelegrini, otherwise known as Guilhem de Pel- latio, witness, being sworn in and summoned to tell the truth as to the said points, which were first read and explained to him, said that his wife Andrea once said to him that Huga was pregnant and had given birth, and that Huga had died in childbirth, because she had not been delivered of the child. He said that he neither knew nor had heard of anything else on this matter.

On the same day Beatrix, wife of Guilhem Gaufrid of Manosque, witness, was sworn in and summoned to tell the truth as to the said points, which were first read and explained. She said that she had, indeed, heard it said that the said Huga was pregnant and it was evident from the way she looked; and the neighbor-women said among themselves that she had given birth and they said that the mother of the said Huga had taken the baby to Lurs. She also said that she had seen the said Master Isaac often speaking to the said Huga, when it was said that she was pregnant. And the rumor among the people was that she was pregnant.

On the same day Aicard Maurell, witness, was sworn in and summoned to tell the truth as to the said points, which were first read and explained. He said that he knew nothing except what was contained in the same point, [namely] that people were saying that the said Huga was pregnant.

In the same year, on 19 November, Alacia Garrella of Manosque was sworn in and summoned [to tell the truth] as to the said points. She said she knew nothing, nor had she heard anything.

On the same day Elisabet, a nursemaid, was sworn in and summoned [to tell the truth] as to the said points. She said she knew nothing, nor had she heard or become aware of anything.

In the same year, on 19 November. Since the said Master Isaac had been put in irons on account of the said accusation and because there were fears for the health of the said Isaac on account of the weakness of his person, therefore brother Imbert de Saliniaco bailiff of Manosque and Lord Hugo Hospitaller, judge of the said court, at the request of Joseph the Jew, who on behalf of the said master [*gap in manuscript*] that they might desire and command that the said master Isaac [*gap in manuscript*] might be detained in the said prison but not put in chains....

In the name of the Lord, amen. In the abovementioned year, on 21 November, Lord Hugo Hospitaller, judge of the said court, set a date for the said Isaac to make his defense within ten days.

The said Master Isaac paid a fine of 50 pounds on account of the said inquiry, which the abovementioned Joseph paid to the lord bailiff, and I, Peire Bisquerra, witness, have written the above.

27 November–8 December 1298

Defense of Master Isaac.
In the name of the Lord. In the above year, on 28 November, Master Isaac, physician, Jew of Manosque, son of Resplanda the Jewess, produced and transmitted in his defense before the inquiry against him the points enumerated below, whose tenor is as follows. In the name of the Lord, amen. Isaac

the Jew, son of Resplanda and son-in-law of Joseph of Alesto, Jew, who is said to be a physician in the town of Manosque, in his defense before an inquiry against him in the court of the Hospital of St John in Manosque, in order to invalidate the intention of the said court and those who oppose him, so that by this inquiry it may appear [*gap in manuscript*] concerning the contents of the inquiry, as follows below. He protests that he is not obliged to prove everything below, but only what suffices for his defense, and also that it was not necessary for him to prove something if the said court could not prove it.

First, that if it was found that Huga, daughter of the late Peire de Die, had been defamed that she was pregnant, and so that the said Huga should not be defamed, at the time she was defamed in the city of Manosque she gave birth to a living child and then died near Lurs. And this is common knowledge.

Also that Madame Cristina, mother of the said Huga, carried the said infant alive to Lurs that it might be nursed and that when [Isaac] was upon the road near the place called "Case Pesoles" and ran into her, he had heard crying like that of an infant and he asked the said Cristina, "What is that?" And then she said, "That is an infant." And then Cristina said to him that the infant belonged to her daughter Huga, and that lest she be defamed, she was carrying it to Lurs to be nursed. And this is common knowledge.

Also that Alasatia, wife of Jean Textor of Manosque, perjured herself in this month of November. And this is common knowledge.

And the said Isaac protested that in what he said or says, he did not say nor does he say anything to injure anyone, but rather to preserve his right.

In this year, on 2 December, Galesius Ordei was sworn in and summoned to tell the truth as to the third point, which was first read and explained to him. He said he did not know whether [Alasatia] had perjured herself or not, nonetheless he said that his lord Mastinus and Simon would have a message in fifteen days with an oath, and hitherto he owed them the said debt. And he knew nothing else.

In this year, on 8 December, Raimon Burla of Manosque, witness, was sworn in and summoned to tell the truth as to the said points, which were first read and explained. He said that he himself had gone surety for the said Alasatia for 13 shillings which she owed to [the said?] Jew, and she promised and swore to him to pay the said 13 shillings. When the time for payment had lapsed and she still owed him the debt, nonetheless he believed that she did not have the pledges. And he knew nothing more.

In this year, on 11 December, Beatrix Guillelmi, witness, was sworn in upon her oath and summoned [to tell the truth] as to the said points. She said that she knew nothing save that she had heard it said that [Huga] was pregnant at that time.

b. Contract between a Jewish Doctor and his Christian Patient

4 August 1310

Raimon Sainerii and Master Isaac, Jew.

In the name of the Lord, amen. In the year of his incarnation 1310, on 3 August: be it known to all both present and to come that Master Isaac, physician of Manosque, promises and enters into an agreement through a solemn stipulation with R[aimon] Saunerii of the same place, he being present and stipulating, that [Isaac] shall, to the best of his own ability and that of the art of medicine, well and faithfully and according to law treat the person of Raimon and his wife and his children from this time forth for four continuous years. And the said R[aimon] Saunerii promised through a solemn stipulation to give and pay out to the said master Isaac, being present and stipulating, at every harvest over the next four years, four *sextarii* of good grain (*annona*) according to the measure of Manosque....

c. A Jewish Surgeon Provides Expert Testimony in a Murder Case

31 January 1342

[Account of the Crime]

Against Peire Gautier of Riez, cobbler living in Manosque ... yesterday evening in the lane in front of the house of Philippe Burlle, notary, [Peire Gautier] struck Peire Honorat, cobbler of Riez, in the belly with a sword and severely or lethally struck or wounded him, from which wound a great effusion of blood came forth, such that he was thought more likely to die than to live....

[The Medical Expertise]

Around the third hour of the same day, when the court learned that the said Peire Honorat had died of the said wound, the noble and pious lord Guilhem of Biterre, vice-bailiff of Manosque, summoned into his presence Master Bonafos, Jew and surgeon, who first saw the man when he was wounded and dressed his wounds and went to the house of the said wounded man and found him dead in his bed. The said vice-bailiff ordered the surgeon to inspect and palpate the wound and, when he had inspected and palpated it, to make a deposition as to whether the man had died of this wound or not. This Master Bonafos, in the presence of myself (the notary) and of the witnesses named below and of the said lord vice-bailiff, examined him with a wax candle and in other ways as he was able. When asked by the said lord vice-bailiff whether he had died from the wound, [Bonafos] said upon his oath that he found the said Peire to be dead, wounded in the left side so deeply that the fat had come out; the wound was in the lower part of the left side and from certain signs it was manifest that the small intestine had been injured and wounded, which injury to the small intestines the authorities in the art of surgery considered fatal. He also said that due to that wound, the wounded man had agonizing pains in the belly and also vomited with pain in the stomach and urinated very frequently, more so than normal, and sprayed his urine, which circumstances are true signs of an injury in the small intestines. For which reason he said and judged it true that the wounded man had died from that very wound.... As a precaution, the lord vice-bailiff asked him to make a public written declaration on this matter.

CHAPTER ELEVEN

WHAT CAN THEY DO? CLINICAL
ENCOUNTERS IN MEDIEVAL EUROPE

Scholastic medicine regarded bedside practice as the assumption of control by the doctor over the patient's life. To diagnose and cure, the doctor had to know in the first instance what the patient's individual *temperament was; this was the product of a complex formula whereby the *"naturals" of *humoral *complexion, body type, age, sex, and so forth were multiplied by the *"non-naturals" of environment and lifestyle. To arrive at this assessment, the physician examined physical signs and interrogated the patient and his entourage. To succeed in treating the patient, however, he had to establish his authority and engage the patient's obedience and trust. After all, much of what the patient was paying for when he hired a learned physician was the coherent and sophisticated explanation the doctor could provide. As we have seen in the previous chapter, empirics assessed disease in much the same way as university-trained practitioners did and offered almost identical therapies. What made the educated doctor special was the explanatory framework within which he managed treatment.

Medieval doctors wrote helpful advice about negotiating these encounters and avoiding situations that might threaten the doctor's authority. Those threats were real, because patients who hired learned doctors knew something about the product they were paying for and had their own ways of determining whether they were getting value for money. Doctors, on the other hand, had resources in case they were challenged. Besides scholastic drug theory, they could also lean on the idea that some treatments worked because of their *specific form. *Theriac was the most famous such remedy. Collectively, these were known as *experimenta or tried-and-true treatments. From the social historian's perspective, they are interesting because their reputation was validated by the status of the patient as well as the authority of the doctor; hence the record of an experimentum *will often include a narrative of who it was used on, and how. Physicians could also dispense diagnoses and treatment plans through letters of advice or* consilia. Consilia *eventually became a formal genre of scholastic medical literature: famous professors would publish their* consilia *and use them to teach practical medicine, as well as to broadcast their social connections and therapeutic prowess.*

Into this intimate world of bedside encounters and customized therapy came the Black Death. It might seem inappropriate to deal with the plague under the rubric of clinical encounters, for it was notoriously not a disease confined to individuals. The main problem the doctors faced in explaining the plague was precisely to account for its pandemic character. But scholastic medicine quickly found its feet and set about domesticating plague as a "distemper" that was ultimately connected to humoral type, environment, and behavior. This chapter closes with a plague-tract, a representative of the most popular form of medical writing of the late Middle Ages. Plague tracts were pitched to individuals and held out the promise that sound naturals and prudent use of the non-naturals would protect even against this universal poison.

78. THE DOCTOR AT THE BEDSIDE (I): PRECEPT ACCORDING TO ARCHIMATTHAEUS

Advice literature of the type presented here was highly stereotyped, and barely changed at all from the early Middle Ages to the fifteenth century (see doc. 93). Nonetheless, the emergence of learned medicine and lay professionals working for a fee did influence expectations of professional medical care. This tract on comportment ascribed to the twelfth-century physician Archimatthaeus should be read in this light. The text describes diagnosis by pulse and urine analysis and gives a detailed picture of the most common therapeutic mode of medieval medicine, namely diet. But the emphasis is on professional decorum, the ritual of the medical visit, and the cultivation of the patient's trust and submission.

Source: trans. Henry E. Sigerist, "Bedside Manners in the Middle Ages: The Treatise *De cautelis medicorum* Attributed to Arnold of Villanova," in *Henry E. Sigerist on the History of Medicine*, ed. Félix Marti-Albañez (New York: MD Publications, 1960), pp. 137–40. Rept. from *Quarterly Bulletin. Northwestern University Medical School* 20 (1946): 135–43. Latin.

Physician! When you shall be called to a sick man, in the name of God seek the assistance of the Angel who has attended the action of the mind and from inside shall attend departures of the body. You must know from the beginning how long the sick [man] has been laboring, and in what way the illness has befallen him, and by inquiring about the symptoms, if it can be done, ascertain what the disease is. This is necessary because after having seen the feces and urine and the condition of the pulse you may not be able to diagnose the disease, but if you announce the symptoms the patient will have confidence in you as in the author of his health and therefore one must devote greatest pains to knowing the symptoms.

Therefore, when you come to a house, inquire before you go to the sick [man] whether he has confessed, and if he has not, he should confess immediately or promise you that he will confess immediately; and this must not be neglected because many illnesses originate on account of sin and are cured by the Supreme Physician after having been purified from squalor by the tears of contrition, according to what is said in the Gospel: "Go, and sin no more, lest something worse happen to you."

Entering the sickroom, do not appear [excessively] haughty or overzealous and return, with a simple gesture, the greetings of those who rise to greet you. After they have seated themselves you finally sit down facing the sick; ask him how he feels and reach out for his arm, and all that we shall say is necessary so that through your entire behavior you obtain the favor of the people who are around the sick. And because the trip to the patient has sharpened your sensitivity, and the sick [man] rejoices at your coming or because he has already become stingy and has various thoughts about the fee, therefore by your fault as well as his the pulse is affected, is different and impetuous from the motion of the *spirits. When it has quieted down on both parts, you shall examine the pulse in the left arm because, although the right side would be satisfactory, yet it is easier to diagnose the motion of the heart in the left arm on account of its vicinity to the heart. Be careful that the patient does not lie on the right side because the compression would hinder the sense motion, nor should he stretch the fingers or make a fist. While you apply the fingers of your right hand you shall support with your left the patient's arm, because from greater sensibility you will distinguish the different and various motions more easily, and also because the patient's arm being, so to say, weak requires your support. If the arm is very full and fleshy you must press your fingers hard so as to get into the depths; if it is weak and lean you can feel the pulse sufficiently on the surface. You must examine the pulse to a hundred beats at the very least, so that you may form an opinion on the various kinds of pulses, and the patient's people should receive your words as the result of a long examination of the heart beat.

Finally you [should] request to have the urine brought, and if the change in pulse indicates that the individual is sick, the kind of disease is still better indicated by the urine, but they will believe you to indicate and diagnose the disease not only from the urine but also from the pulse. While you look at the urine for a long time you [should] pay attention to its color, substance and quantity, and to its contents, from the diversity of which you will diagnose the different kinds of diseases, as is taught in the *Treatise on Urines*, whereupon you promise health to the patient who is hanging on your lips. When you have left him say a few words to the members of the household. Say that he is very sick, for if he recovers you will be praised more for your art; should he die his friends will testify that you had given him up.

Let me give you one more warning: do not look at a maid or a daughter or a wife with an improper or covetous eye and do not let yourself be entangled in female affairs – for there are medical operations that excite the helper's mind; otherwise your judgment is affected, you become harmful to the patient, and people will expect less from you. And so, be pleasant in your speech, diligent and careful in your medical dealings, eager to help. And adhere to this without fallacy.

When you have been invited for dinner you should not throw yourself upon the party and at table should not occupy the place of honor, although it is customary to assign the place of honor to the priest and the physician. Then you should not disdain certain drinks, nor find fault with certain dishes, nor be disgusted perhaps because you are hardly accustomed to appease your hunger with millet bread in peasant fashion. If you act thus your mind will feel at ease. And while the attention is concentrated on the variety of dishes, inquire explicitly from some of the attendants about the patient or about his condition. If you do this the sick will have great confidence in you, because he sees that you cannot forget him in the midst of delicacies. When you leave the table and come to the sick, you must tell him that you have been served well, at which the patient greatly rejoices because he was very anxious to have you well served.

If it is the time and place to feed the sick you will feed him. It is necessary, however, that you set the time for the patient's meals, namely in intermittent *fevers when the sick have a real remission; in continuous fevers when there happens to be a quiet moment because a decline of their fever does not occur before the *crisis. In intermittent fevers they must be fed before the attack and so early that when the attack comes the entire food [will] be *digested, because otherwise nature will have to fight a war on two fronts and it will not be strong enough to digest what has been offered at the wrong moment nor will it be able to defeat the enemy disease. When the attack of fever has begun, wait until it has ceased and then wait for two more hours or for one at least, because the organs are exhausted from the preceding battle and the attack of the enemy and do not want that a burden be imposed on them in the form of food, but after having so to say triumphed over the enemy they wish to have a rest.

You shall feed the sick according to the season of the year and according to the change of seasons and of the disease; and [the] quantity and quality of food must be varied according to the diseases, for you shall give the patient ampler food in intermittent than in continuous fever, more food in winter and spring, less in summer and autumn because they stand it very badly. The [patient's] age must be considered, and you will restore children more often than youths, because their consumption is greater on account of the liquidity of the humors and because they must grow, for it is according to nature to restore where there is a daily loss. Old people you will restore with less food because they have little heat and vigor; and also according to what they are accustomed to eat, because if they are accustomed to use an ampler and coarser diet you will not give them the same kind of food, but rather prescribe a liquid or moderate diet. You must fear constipation of the bowels or *flux, and if there is flux you must start out with coarser food such as quinces, sorb-apples, and medlars, because they constipate through their thickness. If, however, there is constipation you will start out with lighter, liquid foods. Thus you will give prunes and the cooked juice of Damascene prunes because they quickly eject through their heaviness. If the condition of the bowels is between the two, you will begin with a lighter and more liquid diet because this is very useful to the sick and protects against greater harm. If the bowels have moved, give such a diet because it relieves the various organs. Thus you shall give first prunes cooked in water or pomegranates or almond milk that you shall prepare in the following way: almonds removed from the shells shall be put in hot water, whereupon they shall be ground thoroughly and a little cold water shall be added; the whole shall be stirred, strained through a clean linen cloth and given to drink. If however a little bread, that is the soft part of it, is cooked in the pot, that almond milk is better digested than if it is drunk pure. After it has been prepared, a small amount must be poured off, and then one must remove by blowing or with a feather the oily substance that is on the surface because it is a hot matter. After this has been done, give several times chicken broth to drink or water in which the soft part of bread has been dissolved.

You shall also give barley flour and make it in the following way: first wash the barley in cold water, pour it over a stone and rub it so that it loses the skins, whereupon it must be rubbed and ground in a mortar or ground between millstones; then have the finer parts very well cooked and toward the end of the cooking add a little almond milk and present it to the sick. If, however, you wish to have *ptisane, cook the coarser parts of the barley in water and give him ptisane in a drink, or water in which bread has been soaked, cooked or not. And remember that while there is food in the stomach you shall not give diuretic water with syrup because such drinks force the food out of the stomach undigested or retard digestion.

Remember, furthermore, that in the beginning of the disease the physician endeavors to oppose it with digestive remedies, for he is the helper of nature and must aid it. Nature namely proceeds to making the crisis [in order] to triumph over the disease; she wishes to reduce the forces of the disease by changing the condition and quality of the matter and by dispersing it among the organs so that the parts [may] be separated from each other and she may reach her end and more easily than expected with complete results in one weak expulsion. In the same way, the physician in order to drive out the matter that must be driven out, must be prepared to treat the digested matters, according to the aphorism in the first book of Hippocrates. Consideration of the cause of the disease determines the choice of remedies that digest the humors; for if the patient suffers from *cholera you will give him vinegar syrup; if he suffers from a cold humor you will give *oxymel and everything else as I have said in another chapter. Oh physician, thanks be given to God.

79. THE DOCTOR AT THE BEDSIDE (2): PRECEPT ACCORDING TO ARNAU OF VILANOVA

Despite the prestige of his academic training, the doctor could never take his patient's confidence and compliance for granted. He had to cultivate in the patient an attitude of trust – trust in the physician's competence and, beyond that, trust in the claims of scholastic medicine. Scholastic medicine asserted that the physician's academic training enabled him to furnish a rational account of the invisible workings of the body, and that this rational account was the only sure foundation of safe and effective practice. It was important that the patient buy into that claim, not only because it was almost the only thing that distinguished the university-trained physician from the empiric, but also because it was essentially the physician's scientific story about the body that the patient was paying for. On the other hand, the more familiar medieval patients became with learned medicine, the more likely they were to contest the authority of the physician.

Advice literature for doctors seems to assume that patients will find ways to test the competence of their physicians before committing themselves to their care. Uroscopy was both an attractive and an easy target; the consumer recognized that uroscopy symbolized the learned doctor's claim to a special expertise based on theory. This text by Arnau of Vilanova (introduced in doc. 44) shows that doctors had to be on guard against those who would try to probe their credentials by sending a urine sample through an intermediary and asking for a diagnosis. The trick, according to Arnau, is to coax information out of the servant who brings the sample and to assert your expertise by making noncommittal and irrefutable statements. While the public might be skeptical about a particular physician's claim to diagnose from urine, it seems to have accepted the validity of uroscopy itself; otherwise, it would not have bothered to test the physician's skill in this area. But what about the practitioner? Why did Arnau not trust that his training would help him detect a phony sample?

Source: trans. Henry E. Sigerist, "Bedside Manners in the Middle Ages: The Treatise *De cautelis medicorum* Attributed to Arnold of Villanova," in *Henry E. Sigerist on the History of Medicine*, ed. Félix Marti-Albañez (New York: MD Publications, 1960), pp. 134–37. Rept. from *Quarterly Bulletin. Northwestern University Medical School* 20 (1946): 135–43. Latin.

We must consider the precautions with regard to urines, by which we can protect ourselves against people who wish to deceive us. The very first shall consist in finding out whether the urine be of man or of another animal or another fluid; and if it is human urine, it is diagnosed in four ways.

The second precaution is with regard to the individual who brings the urine. You must look at him sharply and keep your eyes straight on him or on his face; and if he wishes to deceive you he will start laughing or the color of his face will change, and then you must curse him forever and in all eternity.

The third precaution is also with regard to the individual who brings the urine, whether man or woman, for you must see whether he or she is pale, and after you have ascertained that this is the individual's urine, say to him: "Verily, this urine resembles you," and talk about the pallor, because immediately you will hear all about his illness. It commonly happens with poor people and those of moderate means that they go to the doctor when they are afflicted very seriously.

The fourth precaution is with regard to sex. An old woman wants to have your opinion. You inquire whose urine it is and the old woman will say to you: "Don't you know it?" Then look at her from the corner of your eye, and ask: "What relation is it of yours?" And if she is not too crooked, she will say that the patient is a male or female relation or something from which you can distinguish the sex. Should she say: "We are not related," then ask what the patient used to do when he was in good health and from the patient's doing you can recognize or deduce the sex.

The fifth precaution is that you must ask if the patient is old. If the messenger says yes, you must say that he greatly suffers from the stomach, and that he spits a lot, and in the morning more than at any other time, for old people have by nature a cold stomach.

The sixth precaution: whether this illness has lasted for a long time or not. If the messenger says that it has, you must say that the patient is altogether irritable and that one can help him, or some such talk. If he says no, you must say that the patient is altogether oppressed because in the beginning of diseases there is much matter that oppresses the organ.

There is a seventh precaution, and it is a very general one; [if] you [can] not find out anything about the case, then say that he has an obstruction in the liver. He may say: "No, sir, on the contrary he has pains in the head, or in the legs, or in other organs." You must say that this comes from the liver or from the stomach; and particularly use the word "obstruction," because they do not understand what it means and it helps greatly that a term is not understood by the people.

The eighth precaution is with regard to conception. An old woman consults you because the patient cannot become pregnant. Perhaps you do not know the cause but say that she cannot hold her husband's sperm, which she could have done very well if she had been well disposed.

The ninth precaution is with regard to a woman, whether she is old or young; and this you shall find out from what is told you. Should she be very old, say that she has all the evils that old women have and also that she has many superfluities in the womb. Should she, however, be young, say that she suffers from the stomach, and whenever she has a pain further down, say that it comes from the womb or the kidneys; and whenever she has it in the anterior part of the head, then it comes from the stomach; and whenever on the left side, then it comes from the spleen; whenever on the right, then it comes from the liver; and when it is worse and almost impedes her eyesight, say that she has pains or feels a heaviness in the legs, particularly when she exerts herself.

The tenth precaution: you must keep yourself very busy spitting or blowing your nose and if the old woman pesters you with the urine say quite casually: "What concern is this of yours?" or "Why do you pester me so much?" If she says: "Yes, it concerns me," then you shall know the sex. If she says, no, ask as has been explained under the fourth precaution.

The eleventh precaution is taken with regard to white or yellow wine. If you have any doubts in this respect, be cautious and put the lid of the urinal down and pour out a little of the content in such a way that the wine in being poured out touches your finger. Then you must give her the urinal and act as if you were going to blow your nose whereby you put the finger that has been dipped in, on or next to your nose; then you will smell the odor of wine, whereupon you must take the urinal again and say to her: "Get away and be ashamed of yourself!"

The twelfth precaution is taken with respect to fluid made from figs and also nettles. Although you could recognize this under the first precaution, yet you will clearly see that the residue extends in the form of a circle touching the urinal and does not make a rotundity or pine cone like a true sediment.

The thirteenth precaution: whenever the old woman asks what disease the patient has, you must say: "You would not understand me if I told you and it would be better for you to ask what he should do." And then she will see that you have judgment in the matter and will keep quiet. But perhaps she will say: "Sir, he is very hot; therefore he seems to have a fever." [You should reply:] "Thus it seems to you and other lay people who do not know how to distinguish between fever and other diseases."

The fourteenth precaution: when you have been called to a patient, feel the pulse before you examine the urine and make them talk so that the condition of the animal *virtue becomes apparent to you. After having recognized these factors you will be able to evaluate the urine better and with more certainty and you may proceed thus.

The fifteenth precaution is: should the patient be in a bad condition so that you think that he may die the following day, do not go to him, but send your servant to bring you the urine or tell them to bring it tomorrow in the early morning because you wish that they prepare for the meal and that after you have seen the urine you will [then] tell what they shall administer. And so from the report of the person who brings the urine you will be able to form an opinion about the patient, whether he is in good or bad condition.

The sixteenth precaution is that when you come to a patient you should always do something new lest they say that you cannot do anything without the books.

The seventeenth precaution is that if by hard luck you come to the home of the patient and find him dead and somebody perhaps says: "Sir, what have you come for?" you shall say that you have not come for that and say that you well knew that he was going to die, but that you wanted to know at what hour he had died.

The eighteenth precaution is that if you have a competitor whom you believe to be a shameless crook, be careful when you go to the house of the patient; perhaps he will stir up the urine for you and you will not be able to form a certain judgment from it.

The nineteenth precaution is the following: if two urines of the same patient are presented to you and you wish to know which was the first, ask at what time of the night he got up, for if he did at dawn or after digestion had taken place that urine which is more digested and red will be the first, if it has sediment. If, however, he got up before midnight or around that time, you may judge that the less digested and less red urine is the first.

No other deception can occur outside of these, but these points must be kept in mind, and you must be cautious because the physician is greatly honored if he knows how to be cautious, for he is asked questions many times.

80. THE DOCTOR AT THE BEDSIDE (3): PRACTICE ILLUSTRATED BY GUILLAUME BOUCHER

The remarkable casebook of the German student who observed Drs Guillaume Boucher and Pierre d'Ausson as they went on their rounds in early fifteenth-century Paris has already been introduced in connection with the treatment of breast cancer (doc. 71). The two cases below show that the reality of the bedside encounter of doctor and patient rarely conformed to the image of total medical control and authority projected by prescriptive texts such as those of Archimatthaeus and Arnau of Vilanova. In the first case, we see Boucher working in partnership with d'Ausson and others on a case of stroke. As intervention after intervention failed to bring improvement, their collaboration started to fracture. Though this is implied rather than stated, it seems that Boucher withdrew and left the case to d'Ausson, who achieved a surprising outcome. In the second case, a feisty patient challenged Boucher's competence as a learned physician.

Source: trans. Faith Wallis from Ernest Wickersheimer, "Les secrets et les conseils de maître Guillaume Boucher et de ses confrères. Contribution à l'histoire de la médecine à Paris vers 1400," *Bulletin de la société française d'histoire de la médecine* 8 (1909): 49–57, 65–66. Latin.

No. 47 A Case of Paralysis

Here follows another [case], against a serious paralysis or light *apoplexy, for a man who was suddenly struck down, so that he could not speak or move, and he was surfeited [with drink?].

Let his diet be warm and dry: roasted pigeons and capons, chickens – but not young ones, because these are very humid. Again, let him drink *mellicratum*, that is honey-water. Again, his vegetables ... can be roasted. Again, the nape of the neck and the paralyzed limbs ought to be anointed with oil of costus or oil of wolf.

Again, against the swelling of his tongue, because he could not move it more than a little bit forward, but he could not extend it because it was paralyzed at the root: take root of yellow iris, Spanish pellitory, anise, and aged *theriac. Put into a small bag, and rub the tongue with it.

Again, everyone agreed that they should make sneezing-powders: take staves acre, preserved Spanish pellitory, and white hellebore. Grind them into a fine powder and introduce this into the nostrils with a feather, and they will cause sneezing....

Again, everyone said that they should insert into the *clysters colocynth mostly, and then agaric, and then centaury along with other suitable ingredients such as mallow, marsh mallow, etc. Again, if he cannot or will not take pills by mouth, they should be dissolved in small pieces in wine and let him take them thus with ground nutmeg. The wine, however, does not hide the taste of the medicine, so let it be given in whey from goats. And in this case it is very appropriate to apply clysters, as Averroes says in *Colliget* book 4, because they draw down [morbid] matter from the upper regions to the greatest degree.

They were of one mind that he should not sleep, because he would immediately die, since there would be a fullness of *phlegm in all the *ventricles of the brain. Again, everyone said that this called for "fetid pills" ... and pills of *hierapigra*, and euphorbia pills; likewise almond milk with barley-meal or oatmeal and, if he wished, let it be made with sugar. Again, he should abstain totally from wine, but let his drink be *hydromel with marjoram, sage or hyssop added.

His tongue should be rubbed vigorously and painfully so that he begins to talk, and with root of yellow iris and with "Alexander's Gold" [*a compound drug made with gold and opium*], and with aged theriac, and with *castoreum, mixed in equal amounts. Again, let there be painful ligatures made at the extremities – that is, the hands and feet – and the arms, in order to divert the [morbific] matter from the head. And as Avicenna advises, let him be gently rubbed on the neck and shoulders with lily root and root of yellow iris.

Because nature began to exert itself and he spat up blood from his throat, and because his vital *powers were weak, they did not advise bloodletting, for he was a good sixty years of age. And they repeated the same clysters and rubbings upon his tongue and neck.

Again, after shaving [the patient's] head, a *decoction was made to *foment the head. Here it is: take two handfuls each of both kinds of sage, both kinds of calamint, marjoram, betony, and Arabian lavender, one handful each of primrose, St John's wort and hyssop, one and one-half handfuls of flowers of senna, a half-quart of yellow iris root, and two handfuls of both kinds of rue, and pound them up.

They agreed that he could sleep a little bit for the sake of restoring his powers, but that he should be instantly aroused with the above-mentioned sneezing powders.

And because the case was desperate, Boucher said that they should limit themselves to the prescribed clysters and the friction of the tongue, because applying so many remedies in a desperate case results in lay-folk defaming the doctor when the patient dies, saying "Look at those doctors! They administered so many remedies that they killed him!" He also said that in a desperate case like this, if the patient insistently demands certain things, like wine or cherries, he should be given them, provided he is not asking for outlandish things that might harm him. No one should actually mention wine or cherries to him, but if he demands them with vehemence, they should be given to him.

Again they were of one accord that he should eat small songbirds, roasted, or something similar. Also, that warming and *resolvent medications should be applied to the muscles of his arms "to arouse the motive nature of the members" (said the Italian, who was the king's physician)....

Again, Boucher said that [the patient] might be so bold as to drink a small amount of wine with water, because it was incumbent upon him (as he said) to keep his strength up. They repeated the remedies continuously, namely the pills and clysters and rubbings, as you saw. Nonetheless, it is difficult to take pills so often....

This disease can be broadly termed a debilitating apoplexy, which is a paralysis that completely disables one whole side [of the body], namely in the right arm and right hand, and in the shin – in short, his whole right side was paralyzed. And so the masters deliberated, saying that this disease is difficult to cure, considering [the patient's] age and *complexion, and his state of repletion. Hence, it is a chronic disease. But there was doubt over the prognosis, namely whether an apoplexy could turn into a paralysis and then back again, going in a circle, because the [morbific] matter, being imbibed by the *nerves, could easily reach the brain, and vice versa. It behooved them to *evacuate with the abovementioned [*purgatives] at intervals, for when the matter reached the brain, [the patient] would die....

D'Ausson [said] that powders should be made of castoreum, yellow iris, mustard, Spanish pellitory, and salt, all [placed] in a sac of fine fabric, so that they would come out as a fine powder. They should be applied to the tongue and rubbed in vigorously. And this little sac should not be rubbed [on the tongue] unless it was first moistened or infused in water, whether distilled alcohol or sage-water; and this was a good idea, because such rubbings with the little sac could dry out [the tongue]. However, d'Ausson wanted these powders to be applied to the tongue directly and not in the little bag, as their action would be stronger. And Boucher only wanted it in the way described above.... [*Boucher seems to quit the case at this point, as he is not mentioned again.*]

Note that when all these things had been prepared, within about eighteen days, [the patient] began to speak perfectly; and always and continuously by repeating the aforementioned regime, but as d'Ausson saw it. Again, d'Ausson compounded the ointment which follows, for anointing paralytic limbs, and it is made thus: take one ounce each of camomile, melitot, tamarisk, cala-mint, mint, wormwood, both kinds of sage, hyssop, paralysis-herb [*that is, primrose*], Arabian lavender, St John's wort, rue, bay leaves, mugwort and betony, a half-quart of yellow iris root, costus and iris root, and one ounce each of common lavender and camel's hay. Make a decoction in one quart of balsam wine until reduced by two-thirds. Strain, and boil the strained [mixture] with the following: take one half-quart each of laurel oil, oil of costus, juniper oil, oil of castoreum and euphorbia, pine oil, and mastic oil. Boil until the wine is evaporated and then add the following aromatics: one half ounce each of sagapenum [*a gum resin*] and opopanax [*resin from the root of* Opopanax chronium], three drams each of castoreum and euphorbia, one dram of pepper, one dram each of fat from a fox, a wolf and a cat, and a suf-ficient quantity of wax. Make an ointment.

When the abovementioned was applied, [the patient] spoke perfectly, and walked about his room, and made some use of his paralyzed arm and paralyzed leg. [After taking an *electuary], he was so much improved that he went to church. But d'Ausson administered clysters to him for fifteen days, so that he took fifteen clysters, excepting the first two, to the glory of God in France.

No. 67 A Quarrelsome Patient with a Phlegmatic *Fever

Here follows another chapter on *phlegmatic fever, in the case of a man of about forty years of age, whose urine was very scorched and quite thick.... [*There follows a recipe for a syrup.*]

[Boucher] prescribed bloodletting, and also a diet, as you know: purée of peas with verjus, almond milk, three chickens (but I am astonished that [he did] not [prescribe] barley-meal), and syrup of endives, because his liver was overheated. Again, [the patient] underwent bloodletting not during the paroxysm, but after. During the paroxysm he drank barley-water, but at dinner and supper three parts wine to two parts water; chicken broth for dinner and "you should eat the wings and legs, with purée"; but for supper, almond milk with washed barley. Because his head was flushed, his forehead and temples were moistened with rose water. Again, he ate some veal, as before. Note that his urine remained clear, and since it never became colored and remained clear, he did not require a laxative medicine. "And so," said Boucher, "let him take the same syrup prescribed in the beginning and let him be under observation (*regatur*) every day, and he can certainly go to church as he did yesterday and the day before and he will get on well." And Boucher prescribed that he eat poached eggs with verjus, if he wished. "O master, dear master," [the patient replied], "they will engender heat." Boucher replied, "Now, look at that! This is why physicians are wise, because everybody teaches them – the old wife, the barber, the layman, the patient, and if it could talk, the pustule itself would instruct us how we should purge it!" Then Boucher asked the patient what he had eaten in the third [hour] and the second. [The patient replied,] "O master, you yourself should know and judge by my urine." Boucher said: "Of course I know, but I want to learn about your appetite and inclinations, and if you are inclining towards something which is harmful for you, I shall forbid it." Again the patient said, "I am too old; I cannot tolerate bloodletting." Boucher replied, "It is just as I said: the patients tell *us* what to do. Those who are rather advanced in years – say, fifty or sixty years of age – or those who are well nourished, are in no danger; indeed, even less so than a young man who is poorly fed, such as poor young men." But this old man got better.

81. TRIED AND TRUE: MEDICAL *EXPERIMENTA* ("PROVEN REMEDIES") BY ARNAU OF VILANOVA

These *experimenta *by Arnau of Vilanova are remedies that he claims to have tested and proven, but whose efficacy cannot be explained by medical theory.* Experimenta *or* empirica *constituted a significant theoretical problem for academic physicians and surgeons: how could they justify using a treatment whose action could not be explained in rational terms? Arnau found a solution in Avicenna's doctrine of* proprietas *or "property." This is sometimes referred to as the* tota species *or "global species" of a substance: a quality that inheres in its overall nature and not in the sum of its elemental parts. Every substance has a* *complexion *that can be described in terms of the four elemental qualities, and its actions can be inferred from this complexion. But besides this complexionate nature, it possessed an independent "property" or specific quality, ultimately derived from astral influences. This* proprietas *could be discovered only by experience (*experimentum*). Even an unlearned "empiric" might stumble across an effective remedy; but a learned physician tested such* empirica *and would reject out of hand any that were based on absurd or superstitious premises, such as sympathetic action at a distance.*

Source: trans. Faith Wallis from the edition by Michael McVaugh, "The *experimenta* of Arnald of Villanova," *The Journal of Medieval and Renaissance Studies* 1 (1971): 107–18. Latin.

Here begins the treatise on the cures of diverse infirmities composed by Master Arnau of Vilanova, the famous doctor, and dedicated to the Lord Pope Clement [V]. And here begins the [dedicatory] letter to the most holy and blessed pope and lord, by divine providence supreme pontiff of the sacrosanct Church of Rome: To your holiness, your servant Master Arnau of Vilanova, among physicians, etc....

7. Another *experimentum* concerning headache. When I was in Lyons, it happened that a certain noble lady of the city of Vienne suffered from very severe headache, so that she could find no repose, neither was any remedy of use. She claimed that the aforementioned infirmity had oppressed her for about a year, and that she had spent much of her wealth in seeking the help of doctors. When she was brought into my presence, she was complaining a good deal and anxious about what would happen to her. And because in other cases the aforementioned infirmity commonly occurs because of *vapors rising into the brain, I caused to be gathered a certain herb called camomile; it is found in the meadows in summer. Having collected a large quantity of this herb, I separated out the flowers and I caused a water to be made from the flowers in the same way as one makes distilled rose water, and

I made her wash her head with this water. Within four days, she felt herself to be completely cured. This water is indeed very good for the brain, and more effective against headache than any other medicine and vapors can readily be expelled from the brain with it....

9. Another *experimentum* for tooth-ache. Once the lord pope had a pain in his jaw; this pain came from his inability to chew food. One of his teeth had a cavity and there a worm tossed to and fro. When the worm stirred within the tooth, the aforementioned lord suffered greatly, so that he could not drink or sleep. After I had carefully inspected it, I easily administered a remedy. For this remedy, I caused to be gathered a certain herb called "camomile" in the vernacular (but which in books is called *quamcularia*). I took the seed of this herb. Now I had a small tile which I applied to the jaw until the tooth became hot, and then I put the seeds on the tile, and immediately smoke went up from the seeds because of the heat of the tile. I made the lord open his mouth so that the smoke went into his mouth. When the smoke entered [the mouth], suddenly the worm which was in the tooth emerged and fell out onto the tile, and thus the tooth-ache completely stopped. And this *experimentum* is highly effective for teeth with cavities in which a worm has been generated. If someone is suffering from tooth-ache for some other reason, the aforementioned remedy will not be effective, but another should be applied, as will be described below....

14. Another *experimentum* against indigestion of the stomach. If someone is suffering from indigestion of the stomach, because of which he feels somewhat upset, let him take a small amount of *aqua vitae* [*distilled alcohol*], which is called "fire-water" in the vernacular, but which is called in medicine "water of life" because of its various virtues. This *aqua vitae* should, however, be mixed with wine; it should not be drunk by itself, for it is exceedingly hot and dessicative, and taken by itself it destroys and annihilates the chest area. But if taken with wine, it is very effective and ends stomach indigestion, and causes the undigested matter to be carried off, and the stomach to be emptied of the aforementioned matter. I cured the lord Cardinal James of the aforementioned infirmity, who often had the aforementioned indigestion. But what causes it is dining at night, particularly when a person goes to bed [directly] after dinner. Drinking too much wine aggravates stomach indigestion, and wine drunk straight aggravates more than wine which has been watered; and pure wine drunk in moderation greatly improves phlegmatic men, but harms *choleric ones, because of its effect and power....

26. An *experimentum* concerning lice. If you have an abundance of lice and wish to be rid of them, take mercury and rub your belt with it. Then know that all the lice, wherever they are lurking on your body, will descend to the aforementioned belt, and the moment they touch it, they will die. This does

not avail unless you rub the belt twice with mercury and in this way you can avoid harm from lice....

32. Another *experimentum* for closing a wound. If you have been wounded in any part of your body, if you want the wound to close quickly, take a certain herb called comfrey; then crush it and afterwards apply it to the wound and within an artificial day [of 24 hours] the wound will be completely closed, so that only a scar will remain. But take care that as much blood as possible comes out before the wound is closed, lest an *aposteme be generated because of the danger of *corrupt blood remaining, and [this aposteme] emerge in another part of the body. Very many doctors fail in this *experimentum*, because it involves going to rather a lot of trouble....

36. Another *experimentum* against aposteme. If you have an aposteme next to the heart, by reason of which you are in imminent danger and you wish to be rid of it, take a certain herb called scabwort and make from it a water, just as they do from roses. And take this water in the morning and drink it on an empty stomach, and continue this for six or seven days, and within that time the entire aposteme that is in your body will drain out through a hidden place and you will be rid of it. This water is extremely powerful, but after it has been distilled, it ought to be placed in direct sunlight; and thence it will be purified and the dregs will go down to the bottom. This *experimentum* should be done at the beginning of spring so that a man may avoid apostemic infirmities, and it should be done as I advised the lord cardinals when I was at the Curia in Rome....

43. Another *experimentum* for retaining hair. If you wish to retain the hair on your head so that it does not [fall out], take anise and a certain herb called nasturtium (in the vernacular, *mastuerco*), coriander prepared with transmarine sage, mint, hyssop, violet flowers; and place all the aforementioned into water and boil vigorously. Afterwards, wash the head with the aforementioned water once a day and continue this for eight, ten or nine days, and if you do this your hair will be strengthened and will stay in for a whole year. And if you want red hair, add orpiment to the above, by virtue of which the hair will appear somewhat red. And this was proven on myself, who progressively lost my hair because of a certain infirmity of continuous fever from which I suffered for a month; and I escaped this condition by virtue of the aforementioned water. And this water fortifies the anterior part of the brain, in which region the hair is wont to fall out more quickly, and from this part it more easily takes root....

56. Another *experimentum* concerning stomach pains. If you suffer from pains in the stomach, which happen at times from a superabundance of inflamed or burning choler, take fennel water and drink it in the morning on an empty stomach, and immediately you will experience some benefit due to

the virtue of this water, and you will be rid of that suffering in the stomach. The aforementioned water is very effective in suppressing choler and in dissolving that matter from which the aforementioned pains are engendered. And this was proven in the case of a certain cardinal of Ostia who bore this affliction, from which he was freed by the aforementioned *experimentum*.

57. Another experiment concerning cleansing of the blood. If you have *putrid and corrupt blood and wish to purify it, take borage and lettuces – not the long ones, but those which are usually wrinkled and curly – and cook them; and everyday eat one bowl of the aforementioned borage and lettuces. And if you continue this for a week, your blood will be purified, and if afterwards you wish to extract a small amount of blood by bloodletting, you will be able to do this once this treatment has been undergone. And if some corrupt blood remains, it goes out through the vein and thereafter you need not dread any infirmity or continuous, *tertian, or *quartan fever, that year. This advice or remedy I gave to my Lord [Pope] Clement, and he made much use of the abovementioned food....

59. Another *experimentum* concerning lethargy. It is necessary to cure this infirmity, which often arises from excessive sleep and is always located in the posterior part of the head; it is a highly dangerous infirmity. A person suffering from it will be as good as dead in two or three days, and will lose his wits and memory, so as to recall almost nothing. This is the remedy to be applied (and it is a very useful one) to cure this infirmity. Take red wine, very strong and as coarse as may be found, and strong vinegar, and flowers of *recemi* [*unidentified plant; racemus means "bunch" or "cluster" and usually refers to fruit*], and white elder flowers, and mix the flowers with the wine and vinegar. Then you shall twice each day, morning and evening, wash this person's head with the aforementioned water, and continue for about a month, and all the above [ingredients] are to be fresh each day. And if you continue, the person suffering from the aforementioned infirmity will be rid of it and the aforementioned *humors impeding the memory will be completely consumed. And this is a very potent remedy for curing the abovementioned infirmity. The abovementioned infirmity is very stubborn; it causes people to die and while it seems to you that the person is asleep, his spirit has departed. I proved this [*experimentum*] in the case of the bishop of Auxerre, who suffered greatly from this disease and could hardly remember anything....

59A. Another *experimentum* for preserving memory. If you have a good memory and you wish to preserve or increase it, lest it be lost for any reason, take a certain very precious substance called *vespetion*; mix it with white wine, the clearest you can find, and wash the head three times a week or more, and continue doing this. And if you do this, you will know for certain that you will preserve your memory and you will be able to retain more, and there is nothing in the world that strengthens the brain more than this. And I have often applied this remedy on myself....

65. Another *experimentum* concerning knitting of the bone. If you have broken your shin or another bone due to a blow or fall and you wish it to knit, take a certain herb called *tamaria*, similar in scent to the herb called St John's wort. Apply this herb to the broken bone; then tie it securely with a linen bandage and make the person (if he has a broken shin) remain in bed, lying down. And continue this for forty days and never let him move from bed or walk about. And if you do this, when you join the middle part of the bone to the bone, and the bone is set, he will be able to walk with ease just as before. And although in medicine many remedies are applied for setting [the bone], nonetheless this remedy is very simple and without danger. And I proved this in the case of a certain messenger of our lord pope who fell from a horse and broke his shin in two places.

82. CUSTOMIZED THERAPEUTICS: THE MEDIEVAL MEDICAL *CONSILIUM* (1)

In chapter 5, Bartholomaeus of Salerno was introduced as a commentator on Joannitius and as the author of works on anatomy and therapeutics. He appears here as a medical consultant to the great and good. It is instructive to contrast his exchange of letters with Peter the Venerable, abbot of the monastery of Cluny, with the medical letters of bishops in chapter 3. Peter displays a rather sophisticated understanding of illness, but now the churchman seeks advice from a teacher and practitioner, not a fellow prelate. Bartholomaeus's response is a precocious example of the consilium *− a letter of advice addressed by a physician to an individual patient with a specific medical problem, offering an analysis of the case and customized remedies.*

Though the energetic head of a far-flung monastic empire, Peter the Venerable suffered from ill health for much of his life. In 1150, he contracted a prolonged head cold that turned into bronchitis and laryngitis. It is not clear where Bartholomaeus was at the time Peter wrote to him. Bartholomaeus was worried that a journey by his socius *(apprentice or associate) Bernard to Cluny and back might take more than a month; this suggests that he is in or near French territory. Another letter of advice by Bartholomaeus addressed to King Louis VII of France (r. 1137−80) indicates that Bartholomaeus was a well-known elite consultant and that he may have resided in France.*

Incidentally, Peter was soon on his feet again: he took a long and strenuous journey to Italy from November 1151 to March 1152.

Source: trans. Faith Wallis from *The Letters of Peter the Venerable*, ed. Giles Constable (Cambridge, MA: Harvard University Press, 1967), Letter 158a–b, pp. 379–83. Latin.

a. Peter the Venerable of Cluny Writes to
Master Bartholomaeus of Salerno

To Doctor Bartholomaeus.

To our beloved Master Bartholomaeus, brother Peter, the humble abbot of Cluny, [sends] greetings and familiar affection.

Ever since I saw you at Cluny last year, I have held you ever in my heart and loved you most affectionately. For I cherished your great knowledge and loved even more that which is more worthy of love in any person, namely, your character, which is of the highest caliber. Hence because (as I said) I love you, I dare to ask you to love me as well. For this reason I bring certain matters to your notice as a friend, because I stand in need of your advice. For almost a year I have been repeatedly afflicted with the disease called *catarrh; I have had it twice already, once in the summer and once in the winter or around that time. This year I came down with it at the end of summer and beginning of autumn. Prior to this, I had had [legal] cases and many meetings with the nobility of our territory. For this reason I was forced to postpone much longer than usual my customary bloodletting, which I normally have at the end of every second month. And because the disease that I mentioned came upon me during that delay in bloodletting, I did not dare to go ahead with it the way I normally would, lest with the blood seizing hold of my body, bloodletting would be dangerous. I had learned from some people that bloodletting during catarrh would cause me to lose my voice entirely or to a very great extent, either permanently or for a long time. They added that if it were done, in some cases a close brush with death would not be out of the question. They also invoked the example of pack-animals who, when they suffer from a similar disease and are bled by ignorant folk, can never or only rarely escape death. I listened to these things, and because I was afraid of what I heard, I postponed bloodletting for almost four months. But when the catarrh did not depart in the manner or at the time that was usual and I began to be dominated by a superabundance of blood or of *phlegm (which I have more of than of any other *humor), I feared that I would come down with some kind of fever. But I did not wish to put off the bloodletting, choosing rather to lose the use of my voice for a time than to incur the loss of my health. So I underwent bloodletting; and because I had put it off longer than usual, it was done twice within three weeks and in very large quantity, and what my prophets predicted came to pass. The catarrh did not recede, nor was my voice able to return to its previous state for three months. Up to that time, [my] nature suffered under these things; and I felt those organs that are adjacent within the chest itself get worse because of I know not what humor, though I suspect it was phlegm. I brought up phlegm from my mouth in large quantities and often I was not able to relieve nature fully. The people whom I mentioned above say, as do the doctors, that [my] nature is suffering these things because in the aforementioned bloodletting, the heat of the blood was drawn off along with the blood itself, and so what was left behind was not able to expel the coldness of the already *corrupted phlegm. The bitter phlegm remained in the places where it was established, and spread through the veins or other vital channels to press down upon the chest, cause pain to the stomach, and block the normally free passage for the voice. But this judgment I leave to you. To counteract this symptom they advised me to use warm and moist things. Although I have obeyed them, they do not deny that the disease has grown greater because of the cold and moist quality. And so they are not satisfied with the consumption of warm and dry things (which is quite reasonable) in order that the medicine might *purge the disease not only in one quality but in both. Nor have they been fully consistent in the opinion they have expressed to me; for they say that the pharynx, the trachea, and other terms which I do not know should be soothed with moist things, not irritated with dry things, at least as far as diet is concerned. As for the rest of the medicine, they said that vitriol can be beneficial, and hyssop, cumin, liquorice, figs – some or all of these with cooked wine, and given as a *potion at bedtime. I tried it often, but all in vain. Again they swore that electuaries would be able to provide some remedy – the ones called *diadragantium*, *diabutyrum*, or preserved ginger. I have not tried these to see whether they would help or hinder. There was much and varied discussion and debate about what to do next among those who then came to help the doctors. And although what they said sometimes seemed not completely reasonable to me, I yielded to them and for almost three months, as I said above, I have used the diet and medicine that they wanted. Up to this point, I see little or no improvement.

You remain, my dearest friend, my last resort; nor is there anyone else who can advise me, because as I have heard from so many about you and as I myself came to know directly from you in our intimate conversations last year, if I cannot have advice from you in these or similar matters, it would be futile for me to seek out another in our France. I would have preferred to tell you these things in person rather than to write them down to be read by your eyes, because although much can be conveyed to your understanding even when you are absent, it would perhaps be more effective if you were present. But because it would not be easy for me to journey to you or you to me, I ask in the meantime that whatever is permitted be done, at least as far as a friend can learn directly from the knowledge of his friend what friendship expects of him. And because it seemed inappropriate to summon you to me right now on this matter, I ask – indeed I call upon you as friend to friend – that you send to me quickly, for it is urgent, our countryman and well-beloved Bernard, your student, in whose reliability and good judgment your prudence confides (or so I hear), armed with your orders and with the medicines required against this plague, so that through him you may carry out effectively what I suppose cannot be done by you in person. Give him instructions as well as to whether I may or should undergo bloodletting in the usual way or put off bloodletting until I have taken the medicine you advise. I have already postponed it from the first of November to the Octave of Epiphany, when I write these things; nor would I give orders to repeat it without your advice. Hence, before postponement or reiteration produces anything worse, command which of the two it would be best to do. And lest you wonder that I am worried not only about recovering my health but also about recovering my voice, you should know that with my health preserved I am capable of remaining silent, by the grace of God, without much trouble, did my office not oblige me [to speak]. For what disadvantage would there be, as far as the salvation of the soul is concerned, if lacking tongue or voice I am not audible by men, but can be heard all the more by God? But because no small amount, indeed, a very large amount of my office consists in my tongue and voice, I cannot fulfill my office if the use of my voice is gone. My voice is necessary not only for reading, chanting, celebrating the heavenly liturgy – which I share with many under my authority – but particularly for preaching the word of God, since it is said to me by God through the prophet, "Cry out, spare not, lift up your voice like a trumpet." [Isa. 58:1] How then can I cry without a voice? To put it plainly and concisely, the use of the voice is necessary to me as to any ruler of the Church of God, for either [rulers] are idle, and hence like "dumb dogs that cannot bark" [Isa. 16:10] or if they are not lazy, they use the voice of John the Baptist: I am "a voice crying in the wilderness." [Isa. 40:3; Matt. 3:1; Mark 1:3]

b. Reply of Master Bartholomaeus

To his venerable lord Peter, by divine dispensation abbot of Cluny: his Bartholomaeus, such as he is, [sends greeting].

Having read the letter from your sublimity, I was grieved to learn that such a great man of the Church, and one so very necessary to her, was violently afflicted by bodily ailments. For I recall the experience of your humility and charity. When I came to Cluny last year, your affection received me, who deserved nothing from you, and even let me share your fraternal company, and in the end sent me home with gifts. Therefore desiring to be worthy of the affection that I have received from you, not by offering words but by performing deeds, I have dropped all other business to acquiesce to your petition. To this end I have not hesitated to send to your sublimity Bernard, our friend and associate – and if I may put it this way, the instrument of our operation – armed against those necessities which I have learned about from your letter. Indeed I myself, when it pleases your discretion and desire, will not refuse to come to you as to my father and lord. Meanwhile, let your discretion consider in advance that I have committed to the aforementioned Bernard oversight of my whole household, my assistants, and the sick [in my care]. For this reason, his absence will entail deprivation of many kinds for me, particularly if it takes more than a month for him to go and come back.

Concerning those things which pertain to your treatment, you may have this. In my view, bloodletting should be postponed until your voice begins to return to its full functioning, unless perhaps – and may this not be the case – necessity supervenes. For your nature is aggravated more by an excess of phlegm than an excess of blood, as I learned from clear indications when I stayed with you for few days last year. It is my opinion that *cautery should be performed for your headache; do not be afraid that it will damage your sight. Furthermore, your doctors were persuaded that you should use moist substances to soften the respiratory channels, and it seemed more beneficial to your discretion to use dry medications against the moist morbid matter. I reply that there is no contradiction here, though there might seem to be. For the same medication can be *actually* moist and *potentially* dry; to speak more plainly, the same thing will dry out and purge the morbid matter and at the same time moisten and soften. This is confirmed by authority: for example, according to the *Book of *Degrees [ascribed to Constantine the African's On Grades]* myrrh is considered dry and hence dries out putrid humors, but nonetheless it is said to smooth the rough channels of the lungs and also the eyelids. It does this from its glutinous and gummy quality. Those medications that dry by purging humor and also soften by moistening the trachea will be conducive to your health, by the grace of God. Furthermore, I have discussed with Bernard concerning baths and steam-baths, *fumigations and *fomentations about the chest, and concerning pills that should be held under the tongue, pills for catarrh, a balsamic potion, gargles and the like. If he gives satisfaction to your reverence and goodness, please do not delay to send word back to us with all speed. If I learn from his account anything concerning your condition which ought to be done differently, I shall undertake diligent treatment.

Farewell, and may you find relief from the mercy of God and from the medications provided by us.

83. CUSTOMIZED THERAPEUTICS: THE MEDIEVAL MEDICAL *CONSILIUM* (2): GENTILE OF FOLIGNO

Gentile of Foligno's career has already been sketched in the introduction to doc. 43. The text below looks rather different from Bartholomaeus of Salerno's letter of advice, because by Gentile's day the consilium *had become a formal genre of scholastic medical writing, laid out according to prescribed conventions. The scholastic* consilium, *even when it was a response to a letter, addressed the patient in the third person. It began with a presentation of the patient and description of his or her symptoms, followed by a diagnosis, prognosis, and a point-by-point program of management, comprising regimen and recipes for medications. In both the* consilia *presented here, the inquiry seems to have been a "referral" from a professional colleague.*

Source: trans. Faith Wallis and Michael R. McVaugh from a transcription of the *consilia* of Gentile of Foligno in Munich, Bayerische Staatsbibliothek MS CLM 77, fols. 18ra–vb, prepared by Michael R. McVaugh. Latin.

Spitting of Blood

Master Angelo of Arezzo writes to Master Gentile of Foligno asking his advice about a certain young man, aged 24, who suffers from spitting up of blood along with other attendant symptoms contained in this account. The young man Angelino de Patiis is frequently troubled by spitting up of a large quantity of frothy blood, with severe cough and raging thirst; [he has] an intermittent *fever which begins with a chill in the evening, and severe pain in the legs, and slight pain in the stomach. Sometimes he vomits, although not much; there is slight pain in the liver and hot *catarrh. It is said that this harmful condition was caused by the weight upon his chest of the burden of his household. May it please your discretion to find effective remedies and to send them back by letter so that we may put them to good use and (with God's honor and yours) reach a satisfactory outcome.

Master Gentile answered with the following remedies. The case is bad and probably fatal. Everything, however, should proceed as follows.

First, with the rectification of his regimen, all flesh should be eliminated at supper and in its place he should take barley *ptisane or barley flour. And in the morning let him eat the commendable meat of partridge or chicken or other things such as will seem [good] to the present master [Angelo] and let other aspects of the regimen be arranged as he judges best.

Secondly, one must plan to divert [the morbific matter] by means of vigorous rubbing before meals, morning and evening, moving downward towards the feet and hands morning and evening and also at any other time, so that the force of the flow will turn back toward these [members]; for this purpose, and [also] to stop the catarrh, let the coronal suture be cauterized, and let it be kept open and discharging *sanies.

Thirdly, one must plan to constrict the flow, be it in the lung or in the chest, and to strengthen the lung lest it take on [morbific] matter and to cleanse it (if any matter is in the vicinity of the ulcer or adjacent parts) of *corrupt or congealed blood retained [therein] or in other members, which the spitting of blood signifies and judgment confirms.... And at the top of one's priorities should be to plan to stop the widening of the ulcer and to plan to make flesh and a scar. So let the following syrup be made: take distilled water, [and] arnoglossa ... And take some of this in the morning, at noon, and at night, the same amount each time, swallowing a little bit. Should any difficulty in breathing manifest itself, let him take a syrup made from a *decoction of liquorice and raisins....

Fourthly, one must plan to reduce the attendant symptoms: the *fever, with what will be seen to be in harmony with the regimen, as I have corrected it; the severe cough, with plain syrup of pepper administered sometimes at bedtime, and rarely, and being on the alert for fresh spitting. The liver should be treated with a poultice of sandalwood, if his urine indicates this; the stomach, with oil of mastic and nard and wormwood, and rose oil; the pain in the legs, with a lotion of water from the decoction of field camomile. And indeed lesser *corrigiola* [*a kind of grass*] is very strengthening....

Melancholy. A *Consilium* of Master Gentile of Foligno for a Man from Arezzo

My dearest friends: the long duration of this disease and its strong resistance to the excellent remedies, along with the other things that I was able to add on (*consuperare*), show that the cause of his headache is matter tending towards natural *melancholy, which is fixed in the upper membranes of the brain in the veins. There the matter is retained in an evil manner because of the way [the veins] are bent, which is different with respect to the arteries from any other part of the body. So now their walls and the substance of the membranes have crushed the aforementioned matter together and the injury is communicated to the marrow of the brain so that it receives every evaporation, and is damaged by the bad ones. Therefore one should regard such a very persistent illness with misgivings, and [pay heed] particularly to good regimen, lest this matter burst out upon the *spirits or the marrow [of the brain] and cause the patient to suffer the symptoms of melancholy – a great distortion of the imagination, for example – or other diseases. Should it travel to other parts, it could lead to epilepsy or spasm or all manner of bad symptoms that originate in the brain, just as we sometimes see in a rotten egg. This should be no cause for surprise, because in melancholic diseases perverse eruptions or violent alarms sometimes happen. And this condition is not resolved by the presence of raw *phlegmatic *humors. Hence my plan is to gently and slowly *evacuate those humors and to correct them with subtle warming and good moistening. And I plan to strengthen his brain, to prevent it from receiving humoral matter or *vapors.

He should be governed by the following regimen. As much as possible, he must avoid extreme [conditions] of the air. He may eat the meat of chickens, hens, capons, partridges, nestlings from the towers complete with their feathers, tiny birds, a castrated and sometimes a lactating [animal], and sometimes soft eggs, cooked almond milk and chopped vegetables like spinach, orach, a tray of borage, parsley and sometimes lettuce of the cooler kind, and occasionally rock fish, roasted or boiled, and sprinkled with a spice powder I shall describe later. Afterwards [he should] eat emmer, well cooked and soft; sometimes turnips, and sometimes cabbage broth with the aforementioned juicy meats, and sometimes broth made from eggs. When the weather is cold, he can occasionally have mustard made with boiled-down new wine, and sometimes a savory made from almonds and marjoram and spices, thinned with weak vinegar or chicken broth or pomegranate juice.

After the meal, he may eat cooked pears or quinces. Let him eat bread that is not very white, and let it be well baked. He should drink wines of the middling sort, refined, and watered down in the approved manner; they should be more dilute in winter. He should avoid any kind of beans, dried meats, flesh of aquatic birds and game – except sometimes the flesh of a young goat, and occasionally the brain of a hare, and once in a while young wild boar: he can have these. He should avoid cheese, especially dry cheese, all sharp foods, vinegar and vinegary foods, except when his appetite needs stimulating. He should avoid raw vegetables except for lettuce, as specified above. He should avoid plums, high-bush mulberries, cucumbers, melons, gourds, serviceberries and medlars, but he can have before meals ripe figs, grapes that have been hung [to dry], and raisins, morning and night. He should exercise as much as he can; but if he is not able [to exercise], at least his thighs, shins and arms should be rubbed in a downward direction. He should not fill himself up with a variety of foods and drinks in single meal or eat until he is stuffed; and he should water down the wine he is going to drink at least one hour before dinner. He should sleep in accordance with his habit and if possible he should observe the standard laid down in the writings of the authorities. In particular, he should not go to sleep right after a meal. When he awakes, let him take care to eliminate all wastes, notably by shaving and blowing his nose. And if his sleep is especially heavy and deep, let him be shaken awake (rubbing will be helpful). Above all he should take particular care not to be alone or to brood about himself, but he should live as free from anxiety as possible and not be anxious about anything concerning his conduct of daily life or other things that happen to him. And therefore he should seek out pleasant company as much as possible and avoid wordy quarrels. In sum, he should apply himself to diverting his mind and so it would do him good to travel. He should avoid sex.

In this present month of November, he should take this syrup: take 2 pounds each of distilled water of melissa and distilled water of bugloss; one half-pound of water distilled from borage; grind into them 1 dram of crocus and add in 6 ounces of senna, 2 drams each of cinnamon flowers, cinnamon and mastic, and let it stand for a day and a night. Then boil away one-quarter of the volume, strain it and make it into a syrup with 1 ½ pounds of sugar. He should take this syrup for ten days, taking up to 2 ounces every morning with hot water, and then he should stop for a few days, particularly if he finds it repugnant, and then go back to the syrup and continue for a whole month. Let the following pills be made and let him take two with the syrup, fifteen times. Take one dram each of turpeth, epithymum, senna, and lapis lazuli which has been artificially liquefied; one scruple each of Arabian lavender, ginger and *diagridium* [*a compound medicine*]; 2 drams of *hierapigra; mix them with fennel juice and coat them with gold leaf. And when he has taken the aforementioned syrup for another fifteen days, let him take another dram of the pills, unless a violent chill has come upon him. If he finds the pills distasteful, dissolve the quantity specified above in warm water and let him drink it first thing in the morning; and if he wants it to be sweetened, dissolve sugar-water in it. From the month of December to the month of April he should stay away from [laxative] medicines.... He can have the *clyster he is used to from time to time, but always with a increasing interval between one clyster and the next....

The following is the powder he can use on his foods: take one dram each of cinnamon, cloves, cardamom, white pepper and ginger, and ½ dram of crocus, and make a powder. But because *cautery does not seem to produce any evident effect, either because the humors are so firmly fixed in the members or because of the particular arrangement of the cranial sutures (which are unknown) or because [the sutures] are very tight, I would advise washing the head once a week with mild soap in which Arabian lavender has been boiled.

84. THE SPECIAL CHALLENGES OF PLAGUE (1): THE REPORT OF THE PARIS MEDICAL FACULTY, OCTOBER 1348

In 1348, the Black Death rolled over France like a tidal wave. Doctors were baffled by the plague: no disease like it was recorded in the ancient or Arabic medical literature, and its universal scope defied Galenic logic. Everyone knew that disease could be generated from the interaction of the *naturals and the *non-naturals, but even the most generic of non-naturals, like air or food, were normally circumscribed by region or season. How could one explain the fact that so many people all over the known world were falling ill and dying at the same time?

Physicians who witnessed the first wave of the plague were frank about their in-ability to save lives, but confident that they could answer these difficult questions and so furnish some reassurance and resources for future planning. King Philip VI commissioned the Faculty of Medicine of Paris to draw up a report on the plague and make recommendations. The resulting document was in two parts: one on the causes of the plague, the other on remedies and prophylactic regimen. Part one is reproduced below.

The Report reflects the anguish and dismay of contemporaries, and yet it remains a recognizably scholastic production. It is, in fact, structured like a consilium, *with a diagnosis and a management plan. But because it is a diagnosis of a collective – indeed, pandemic – disease, it also draws on medical astrology to explain the relationship between the cosmos and health events on earth (see chapter 8). Above all, the Report illustrates the value to medieval people, even at a time of extraordinary emergency, of scholastic medicine's most characteristic product: rational explanations of cause and effect. The opening words, written in the midst of such horror, are a touching declaration of faith in the human mind to comprehend and thus master even global catastrophe.*

Source: trans. Rosemary Horrox, *The Black Death*, Manchester Medieval Sources Series (Manchester and New York: Manchester University Press, 1994), no. 56, pp. 158–63. Latin.

Seeing things that cannot be explained, even by the most gifted intellects, initially stirs the human mind to amazement; but after marveling, the prudent soul next yields to its desire for understanding and, anxious for its own perfection, strives with all its might to discover the causes of the amazing events. For there is within the human mind an innate desire to seize on goodness and truth. As the Philosopher [Aristotle] makes plain, all things seek for the good and want to understand. To attain this end we have listened to the opinions of many modern experts in astrology and medicine about the causes of the epidemic that has prevailed since 1345. However, since their conclusions still leave room for considerable uncertainty, we, the masters of the Faculty of Medicine at Paris, inspired by the command of the most illustrious prince, our most serene lord, Philip, king of France, and by our desire to achieve something of public benefit, have decided to compile, with God's help, a brief compendium of the distant and immediate causes of the present universal epidemic (as far as these can be understood by the human intellect) and of wholesome remedies; drawing on the opinions of the most brilliant ancient philosophers and modern experts, astronomers as well as doctors of medicine. And if we cannot explain everything as we would wish, for a sure explanation and perfect understanding of these matters is not always to be had (as Pliny says in book 2, chapter 39 [of the *Natural History*]: "some accidental causes of storms are still uncertain, or cannot be explained"), it is open to any diligent reader to make good the deficiency.

We shall divide the work into two parts, in the first of which we shall investigate the causes of this pestilence and whence they come, for without knowledge of the causes no one can prescribe cures. In the second part we shall include methods of prevention and cure. There will be three chapters in the first part, for this epidemic arises from a double cause. One cause is distant and from above, and pertains to the heavens; the other is near and from below and pertains to the earth, and is dependent, causally and effectively, on the first cause. Therefore the first chapter will deal with the first cause, the second with the second cause, and the third with the prognostications and signs associated with both of them. There will be two treatises in the second part. The first will deal with medical means of prevention and cure and will be divided into four chapters: the first on the disposition of the air and its rectification; the second on exercise and baths; the third on food and drink; the fourth on sleeping and waking, emptiness and fullness of the stomach, and on the emotions. The second treatise will have three chapters: the first on universal remedies; the second on specific remedies appropriate to different patients; the third on antidotes.

Chapter 1 of the First Part.
Concerning the Universal and Distant Cause

We say that the distant and first cause of this pestilence was and is the configuration of the heavens. In 1345, at one hour after noon on 20 March, there was a major conjunction of three planets in Aquarius. This conjunction, along with other earlier conjunctions and eclipses, by causing a deadly *corruption of the air around us, signifies mortality and famine – and also other things about which we will not speak here because they are not relevant. Aristotle testifies that this is the case in his [*pseudonymous*] book *Concerning the Causes of the Properties of the Elements*, in which he says that mortality of races and depopulation of kingdoms occur at the conjunction of Saturn and Jupiter, for great events then arise, their nature depending on the trigon [*that is, the set of three signs of the zodiac which are "in trine"*] in which the conjunction occurs. And this is found in ancient philosophers, and Albertus Magnus in his book, *Concerning the Causes of the Properties of the Elements* (treatise 2, chapter 1) says that the conjunction of Mars and Jupiter causes a great pestilence in the air, especially when they come together in a hot, wet sign, as was the case in 1345. For Jupiter, being hot and wet, draws up evil vapors from the earth and Mars, because it is immoderately hot and dry, then ignites the vapors, and as a result there were lightnings, sparks, noxious vapors, and fires throughout the air.

These effects were intensified because Mars – a malevolent planet, breeding anger and wars – was in the sign of Leo from 6 October 1347 until the end of May this year, along with the head of the dragon [*the highest point of the Moon's apparently undulating path around the ecliptic*], and because all these things are hot they attracted many vapors; which is why the winter was not as cold as it should have been. And Mars was also retrograde and therefore attracted many vapors from the earth and the sea which, when mixed with the air, corrupted its substance. Mars was also looking upon Jupiter with a hostile aspect, that is to say, quartile [*at 90 degrees of arc with respect to the zodiacal circle*], and that caused an evil disposition or quality in the air, harmful and hateful to our nature. This state of affairs generated strong winds (for according to Albertus in the first book of his *Meteora*, Jupiter has the property of raising powerful winds, particularly from the south) which give rise to excess heat and moisture on the earth; although in fact it was the dampness which was most marked in our part of the world. And this is enough about the distant or universal cause for the moment.

Chapter 2 of the First Part.
Concerning the Particular and Near Cause

Although major pestilential diseases can be caused by the corruption of water or food, as happens at times of famine and infertility, yet we still regard illnesses proceeding from the corruption of the air as much more dangerous. This is because bad air is more noxious than food or drink in that it can penetrate quickly to the heart and lungs to do its damage. We believe that the present epidemic or plague has arisen from air corrupt in its substance, and not changed in its attributes. By which we wish it to be understood that air, being pure and clear by nature, can only become *putrid or corrupt by being mixed with something else, that is to say, with evil vapors. What happened was that the many vapors which had been corrupted at the time of the conjunction were drawn up from the earth and water, and were then mixed with the air and spread abroad by frequent gusts of wind in the wild southerly gales, and because of these alien vapors which they carried the winds corrupted the air in its substance, and are still doing so. And this corrupted air, when breathed in, necessarily penetrates to the heart and corrupts the substance of the spirit there and rots the surrounding moisture, and the heat thus caused destroys the life force, and this is the immediate cause of the present epidemic.

And moreover these winds, which have become so common here, have carried among us (and may perhaps continue to do so in the future) bad, rotten and poisonous vapors from elsewhere: from swamps, lakes and chasms, for instance, and also (which is even more dangerous) from unburied or unburnt corpses – which might well have been a cause of the epidemic. Another possible cause of corruption, which needs to be borne in mind, is the escape of the rottenness trapped in the center of the earth as a result of earthquakes – something which has indeed recently occurred. But the conjunctions could have been the universal and distant cause of all these harmful things, by which air and water have been corrupted.

Chapter 3.
Concerning Prognostication and Signs

Unseasonable weather is a particular cause of illness. For the ancients, notably Hippocrates, are agreed that if the four seasons run awry, and do not keep their proper course, then plagues and mortal passions are engendered that year. Experience tells us that for some time the seasons have not succeeded each other in the proper way. Last winter was not as cold as it should have been, with a great deal of rain; the spring windy and latterly wet. Summer was late, not as hot as it should have been, and extremely wet – the weather very changeable from day to day and hour to hour; the air often troubled, and then still again, looking as if it was going to rain but then not doing so. Autumn too was very rainy and misty. It is because the whole year here – or most of it – was warm and wet that the air is pestilential. For it is a sign of pestilence for the air to be warm and wet at unseasonable times.

Wherefore we may fear a future pestilence here, which is particularly from the root beneath [that is, the terrestrial causes], because it is subject to the evil impress of the heavens, especially since that conjunction was in a western sign. Therefore if next winter is very rainy and less cold than it ought to be, we should expect an epidemic round about late winter and spring – and if it occurs it will be long and dangerous, for usually unseasonable weather is of only brief duration, but when it lasts over many seasons, as has obviously been the case here, it stands to reason that its effects will be longer-lasting and more dangerous, unless ensuing seasons change their nature in the opposite way. Thus if the winter in the north turns out to be cold and dry, the plagues might be arrested.

We have not said that the future pestilence will be exceptionally dangerous, for we do not wish to give the impression that it will be as dangerous here as in southern or eastern regions. For the conjunctions and the other causes discussed above had a more immediate impact on those regions than on ours. However, in the judgment of astrologers (who follow Ptolemy on this) plagues are likely, although not inevitable, because so many exhalations and inflammations have been observed, such as a comet and shooting stars. Also the sky has looked yellow and the air reddish because of the burnt vapors. There has also been much lightning and flashes and frequent thunder, and winds of such violence and strength that they have carried dust storms from the south. These things, and in particular the powerful earthquakes, have done universal harm and left a trail of corruption. There have been masses of dead fish, animals and other things along the sea shore, and in many places trees covered with dust, and some people claim to have seen a multitude of frogs and reptiles generated from the corrupt matter; and all these things seem to have come from the great corruption of the air and earth. All these things have been noted before as signs of plague by numerous wise men who are still remembered with respect and who experienced them themselves.

No wonder, therefore, that we fear we are in for an epidemic. But it should be noted that in saying this we do not intend to exclude the possibility of illnesses arising from the character of the present year – for as the aphorism of Hippocrates has it: a year of many fogs and damps is a year of many illnesses. On the other hand, the susceptibility of the body of the patient is the most immediate cause in the breeding of diseases, and therefore no cause is likely to have an effect unless the patient is susceptible to its effects. We must therefore emphasize that although, because everyone has to breathe, everyone will be at risk from the corrupted air, not everyone will be made ill by it but only those, who will no doubt be numerous, who have a susceptibility to it; and very few indeed of those who do succumb will escape.

The bodies most likely to take the stamp of this pestilence are those which are hot and moist, for they are the most susceptible to putrefaction. The following are also more at risk: bodies bunged up with evil *humors, because the unconsumed waste matter is not being expelled as it should; those following a bad life style, with too much exercise, sex and bathing; the thin and weak, and persistent worriers; babies, women and young people; and corpulent people with a ruddy complexion. However those with dry bodies, *purged of waste matter, who adopt a sensible and suitable regimen, will succumb to the pestilence more slowly.

We must not overlook the fact that any pestilence proceeds from the divine will, and our advice can therefore only be to return humbly to God. But this does not mean forsaking doctors. For the Most High created earthly medicine, and although God alone cures the sick, he does so through the medicine which in his generosity he has provided. Blessed be the glorious and high God, who does not refuse his help, but has clearly set out a way of being cured for those who fear him. And this is enough of the third chapter and of the whole first part.

85. THE SPECIAL CHALLENGES OF PLAGUE (2): GUY OF CHAULIAC ON THE BLACK DEATH

The Inventarium *or* Great Surgery *of Guy of Chauliac (see doc. 60) also included a first-hand account of the Black Death and of the controversy surrounding its cause and cure. Mainstream medical opinion considered plague to be an outbreak of "pestilential fever" caused by poisoned air, which entered the body and attacked the heart or lungs, causing overheating. But this theory did not entirely account for either the* *apostemes or swellings ("buboes"). Debate ensued between those who identified plague with pestilential fevers, and those who classed it with the apostemic diseases, treating the* *fever as an ancillary symptom. Guy of Chauliac sided with the "aposteme group." Later medieval writers tried to go beyond this dichotomy by creating a broader category of pestilential disease encompassing both fever and morbid swellings. In attempting to negotiate the old categories in order to make sense of their own experience, these doctors acknowledged – some reluctantly, others proudly – that the "moderns" were expanding medicine into frontiers unknown to the ancient authorities.*

Source: trans. Michael R. McVaugh from Guy de Chauliac, *Ars chirurgicalis Guidonis Cauliaci medici* (Venice, 1546), in *Sourcebook in Medieval Science*, ed. Edward Grant (Cambridge, MA: Harvard University Press, 1974), pp. 773–74 (no. 107). Latin.

Internal apostemes, especially those near the principal members [that is, the liver, heart and brain], are dangerous. We saw this clearly in the great and unprecedented mortality that appeared to us in Avignon in the year of our Lord 1348, in the sixth year of the pontificate of Pope Clement VI, in whose service, by his favor, I unworthily then was. Let it not displease you if I tell of it, since it was so remarkable, and as a guide in case it comes again. The mortality began with us in the month of January and lasted for seven months. It was of two kinds. The first lasted for two months; it was characterized by a continuous fever and a spitting of blood, and men died of it within three days. The second lasted for the rest of the time; it too was characterized by continuous fever and by apostemes and *carbuncles and tumors in the external parts, mainly the armpits and groin; and men died of it within five days. It was so contagious (especially that which involved spitting of blood) that one man caught it from another not just when living nearby but simply by looking at him; so much so that people died without servants and were buried without priests. Father would not visit son, nor son, father; charity was dead, and hope prostrate.

I call it great because it engaged all the world, or nearly. For it began in the east, and shooting out into the world, passed through our region toward the west. It was so extensive that it left scarcely the fourth part of the population alive. And it was unprecedented, since, though we read in the *Epidemics* [of Hippocrates] of the mortality in the city of Thrace, and in Palestine, and of another which occurred in Hippocrates's time, and (in the *Euchymia*) of that which afflicted the Romans' subjects in Galen's time, and of that of the city of Rome in the days of [Pope] Gregory [I], none of these was as great as this one. For they affected only one area; this one, the whole world; they were curable in one fashion or another; this one, in none. Because of this physicians felt useless and ashamed, inasmuch as they did not dare visit the sick for fear of *infection; and when they did visit them they could do very little and accomplished nothing, for all the sick died except for a few towards the end, who escaped with matured buboes.

Many have speculated on the cause of this great mortality. In some places they believed the Jews had poisoned the world, and so they killed them. In others, they believed it was the mutilated poor, and so they drove them away. And in still others, that it was the nobles, so that they feared to travel in the world. Finally it came to the point that a watch was kept in cities and towns, forbidding entry to anyone who was not well known. And if they found anyone with powders or ointments, they made him swallow them, fearing that they might be poisons.

But whatever the people said, the truth is that the cause of this mortality was twofold: one active and universal, one passive and particular. The active, universal cause was the disposition of a certain important conjunction of three heavenly bodies, Saturn, Jupiter, and Mars, which had taken place in 1345, the 24th day of March, in the fourteenth degree of Aquarius. For (as I have said in my book on astrology) the more important conjunctions presage marvelous, mighty, and terrible events, such as changes of rulers, the advent of prophets, and great mortalities; and they depend on the [zodiacal] sign and the aspects of the bodies in conjunction. It should not amaze you, therefore, that such an important conjunction signified a marvelous, awful mortality, for it was not just one of the greater ones but one of the greatest. Because the [zodiacal] sign was a human one [*Aquarius is represented as a young man pouring water from a jar*], it foretold grief for humanity; and because it was a fixed sign, it signified long duration. For [the mortality] began in the east, a little after the conjunction, and it was still abroad in the west in [13]50. It so informed the air and the other elements that, as the magnet moves iron, it moved the thick, heated poisonous *humors; and bringing them together within the body, created apostemes there. From this derived the continuous fevers and spitting of blood at the outset, when this *corrupt matter was strong and disturbed in the natural state. Then, as this lost its strength, the natural state was not so troubled, and expelled what it could, mainly in the armpits and groin, and so caused buboes and other apostemes, so that these external apostemes were the effects of internal ones. The particular, passive cause was the disposition of each body, such as cachochymia [bad *digestion], debility, or obstruction, whence it was that the working men or those living poorly died.

Men looked for a preventative treatment before the attack and for a curative one thereafter. For prevention nothing was better than to flee the area before becoming infected; and to *purge oneself with pills, to diminish the blood by *phlebotomy, to purify the air with fire, and to strengthen the heart with *theriac, fruits, and good-smelling things; to fortify the humors with *Armenian [bole], and to resist decay with sharp[-tasting] things. For a cure men tried bleedings and *evacuations, electuaries and cordial syrups. The external apostemes were brought to a head with figs and cooked onions mixed with yeast and butter; then they were opened and treated as ulcers. The tumors were *cupped, *scarified, and *cauterized.

I myself did not dare to leave lest I lose my good name, but in continuous dread kept myself healthy as well I could, using the remedies above. Nevertheless, toward the end of the mortality I fell into a continuous fever, with an aposteme in the groin; I was ill for six weeks, in such great danger that all my friends believed I would die; but the aposteme *ripened, and was treated as I have described, and by God's will I survived.

Afterwards, in [13]60, the eighth year of the pontificate of Pope Innocent VI, the mortality returned to us on its way back from Germany and the northern lands. It began toward the feast of St Michael [29 September], with swellings, fevers, carbuncles, and tumors, growing little by little, sometimes even dying away, until the middle of [13]61. Then it raged for the next three months, so furiously that in several places it left less than half the population. It differed from the earlier one in that more of the populace died in the first, while in the second more of the rich and noble died, innumerable children, and few women.

86. THE SPECIAL CHALLENGES OF PLAGUE (3): JOHN OF BURGUNDY'S *TREATISE ON THE EPIDEMIC*

The Black Death created a new genre of medical literature: the "plague tractate." Like the Paris report (doc. 84), plague tractates were essentially generic consilia that offered scientific explanations of the pestilence and advice for avoiding, or if necessary treating, the disease. Countless plague tractates were composed in the centuries following the first onslaught of 1347–50, but few could rival John of Burgundy's Treatise on the Epidemic *(De epidemia or De pestilentia) in popularity. Apparently composed around 1365 by an otherwise unknown medical practitioner of Liège (in modern Belgium), the* Treatise *survives in more than a hundred manuscripts. The original Latin text was translated into English, French, Dutch, and Hebrew; the author's shadowy identity was hidden under other ascriptions, including that of Medical Faculty of Bologna, and the text was frequently modified by abbreviation or interpolation. As is the case with the medical literature of the Early Middle Ages, the more popular and useful a late medieval plague tractate was, the more vulnerable it was to manipulation and "piracy."*

Source: trans. Rosemary Horrox, *The Black Death*, Manchester Medieval Sources Series (Manchester and New York: Manchester University Press, 1994), pp. 184–93. Latin.

Everything below the moon, the elements and the things compounded of the elements, is ruled by the things above, and the highest bodies are believed to give being, nature, substance, growth, and death to everything below their spheres. It was, therefore, by the influence of the heavenly bodies that the air was recently corrupted and made pestilential. I do not mean by this that the air was corrupted in its substance – because it is an uncompounded substance and that would be impossible – but it is corrupted by reason of evil vapors mixed with it. The result was a widespread epidemic, traces of which still remain in several places. Many people have been killed, especially those stuffed full of evil *humors, for the cause of the mortality is not only the corruption of the air, but the abundance of corrupt *humors within those who die of the disease. For as Galen says in his book on *fevers, the body suffers no corruption unless the material of the body has a tendency toward it, and is in some way subject to the corruptive cause; for just as fire only takes hold on combustible material, so pestilential air does no harm to a body unless it finds a blemish where corruption can take hold. As a result, cleansed bodies, where the *purgation of evil humors has not been neglected, remain healthy. Likewise those whose complexion is contrary to the immutable complexion of air remain healthy. For otherwise everybody would fall ill and die whenever the air is corrupted.

It follows that corrupt air generates different diseases in different people, depending on their different humors, because it always develops according to the predisposition of the matter it has entered. And therefore there are many masters of the art of medicine who are admirable scholars, well-versed in theories and hypotheses, but who are too little experienced in the practicalities and are entirely ignorant of astrology: a science vital to the physician, as Hippocrates testifies in his *Epidemics*, where he says that no one ought to be put under the care of any physician who is ignorant of astrology. For the arts of medicine and astrology balance each other, and in many respects one science supports the other in that one cannot be understood without the other. I am as a result convinced by practical experience that medicine – however well it has been compounded and chosen according to medical rules – does not work as the practitioner intends and is of no benefit to the patient if it is given when the planets are contrary. Thus if medicine is given as a laxative it should be with reference to the planets if the patient is to empty his bowels successfully, and also if he is not to have an adverse reaction to the medicine. Accordingly those who have drunk too little of the nectar of astrology cannot offer a remedy for epidemic diseases. Because if they are ignorant of the cause and quality of the disease they cannot cure it; for as [Galen] the prince of doctors says: "How can you cure, if you are ignorant of the cause?" And Avicenna in *Concerning the Cure of Fevers* emphasizes: "It is impossible that someone ignorant of the cause should cure the disease." Averroes also makes this point, saying: "It is not to be understood, except by grasping the immediate and ultimate cause." Since, therefore, the heavens are the first cause, this is the cause it is necessary to understand, since ignorance of the highest cause entails ignorance of the subsequent cause, and also because the primary cause has a greater impact than the secondary cause.

It is accordingly obvious that [medicine] is of little effect without astrology and as a result of a lack of advice many succumb to disease. And therefore I, John of Burgundy, otherwise known as Bearded John, citizen of Liège and practitioner of the art of medicine, although the least of physicians, produced a treatise at the beginning of this epidemic on the causes and nature of corrupt air, of which many people acquired copies. I also published a treatise on the difference between epidemic and other illness. Anyone who has copies will find many things in these treatises about lifestyles and cures – but not everything about cures. Because the epidemic is now newly returned and will return again in future, because it has not run its course, and because I pity the carnage among mankind and support the common good and desire the health of all, and have been moved by a wish to help, I intend, with God's help, to set out more clearly in this [brief work] the prevention and cure of these illnesses, so that hardly anyone should have to resort to a physician but even simple folk can be their own physician, preserver, ruler and guide.

Concerning Prevention

First, you should avoid over-indulgence in food and drink, and also avoid baths and everything that might rarefy the body and open the pores, for the pores are the doorways through which poisonous air can enter, piercing the heart and corrupting the life force. Above all sexual intercourse should be avoided. You should eat little or no fruit, unless it is sour, and should consume easily-digested food and spiced wine diluted with water. Avoid mead and anything else made with honey and season food with strong vinegar. In cold or rainy weather you should light fires in your chamber and in foggy or windy weather you should inhale aromatics every morning before leaving home: ambergris, musk, rosemary and similar things if you are rich; zedoary, cloves, nutmeg, mace and similar things if you are poor. Also once or twice a week you should take a good dose of *theriac the size of a bean. And carry in the hand a ball of ambergris or other suitable aromatic. Later, on going to bed, shut the windows and burn juniper branches so that the smoke and scent fills the room. Or put four live coals in an earthenware vessel and sprinkle a little of the following powder on them and inhale the smoke through mouth and nostrils before going to sleep: take white frankincense, labdanum, storax, calaminth, and wood of aloes and grind them to a very fine powder. And do this as often as a fetid or bad odor can be detected in the air, and especially if the weather is foggy or the air tainted, and it can protect against the epidemic.

If, however, the epidemic occurs during hot weather, it becomes necessary to adopt another regimen and to eat cold things rather than hot and also to eat more sparingly than in cold weather. You should drink more than you eat and take white wine with water. You should also use large amounts of vinegar and verjuce in preparing food, but be sparing with hot substances such as pepper, [ginger]; or grains of paradise. Before leaving home in the morning smell roses, violets, lilies, white and red sandalwood, musk, or camphor if the weather is misty or the air quality bad. Take theriac sparingly in hot weather and not at all unless you are a *phlegmatic or of a cold *complexion. *Sanguines and *cholerics should not take theriac at all in hot weather, but should take pomegranates, oranges, lemons, or quinces, or an *electuary made of the three types of sandalwood, or a cold electuary or similar. You should use cucumbers, fennel, borage, bugloss, and spinach, and avoid garlic, onions, leeks and anything else that generates excessive heat, such as pepper or grains of paradise, although ginger, cinnamon, saffron, cumin, and other temperate substances can be used. And if you become extremely thirsty because of the hot weather, then drink cold water mixed with vinegar or barley water regularly, for this is particularly beneficial to people of a cold and dry complexion and to thin people, and thirst should never be tolerated at such times.

If you should feel a motion of the blood like a fluttering or prickling, let blood from the nearest vein on the same side of the body; and the floor of the room in which you are lying should be sprinkled two or three times a day with cold water and vinegar or with rose water, if you can afford it. The pills of Rhazes, if taken once a week, are an outstanding preventative and work for all complexions and in all seasons, but Avicenna and others recommend that they should be taken on a full stomach. They loosen the bowels a little, but the corrupt humors are expelled gradually. They should be made as follows: take socotra aloes, saffron, myrrh and blend them in a syrup of fumitory. Anyone who adopts this regimen can be preserved, with God's help, from pestilence caused by corruption of the air.

Concerning the Cure of the Swelling

Now if anyone should contract epidemic disease for lack of a good regimen it is necessary to look at remedies and at how he should proceed, for these epidemic diseases take hold in twenty-four hours and it is therefore vital to apply a remedy immediately. But first it should be understood that there are three principal members in the human body: the heart, the liver, and the brain, and that each of these has its *emunctory, where it expels its waste matter. Thus, the armpits are the emunctories of the heart, the groin for the liver, and under the ears or beneath the tongue for the brain. Now it is necessary to know that it is the nature of poison to descend from the stomach, as is shown by the bite of a serpent or other venomous creature. And thus poisonous air, when it has been mixed with blood, immediately seeks the heart, the seat of nature, to attack it. The heart, sensing the injury, labors to defend itself, driving the poisoned blood to its emunctory. If then the venomous matter finds its way blocked, so that it cannot ascend back to the heart by some other path, it seeks another principal member, the liver, so that it can destroy that. The liver, fighting back, drives the [poisonous] matter to its emunctory. In the same way it lays claim to the brain. By means of these events, which are signs to the physician, it is possible to tell where the poisonous matter is lurking and by what vein it ought to be drained.

For if the *infected blood is driven to the armpits it can be deduced that the heart is oppressed and suffering, and so blood should be let immediately from the cardiac vein, but on the same side of the body, not the opposite side, for that would do double damage: firstly, the good and pure blood on the uncorrupted side would be drained away; secondly, the corrupt and poisoned blood would be thereby drawn to the healthy side of the body, with the result that the blood on both sides would be corrupted. What is worse, in the process the venomous blood would pass through the region of the heart and infect it, and thereby cause the rapid onset of illness. If, however, the patient feels prickings in the region of the liver, blood should be let immediately from the basilic vein of the right arm (that is the vein belonging to the liver, which is immediately below the vein belonging to the heart) or in the cephalic vein of the right hand, which is between the third and little fingers.

If the liver expels matter to the groin and it becomes visible next to the privy member towards the inside of the leg, then a vein should be opened in the foot on the same side of the body, between the big toe and the toe next to it, for if blood was let in the arm it would again draw the matter to the heart, which would be a major error. If the poison manifests itself more toward the flank, and further from the genitals, then open a vein in the foot on the same side of the body between the little toe and the toe next to it, or the vein next to the ankle or heel of that foot, or *scarify the leg next to the tumor with pitch. If the poison appears at the emunctories of the brain, let blood from the cephalic vein above the median vein in the arm on the same side of the body, or from the vein between the thumb and index finger, or scarify the flesh with pitch between the shoulder blades.

When the blood has been extracted in this way and the principal members purged, strengthen them with a cold electuary to offset any febrile cardiac inflammation. Make an electuary thus: take a preparation of roses including the three kinds of sandalwood, cold tragacanth, powder to encourage moistness, add candied rose petals, and make an electuary in pill form, which should be taken several times by day and night. If you are poor, make a distilled water from dittany, pimpernel, tormentil, and scabious by blending the herbs and mixing them with an equal quantity of water, and a spoonful of the mixture should be taken in summer. If the patient is choleric or sanguine, stir a pennyweight of camphor into the water until it is dissolved. If he is weak, six spoonfuls should be taken in twenty-four hours as soon as he feels himself gripped by illness. In illnesses of this kind, this is the very best and surest medicine.

Diet in these illnesses should be as in the case of fevers, since the illness is always accompanied by fever. Therefore no meat should be eaten, except occasionally a small chicken poached in water and verjuce. Patients should eat small scaly fish, grilled on a gridiron with vinegar or verjuce, and soup of almonds, and drink barley water or small ale. If the patient demands wine, he should be given vinegar mixed with plenty of water. Occasionally, however, he can be given, to cheer him up, white wine diluted with plenty of water.

Place this plaster, called Emanuel, on the tumor. Take the root of the greater valerian, ammoniac, the root of dwarf elder, the root of *somerib* [*unidentified herb*], seeds of rue and oil of camomile. They should be bound together with a little wax and a touch of pine resin. And let the plaster be made like an ointment, but not too runny, and let it be renewed two or three times a day. For this ointment draws the venomous matter to itself, coagulates it and *mortifies it, so that the matter is kept from approaching the principal members and harming them. If the tumor remains there for a lifetime, it would do no harm once it had been mortified. But if someone wants the swelling removed entirely let him place on it *ripening and dissolving agents, with which all surgeons are amply provided.

Also anyone who wishes can use this powder, which is a powerful preventative, and is the very best medicine and cure, stronger in this respect than theriac. It is called the imperial powder, because [pagan] emperors used it against epidemic illness, poison, and venom, and against the bite of serpents and other poisonous animals, and in Arabic it is called Bethzaer, which is to say "a freeing from death." Make this powder from these herbs: take St John's wort, dittany, tormentil, pimpernel, scabious, philadelphia, ammoniac, medicinal earth from Lemnos. Concerning this powder, I can say this, that I have proved it a hundred times and that however it was used – whether it is simply rubbed on or drunk in wine – it immediately clears the poison and expels it through the bite. Anybody can protect himself from all poisons and cure himself of snakebite as effectively as emptying the veins of blood. But few apothecaries are aware of these herbs, and nor do our authors make more than a brief mention of them, because they are not expert in such matters. And all the [pagan] physicians agree that however this powder is used, it makes it impossible to die of poison.

Statement of the Times for Blood-letting

Certain lords have sought from me a schedule of what ought to be known to perform bleeding, and whether it should be done immediately or on the first or second day, and they are the people to whom I have addressed these things concerning the onset of illness.

I say that these pestilential illnesses have a short and sudden beginning and a rapid development, and therefore in these illnesses those who wish to work a cure ought not to delay, and bleeding, which is the beginning of the cure, should not be put off until the first or second day. On the contrary, if someone can be found to do it, blood should be taken from the vein going from the seat of the diseased matter (that is, the place where morbidity had appeared) in the very hour in which the patient was seized by illness. And if the bleeding cannot be done within the hour, at least let it be done within six hours, and if that is not possible, then do not let the patient eat or drink until the bleeding is done. But do not by any means delay the bleeding for longer than twelve hours, for if it is done within twelve hours, while the poisonous matter is still moving about the body, it will certainly save the patient. But if it is delayed until the illness is established and then done, it will certainly do no harm but there is no certainty that it will rescue the patient from danger, for by then the bad blood will be so clotted and thickened that it will be scarcely able to flow from the vein. If, after the *phlebotomy, the poisonous matter spreads again, the bleeding should be repeated in the same vein or in another going from the seat of the diseased matter. Afterwards three or five spoonsful of the herbal water, made as above, should be administered.

And if not as much as that is available, let one spoonful be given morning and evening, and one spoonful should always be given after consumption of the electuary described above, whether by day (when it can be given at any hour) or by night. Or let the patient be given this confection, which strengthens the heart, expels harmful flatulence from it and quenches fever. Take conserves of violets, roses, bugloss, borage and oranges, powdered roses and sandalwood, cold tragacanth, an electuary of the three sandalwoods, powder to encourage moistness, a cold electuary, camphor and candied roses, mix them together without applying heat and place them in a box, and if the patient is of a hot complexion or if the fever is intense, add six or seven grains of camphor. If the patient is rich and can afford it, pearls, gold leaf, pure silver, jacinths, emeralds, and the bone from the heart of a stag should be added. In the course of more than twenty-four years of experience in places where the epidemic held sway it has been certainly and frequently demonstrated that such an electuary, together with the prescribed regimen, can save the patient from death. And many people have been cured by one bleeding alone, performed at the right time, without any other medicine. But where people delay bleeding beyond the development of the disease, it is doubtful whether it will lead to a cure or not. For while nature keeps the matter in motion, and the heart by its expulsive *virtue drives out the noisome and infected blood to its emunctory, phlebotomy should be performed because it helps nature, in that the extraction and *evacuation of the blood strengthens the expulsive virtue of the heart and diminishes the quantity of unhealthy matter, whereby nature is made more powerful against what remains and medicine becomes more efficacious.

I have never known anyone treated with this type of bleeding who has not escaped death, provided he has looked after himself well and has received substances to strengthen his heart. As a result I make bold to say – not in criticism of past authorities, but out of long experience in the matter – that modern masters are more experienced in treating pestilential epidemic diseases than all the doctors and medical experts from Hippocrates downward. For none of them saw an epidemic reigning in their time, apart from Hippocrates in the city of Craton, and that was short-lived. Nevertheless, he drew on what he had seen in his book on epidemics. However, Galen, Diocorides, Rhazes, [John] Damascenus, Geber, Mesue, Copho, Constantine, Serapios, Avicenna, Algazel and all their successors never saw a general or long-lasting epidemic, or tested their cures by long experience; although they draw on the sayings of Hippocrates to discuss many things concerning epidemics. As a result, the masters of the present day are more practiced in these diseases than their predecessors, for it is said, and with truth, that experience makes skill. Moved by piety and by pity for the destruction of men, I have accordingly compiled this compendium and have specified and set out the veins to bleed in these epidemic diseases, so that anyone may be his own physician. And because these illness[es] run their course very quickly and the poisonous matter rages through the body, let the bleeding be done without delay according to my advice, for in many cases delay brings danger.

I have composed and compiled this work not for money but for prayers, and so let anyone who has recovered from the disease pray strongly for me to our Lord God, to whom be the praise and glory throughout the whole world for ever and ever, amen.

Here ends the valuable treatise of Master John of Burgundy against epidemic disease.

CHAPTER TWELVE

THE ETHICS OF MEDICAL CARE (1):
CONSCIENCE AND THE LAW

Medical care exemplifies Christian morality. Christ's miracles of healing are not only signs of salvation, but examples of unconditional love or caritas, *the axis on which all Christian ethics turn. Jesus' parable of the Good Samaritan depicts treating wounds and furnishing nursing care as the ideal demonstration of love of one's neighbor. All Christians are enjoined to care for the sick, as well as to feed the hungry, relieve the thirsty, clothe the naked, house the stranger, and visit the imprisoned. To perform these "acts of mercy" on behalf of anyone is to minister to Christ himself (Matt. 25:35–37).*

That being said, medieval Christian physicians had special ethical obligations and confronted unique ethical dangers. Once again, medicine's academic turn in the twelfth century marks a watershed. The early medieval texts presented in this chapter are direct heirs of the classical tradition of advice and precept written by physicians, for physicians. Though reframed in Christian terms, the moral syntax, so to speak, is that of the Hippocratic Oath. The focus is on the character traits of the doctor himself. After the twelfth century, however, the accent falls more on codifying obligations, because practicing medicine was now a matter of legalized privilege. At the same time, the reformed Church undertook to Christianize Europe, not merely by indoctrinating the faithful, but by furnishing every rank and estate within society with customized guidelines for living their lives according to the teaching of the Gospels. This mission culminated in the Fourth Lateran Council of 1215, which obligated Christians to confess their sins at least once a year. In the wake of Lateran IV, both the faithful and their priests had to be trained in a new kind of ethical reflection. For centuries, confession had been compared to the diagnosis of spiritual illness, but now the confessor (not unlike the scholastic doctor) was expected to inquire into particular circumstances, and tailor his therapy to the individual condition of his patient. Manuals for confessors even catalogued "cases of conscience," which take on a special interest when the "patient" is a physician (doc. 89). As the Church struggled to define its position with regard to the new money economy, it also had to rethink the problem of the doctor's fee.

Secular governments also weighed in. Academic medicine claimed that the practice of medicine should belong only to the duly qualified; in the eyes of kings and rulers, that privilege, like any other privilege, should be defined, protected, and supervised by the law. The revival of the study of Roman law, the growth of the managerial machinery of government, and the demand for accountability from below, worked in concert to make public licensing and supervision of medical practitioners increasingly desirable.

87. PROFESSIONAL CHARACTER IN THE EARLY MIDDLE AGES: VARIATIONS ON HIPPOCRATIC THEMES

The original Hippocratic Oath was not a code of professional ethics, but a personal prayer for virtue, good reputation, and sound practice. In late antiquity, however, it was recast as an exhortation to professional morality. The process began in Rome and intensified when Christianity and Islam became the dominant religions in the former empire. The Greek text of the Oath was "Christianized" by the middle Byzantine period at the latest; it was reformulated in Hebrew around 500 and adapted by the ninth century for a Muslim audience. Indeed, the Oath seems to have attracted more consistent attention in the Middle Ages than in antiquity, perhaps because its particular injunctions concerning abortion (for example) were more congenial to Christian, Jewish, and Muslim values than to those of paganism.

One such adaptation – a letter addressed to a certain Nepotian by his father or teacher Arsenius – circulated in Latin manuscripts dating from the late eighth to the eleventh centuries. Nothing is known about Arsenius; he may even be a literary fiction. While the Hippocratic Oath is implicitly present – notably in the injunctions to respect confidentiality – much more space is accorded to positive exhortations to love wisdom, to treat all without regard for pecuniary gain, and to exhibit honesty, humility, patience, and strongmindedness. There is a marked emphasis on the moral duty to be competent, particularly through diligent reading and study. The Letter of Arsenius *also links skill in the art with religious qualities of love and reverence.*

The Art of Medicine *is an early medieval composite text similar to* The Wisdom of the Art of Medicine *(doc. 4). It contains, inter alia, a character-sketch of the ideal medical student, followed by a truncated summary of the Oath. An even closer paraphrase of the Oath – although not identified as such – is found in Constantine the African's translation of 'Ali ibn al' Abbas al Maĝūsi's* Pantegni. *It contains additional elements that seem to have a religious flavor, such as not curing or even teaching for gain, and living a frugal, abstemious life. Once again, the requirement to study diligently, as well as to seek out experience, is a Galenic touch, though it also resonates with Muslim piety.*

a. The *Letter of Arsenius to Nepotian*

Source: trans. Loren MacKinney, "Medical Ethics and Etiquette in the Early Middle Ages: The Persistence of Hippocratic Ideals," *Bulletin of the History of Medicine* 26 (1952): 11–12. Latin.

Arsenius to Nepotian, his sweetest son, greeting…. I shall point out what you earnestly desire to know as to what sort of person a physician ought to be. First, he should test his personality to see that he is of a gracious and innately good character, apt and inclined to learn, sober and modest; a good conversationalist, charming, conscientious, intelligent, vigilant and affable, in all detailed affairs adept and skilful. Humility ever seeks knowledge, ever accumulates, and never goes to excess or offends. Good will restores sweetness, inspires sagacity, maintains remembrances in the heart, love in the soul, discipline in obeying, wisdom imbued with fear and diligence, and respect, for he who loves not honors not and will not be skilful or sure in his work. [The physician should] not be hesitant or timid, turbulent or proud, scornful or lascivious, or garrulous, a publican, or a woman-lover; but rather full of counsel, learned, and chaste. He should not be drunken or lewd, fraudulent, vulgar, criminal or disgraceful; it is not right for a physician to be taken in a fault or blush for shame in the presence of his people. Even as love of wisdom reveals itself in manners, so let him be irreproachable for he is chosen to a higher honor. Medicine is not to be scorned, but invoked. Inasmuch as the physician has high honors he should not have faults, but instead discretion, taciturnity, patience, tranquility, and refinement; not greed but more of restraint and subtilty, rationality, diligence, and dignity. One of the virtues of this art is zeal in the acquisition of wisdom, long sufferance, and mildness. [The physician should strive for] a cheerful pleasant approach; for even as light illuminates a home and makes men see in dark shadows, so a cheerful physician turns sorrow and sadness into joy, and comforts all of the members of his patient, and restores his spirits. According to the secret teachings that should be pursued in medical instruction, let the physician be cheerful because he is the gentle helper [of his patients]....

b. The *Art of Medicine*

Source: trans. Faith Wallis from Rudolf Laux, "Ars medicinae. Ein frühmittelalterliches Kompendium der Medizin," *Kyklos* 3 (1930): 419–20. Latin.

Therefore, before transmitting the Hippocratic Oath it behooves us to describe the student of medicine. First, he should be free-born, noble in his faculties, a youth, moderate in size, strong, capable of anything, sensitive in body and soul, of good counsel, benign, manly, benevolent, chaste, and in particular, diligent of mind, bold without being hot-tempered, not stubborn, quick to grasp and understand what is being taught, trained to speak concisely, pure, endowed with a good memory, and not lazy. First, then, he is to be taught the art of grammar and astronomy and arithmetic and geometry and music. He should abstain from rhetoric so that he does not become loquacious. But philosophy should be taught along with medicine. His hair-cut should be sober and even; he should not wear his hair too long or curled in ringlets, and his beard should be such as is becoming to a young man. He should not be wanting nails on his hand, nor should he allow them to grow over the ends of his fingers. He should dress in white clothes or clothes which are close to white. His dress should be soft and he should walk with an even pace, neither rushing along nor [too] slowly, for gravity signifies great mental endowment. Let him enter the sickroom with steady gait and not in a rush, looking about him and observing silence until he reaches the patient's bed. And let him suffer injuries with patience, for those who are taken with a *melancholic or frenetic passion let fly malign words and actions which it behooves us to ignore. For these men harbor no ill-will, but rather [labor under] natural illnesses and sufferings.

One who is of such a constitution swears the Oath of Hippocrates according to his precept, so that whatever house he goes into, he shall enter without any will to do harm or corrupt. For no fatal medicament should be given, nor should an abortive agent be given under pressure from women, nor should he be party to such a scheme, but he should remain spotless and holy. He should abstain from sexual congress, from serving-maids and freedwomen, from married women and virgins. And he should treat as secret whatever he hears or sees in the course of his treatment which ought not to be revealed.

c. The *Pantegni* Paraphrase of the Hippocratic Oath

Source: trans. Faith Wallis from *Pantegni theorica* 1.1, in *Omnia opera Ysaac* (Lyons, 1515), vol. 2, fol. 1rb. Collated with MS Cambridge Trinity College R.14.34 (906), fol. 1v–2r, where it is chapter 2 of book 1. Latin.

He who wishes to attain the status of a physician ought to reverence his teacher, earn his praise, and obey him just as he would his own parents. For reverence should be displayed to one's parents, because our very existence comes from them. The master should be held in reverence, for he gives shape to what is shapeless and crude. Whoever is accepted by a teacher in order to be instructed should see to it that he is a worthy pupil; and the teacher should teach worthy pupils without a fee, and without expecting any future remuneration. And [the teacher] should make it his business to drive off all who are unworthy of this knowledge. The physician should exert himself to recover the health of the sick, nor should he do this for hope of gain, or give greater consideration to the rich than to the poor, to nobles than non-nobles. He himself should not teach [how to make] a [harmful] *potion, nor be complicit in teaching [such a thing], lest some ignorant person overhear, and on [the teacher's] authority mix a deadly potion. Nor should he teach how to bring about an abortion. When he visits the sick, let his heart not incline to [the patient's] wife, maidservant or daughter, [for women] blind a man's heart. He should keep to himself what he learns about the illness, for sometimes a patient will reveal to his physician things that he would blush to confess to his own parents. Let him flee from lust. Let him avoid worldly delights and drunkenness. These things perturb the mind and encourage the vices of the body and cause God's help to be withdrawn. Let him love to apply himself with zeal to defending the health of the body, and let him not grow weary of diligent reading, so that memory may come to his aid when books are not at hand. He should never disdain to visit the sick, for experience will make him more effective. He should be pure, humble, gentle, amiable, and put his trust in divine assistance.

88. ETHICS OF CARE IN THE EARLY MIDDLE AGES: CHRISTIAN REFLECTIONS

This poem from the Lorsch Leechbook *(doc. 23) presents a picture of the mutual obligations of patient and physician within the framework of Christian justice and charity. It begins by invoking the Christian saints Cosmas and Damian (see doc. 15) along with the medical giants of pagan antiquity, Hippocrates and Galen, as exemplary physicians. Galen and Hippocrates stand for the professional who heals for a fee and who is worthy of his hire. But Cosmas and Damian, who never took money for their services, remind the Christian physician of his obligations toward the unfortunate. The rich patient who can pay can be charged without injustice, but the poor should be treated without remuneration. The poem then moves to a related theme: the dichotomy between expensive imported* materia medica *and locally grown herbs that are just as efficacious, and not as costly. There is an implicit lesson here, namely that God furnishes immediate help for the poor and that the doctor should take advantage of what lies close at hand. One catches echoes of Walahfrid Strabo's encomium of the medical value of European plants (doc. 25) and, in the final line of the poem, of the Hippocratic Oath as well.*

Source: trans. Faith Wallis from *Das 'Lorscher Arzneibuch'. Ein medizinisches Kompendium des 8. Jahrhunderts (Codex Bambergensis medicinalis 1). Text, Übersetzung und Fachglossar*, ed. Ulrich Stoll, Sudhoffs Archiv, Beiheft 28 (Stuttgart: Franz Steiner, 1992), p. 64. Latin.

Cosmas, Damian, Hippocrates, and Galen,
whom Medicine celebrates as masters, famous throughout the world:
the pages of this book single out these men as distinguished.
To the doctor belongs his fee – as long as the patient is ailing,
But the moment he is on his feet again, no bottle of wine is forthcoming
　　[for the doctor].

O patient, give the doctor what you owe, lest worse befall,
or else the doctor may not call again.
O doctor, take heed of the poor man's resources, and those of the rich:
different circumstances require different standards.
If he is rich, this is a righteous opportunity for gain;
if he is poor, be content with a token payment.
The perfumes that Arabia bears or India,
whatever the waves of the ocean convey,
cinnamon, myrrh, leaf [of nard], bright cassia,
balsam, frankincense, calamus, Corycian saffron –
these spices avail great things,
and a house overflowing with immense wealth.
But we take delight in the common meadow herbs,
which lowly plain and lofty mountain bear.
So hail! holy mountains and fields of the West!
for your gifts contribute to many cures.
Here lie and breathe forth fragrant cinnamon and frankincense,
everything that China and Saba bear.
Of all the kinds of unguents, be they never so fine,
none can be sweeter than nard and resin of myrrh;
of all the kinds of unguents, be they never so fragrant,
none can be more delightful than the rose and the violet.
You see the many unguents Greece sends:
but many of us [herbs and flowers] are from the West.
We fill drug-jars with finely powdered spices blended,
and give no poisoned drink.

89. PROFESSIONAL CONDUCT IN THE LATE MIDDLE AGES: FROM CHARACTER TO CODE

Handbooks for confessors were wont to compare scrutinizing a sinner's conscience to a physician probing a wound. This is certainly true of the Summa Theologica *of Antoninus Pierozzi (1389–1459), Dominican friar, archbishop of Florence, and author of one of the most influential guides to moral theology for confessors of the late medieval period. His* Summa *can be likened to a physician's* practica: *it is a reference manual where the confessor could look up the condition and status of the penitent and find a compendium of occupational vices that might require attention. Antoninus grouped doctors with lawyers, merchants, courtiers, and cooks as people whose way of life, though not inherently disreputable, was filled with temptation. In particular, there was some doubt about what the learned doctor actually was being paid for, since he sold a service rather than a product. If he sold his learning and judgment, then the confessor was obliged to look into the matter of his competence.*

Antoninus paid very close attention to one of the principal pieces of ecclesiastical legislation addressed to doctors, namely canon 22 of the Fourth Lateran Council of 1215, "Because bodily infirmity...." This canon obliged physicians who were summoned to a patient's bedside to admonish the patient to confess before receiving treatment. It was copied into most of the important decretal collections of the later Middle Ages, such as the Decretals *of Pope Gregory IX and the* Liber sextus *of Pope Boniface VIII.*

Source: trans. Faith Wallis from Antoninus of Florence, *Summa theologica* (Verona: ex typographia Seminarii, 1740; rept. Graz: Akademische Druck- und Verlagsanstalt, 1959), pp. 281–92. Latin. Antoninus's internal references to decretals and canon law authorities have largely been omitted; these omissions are signaled by ellipses.

Part 3, Title 7, Chapter 2. The Diverse Vices of Physicians and Their Salaries

In the practice of their art, physicians are wont to commit offences in many ways. First, in the bodily care of the sick: here they offend from ignorance, from negligence, and sometimes from malice.

Therefore one must first look into whether the physician is expert in the art, such that he would generally be considered competent by those who are experts in this field. It is not sufficient for him to hold a doctoral degree, because these days many unworthy people are masters and doctors in every field, to their own damnation and also of those who promote them [for the degree]. Subsequently, when they harm their patients through their treatments because of conspicuous ignorance, they always commit a mortal sin.... Nor can they excuse themselves by claiming that they did not intend [to do harm], because they voluntarily put themselves in that position ... and even if the outcome is healing, they are not excused from sin, because they have exposed themselves to the danger of mortal sin by an act that can result in significant harm to one's neighbor.

Secondly, a physician must exercise due diligence, for however great his expertise, if he is conspicuously negligent in consulting his books, in visiting the sick, or in [assuring] the quality of medicinal products, and death results, he has sinned mortally and acted irregularly. And even if the result is a considerable worsening of the illness, and not actual death, he is not excused from mortal [sin]. And therefore ... he should exercise diligence. He is said to do this when he follows the traditions of the art, and when he visits the patient in person, and when he prescribes [the patient's] diet and regimen himself, but he is not bound to keep him under continuous personal observation, as Hostiensis says. And [the doctor] does ill by administering a medication if there is any doubt as to whether it might harm or be of benefit; for according to the dictum of Innocent [III?], in a doubtful situation, one ought rather to leave the patient in the hands of the Creator than to expose him to a medication one does not know about.

Thirdly, a physician should treat the patient as expeditiously as possible. Whence, if he deliberately omits a medication which is suitable and which would bring about a quick cure, so that [the patient] continues to be sick, in order to increase his earnings, then he sins gravely and what he has earned has been by theft. And likewise if in making up a medication he allows the apothecary to put in old spices and other things of this kind, which have no efficacy, to profit [the apothecary], when he can and ought to put in other things, he sins gravely. And if anything detrimental happens to the patient, the blame lies with both of them. In fact, a physician should not confide the compounding of medications to an apothecary, unless he knows him to have a scrupulous conscience and to be well taught and practiced in this kind of thing; rather, he should have [the medication] made up in his presence, and closely observe what goes into it.

Physicians also commit mortal sin if they give any advice or remedy for the health of the body that imperils the soul – for example, [advice] to do something against the divine law, for instance, to know a woman carnally outside matrimony, or to get drunk, or the like…. [I]t is a mortal sin for both the physician and the patient, for it is against the order of charity according to which the health of the soul takes precedence over that of the body…. And a physician who says to the patient, "I do not advise this, but were you to have sex with a woman, you would get better," transgresses this law. For when I sell you something, adding, "I do not wish to be held accountable if it is dangerous and harmful," when I know it is such, I am accountable. The physician should, therefore, beware of what he says, lest in assigning a cause to the disease he incite [the patient] to do something evil.

Again, there are some doctors who, when it comes to themselves and even to other healthy people, have a coarse conscience concerning the Church's fasts; they claim that [fasts] destroy the body, which is most false, because the Church is governed by the light of the grace of the Holy Spirit in its ordinances, and grace does not destroy nature…. Also, they ought not to persuade the sick or weakly to break the fast without cause or reason or to eat meat on days when this is prohibited, because they lay sin to their charge. Nevertheless, in doubtful cases the patient may be excused if he was following his doctor's advice.

Physicians or others commit mortal sin in giving medicine to pregnant women to procure abortion and still-birth in order to conceal sin. But if they do this to preserve the pregnant woman from peril of death during childbirth, then according to Giovanni of Naples ... a distinction should be made concerning the fetus, because either it was animated with a rational soul or it was not yet animated. And if it was animated, the physician commits a mortal sin in giving such a medicine. The reason is because it is the cause of the death of the fetus both corporeally and spiritually. But by not giving a medicine, [the physician] cannot be said to be the cause of death; rather, the illness [will be the cause of death]. For he is not directly the cause, because he did not kill by his action; nor is he indirectly the cause, the way a sailor is said to be indirectly the cause of the sinking of a ship. And although in giving the medicine he might have saved the mother from death, nonetheless he is not held accountable [for her death] if he does not do it, and indeed he ought not to do it, because in giving [the medicine] he would be the cause of the child's death.... But if the fetus is not yet animated with a rational soul, [the doctor] then can and should give such a medicine, because although he will impede the animation of the fetus, nevertheless he will not be the cause of any human being's death. And good will result from this, because he will free the mother from death. Therefore in this case he should give it, but not in the first. If there is any doubt as to whether the fetus is animated with a rational soul or not, it would seem that in giving such a medicine, [the physician] would commit mortal sin, because he exposes himself to the danger of mortal sin, that is, of homicide.... Hence in such a case he ought not to give it.

[A physician] may justly claim a salary or wage for his labor, as is evident from Luke 10[:7]: "A workman is worthy of his hire." ... Doctors are either salaried by the community, in which case they should take nothing from the sick; or they are not salaried, but limited by the law of the community or the lord so that they can only accept so much; or they are neither salaried nor limited. And in the first case, they cannot accept [a fee]; and if their salary is insufficient, the blame lies on him with whom they entered into the agreement. For by a mutual compact they accept the law.... In the second case, they should take no more than what is in the statute, unless this statute is abrogated by a contrary law.... In the third case, they can accept and should exact a moderate salary. What is "moderate" is determined by the quality of the treatment, the labor, diligence and conscientiousness of the physician, the means of the patient, and the custom of the region.

But the question arises: when a contract has been made with the physician for a certain fee payable upon recovery, is [the physician] obliged to treat for the same fee a patient who has recovered and afterwards suffers a relapse? [Legal authorities] draw a distinction between a disease that rapidly recurs, in which case [the physician] is obliged (since it seems that a disease that immediately comes back never actually went away, nor was [the patient] fully freed), and [a disease] that recurs after a space of time, in which case [the physician] is not obligated. Or they say that if the relapse occurs because of the patient's fault, [the physician] is not obligated because such an outcome ought not to be laid to his charge....

Physicians are also obliged to observe the decretal ... which states, "Because bodily infirmity not infrequently is the consequence of sin – the Lord himself saying to the invalid whom he had healed, 'Go and sin no more, lest something worse befall you' – we legislate by the present decree and strictly command the doctors of the body, that when they are summoned by the sick, they shall before anything else warn and persuade them to call for physicians of souls [that is, priests] so that after provision has been made for the health of the patient's soul, the remedy of bodily medicine may be applied to better effect, because when the cause ceases, so does the effect." ... And in the same decretal, this follows: "If anyone transgresses this constitution after it has been proclaimed by the presiding clergy of the region, he shall be barred from entering the church until he has made adequate satisfaction for his transgression." ... And note that some physicians observe this [decree] in dealing with their patients when they see that the sickness is fatal and not otherwise. But these people do not fulfill the decree, as is evident from the text of the decretal itself. It is said there, at the beginning of the paragraph cited above, "The reason for this edict is that some lying in the sickbed, when they are encouraged by the doctors to look to the health of their souls, fall into despair, and hence incur more readily the danger of death." To which Johannes Andreas [*authority on canon law*] says, "Indeed, if patients know that doctors say this in every illness, mortal or not, because of the commandment, fear and danger will cease."

Note as well that physicians must observe this precept "before all else" (as the decretal says) – before [the doctor] begins treatment, or contracts for the fee, according to Johannes Andreas. But it is a doubtful point whether it is enough for physicians to admonish their patients to call the doctors of souls, that is, the confessors, to whom they should confess, or whether they should require them [to do so].... Hostiensis is of this opinion.... But this opinion seems harsh, since according to the order of charity help should be given in a situation of danger even against the laws; nor does the text [of the decretal] say this. Petrus de Palude says only that physicians are obliged to warn. Is the physician who knows that the death of the patient he is treating is near obliged to announce this to him? On this matter, Johannes Neapolitanus.... makes the following distinction: either the physician believes it likely that such an announcement of death would greatly benefit the sick man with respect to the salvation of his soul and the disposition or ordering of his affairs or he believes the opposite, namely, that it would not be of benefit, or he hesitates between the two. In the case where he believes that it would be beneficial – for instance, because he believes the patient is in a state of mortal sin, and that he has not put his affairs into any order, and that these would be in disarray after his death, and this could cause serious dissention among his heirs; and that were he to hear that death was near the patient would dispose himself to make a good death and to order his affairs well – in that case he is obliged by the law of charity to make this plain to the patient either by himself or through another and he would commit a mortal sin by not doing so. And the reason for this, is because he would bring great loss upon his neighbor both with respect to the salvation of his soul and with respect to his temporal affairs, not indeed by doing him harm directly through his action, but indirectly, because he does not impede harm when he could do so and ought to do so.... But if the physician believes the opposite to be probable, namely, that such an announcement of death would do little or no good to the patient, and believes on the contrary that his silence would do little or no harm because he believes [the patient] to be in a good [spiritual] state, and to have put his affairs into good order, then the physician is not obliged to announce death in advance.... Nonetheless, he would do better to announce it. And the reason is that however much the patient may believe himself to be in a good [spiritual] state and to have disposed his affairs well, he can make improvements in both these things; and it is probable that having heard that death is near he would dispose himself more thoroughly. But if the physician believes neither of the two things mentioned above, but is in doubt, then he is obliged to announce the approach of death. The reason is that in cases of doubt, a man is obliged to avert notable harm to his neighbor if he can. In this case, the harm of eternal damnation and harm to temporal good will follow. Now Galen says that, however much a physician may despair of the patient's health, he should always comfort the patient and promise him health. Johannes [Neapolitanus] says that Galen is no guide to what is the best thing to do – as Ambrose says in *On Consecration*: "The precepts of medicine are contrary to the ardently divine cognition." Or it could be said that Galen's dictum can be followed when one would do serious harm by announcing death and no harm by keeping silence. But under no circumstances should a doctor tell a lie.... If it is asked whether the patient would sin by not obeying the physician, Innocent [III] replies that it would seem not, because [the physician] is not his ruler, nor one whose commands he is obliged to obey. He cannot command [the patient] because he has no jurisdiction over him, but he can advise or exhort him.... Nonetheless, it is good for him to believe [the physician], for as the Philosopher [Aristotle] says in book 1 of the *Posterior Analytics*, one who is expert in his art should be believed. If the patient

a license. One should commit the care of one's body to practical, rather than theoretical physicians. Hence the Philosopher says in book I of the *Metaphysics* that those who have the art and science of medicine are more knowledgeable than those who have experience. Nonetheless we should choose experienced doctors to treat us, rather than those who have knowledge without experience.... I consider it better and safer to commit oneself for treatment to practical physicians rather than theoretical ones. If there are doctors who want to apply one medicine to all diseases without consideration of the cause and the application of particulars, these should not be called expert or knowledgeable doctors, because these men only cure sometimes, and in some people, and by chance.... Those uneducated (*idiotae*) doctors should also be avoided who are sometimes wont to mix superstitions with certain natural remedies; one should abstain completely from these. For these people and the doctors who use such superstitious medicines are guilty of sin.... It is also forbidden to follow the superstitious teaching of the pagans, who consider certain times to be lucky or unlucky and who follow the constellations, not with respect to the natural effects of the stars or elements, but in accordance with divination and the fallacies of demons. For it is certain and true that just as human bodies are by necessity subjected to the influence of the heavenly bodies, so also by necessity the influence of the appropriate sign is required in the cure of ailing bodies. Hence if physicians give [*purgative] medicine in *choleric signs, it will do little good, because the body will be moved little or not at all. If in *phlegmatic signs, the medicine, when it is taken, will easily relax the body. Because of this, just as physicians in treating the sick observe the *critical days which are determined by the sun and moon, so in giving medications they should observe the appropriate signs of the stars. Thus Alexander the Great was advised not to take medicine without the advice of someone with expertise in the art of the stars. And although it is useful for a physician to have expertise in this subject, it is nevertheless not necessary for him to be an astrologer himself, but [only] to know certain basics that pertain to the suitable administration of medicines.

It is not illicit for physicians to receive a salary or fee for an illness which they know is incurable. Augustine of Ancona explains that this is because the physician is the instrument of nature. The instrument of medicine is not to be totally withdrawn from the patient as long as nature has not succumbed. Therefore, the physician does not sin in taking a fee for treating an illness that he believes to be incurable by the principles of the art of medicine, except perhaps by maliciously concealing this from his patient, or giving him superfluous things, or promising to cure him completely. But if he tells the truth as he knows it concerning the treatment of the illness, he may with justice accept his fee as long as he displays faithful ministration and true advice in his treatment.... Because the physician does not know what God has in mind for the patient, whether he will live or die (although according to the art of medicine [the patient] is going to die); he may, therefore, legitimately pursue the treatment and accept his fee to the end, or almost. But for the patient, it is safer and better for his treatment if he has a number of doctors rather than just one, if he can afford it. Hence the Philosopher said in his letter to Alexander [the Great], "You should not rely on one doctor, because a single doctor has great power to do harm, and will readily dare to take upon himself some evil deed. And if medicines are to be consumed, do not consume them save on the advice of many."

On this subject, Augustine of Ancona says, "In the treatment of illness one should consider the condition of the art of medicine, the condition of the illness, and the condition of the patient."

As to the first, it is clear that medicine, like any art, was discovered so that people could help one another, and to help those who will come after, for those who follow always add to those who came before, according to the Philosopher in *Metaphysics* book 2. Hence, just as what adds to the art of medicine is discovered by the experience of many, so what adds to the treatment of illness should be made rationally, through the discussion and knowledge of many physicians.

As to the second, that is, the condition of the illness: this is sometimes hidden from one physician in the manifest symptoms, but another [physician] is able to know its cause, either through these same symptoms or through others.

As to the third, that is the condition of the state of the patient, it is evident that the higher the station, the greater the danger in which he finds himself. Lords are hated and envied by many, both because of the dignity which they enjoy, of which many are jealous, and because of the justice they administer in disputes, which inspires malice. Hence we read in the letter to Alexander that the queen of the Indies sent him many precious gifts and among them a most beautiful virgin, who had been brought up on a diet of poison and who had been transformed into the nature of a poisonous serpent. This was done so that when Alexander had sexual relations with her, he would be poisoned and would die. But being warned in advance, he abstained from her. And thus for the sake of administering more diligent treatment and to remove all suspicion, it is safer if great men have many physicians rather than one. Those who cannot have many, and can only employ one, must be content with one.

Note briefly the grave sins of physicians. First, if they exercise the important art of medicine when they are ignorant of it, the death or deteriorating condition of their patients will be imputed to them.... Secondly, when they are summoned, either because they are negligent or because they are busy elsewhere, they do not consult their books, or diligently provide the things that should be provided. Thirdly, when they give medicine and remedies that are contrary to the salvation of the soul, for example to procure an abortion or to persuade to some other evil deed.... Fourthly, when they do not induce the patient to summon a priest to make a confession.... Fifthly, when they do not visit the sick poor of their acquaintance, because they cannot pay them.... Sixthly, when the physician, foreseeing the death of the patient, does not advise him or his relatives or his confessor, that they might provide for the sacraments, or a will if this is required, and so forth, out of fear that [the patient] would feel worse or that he or his people would be displeased.... Seventh, when he does not exercise diligence in compounding medications, unless he has certain experience of the skill and faithfulness of the apothecaries, who add many adulterated things into [medicines]. Eighth, when they keep the patient sick for a longer period of time so that they can profit from attending him, when he could well be cured more quickly. Ninth, when they induce the weak to break the fasts of the Church without reasonable cause or to eat meat on prohibited days, and even more, when they themselves denigrate the fasts and abstinences of the Church. Tenth, concerning their jealousy of one another, by which they vaunt their own treatments and put down their colleagues by finding fault with their treatments.

90. LICENSING AND ACCOUNTABILITY (1): MALPRACTICE IN CRUSADER PALESTINE

One of the earliest western legal texts to consider malpractice in detail comes from the expatriate European communities of Crusader Palestine. The Assises of the Court of the Bourgeois *(Livre des Assises de la Cour des Bourgeois) is a commentary on the laws of the Latin Kingdom of Jerusalem, as applied in the courts for free non-nobles (the nobility had their own system of courts). It was composed in Acre around 1240–44.*

Though the text offers no hint of Islamic influence, the manner in which licensing and medical responsibility are handled bears the strong impress of Muslim governmental and policing institutions, notably the office of the muhtasib *or overseer of standards in public life. Historians are divided over whether European licensing laws in places such as Sicily or Valencia (docs. 91–92) were shaped by these Crusader experiments, or whether they absorbed Islamic influence independently. In all three cases, the rules for examining practitioners and apportioning blame for medical mishaps seem to blend Muslim administrative practice with Roman property law. Almost all the cases discussed below involve redress for damage to property (servants or slaves) in a legal culture familiar with cure contracts. Only if the victim were a Christian or a free person did the issue of criminal liability arise. The author of the commentary was quite familiar with the conceptual system of Galenic medicine (for example, the idea of hot and cold members and remedies; the purpose of urine inspection, bleeding etc.) and assumed that the doctor's competence would be judged in accordance with this knowledge. Urine inspection was literally the badge of the professional doctor, who, if he was guilty of murdering his patients, was beaten through the streets with his urine flask in his hand.*

Source: trans. Vivian Nutton, in Piers D. Mitchell, *Medicine in the Crusades: Warfare, Wounds and the Medieval Surgeon* (Cambridge: Cambridge University Press, 2004), pp. 232–37. Middle French.

Chapter 231. The Law Regulating Surgery

Here you will have an account of all doctors, usually of wounds, who medicate or cut an injured person other than one should, and hence the injured person dies, what right one has of that doctor.

If it happens that I accidentally injure my servant, man or woman, or someone else injures them and I bring in a doctor and that doctor contracts with me for a fixed sum and tells me on the third day after seeing the wound that he will cure it without fail; and it happens that he cuts it badly or cuts for something that should not be cut and then he dies; or if he should have cut the wound along the lips or along the swelling and he makes a cross cut, so that he dies; reason judges and commands us to judge that that doctor must pay for the servant, male or female, the value on the day he was injured or the price for which he was bought, for this is the law and reasoning of the Assise. And the court should order the doctor to leave the town where he effected that bad treatment.

Likewise, if my servant had a wound in a hot place or in a place to which hot things are appropriately applied, like the brain or the *nerves or on joints which are of a cold nature, and he always applies cold things and the slave dies, reason judges and commands us to judge that he is obliged to pay for that slave, man or woman, for that is right and reasonable....

Likewise, if my servant has a head wound with the bone broken and he doesn't know how to remove the pieces, so that the broken bone pierces the brain so that he dies, reason adjudges that he is legally bound to pay for the servant....

Likewise, if the doctor can show in court, with good guarantee, that he whom he treated lay with a woman or drank wine or ate some bad food that he had forbidden him, or did anything other than he should, reason judges and commands to judge that even if the doctor should still have treated him differently from what he should have done, he is not held liable to pay compensation, for the most expert argument is that he died from doing what was forbidden him, not through a poor doctor, and that is the reason and judgment of the Assise. But if a doctor had not stopped him from eating or drinking, or touching a woman and he did so, or ate and drank when he ought not and he dies, reason adjudges that the doctor is rightly held to pay compensation since the doctor is rightly liable, on seeing the sick [individual], to tell him what to eat and what not; and if he does not and an accident happens that is the doctor's responsibility.

But if the doctor himself, once taking over the care and treatment himself met with misfortune, being captured by the Saracens or falling ill or something else that prevented him from visiting the sick and he died, reason adjudges that in law the doctor is not liable for compensation.

And if a doctor had wrongly treated, as above, a free man or woman who died, reason adjudges that the doctor should be lawfully hung and his property should belong to the lord. But if he had received anything from the dead man, the doctor's property should be handed over to the deceased's relatives, for that is right and reasonable.

Likewise, if the doctor treated a servant, male or female, for a broken arm or leg and said that he would cure it completely, as would be the case if he had acted properly, and he made a solemn covenant but then broke it and acted badly, applying useless plasters which left men forever crippled, reason judges that the doctor is liable to take the servant and pay his master what he cost. If he cannot pay all, reason adjudges further that he must leave the servant with his lord or lady and instead should pay as much as the value of that servant, male or female, has fallen, for he has been left injured by his intervention. If he crippled a Christian man or woman, reason adjudges that he should lose his right thumb and owe no further damages so long as he took nothing for the treatment, otherwise he is rightly responsible for giving it back....

Chapter 233. The Law Regulating Physic

Here you will have the reason and law of medicines and of the activities of physicians who give the sick a syrup, drug or *electuary from which he dies as a result of bad treatment.

If it happens by misadventure that my slave, man or woman, falls ill and a doctor goes to his lord or lady and says he will cure him and agrees [on] a fee with the lord, and then if the doctor gives laxatives or heating substance by which the seat of the disease is *putrefied and he betakes himself to bed; and if he should have given him astringents and cold substances and did not, with the result that he died, reason judges and commands to judge that the doctor is liable to give me another servant or the amount he was worth on the day he died, and that is the law and judgment of the Assise.

Likewise, if my servant should be ill with *fever so that he has great heat within his body, and the doctor bleeds him before the due time and removes too much blood so that, both by the weakness of the fever that he has so disturbed and by the bleeding, the fever climbed into the head of the patient, he relapsed and died, reason commands to judge that the doctor is held liable in law and by the Assise to pay compensation to the value of the servant, male or female, on the day of death, or what he cost when first bought, for this is the right and judgment of the Assise.

Item, if my slave should become cold and have a cold disease and a doctor comes and says to his lord, "I'll cure him," and contracts with his lord and takes up the cure, and if it happens that he is bled for his coldness and this happens because of his ignorance of urine, and failure to judge, and the patient becomes entirely dry, loses his voice or is dried worse because of his previous chill and by the bleeding which had been done, and he dies, reason adjudges and commands that he should be liable to pay to the lord or lady in law as much as he had cost, for this is the reason and judgment of the Assises....

Likewise, if my slave was ill with a *quotidian fever, hot and cold, and a doctor comes to his lord or lady and says he will cure him by the application of a drug and agrees with the lord to do so and takes the servant into his care, and then he gives the drug at prime [6 *a.m.*] or midnight, and in this drug there is so much *scammony that it was so strong that he died, just as if he had drunk it; or if he went to the toilet before it was day and vomited all he had in him, heart, bowels, and lungs, and died; or if the doctor had not diagnosed the illness as he should but gave him medicine and he could not go out, reason adjudges that he died of the aforesaid signs and that the doctor must pay compensation in law and by the Assise....

Likewise, if my servant has a bowel disease and a doctor undertakes the cure, and if he takes a very hot iron and wants to cure the hemorrhoids from which the illness comes, and he does not know how to do it so that he burns and makes an end of the bowel damaged at the rectum, so that the bowel constricts itself and closes with the *cauterisation so that he can no more open his bowels and dies, reason judges and commands to judge that the doctor is bound to pay compensation for that servant, lawfully, for what the lord paid for him.

Item, if my slave is ill with measles, or a dry ulcer, or some other disease and I come to a doctor and contract for his cure so that half of the money for which he is sold will be his and the other is that of the owner, and the doctor undertakes the cure and does what he can, to no avail, and he dies, reason judges that the doctor is not liable to pay compensation for the servant, male or female, since he loses all his work in the first place and all that he was going to have; and that is the right and judgment of the Assise.

Likewise, if a doctor has treated in this way a free man or woman, reason judges and commands that the doctor be hung, even when he is the doctor to the lord of the land. But before he is hung, he must be beaten through the town, urine flask in hand, for that is right and reasonable, to warn others of his crime, for that is the right and reason of the court.

Know well that in all these crimes there should be witnesses, so that if the doctor is accused, if he denies having acted in the above way, these witnesses will swear by the saints that they saw him before them treat this patient with these drugs or syrups and that this is why the patient who had another disease died, and they heard the patient say that because the doctor had given him such things he felt strongly in his body that he would die. Then the doctor ought to be tried for the murder either of the servant, for which he should pay compensation, or of a Christian, for which he should be hung, as said above, for that is right. For otherwise the doctor ought not to be tried on the unsupported word of people or of the patient.

Besides, no foreign doctor, that is one coming from Outremer or pagan [that is, Muslim] lands, should practice as a urine doctor until he has been examined by other doctors, the best in the land, in the presence of the bishop of the place wherein this is to be done. If it is recognized that he can correctly practice medicine, the bishop will give him a license to treat in that particular town where he will see, from the bishop's letter which he will have as testimony, that doctors are proven and can rightly treat by means of urine. And that is the right and reason of the Assise of Jerusalem.

Likewise, if it turns out that he is a poor doctor who cannot practice, reason adjudges that the bishop and court should order him to leave the city or if not, that he should remain without practicing on anyone. If it happens that a doctor practices in the town without the leave of the court or bishop, the court should arrest him and beat him out of town, according to the law and decision of the Assise of Jerusalem.

91. LICENSING AND ACCOUNTABILITY (2): LEGISLATION GOVERNING DOCTORS IN THE THIRTEENTH-CENTURY KINGDOM OF SICILY

The rise of the new academic medicine coincided with important changes in the political culture of medieval Europe. Towns sought self-government; kings began to overhaul legal codes; rulers hired bureaucrats and recorded their decisions in writing; and in the schools, a new class of "clerks," who would find employment in royal and ecclesiastical courts, were imbibing classical concepts of the state by reading the works of Cicero and

Aristotle. That governments might have some responsibility for protecting and promoting the health of subjects was still a rather embryonic notion, but it was one whose outlines are visible in the Constitutions of Melfi, *promulgated in 1231 by the emperor Frederick II for his kingdom of Sicily. The* Constitutions *was a pragmatic law code designed to stabilize the government of the kingdom; it was neither comprehensive in scope nor driven by ideology. Yet Frederick's laws show how government involvement helped to shift the focus of medical ethics away from the old private and subjective criteria of character and toward new public and objective standards of competence. According to the* Constitutions, *no one, whatever his intent and regardless of the outcome, could practice without publicly sanctioned credentials, backed by formal educational requirements. Though they were not yet organized as a university, the schools of Salerno were co-opted by the king to administer these requirements, which not surprisingly coincided with the scholastic medical curriculum. The ethical duty of doctors was subordinated to the ethical duty of the king to protect the subject; hence Frederick could even mandate treatment guidelines and define a medical conflict of interest.*

Source: trans. Edward F. Hartung, "Medical Regulations of Frederick the Second of Hohenstaufen," *Medical Life* 41 (1934): 592–94. Latin.

Book 3, Title 46. Concerning Doctors

Because the science of medicine can never be known unless some knowledge of logic is first acquired, we decree that no one shall study medical science unless he has first studied the science of logic for at least three years; after this period of three years, if he wishes, the student may advance to the study of medicine to which he must devote five years, in such wise that he shall within the prescribed period of study, learn in addition that field of medicine which is called surgery. After this and not before, he will be granted a license to practice as a doctor, provided he has first attended an examination of a form prescribed by the government and has also received a testimonial from his master, certifying that he has completed the prescribed period of study.

A doctor shall swear that he will observe the regulations fixed by the government up to this time; that, in addition, he will denounce to the authorities any pharmacist who, [to] his knowledge, prepares drugs under the required strength, and that he will give freely of his advice to the poor.

A doctor shall visit his patients at least twice a day and, at the request of the patient, once during the night; he shall receive from the patient for a day-visit, provided he has not been called beyond the city or village limits, not more than half a *tarenus* of gold. If he has been summoned beyond the city limits, he shall receive not more than three *tareni* if the patient pays the expenses. A physician may not make contracts with pharmacists or receive any of them under his patronage for the payment of a fixed sum, nor may he have his own shop. Pharmacists are to prepare a concoction at their own expense and must have a prescription from the doctor in accordance with our regulations, nor shall they be allowed to keep preparations unless they have taken an oath; they shall prepare all their medicines in the prescribed form without fraud. Moreover, the shop-keeper shall be paid for his medicines in the following manner: For compounds and *simple medicine which are usually kept in stock not longer than a year from the time of purchase, for any ounce he shall be empowered and permitted to receive three *tareni*. For others, which because of the nature of the drugs or for some other reason must be kept in stock longer than a year, for any ounce he shall be allowed to receive six *tareni*. Shops of this kind shall not be allowed everywhere, but only in certain cities throughout the kingdom as shall be described below.

No doctor shall practice after the completion of the five-year period who has not practiced for an entire year under the direction of an experienced doctor. During the period of five years the masters shall teach in the schools the authenticated books of both Hippocrates and Galen, and shall instruct in the theory as well as in the practice of medicine. Moreover, we decree as a measure for public health that no surgeon shall be admitted to practice who does not present testimonials from masters in the faculty of medicine, stating that he has studied for at least a year in that field which develops skills in surgery, in particular, that he has learned in the schools the anatomy of human bodies, and that he is proficient in that field of medicine without which incision cannot be safely made nor fractures healed.

Book 3, Title 47. Concerning the Number of Faithful Men to Be Appointed over Electuaries and Syrups

In every land of our empire subject to our jurisdiction we decree that there be appointed two men cautious and worthy of confidence, who, upon swearing a formal oath, shall be retained and their names submitted to our court. Under the supervision of these men, electuaries and syrups and other medicines shall be legally prepared, and, when so made, may be sold. At Salernum [*Salerno*] in particular, we wish these medicaments to be tested by masters of *physic. By the present enactment, we likewise decree that no one (in the kingdom) except at Salernum (or Naples) shall lecture in medicine or surgery, or assume the title of master, unless he has been carefully examined in the presence of our officers and of masters of the same art. Moreover, we desire those who prepare medicine to bind themselves solemnly by oath that they will prepare them conscientiously in accordance with their best knowledge and, so far as possible, in the presence of the inspectors. But if they do otherwise, they shall be sentenced to be deprived of all their chattels. Furthermore, if the appointed men to whose trust the aforesaid matters have been consigned are convicted of fraud in the operation of the entrusted office, we hold that they are to be punished with the extreme penalty.

Book 3, Title 65. That No Man Shall Practice until He Has Been Officially Certified in the Convention of the Masters of Salernum

We secure advantage to the individual whenever we provide for the health of our faithful subjects. Accordingly, being mindful of the heavy loss and irreparable harm that can result from the inexperience of doctors, we order that in future no one alleging the title of doctor shall dare to practice in any other manner or even to heal, unless he shall first be certified by the judgment of the masters in the public convention at Salernum, and licensed by testimonials as to his trustworthiness and sufficient science from his masters and from our representatives, in our presence, or, if we be absent from the kingdom, in the presence of our viceroy, [having been appointed, he shall draw near] and shall receive from our viceroy a license to practice; the penalty of confiscation of goods and a year's imprisonment shall await those who in future venture to practice in defiance of this ordinance of our serene majesty.

92. LICENSING AND ACCOUNTABILITY (3): EXAMINING AND SUPERVISING PRACTITIONERS IN FOURTEENTH-CENTURY VALENCIA

After it was reconquered from the Muslims in 1238, the kingdom of Valencia on the Mediterranean coast of Spain was joined with Catalonia and Aragon to form the united kingdom of Aragon. The capital city, Valencia, was a prosperous port and a center of textile manufacturing. It also became the site of a well-documented experiment in medical licensing, inaugurated by the furs (law code) proclaimed by King Alfons IV in the corts (political assembly) of 1329.

Adopting academic education as the benchmark of competence did more than solve the practical problem of accreditation; it also proclaimed society's conviction that learned doctors offered the best care, and that it was to the public's advantage to promote these standards. The furs of 1329 went beyond previous legislation by requiring, for the first time, a university degree in order to practice as a doctor (the University of Lérida was founded in 1300); barbers, surgeons, and apothecaries also had to be approved by the medical examining board. The public seems to have appreciated the new regulations: even towns of modest size wanted the best in medical care, and the municipal authorities not only gave the license but chose the panel of examiners.

The two documents presented here set out the program of the Valencia reforms and illustrate its limits in practice. The furs *of 1329 stipulated the new conditions for practice. The account of how Bernat Giner received his conditional license in 1383 shows that the rules (in this case, the requirement for university learning) could be waived. Bernat's written testimonial may have descended from the Islamic* ijaza, *originally a document from a master testifying that its bearer had studied certain medical books and was qualified to teach, but which with time came to include confirmation of clinical training. His case also shows that many who applied for the license were already practicing. Whole categories of healers – notably Muslim women practitioners or* metgesses *– were simply ignored by the authorities. For as Valencia learned to its cost, licensing was a two-edged sword: high standards for practitioners increased consumer demand but exacerbated the shortage of practitioners. Hence, some elasticity had to be built into the system.*

Source: trans. Luis García-Ballester, Michael R. McVaugh and Agustín Rubio-Vela, *Medical Licensing and Learning in Fourteenth-Century Valencia*, Transactions of the American Philosophical Society 79, part 6 (Philadelphia: American Philosophical Society, 1989), appendix II, no. 2, pp. 60–61 and no. 11, pp. 94–95. Latin.

a. The *Furs de València* of 1329, Promulgated by King Alfons IV el Benigne

Concerning Medical Practitioners

1. We command and ordain that the justiciar and the *jurats* [*members of the town's executive council*] elect every year, three days before Christmas, two leading physicians who shall be examiners of all the practitioners of *physic who have recently come to practice in the city or in the towns of the kingdom; and those whom they find competent, and who have followed the art of medicine for at least four years in a *studium generale*, shall be admitted to practice the said art, and if not they shall not be admitted. And if they practice without the said examination and license, they shall be liable to a fine of 100 gold morabatins for each occasion, of which a third part shall go to the court, a third to the town, and a third to the accuser. And under the same penalty, allotted as above, no physician shall share in the fees of apothecaries, and each year they shall swear an oath the day after New Year's promising to set apothecaries' fees moderately, as often as necessary. And if any physician shall be assessed the said fine and not be able to pay, let him be expelled from the town forever.

2. Practitioners who are now practicing physic or surgery shall be examined, and those who are found competent may remain in practice but not the others, under a fine of 100 gold morabitins allotted as above.

3. No woman shall practice medicine or give *potions, under penalty of

being whipped through the town; but they may care for little children and women – to whom, however, they may give no potion.

4. Every surgeon who has a wounded patient in his care shall be required to state an oath [whether the wound was the result of a crime], for no fee and as often as he shall be asked, whether the patient is out of danger or not.

5. No barber shall practice medicine or surgery if he has not been examined by the examiners of practitioners and found competent. And if he should practice without their examination and license, he shall pay a fine of 50 gold morabatins every time he transgresses, of which the court shall receive a third, the town a third, and the accuser a third.

6. Every practitioner, whether of physic or surgery, shall swear each year before the justiciar at the beginning of his term that he will not treat anyone who is seriously ill or wounded, man or woman, if the patient has not first made confession – except in a potentially fatal case where a delay would be dangerous, and then he will not make a second visit until the patient has confessed.

7. Practitioners, both physicians and surgeons, shall give prescriptions for medicines in the vulgar tongue, naming herbs and other medicinal things by their common or popular names. Likewise they shall give weights and measures of the said things in a manner that can be readily understood by the ordinary people. And whosoever shall disobey shall pay each time a fine of 10 gold morabatins, of which the court shall receive a third, the town a third, and the accuser a third.

b. Bernat Giner Receives His License (1383)

In the year of our Lord 1383, Monday the 9th of February, appeared Bernat Giner, alias Fuster, physician-surgeon, before the honorable Johan de Cervató, civil justiciar of the city of Valencia; and he presented him with a letter from the honorable Jacme Maderes and Pere Gironés, examiners for the current year of surgeon-practitioners in the said city, whose tenor was as follows:

> To the honorable lord civil justiciar of the city of Valencia, or his lieutenant; from us, Jacme Mederes, master in arts and in medicine, and Pere Gironés, bachelor in medicine, citizens of the said city, examiners appointed for the current year to practitioners newly arrived and wishing to practice medicine and surgery in the said city and kingdom of Valencia; health and honor. We inform your lordship that Bernat Giner, alias Fuster, has appeared before us and has asked us that we examine him in medicine and in surgery; we have examined him in the said skill in the customary manner and have found that the said

Bernat Giner is not learned, but has long practiced in medicine and in surgery; and given the long involvement he has had with practicing physicians and in this skill, as a number of practitioners of long standing have certified in a public document that we have seen, we judge the said Bernat Giner to be competent to practice medicine and surgery in the said city and kingdom of Valencia – with the restriction that he not engage in surgery on dangerous wounds (as wounds of the head, the chest, the intestines, and other dangerous wounds) or in medicinal treatment of dangerous illnesses ([such as] continued *fevers and frenzy and other acute diseases) unless he is assisted by another expert physician or physicians of authority, under the penalty prescribed by the *fur*. Wherefore, at the request of the said Bernat Giner, notifying you, honored justiciar, or your lieutenant, of the said things, we send on the said Bernat and request that you grant permission to him ... to exercise, employ, and practice the said skills of medicine and surgery within the said city and kingdom in the manner set out above, taking oath from him that he will fulfill and not contravene it....

When this letter had been presented, the said honorable [justiciar] took the oath of the said Bernat Giner on the holy Gospels that he would engage well and loyally in the said practice of surgery and physic, with the restriction imposed above by the said examiners. And furthermore he commanded that the following certificate be drawn up for him: [*the text of the certificate follows, which reiterates the conditions laid down in the examiners' letter.*]

93. JOHN ARDERNE'S ADVICE ON HOW TO DETERMINE THE FEE, AND OTHER MATTERS OF MEDICAL ETIQUETTE

John Arderne (1307–after 1377, perhaps ca 1380/92) was an innovative and enterprising English surgeon. There is no evidence that he ever attended a university, yet he wrote in Latin (admittedly rather inexpert Latin) and seems to have acquired a considerable medical education. He vigorously promoted surgery in the "rational" tradition against the claims of lesser practitioners such as barbers, yet he was fundamentally a surgical entrepreneur. He developed a successful technique for treating fistula in ano, *a tubular ulcer that forms on the inside of the anus and eventually perforates the flesh and skin of the buttocks or the region around the anus. Fecal matter drains through the *fistula along with blood and pus, causing great discomfort and distress. One cause of anal fistula seems to be spending long hours on horseback, and hence it was a disease associated with the military aristocracy. John Arderne devised a procedure to ligature and* *drain the fistula, thus allowing it to heal. His prologue reveals much about the ethics and economics of a successful surgical career in late medieval England.*

Source: trans. Faith Wallis from *Treatises of Fistula in Ano, Haemorrhoids, and Clysters by John Arderne*, ed. D'Arcy Power (London: Kegan Paul for the Early English Text Society, 1910), pp. 1–8. Middle English.

Of the Wound of *Fistula in ano*, and of the Physician's Behavior, and of the Instruments Necessary for the Fistula

I, John Arderne, lived in Newark in Nottinghamshire from the first pestilence that was in the year of our Lord 1349 to the year of our Lord 1370, and there I treated many men for *fistula in ano*. Of these, the first was Sir Adam Everingham of Laxton-in-the-Clay near Tukesford; which Sir Adam, forsooth, was in Gascony with Sir Henry, at that time earl of Derby and afterwards made duke of Lancaster, a noble and worthy lord. The aforesaid Sir Adam, suffering from *fistula in ano*, asked the advice of all the physicians and surgeons that he could find in Gascony, at Bordeaux, at Bergerac, Toulouse and Narbonne, and Poitiers, and many other places. And all abandoned him as incurable. When he saw and heard this, the aforesaid Adam hastened to return to his own country. And when he had come home, he took off all his knightly clothing and put on mourning garments, because the dissolution or loss of his body was drawing nigh. At last I, the aforesaid John Arderne, was sought out, and when an agreement had been made, I came to him and cured him and with the Lord's intervention I healed him perfectly within six months. And afterwards, whole and sound, he led a gladsome life for thirty years and more, for which cure I obtained much honor and affection throughout all England. And the aforesaid duke of Lancaster and many other gentlefolk were amazed at this. Afterwards I cured Hugo Derling of Fowick of Balne by Snathe. Afterwards I cured John Sheffield of Brightwell near Tekyll. Afterwards I cured Sir Reynald Grey, lord of Wilton in Wales and lord of Sherland near Chesterfield, who asked for advice from the most famous doctors in England, and none could avail him. Afterwards I cured Sir Henry Blackburn, clerk, treasurer of the lord Prince of Wales. Afterwards I cured Adam Humfrey of Shelford near Nottingham, and Sir John, priest of the same town; and John of Holle of Sherland; and Sir Thomas Hamelden, parson of Langar in the Vale of Bevare. Afterwards I cured Thomas Gunny, custodian of the Friars Minor of York. Afterwards, in the year of our Lord 1379, I came to London, and there I cured John Colyn, mayor of Northampton, who had asked for the advice of many doctors. Afterwards I healed or cured Hugh Denny, fishmonger of London in Bridgestreet; and William Pole and Ralph

Double; and someone called Thomas Brown, who had fifteen holes out of which went wind with excremental odor; that is to say, eight holes on one side of the arse and seven on the other, of which some holes were distant from the [anus] by the space as wide as a man's hand, so that both his buttocks were so ulcerated and putrefied within that every day a quantity of filth exuded such as would fill an egg-shell. Afterwards I cured four Friars Preachers, that is to say John Writtel, Friar John Hackett, Friar Peter Brown, Friar Thomas Apperly, and a young man called Thomas Voke. Of these, some had only one hole distant from the [anus] by one inch, or two, or three. And others had four or five holes reaching down to the scrotum, and many other circumstances difficult to relate. All these I cured before writing this book. Our Lord Jesus, blessed God, knows that I do not lie, and therefore let no man doubt this, though famous men of old and very distinguished in learning have confessed that they could find no way to cure this disease. For God, who metes out and rewards wisdom, has hid many things from wise and clever men that he later vouchsafed to show to simple men. Therefore, let all who come after me know that the old masters were not energetic and diligent in seeking out and searching for this cure. Rather than confront its difficulty directly, they neglected it completely. Some of them, forsooth, deemed it completely incurable; others held doubtful opinions. Therefore, in difficult matters, it profits students to persevere and persist and to apply their intelligence to the matter at hand, for it is revealed not to those who pass it by, but to those who persevere. Therefore, honor Almighty God who has revealed understanding to me so that I should find treasure hidden in the field of studies, who for a long time and with panting breast have sweated and travailed energetically and pertinaciously. As my skill suffices, without fine rhetoric, I have come to the point of revealing it openly to those who will come after, our Lord and this book being the intermediary. [I do so] not to display myself as more worthy of such a gift than any other person, but so as not to grieve God, or be accused of treachery by him for the sake of the talent he has given me [Matt. 25:14–29]. Therefore I pray that the grace of the Holy Spirit may be upon this work, that he may vouchsafe to prosper it, so that I may plainly explain in this little book those things which, to be sure, I am often very expert in carrying out. And I say this: that I know not in all my time, nor have heard in all my time of any man in England or abroad who can cure *fistula in ano*, except for one Franciscan that was with the Prince of Wales in Gascony and Guyenne, who boasted that he had cured the aforesaid illness. And he deceived many men in London and when he could not cure someone, he suggested to him that no man could cure him, and he affirmed with an oath that if the fistula were dried, that the patient could not escape death; which [patients], forsooth, having been abandoned and forsaken by [the friar], I cured perfectly.

and you fart where you don't want to fart." And it is said in another place: "Cunning speech corrupts good manners." When sick folk, or anyone else, come to a doctor to ask his help and advice, he should neither be too gruff with them, nor too familiar, but moderate his bearing according to the person who is making the inquiry: to some, reverent, to others, familiar. For according to wise men, excessive familiarity breeds contempt. Also it is expedient that he have some plausible excuses for not answering their request, without insulting or arousing the indignation of a great man or a friend. [He should plead] some necessary occupation, or injury, or sickness, or some other conceivable cause why he may be excused. If he grants someone's request, he should draw up a contract for his work and take it beforehand. The doctor should be careful to give no certain answer in any cause before he sees the disease itself and its circumstances. When he has seen and inspected it, even though it seems to him that the patient will recover, nevertheless he shall prognosticate to the patient what perils shall come if the treatment is deferred. And if he sees that the patient cooperates assiduously in the cure, then when the state of the patient allows it he should ask boldly for a greater or lesser [increase of the fee]; but always beware of asking too little, for asking too little diminishes the value of the market and the product. Therefore, for the cure of *fistula in ano*, when it is curable, he should ask from a great and worthy man 100 marks or 40 pounds, with robes and an annuity of 100 shillings per annum for life. From a lesser man, he should ask 40 pounds or 40 marks without annuity; and let him not take less than 100 shillings. For I never in all my life took less than 100 shillings for curing that disease. Nonetheless, let another do whatever he thinks is better and more expeditious. And if the patients or their friends and servants ask how much time he thinks it will take to cure it, let the doctor always say that it will take twice the time he thinks it will; that is, if the doctor thinks he will cure the patient in twenty weeks (for that is the common course of the cure), he should add as many again. For prolonging the cure causes patients to despair at a time when trusting the doctor offers the best hope of health. And if the patient should consider or wonder or ask why he thought the cure would take so long, when he was healed in half the time, he should answer that it was because the patient was of a strong constitution, and bore with the pain so well, and that he was of good *complexion and had flesh that was able to heal; and let him feign other causes agreeable to the patient, for patients are proud and delighted at such words. Also, the doctor should dress respectably, not resembling a minstrel in his apparel or bearing, but emulating the clergy in dress and bearing. Why? Because any well-behaved man dressed like the clergy can sit at a gentleman's table.

The doctor should also have clean hands and well-filed nails, cleansed of all dirt and filth. And he should act courteously at the tables of lords, and

CHAPTER THIRTEEN

THE ETHICS OF MEDICAL CARE (2):
HOSPITALS AND THE PROVISION OF
CHARITY

The Church's project to Christianize medieval society and the interest of governments in overseeing health care created a context for the emergence of the hospital as an expression of Christian caritas. *The hospital is the creation of late-antique Christianity in the eastern Mediterranean. Its origins lie with the hostels created by bishops such as Basil of Caesarea (d. 379) for the poor, and its vocation was fundamentally religious. In the medieval West, hospitals were "God's House,"* maison-dieu *or* Hôtel-Dieu. *The hospital was a "house" because it was always a built space of some kind, a shelter or refuge, and also because it was organized as a religious community, a "household" whose head was God. The community did God's work, which was charity. Charity could take many forms: a hostel for the wayfarer, a hospice for the dying, an almshouse for the elderly poor, an orphanage for foundlings, a hospital for the sick poor, or any combination of the above. In addition, hospitals frequently provided food and fuel or operated as "micro-loan" agencies to help local people in need.*

*From the twelfth to the early sixteenth centuries, places called "God's House" multiplied all over western Europe. In part, this was a response to the social stress consequent on the increasing wealth and complexity of medieval society – the same forces, in fact, that created the universities and the learned medical profession. But the hospital also points to the desire for individuals and groups to gain spiritual merit through conspicuous philanthropy. Hospitals and patrons engaged in a symbiotic exchange of benefits: gifts and endowments by the patron were repaid by the uniquely precious prayers of "the poor" for the souls of their benefactors. The poor were often identified as the "sick poor" (*infirmi pauperi)*, yet even hospitals with strongly articulated medical vocations rarely had professional staff in our sense of the term. Doctors and surgeons could be summoned at need, but the medicine of the hospital was organized and carried out by dedicated religious personnel. It was their knowledge and their ethos that defined health care in the hospital setting.*

94. THE ORGANIZATION AND ETHOS OF A MEDIEVAL HOSPITAL (1): THE JERUSALEM HOSPITAL

The Order of the Hospital was founded in the wake of the First Crusade by a confraternity of laymen attached to an older Latin Christian hospice in Jerusalem. Its modern lineal descendent is the Order of St John of Jerusalem (the Knights of Malta). The Order was formally recognized by Pope Paschal II in 1113, and a distinctive Rule was drawn up by Master Raymond du Puy (1120–60), based on the Rule of St Augustine (a rule for secular clergy living a common life, frequently used as the basis for hospital rules). Before the fall of the kingdom of Jerusalem to Saladin in 1187, they also operated field hospitals (a rarity in the twelfth century), transporting wounded Crusaders to Jerusalem for extended care. After the fall of Jerusalem, the Order established hospitals in Acre, Rhodes, and Cyprus, and in some major port cities of the Mediterranean through which pilgrims passed.

The Jerusalem Hospital was certainly novel and impressive by western standards and probably owed a considerable debt to Byzantine and Muslim models. Its size (between 1,000 and 2,000 beds and a staff of almost 150, according mid-twelfth-century witnesses), its emphasis on the sick poor, and its provision for professional medical care and drugs reshaped the western perception of what a hospital should be. The Jerusalem Hospital was not typical, yet it was what every medieval hospital had in mind as the perfect exemplar of the charitable ideal. That ideal now contained a substantial medical component.

Older historical accounts hold that the Order was a major conduit for the importation of Arabic medical knowledge and hospital organization into the West, but more recent analyses have qualified this claim. The Jerusalem Hospital never copied the Muslim division of wards according to medical condition, for instance, and the number of physicians was low by Byzantine or Muslim standards. More importantly, the ethical mainspring of the Hospital remained religious. This ethos is embodied in the Rule of Raymond du Puy, the first document presented here. The second document, the Statutes promulgated at the Chapter-General of 1181 or 1182, paints a more detailed picture of the inner organization of the Jerusalem Hospital. The poor were to be treated like lords, because they embodied Christ, and their caregivers were their servants. Finally, the Jerusalem Hospital, like its humbler European counterparts, also furnished non-medical charity. Indeed, the Jerusalem Hospital bears a closer resemblance to the new houses of regular canons that sprang up in northern European centers in the wake of the eleventh-century Reform than to the Pantocrator Hospital of Constantinople or the Nûr al-Dîn of Damascus.

Source: trans. E.J. King, *The Rule, Statutes and Customs of the Hospitallers, 1099–1310* (London: Methuen, 1934): Rule of Raymond du Puy, chapters 1–2, pp. 20–21, and 16, pp. 26–27; excerpts from the Statutes of 1181, pp. 34–40. Middle French and Latin.

a. The Rule of Blessed Raymond du Puy (1120–60)

This is the Constitution ordained by Brother Raymond. In the name of God, I, Raymond, servant of Christ's poor and warden of the Hospital of Jerusalem, with the counsel of all the Chapter, both clerical and lay brethren, have established these commandments in the House of the Hospital of Jerusalem.

1. **How the Brethren should make their profession**. Firstly, I ordain that all the brethren, engaging in the service of the poor, should keep the three things with the aid of God, which they have promised to God: that is to say, chastity and obedience, which means whatever thing is commanded them by their masters, and to live without property of their own: because God will require these three things of them at the Last Judgment.

2. **What the Brethren should claim as their due**. And let them not claim more as their due than bread and water and raiment, which things are promised to them. And their clothing should be humble, because our Lord's poor, whose servants we confess ourselves to be, go naked. And it is a thing wrong and improper for the servant that he should be proud, and his Lord should be humble....

16. **How our Lords the sick should be received and served**. And in that obedience in which the master and the chapter of the Hospital shall permit, when the sick man shall come there, let him be received thus, and let him partake of the Holy Sacrament, first having confessed his sins to the priest, and afterwards let him be carried to bed, and there as if he were a lord, each day before the brethren go to eat, let him be refreshed with food charitably according to the ability of the house....

b. Statutes of Roger of Moulins (Master of the Order 1177–87), Promulgated at the Chapter-General of 1181

... 2. And secondly, it is decreed with the assent of the brethren that for the sick in the Hospital of Jerusalem there should be engaged four wise doctors, who are qualified to examine urine, and to diagnose different diseases, and are able to administer appropriate medicines.

3. And thirdly, it is added that the beds of the sick should be made as long and as broad as is most convenient for repose and that each bed should be covered with its own coverlet (*covertour*), and each bed should have its own special sheets.

4. After these needs is decreed the fourth command, that each of the sick should have a cloak of sheepskin (*pelice a vestir*), and boots for going to and coming from the latrines, and caps of wool.

5. It is also decreed that little cradles should be made for the babies of women pilgrims born in the House, so that they may lie separate, and that the baby in its own bed may be in no danger from the restlessness of the mother.

6. Afterwards is decreed the sixth clause, that the biers of the dead should be concealed in the same manner as are the biers of the brethren, and should be covered with a red coverlet having a white cross.

7. The seventh clause commands that wheresoever there are hospitals for the sick, that the Commanders of the houses should serve the sick cheerfully, and should do their duty by them, and serve them without grumbling or complaining, so that by these good deeds they may deserve to have their reward in the glories of heaven....

8. It was also decreed, when the council [*that is, the Chapter-General*] of the brethren was held, that the prior of the Hospital of France should send each year to Jerusalem one hundred sheets of dyed cotton to replace the coverlets of the sick poor, and should reckon them in his Responsion [*portion of annual revenue from the Order's estates transmitted to the common Treasury*] together with those things which shall be given in his Priory to the House in charity.

In the self-same manner and reckoning the prior of the Hospital of St. Gilles [in Provence] should purchase each year the [same] number of sheets of cotton and send them to Jerusalem, together with those things that shall be given in his Priory for the love of God to the poor of the Hospital.

The prior of Italy each year should send to Jerusalem for our lords the sick two thousand ells of fustian of diverse colors, which he may reckon each year in his Responsion....

9. ... The prior of Mont Pelerin [*Tripoli in Lebanon*] should send to Jerusalem two *quintals of sugar for the *syrups, and the medicines and *electuaries of the sick.

For this same service the bailiff of [Tiberias] should send there the same quantity.

The prior of Constantinople should send for the sick two hundred felts.

10. Moreover, guarding and watching them day and night, the brethren of the Hospital should serve the sick poor with zeal and devotion as if they were their lords, and it was added in Chapter-General that in every ward (*rue*) and place in the Hospital, nine serjeants should be kept at their service, who should wash their feet gently, and change their sheets, and make their beds, and administer to the weak necessary and strengthening food, and do their duty devotedly, and obey in all things for the benefit of the sick.

The Confirmation by the Master Roger of the Things
That the House Should Do

Let all the brethren of the House of the Hospital, both those present and those to come, know that the good customs of the House of the Hospital of Jerusalem are as follows:

1. Firstly the Holy House of the Hospital is accustomed to receive sick men and women and is accustomed to keep doctors who have the care of the sick, and who make the syrups for the sick, and who provide the things that are necessary for the sick. For three days in the week the sick are accustomed to have fresh meat, either pork or mutton, and those who are unable to eat it have chicken....

3. And all the children abandoned by their fathers and mothers the Hospital is accustomed to receive and nourish. To a man and woman who desire to enter into matrimony and who possess nothing with which to celebrate their marriage, the House of the Hospital is accustomed to give two bowls (*escuels*) or the rations of two brethren....

5. And the almoner [*officer in charge of distributing charity*] is accustomed to give twelve deniers to each prisoner, when he is first released from prison.

6. Every night five clerics are accustomed to read the psalter for the bene-factors of the House.

7. And every day thirty poor persons are accustomed to be fed at table once a day for the love of God, and the five clerics aforesaid may be among those thirty poor persons, but the twenty-five eat before the Convent and each of the five clerics shall have two deniers and eat with the Convent.

8. And on three days in the week they are accustomed to give in alms to all who come there to ask for it, bread and wine and cooked food.

9. In Lent, every Saturday, they are accustomed to celebrate maundy [*washing the feet of the poor in commemoration of Christ's washing of his disciples' feet at the Last Supper*] for thirteen poor persons, and to wash their feet, and to give to each a shirt and new breeches and new shoes, and to three chaplains, or to three clerics out of the thirteen, three deniers and to each of the others, two deniers.

10. These are the special charities decreed in the Hospital, apart from the Brethren-at-Arms [*the military brethren*] whom the Hospital should maintain honorably, and many other charities there are which cannot be set out in detail each one by itself....

95. THE ORGANIZATION AND ETHOS OF A MEDIEVAL HOSPITAL (2): THE HÔTEL-DIEU IN PARIS

The Book of the Active Life of the Hôtel-Dieu *was written for the dedicated religious women who ran the great hospital of Paris by Jehan Henry (d. 1482), canon and cantor of Notre-Dame de Paris, member of the king's council, and president of the Chambre des Enquêtes or exchequer. From 1471–79 and 1482–84, he served as* proviseur *or external overseer of the Hôtel-Dieu, as part of an initiative to clean up the hospital's finances. In his latter capacity, he exercised spiritual and temporal authority over the personnel and property of the hospital. Given that the poem was written at a time when the reputation of the Hôtel-Dieu was stained by scandal and mismanagement, it is tempting to see the author as a reformer. On the other hand, Henry's dedication and* envoi, *addressed to the sub-prioress Sister Perrenelle Hélène, radiate genuine admiration and tenderness. He saw himself as part of the hospital community; in the author portrait in the principal surviving manuscript, he is shown presenting his book to Sister Mercy and being anointed with her "ointment of pity" to carry out his functions as* proviseur.

The Book of the Active Life *is a series of allegories in which the hospital symbolizes the Church and the Church symbolizes the hospital. It illustrates the complex exchanges of spiritual benefits between caregiver and "sick poor" that fueled medieval charity. The illustrations (reproduced here from the Hôtel-Dieu's own copy, now in the Musée de l'Assistance Publique in Paris) are an integral part of the work.*

Source: trans. Faith Wallis from Jehan Henry, *Livre de vie active de l'Hôtel Dieu de Paris* (ca 1482–83), in Marcel Candille. *Étude du Livre de vie active de l'Hôtel Dieu de Paris de Jehan Henry XVe siècle* (Paris: S.P.E.I, 1964), pp. 20–24, 33–34; illustrations pp. 45 and 57. Middle French.

This is the *Book of the Active Life*, by Master Jehan Henry, counsellor of our lord the king and president of the court of the Parlement, canon of the church and *proviseur* of the Hôtel-Dieu of Paris. Its subject is the offices of the said Hôtel-Dieu, wherein are exercised the principal operations of the active life, which consist in the accomplishing of the works of mercy....

In his prologue, the author explains that his treatise is divided into four books, because the maison-Dieu (book 1) is the symbol of three other houses: the Church (book 2), the rational soul (book 3), and paradise (book 4). He begins with an exegesis of the opening illumination.

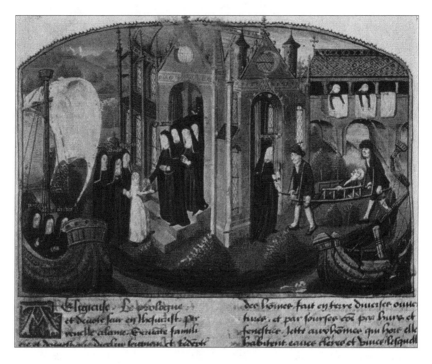

In the first part we shall treat principally of the religious house of hospitality, specially dedicated to the exercise of the works of corporal mercy, which are exercised with compassion and charity, night and day, by holy religious persons on behalf of the poor sick members of Jesus Christ. And this first part will contain the description, effect, and usefulness of Mercy, demonstrating thereby that without [Mercy] the active life cannot exercise its function in the house of righteousness and public prayer. Mercy has her principal residence and permanent home in the house of her daughter Almsgiving, who applies the ointment of compassion, which Mercy carries enclosed in the container of her heart. You see also that this house of Almsgiving is a religious house of hospitality, located on an island surrounded by the water of tears and compassion, which is a river of salubrious water [*"saine eaue," a pun on the name of the river Seine*] of grace, which one must cross in order to enter this house of hospitality. The holy religious persons arrive there by the ship of Profession of the Rule, which holds Virginity, Poverty, and Obedience. The Holy Spirit is the patron of this ship, who by the wind of grace moves and transports them on this ship to the port of salvation. A little skiff is tied to this ship by the cord of mercy, and it carries the *proviseurs* of the house, who do not have the grace to enter the ship of Profession, but who nonetheless for the love of God intend to be of assistance to those in the ship and to the sick poor. In this hospitable house, there are two doors of olive wood, which symbolize compassion. Through one, which is the door of passive compassion, enter the sick who are suffering from their several illnesses; through the other, called the door of active compassion, enter the holy persons who suffer in their heart for the illness of others. Faith constitutes the foundation of this house, so deep that it reaches to the center of the earth where Hell lies. Hope constitutes the walls, so high that they reach above the heavens. And charity constitutes its summit and roof, so wide that it suffices by itself to cover all the sick who ever have been or will be.

Part Two develops an allegory of the Church as spiritual hospital but also allows us to catch a glimpse of the topography and routine of the actual Hôtel-Dieu. The portress acts as a triage nurse, assigning patients to the New Hall if they require intensive care, the Hall of St Denis if the condition is not life-threatening, and the lying-in ward if they are destitute women about to give birth.

In the second principal part, which treats of the works of corporal mercy that are exercised in this religious house of God, mention will be made of the works of spiritual mercy which are exercised in the second house of God, called the Church, and symbolized by this house of mercy. And to this end, in describing how those who are sick with bodily ailments are received, given treatment and bandaged in the house of alms, it will be declared how those who are sick with spiritual ailments, be they mortal, venial, or original [*that is, sin*] are received, given treatment, and brought back to spiritual health in this Church and house of God by religious men and holy ministers. And see here how human spirits, ailing from spiritual ailments, arrive by a light and fragile vessel called the human body, badly equipped, and shattered by the violent agitation of the waves and storms of the sea of this world, from the western sea, and steer to the east along the coast, by the salubrious water of Grace. And [see] how they are received in the merciful house of God, which is the Church, whose doors are always open to receive those who, coming from the west, return to the east along the salubrious water of Grace from the sea of this world. And there they find Hospitality the portress, who through Conscience, who accompanies the sick with all discretion, knows at a glance and discerns the types and qualities of the sick. According to whether they are grievously or slightly ill, she assigns them room and lodging in the said hostel. For if they are smitten with mortal illness, she sends them to the infirmary hall, to the low bed of humility, called the New Hall, so that there the sick can be renewed and recover from their state of spiritual sickness to a state of spiritual health through the ministry of the *chevetaine* [*sister who supervises the ward*] Penitence, accompanied by the sisters

Contrition and Satisfaction, who in this infirmary minister drugs from the pharmacy of Grace to the sick, by which they are restored to spiritual health. Contrition dresses the wounds of the sick with her heart, Confession with the mouth, and Satisfaction with the works of reparation. Confession treats with *purgative medicines through the mouth; Satisfaction, by fasting and prayer, by alms and other works both virtuous and difficult, serves restorative and strengthening *electuaries. And if shortness of time does not suffice for the operation of these electuaries, so that the penitent when he leaves this hostel of God is not detained in purgatory and can be taken directly to the place of repose of the Holy Innocents [*the main cemetery in Paris*], Satisfaction, by a full apostolic indulgence, borrows from the coffer of the treasury of the house of God syrups and restorative medicines made principally from the precious blood and merits of Jesus Christ and generally from the merits of all the holy people who have ever been in the house of God. And if the sick who arrive at the door of the hostel of God are sick with a light and venial sickness, which is not a deadly disease, the portress directs them to the Hall of St Denis. Fervent Devotion presides there, and she heals such light and venial diseases. As for those who are sick with original disease [*that is, original sin*], who are carried, as in a hood, in their mother's womb by poor mothers who know not where to empty the contents of their hood, the portress sends them to the Hall of Birthing Mothers. There Baptism is in charge, who heals them each and all of original sin by a bath. At the entrance of the hostel of God are two ladies, Holy Prayer and Oblation (in charge of triage), who help the sick by directing them to the Hall of Penitence. And Examination of Conscience, the ladies' servant, draws the water of tears from the well of the heart, and with his broom of recollection of the sick, gathers together the dirt of the hostel, in order to throw it out of the house. See there the office of Revulsion-against-Guilt, the keeper of the accounts; she puts the sheets and bedding of affliction, on which the sick have rested in their illness, into the hands of Compunction, mistress of the great laundry, to be scrubbed clean in the hot water of tears, mixed with the ashes which bring remembrance of death.

Part Three compares the Hospital to the rational soul. This is the subject of the second large illumination in the manuscript, which shows the sisters being instructed by the Cardinal Virtues. They are Supervising Sisters over the four wards of the hospital, each devoted to the cure of a particular faculty of the soul that is stricken by vice. The divisions of the soul are Platonic: reason, concupiscibility or desire, irascibility or arousal, and will.

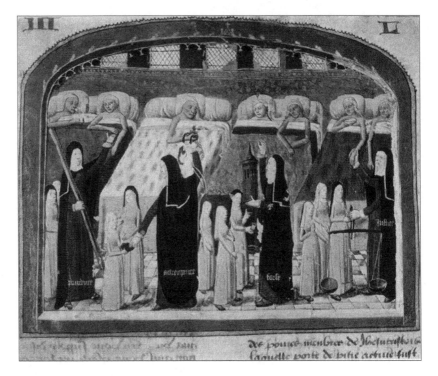

In the third principal part, the house of God, which contains the sick and the healthy, will be understood to represent the rational soul, which in its four parts was wounded and made sick by the guilt of the first father [Adam], from whose seed springs the whole human race. In the first division of this house of God is Reason, sick with the disease of ignorance; over this division presides Prudence, principal *chevetaine*, with her rule, accompanied by many ladies. In the second division of this house of God is Concupiscibility, sick with the disease of disordered concupiscence for mutable goods. And there Temperance, second principal *chevetaine*, presides, accompanied by many ladies. In the third division lies Irascibility, sick and infirm, so feeble that he cannot tolerate anything that discourages him and flees every kind of danger, even death. But there is Courage, the principal *chevetaine*, accompanied by many ladies who heal him of this infirmity. In the fourth division is Will, ill with the disease called malice which craves what is contrary to it, rather than what is to its benefit and advantage. But Justice, the fourth *chevetaine*, who measures all in her just scales, brings him back to health.

While Jehan Henry's approach is resolutely contemplative and allegorical, he provides his reader with some touching vignettes of the work of the real nursing sisters.

When one sees the [sisters] hold poor sick folk, one hand on their head and another on their back, as they use the toilet, and who clean the chamber pots, and wash their dirty feet and their dirty underclothes, pare their nails, cut their hair and carry them, stinking as they are, from one bed to another, and often bury the dead....

Daughter, know that the work of this house is very difficult, for day passes into night and night into day as one watches over the sick poor, to wash their feet, pare their nails, cut their hair, take them to the toilet, clean them, help them to their feet, lay them down, bathe them, wipe them, feed them, give them drink, carry them from one bed to another, cover them up again and again, re-make their beds, rinse every day their underclothes, warm the linen that goes on their feet, launder eight or nine hundred sheets every week, rinse them in clear water, boil them in the tub, collect ashes, stoke the furnace with wood, wash the sheets in the Seine in frost, wind, or rain, spread them out to dry on the galleries in the summer, and in the winter before a great fire, fold them, bury the dead, and innumerable other laborious and difficult services....

96. THE ORGANIZATION AND ETHOS OF A MEDIEVAL HOSPITAL (3): A TWELFTH-CENTURY ENGLISH LEPER HOSPITAL

The century following the First Crusade coincided with a period of spiritual experimentation and enthusiasm for the "apostolic life" that affected every level of society. One consequence was the foundation of hospitals in western Europe as agencies of practical charity and embodiments of the desire for the consecrated life of service. The statutes of the leper hospital of St Mary Magdalene in Dudston, west of Gloucester, may be the oldest surviving statutes of an English hospital; formerly dated to 1155, they are now thought to have been composed at the end of the century at the earliest. Dudston is both like and unlike the Temple hospital, in that its patients constitute a stable quasi-monastic community of resident "brothers and sisters." The statutes claim, without foundation, to be modeled on those devised by Bishop Ivo of Chartres (d. 1115). It should be noted that there is no concern with communicability of the disease, and no moral commentary on the leper's condition (see doc. 69).

Source: trans. Edward J. Kealy, *Medieval Medicus: A Social History of Anglo-Norman Medicine* (Baltimore and London: The Johns Hopkins University Press, 1981), pp. 108–9 (original Latin text on pp. 200–201).

This is the rule of the sick of Dudston prepared by Ivo, the great bishop of Chartres, a man of finest judgment.

1. Before all and above all obedience, patience, chastity, and common property must be observed by the sick.

2. The men should be separated from the women and not go into the house of the women, nor the women into that of the men without permission of the master.

3. On feast days a chapter should be held for the sick about noon time where faults can be corrected.

4. On Sundays, Tuesdays, and Thursdays let them eat meat, if possible. However, on other days they should abstain, unless the celebration of a feast supervenes.

5. However, if anyone should murmur about an insufficient supply of food or drink, let him be rebuked up to the third time. Afterwards, if he complains, let his draught of beer be withheld from him until he makes satisfaction, because on account of complaining the sons of Israel died in the desert.

6. Even if the brothers and sisters possess more than two sets of clothing, let those also be of one color, namely black, white, or russet, not several colors.

7. Those who are accepted as brothers and sisters should promise stability in the house and obedience to the master who presides.

8. The sick should not go outdoors alone, nor should they wander about the streets, but let them go with a servant or companion in good order where they have been instructed to go.

9. The sick should not talk after compline [*the final office of prayer of the evening*], except for those who are altogether bedridden.

10. They should not talk in the church, except in the chapter when business affairs are being transacted.

11. If someone is denounced, prostrate let him seek pardon and humbly confess if he admits the complaint, or deny it if he is not guilty.

12. For the customary discipline of the master in such a case, let him impose a penance of beatings or fasting. However, if anyone refuses to accept discipline, as it is in the Cistercian Order, let him be expelled from the community.

13. If anyone falls into open fornication, let him be expelled from the community without any mercy.

14. If anyone is quarrelsome with the master, let him be sternly corrected; if he does this habitually, he should be thrown out.

15. Guests who are sick should be received charitably and entertained for one night according to the ability of the house.

16. At dawn everyone should rise for divine office and hear the matins of the day and of Saint Mary.

17. However, in place of matins laymen can say twenty-four Our Fathers. For each hour let them say the Our Father five times; instead of vespers, seven times; in place of compline, five times.

18. They should eat twice a day except on principal fasts, but at the proper time. All should know the Our Father, Hail Mary, and Apostles' Creed.

19. If anyone who is in good health should dedicate himself to the service of the sick, let him promise obedience and chastity and live as the warden of the sick directs.

20. No one should speak at table, unless about necessary things, nor should anyone presume to talk after compline except about necessary business of the house.

21. No one should go out into the town or village without the permission of the master and the master should carefully inquire into the business for which such a person goes.

22. And if anyone goes out before breakfast, he should come back for breakfast. And if he goes out after breakfast he should return for vespers. Whoever will not accept this regulation, should lose his special meal treat for twenty days.

23. No brother should be found with any sister, nor sister with any brother, in the cellar, or in the larder, or in the orchard, or in the field, under similar mealtime penalty of forty days.

Thus ends the rule of the sick prepared by Ivo, the great bishop of Chartres.

97. MEDICAL CARE IN A MEDIEVAL HOSPITAL (1): THE JERUSALEM HOSPITAL

The great Hospital established in Jerusalem after the First Crusade under the supervision of the Order of the Hospital of St John was a source of admiration throughout the Latin world (see doc. 94). Several twelfth-century pilgrims to the Holy Land have left us descriptions of the physical arrangement of the Hospital and its medical and religious routine. This document is an anonymous tract by a cleric, who probably visited the Holy Land shortly before 1187. The text is divided into three "distinctions." The first is an encomium of charity, the second a description of the Jerusalem Hospital, and the third breaks off in the middle of a tirade against wealthy pilgrims who exploit the free accommodation offered by the Hospital.

The tract reveals many intriguing details about the Hospital: for example, it accepted patients with any condition except leprosy and also took in Muslims and Jews. The medical services of the Hospital are described in terms of the new twelfth-century medicine. The doctors are described as learned in physica — *text-based medical doctrine grounded in the principles of natural philosophy; they are even (and rather unusually) called "theorists"* (theorici, theoretici) *and distinguished from the surgeons and phlebotomists. The author is particularly struck by the advantages of having the medical staff salaried by the Hospital: hospitals in the West, even in the late Middle Ages, almost never kept doctors on staff, and doctors who attended in the hospitals frequently did so* gratis.

Source: trans. Faith Wallis from the transcription of MS Munich, Bayerische Staatsbibliothek CLM 4620 fols. 132v–139v by B.Z. Kedar, "A Twelfth-Century Description of the Jerusalem Hospital," in *The Military Orders II: Welfare and Warfare* (Aldershot: Ashgate, 1998), pp. 20–22. Latin.

Here Begins the Second Distinction, Which Shows What and How Much and What Kind of Attention Is Given to the Sick in the Hospital

In the first place, the sick poor hold the highest rank in the aforementioned Hospital, whatever infirmity they suffer from. Only leprosy is excluded, which because of some inexplicable repugnance felt by all humanity, is shunned as hateful and, denied community with others, is segregated in the by-way, as it were, of solitude. But for everyone else, tormented by the suffering of whatever infirmity and needing the care of a stranger so that they can recover, or the service of another so that they may eat, or the support of another so that they may walk — indeed, for anyone who is deprived of the functioning of their natural strength, whether in their whole body or in any part, divine aid is tenderly provided. And just as "God is no acceptor of persons" [Acts 10:34] the sick are gathered together in this House out of every nation, every social condition, and both sexes, so that by the mercy of the Lord the number of lords increase in proportion to the multitude of languages. Indeed, knowing well that the Lord invites all to salvation and wishes none to perish [Ezek. 18:32], men of pagan religion find mercy within this holy House if they flock thither and even Jews, for whom the Lord prayed even as they were torturing him, "Father, pay no heed to them, for they know not what they do." [Luke 23:34] ... Again, if the vital energies of the sick poor are so exhausted that they cannot go to the Hospital of St John by their own efforts, they are charitably sought out within the city, and humbly transported by the Hospital servitors. The sick who flock to the holy Hospital are first offered the divine remedy: for the rash of their sins having been revealed and the health-giving medicine of penance having been received from the priests who reside there, they are refreshed with heavenly food [of the Mass]. Then they are admitted to the *palacium* by one of the brethren of the Hospital. For one brother is appointed to receive the sick with patience and kindness, according to the word of the Apostle: "Receive the sick, and show patience towards all." [1 Thess. 5:4] When they are brought into the *palacium*, they are laid down on feather cushions on beautifully wrought beds and lest they be troubled by the coldness or hardness of the pavement, they are placed between white linen sheets, with sewn cushions, and are covered with fleecy blankets. And lest they be harmed by the roughness of other coverings or constricted by the cold, cloaks are handed out to them … which they can wear when they must attend to the call of nature, and goat-skin slippers, lest any dirt stick to their feet when they arise or the cold marble do harm to their soles.

Concerning the Masters of the Wards, and the Attendants [*clientes*]

The *palacium* of the sick is divided into eleven wards, sometimes augmented by two additional ones. For it has happened on a number of occasions that when the space within the *palacium* proves insufficient for the multitude of the suffering, the dormitory of the brethren is taken over by the sick and the brethren themselves sleep on the floor. Each ward is under the supervision of one of the brethren, who humbly receives the sick as they arrive, puts them into bed in the manner described above, and diligently takes care of each patient's personal effects, which are handed back to the sick when they recover. But human inadequacy makes it impossible for a single person to handle so many tasks, and so twelve supporting attendants are assigned to the brethren who preside over the wards. For every ward, there is a brother who is master over it and a "follower." These twelve attendants are supported by the revenues of the House for as long as they serve within it and when they leave, they are gratified with money. Their job is to watch over their patients with diligent care in such a way that not even one of them so much as goes forth from the door of the *palacium* without the permission of his master. They have to make the beds of the sick, that is, to plump up the pillows by turning them over, because the feathers become hard when they are pressed together. They must spread out the sheets, put the sick to bed, cover them, get them up, transfer the weaker ones to other beds; carry them hither and yon under the arms as often as needful; minister water to the hands of the sick with a towel in a respectful manner; lay out the food which is to be eaten on felt [mats]; bring bread in baskets, which by the brethren of the house is laid out for the sick in equal portions, namely two loaves for each two [people] – one ordinary, for all who are residing in that House in separate communion, another particular one made for the use of the sick…. Wine is brought to them by the brethren, the servitors adapting the vessels into which it is poured, and the servitors are also called upon to prepare delicate dishes in the private kitchen. For the sick have two kitchens, one common to both male and female patients, and the other private. In the common kitchen, the coarser dishes are prepared, such as pork, mutton, and the like, on Sunday, Tuesday and Thursday throughout the seasons, when they eat meat by the indulgence of our law.

A detailed description of the diet of the sick follows.

Concerning the Four Learned Physicians [*theoretici*] on Staff

But because those who are ignorant of *physica* of the lower world can certainly not, unless by blind chance, determine the *temperament of many things ... the holy Hospital convent commits its sick to the faithful skill of the learned (*theoreticorum*) and the care of practitioners (*practicorum*) in a manner both holy and prudent. Holy: lest in this house of God anything be wanting for the ailing human capability fail to be furnished for their advantage. Prudent: lest curable diseases become incurable by persisting in similar things or by harmful contrary things and thus the patient find in these [things] kindling for feebleness or causes of death, where he hoped for the means of healing. For the sake, then, of avoiding notorious danger, there are in the hospital four doctors learned in *physica*, salaried by the House, so that they not presume any unconventional treatment upon the sick of the Hospital; and they are bound by an oath that they should look to the Hospital for whatever they think necessary for the wellbeing of their patients, whether it be *electuaries or other medicines, regardless of anyone else's suggestion or dissuasion. For on his own [account] the doctors supply no medications to the sick, but supply everything to them from the House. The physicians are dispersed throughout the wards so that each knows individually the patients he has to treat − lest one of them should despise the tedious multitude of one ward with respect to another or else lest by a confused commingling in the same ward they constantly run up against one another, or else pass over [a patient] without treating him on a certain day because they relied on another to do it. They are obliged to visit their patients every day in the morning and the late afternoon, and to inspect the urines and the qualities of the pulses according to the principles of their art. When they arrive to visit the patients, each of them brings along two "followers" from the ward which he is about to perambulate and when he has perambulated the first [ward] he takes another two from the next, and so on, so that one can carry the syrup, *oximel, *electuaries, and other medicines administered to the poor, and the other can show the urines, discard them after they have been judged, clean out the urine flasks, diligently learn (along with his servant) what diet the physician has prescribed for each [patient], and accompany the *phlebotomist to his patients or his patients to the phlebotomist.

The Phlebotomists of the Sick

The patients have their own phlebotomist, who is supposed to bleed them every day, at any hour. These are salaried by the blessed House, just as the physicians are. In the same way, the sick take food which is pre-assigned to them, but also much more, following the considered discretion of the physicians. For which reason, according to the general prohibition of the doctors, certain foods are never offered to those who are in the Hospital, such as beans, lentils, squills, murena, or even breeding-sows. For as the common assertion of the physicians holds, meats from the female of the more humid animals, compared to those from males of the same species, are found to be tougher, coarser, more viscous, and less digestible. Hence it happens that while meats of this kind can be administered to the healthy, they ought never to be given to the sick, which is redolent of the divine mercy towards all.

The Surgeons of the Hospital

And so that the glorious Hospital may never cease to display the manifold grace of piety towards its patients, it has (besides the above mentioned learned doctors) salaried surgeons, so that they may have the care of as many of the wounded as may resort thither. And truly, they do resort, because not only in Jerusalem, but also indeed whenever the Christian people of Jerusalem set forth on an expedition against the pagans, those wounded in [battle] take refuge in hospital tents as if claiming the right of asylum. There they receive full treatment, insofar as this is possible in that place. And those not cured there are transported on camels, horses, mules, and donkeys to the Hospital in Jerusalem or to a shelter closer at hand where they are taken care of as if in the Hospital. And if the beasts of burden belonging to the Hospital are insufficient for transporting the wounded, the wounded mount the horses of the brethren themselves, while the brethren, even those of noble birth, accompany them on foot due to this critical necessity, so that thus openly they might demonstrate that they appropriate nothing to themselves, but that all they have is at the disposal of the sick. According to this course, with this piety, with this instinct of charity, the blessed Hospital retains salaried practicing physicians (*practicantes theoricos*), as well as surgeons and phlebotomists....

98. MEDICAL CARE IN A MEDIEVAL HOSPITAL (2): JOHN OF MIRFELD AT ST BARTHOLOMEW'S HOSPITAL, LONDON

The Breviary of Bartholomew *(*Breviarium Bartholomei*) of John of Mirfeld (d. 1407) is a scrapbook of extracts from Galen, Hippocrates, John of Gaddesden, Bernard of Gordon, Avicenna, Platearius, Gilbert the Englishman, and Mesue, assembled for use by the staff of St Bartholomew's Hospital in Smithfield, London. It covers nearly every aspect of medicine and surgery, including the diseases of women and children. The staff of St Bartholomew's were not formally trained doctors, and neither was John. He may have been a chaplain, and what he reveals of his attitude toward his project is consonant with the distinctive vocation of the medieval hospital. The preface of the* Breviary *reproduced below stresses the charitable orientation of hospital care, but one can also hear echoes of the origins of monastic medicine in the self-sufficiency of the Roman gentleman and householder (see doc. 8). The chapter on prognosis illustrates the abiding concern of medieval caregivers with recognizing the signs of impending death, so that the appropriate rites of confession and reception of the sacrament might be administered in time (see doc. 11). It is in the main a suite of extracts from Hippocrates's* Prognosis, *Rhazes's* Book for Almansor *10.21, and Avicenna's* Canon *4.2.1, interlarded with verses from the* Salerno Regimen of Health *(doc. 99). But it closes with some empirical, and even "magical," prognostic techniques.*

The Breviary's *companion volume, the* Flower-Garden of Bartholomew *(*Florarium Bartholomei*) is a theological compendium – a handbook of spiritual health.*

Source: trans. Percival Horton-Smith Hartley and Harold Richard Aldridge, *Johannes de Mirfeld of St Bartholomew's, Smithfield; His Life and Works* (Cambridge: Cambridge University Press, 1936), pp. 47–53, 55–63, 67–69. Latin.

Preface

In the beginning of this compilation, as in all our labors, let us offer to God the thanks due to his excellent greatness and to the multitude of his mercies; in whose goodness confiding, I have found and gathered together certain noteworthy matters of a medical nature culled from various sources, such as texts and glosses of the art of medicine, as well as the works of many writers who have treated of this science skillfully and fully; and, since I now merely retain these things in my mind, from whence they are prone to slip away, I have endeavored, at the instigation of certain of my friends, and according to my ability, to collect them together and to set them down in an abridged form; partly because if once they are allowed to slide away from my aforesaid short memory they cannot easily be recovered again by so unskilled a student as myself, and partly because when once brought together, as it were, into a storehouse of moderate size, they may easily be found....

Peradventure, however, somebody will say to me, "How can you make ready to write about a subject in which you have not received proper instruction, and have not known hitherto what it means to occupy the position of a pupil? From this you would appear to heed not the words of the Commentator on the *Viaticum* [of Constantine the African] when he says, 'The art of healing is the only one which all men everywhere appropriate to themselves, and which they all pretend to know, mangle, and expound!' You should consider, therefore, what the blessed Jerome says, when, writing to the monk named Rusticus [*Letter* 125], he thus addresses him: 'Do not speedily blossom forth as an author, or be led away by your light-minded enthusiasm; but receive instruction for a long time, so that you may be able to teach what is correct!'"

I can, indeed, briefly and truthfully reply to this objection, by admitting my own shortcomings; for it is not fitting that I should write in the manner of one about to teach: but if in order to provide a support for my unreliable memory, I should desire to gather together certain noteworthy medical facts and to write them all together into one breviary so that this may serve as a repository for me, I do not believe that anybody ought reasonably to look askance at me upon such an account....

There is also another reason for writing this book. It has frequently happened that I have experienced the fraudulent practices of modern physicians, either when I myself needed their services, or when my friends were ill. Some of these practitioners were led by avarice to promise that they would cure a disease concerning which they were ignorant. Some impudently exacted a high price for medicines of little efficacy or intrinsic value: whilst others of the breed protracted the treatment over a considerable period, in cases where the infirmity could have been healed within a few days, just in order that they might have their patients as tributaries for a long time. Wherefore it seemed to me that it was both necessary as well as useful that I should (as has been said above) write down within one breviary the various remedies applicable to each disease; so that, wherever I might come, I might by this means be able to escape impostors of this kind, and might be able to relieve not only myself, but all the other poor followers of Christ, who should happen to be afflicted by those diseases that are not serious but curable. Nor should one omit here the consideration of how the action of a medicine is frequently changed according to the peculiar nature of the subject for treatment: therefore I propose, in a good many cases, to set down in this compilation several medicines for one and the same disease, since it is a peculiarity of medicaments that at one time they are beneficial, and at another time they are not – a fact which is a matter for wonder! This diversity of effect is perhaps due to the influence of a man's natal planet.

Moreover, I wish it to be known, that in many instances in this compilation, I propose to make use of *experiments, both because they are speedy in operation, and because many patients in these modern days are particularly impatient, and are unwilling to wait until the fourth or fifth day or more for the morbid matter in the body to be *digested and usefully *evacuated, as was the custom in the olden days: for in truth, unless such people feel relief immediately on the first day, they distrust their physician and despise and reject his prescriptions.

And note that the significance of the word "experiment" is twofold, namely, an experiment deriving its strength from reason or one which lacks this quality. Of the former it is said that an experiment is that which has been discovered by the intelligence of prudent men and it is with this type alone that we propose to deal here: but an experiment, which has not been thus approved, is fearsome and deceptive, as both Hippocrates [in *Aphorisms* 1.1] and John Damascene [in his *Aphorisms*] maintain.

Since, indeed, in any kind of treatise, prolixity begets aversion, dulls the acuteness of the intellect, and confuses the memory; and since, moreover, the nature of anything becomes more obvious by its division into sections; and, as the Philosopher [Aristotle] says in his book *On Memory* [2, 452a], those things, which possess an ordered arrangement, are easiest recalled to mind: therefore, I have considered it advisable to divide this present compilation (which I desire should be known as the *Breviary of Bartholomew*) into fifteen principal parts, and to subdivide each of these into appropriate chapters, so that whatever is sought may the more readily be found.

Wherefore, in the first part, I shall, with the grace of Christ helping me, treat of *fevers: in the second, of all the other general diseases that attack the whole body, or at least, the greater portion of the body. The third part will deal with the infirmities of whole of the head, neck, and throat, as far down as the upper part of the chest; and the fourth part with diseases of the innermost parts of the chest and its contents; also with the arms and hands. The fifth part will deal with affections of the body in the regions situated between the chest and the genitals; the sixth part being concerned with these latter. The seventh will treat of all troubles from the anus downwards to the extremities of both feet. Part eight will deal with abscesses; part nine with wounds and all that pertains to them; part ten with fractures of the bones; and part eleven with dislocations of the joints. In part twelve we shall treat of *simple, and in part thirteen of compound medicines. Part fourteen will be concerned with laxatives and *purgations for the noxious *humors; whilst in part fifteen will be found advice on *phlebotomy, the regimen of health, and many other things, as will appear later....

Part 1, Distinction 6, Chapter 19. Concerning the Signs of Evil Portent Appearing in Feverish and Other Types of Patients

When you visit your patient, you must bear in mind first of all the matters to which you should give heed, such as paying due regard to his countenance, and opening his mouth and looking at his tongue; moreover, his eyes and nails must be inspected, and consideration must be given to many other matters connected with him, which will be set forth below. Wherefore, indeed, it should be known that of those signs of evil portent that manifest themselves in the eyes and features of the sick, some appear within the three first days of the onset of the disease, and others appear later.

Of such evil symptoms, those that sometimes appear within the first three days are these: the eyes are hollowed, the temples sunken, the forehead dry and tense; the nostrils pinched; the ears cold, with the lobes turned outward and contracted; the color livid, greenish or black, or something similar. If these symptoms appear at the commencement of the disease, and by reason of the virulence of the malady itself, then death is signified, especially if the stools be very loose and the urine oily: but this is not the case if they appear later. If, however, the appearance of these signs in the opening stages is due, not to the severity of the disease itself, but rather to its accidents, such as sleeplessness, or frequency of stools, lack of food, and the like, then evil is not thus portended. Moreover, if all these aforesaid symptoms appear after the first three days and result from the disease itself, or if they develop a good deal later during its course, then they are not of ill omen; because if they do not make an appearance until after a considerable lapse of time, then this is a matter neither of wonderment nor of concern. It must, however, be understood, that if such symptoms do appear after the commencement of the disease and accompanied by pronounced weakness, death may thus be signified, although not so effectually as when the appearance occurs at the beginning: for it is reasonable to assume that the body of the patient has been wasted away owing to the process of time; and it would, indeed, be a bad sign if such were not the case.

Of those signs of evil import, which appear in the features of the patient, there are some that show themselves later than the outset of the disease, such as on the fourth day or afterwards. They are as follows. The patient cannot bear to gaze upon a lighted candle and he sheds involuntary tears, whilst the eyes appear to squint and one seems smaller than the other: or the whites of the eyes appear bloodshot and the veins black, swarthy, or sallow, the eyes inflamed, and the eyeballs protruding or sunken, whilst the whole aspect of the face is unsightly and horrible to look upon. These symptoms, I say, all signify death in most cases and they are of worse import than those mentioned in the first place; they can also appear at the outset, but this, however, rarely happens.

We may, therefore, it would seem, conclude that whenever and wherever, at the outset or later, all these last-mentioned symptoms appear on account of the fury of the disease and the weakness of the constitution, then most assuredly death is betokened. And to the aforesaid we may add some other indications of death; namely, if the whites of the patient's eyes appear during sleep, without his being able to see anything; if he has lost all his sense of taste and is totally unable to discern those things, which he was once accustomed to perceive; and if he can smell nothing; and if the teeth also, as well as the tongue, appear dry. These and similar tokens portend not merely an approaching death, but death within the doors. With such cases, therefore, do not meddle. Let your prognosis be given and then retire.

Taken note of the following verses [from the *Salerno Regimen of Health*] indicative of a fatal termination:

> When all these various symptoms in the patient do appear
> Then you may safely prophesy that death at hand is near!
> Dusky glows the brow, first the soles of the feet wax cold,
> The dreadful hour of death is by the unwished tears foretold!
> Downward sags the chin; then pales to its tip the nose,
> The belly rigid turns; the left pupil smaller grows.
> Watch too for signs in sleep; for you can surely tell,
> That Death doth strike a grey-beard who sleeps too sound and well,
> Likewise the youth who night and day gains no repose at all,
> Or if perchance priapism holds the sufferer in its thrall!
> If white the urine be, when *tertian, *synocha, or *causus rages,
> In pleurisy or frenzy too, this death, alas, presages!
> And when the sick be stricken with paralysis or *dropsy,
> With *consumption, *apoplexy, or with dysentery as well,
> Then if the urine red appear of patients thus afflicted,
> Alas, their plight is hopeless; you can merely death foretell!

Moreover, if the patient lies prostrate on his back, it is the worst possible sign and indicates a vitality at its lowest ebb. Likewise it is a bad sign to find the patient lying face downwards, for this indicates either excessive pain or delirium. And if he should lie with arms and feet rigid, this is an evil omen because it points to the presence of spasm. And if, after a sleep, or at other times, he suddenly turns himself about in a disorderly fashion, changing for example from the head to the foot of his bed, this shows delirium and bodily weakness; and if he lies stretched out with his mouth open and his feet twisted, this is grave, because it indicates spasm. And if he is suddenly constrained to rise up or to stand erect, this is grave, because it is due to suffocation arising from constriction of the respiratory passages. And if his hands are continually trying to pull straws or hairs or the like out of the bedclothes or from the wall – especially if his reason be affected, so that he is unaware of what he is doing – then this is the worst possible sign, for it signifies the final consuming and *mortification. Again, a drawing up of the lips, hands, or penis is bad, because this indicates spasm. Also, since the nails are generated from the *vapors coming forth from the heart, the vigor or decline of the latter organ may be ascertained most readily by an examination of the former of these members: for if the heat in the heart be insufficient, then the nails grow black, pale, or livid; so that by their change or contraction they present and show forth the withdrawal of the heat, and the departure of life. Wherefore it is said that a black or greenish color in the nails, accompanied by other grave symptoms, and occurring before the signs of maturation [*the* *"ripening" of the diseased matter*], is an evil thing and denotes death.

Again, if the respiration be feeble and shallow, or if it be labored and hurried, or accompanied by sounds within the chest, this is a bad symptom and points to death. When, however, a black vomit appears at the beginning of a disease, most assuredly death is signified. All vomiting of whatever description, if it occur after the symptoms of the maturation of the disease, and which brings alleviation to the patient, is good and praiseworthy, since it comes as a cleansing agent; therefore any natural vomiting, which thus alleviates, should not be checked, unless it be excessive. Vomiting of blood, however, accompanied by continual fever, is the worst possible symptom and is also mortal. Again, if live worms appear in the stools at the commencement of the disease, this is an evil symptom, because it signifies that the corruption of the body is so great that the worms have been unable to bear with it, and have taken to flight; if the worms be dead, then this is a good sign, because it would seem that their appearance is the result of a cleansing. If, however, the worms arrive dead at the close of the illness, then this is a grave matter, for they would seem to have been done to death by the malignity of the disease: if they be alive in such a case all is well, for they would seem to burst forth as a result of the cleansing of the patient. Again, perspiration supervening in a case of fever before the signs of maturation, is of evil import; likewise death is portended by a cold sweat, which appears in an acute disease: if it occur in a lengthy illness, it signifies that death is afar off....

Another mortal sign is the appearance upon the patient's knee of a black pustule, that is, one with a blackish edging. Moreover, it is significant of evil when those actions which normally occasion embarrassment, such as the uncovering of the pudenda or the audible expulsion of flatus from the bowel by the patient, occur [without perturbing him]. ʼQuinsy, again, with very acute fever, is most harmful.

Again, another symptom of death is when the eyes are dull and the eyelids not properly closed. Another sign of ill omen is the uttering by the patient of the names of those no longer living; and if hiccoughs follow, the result will be lamentable. Moreover, if the eye suddenly turns yellowish or black; or if the patient is choked so that he cannot swallow his saliva; then these symptoms are fateful. And when grains the size of a chick-pea appear on the tongue in conjunction with very acute fever, the patient will die at dawn on the following day....

Also, Avicenna advises the physician that, when he visits his patient, he should carry in his hand a twig of vervain and enquire of the patient, "How does this feel to you?" If he shall answer, "It is pleasant to me," then he will recover; but if, on the contrary, he shall say, "It is bad," then he will not escape. Also, the Experimenter [*Rhazes*] states that if, unknown to the patient, artemisia [*mugwort*] be placed underneath his head, then, if he shall sleep, he will live; if he do otherwise, he shall die.

Again, if the hand of the patient be rubbed with yeast, and then this be offered to a dog, if the dog eats it, then the patient will be restored to health; if not, he will die....

Again, carefully anoint all over the sole of the patient's right foot with lard and then throw the lard to a dog. If the dog eats it without vomiting, then the patient will live, but if the dog returns it or makes no attempt to eat it, then the patient will die. Again, mix the patient's urine with the milk of a woman who has brought forth a male child: if the milk and urine mix well together, then the patient will live, but if, on the contrary, they remain separate, then he will die. Also, if the urine of the patient be poured over a green nettle, and if the nettle remain green on the next day, then the patient will live; if not, he will die very shortly....

Likewise take gum ladanum [*made from the lada shrub,* Cistus creticus] and aloes, grind up the aloes and mix with the ladanum and then make therewith a candle, and place it to the nostrils of the dying patient; who, when he feels the heat penetrate through to his brain, will open his eyes; then ask him whatever you desire, and he will speak to you, whilst he retains consciousness. But of this I have not made proof....

Moreover, if there is any doubt as to whether a person is or is not dead, apply lightly roasted onion to his nostrils, and if he be alive, he will immediately scratch his nose.

CHAPTER FOURTEEN

THE CULTIVATION OF HEALTH: LIFESTYLE, REGIMEN, AND THE MEDICAL SELF

One of the most widely copied works of English literature in the fifteenth century was the verse Dietary *of John Lydgate (ca 1370–ca 1451). Compared with Lydgate's vast output of imaginative poetry, the* Dietary *seems pedestrian and unoriginal – it is basically a highly condensed translation of the* Salerno Regimen of Health *(doc. 99) – but its readers evidently thought that the work was interesting and valuable. The fortunes of the* Dietary *illustrate the robust appetite of late medieval people for advice on how to live a healthy life. This regimen literature is a truly medieval genre. Both the Galenic and the Hippocratic corpora contain treatises on preventive medicine, but there is little evidence that doctors actually prescribed health management plans until late antiquity. The early regimens were addressed to individuals, usually a ruler such as the Frankish king Theuderic (doc. 19).*

The great changes that overtook western medicine after the twelfth century turned this intimate genre into mass-market literature. The new regimens were grounded in the Galenic medical theory that the *"non-naturals" were causes of health as well as disease. Moreover, when diffused from the university, pronouncements of learned doctors on health went beyond mere advice: they were authoritative prescriptions for living. A money-based economy, greater social diversification, and rising literacy all drove demand for these treatises. But the demand was also connected to the religious transformations of the post-Investitures period. After the Fourth Lateran Council of 1215 mandated compulsory annual confession, clergy had to be trained to guide, interrogate, and prescribe suitable penance for individual souls. The laity, conversely, had to be instructed through sermons and handbooks concerning the nature of the virtues and vices and the steps to be taken to order their lives on Christian principles. The medicalization of daily life is the secular counterpart of the moralization of daily life; indeed, Lydgate's Dietary *addressed both dimensions. The preachers had their seven virtues and seven sins, and the doctors their six non-naturals. Canon law, the confessional, and the flowering of private piety encouraged all Christians, and not only monks, to live their lives according to rule; likewise the food one ate, the house one lived in, how one slept, exercised, made love, and even expressed emotions, were all subject to regimen. Sermons were directed to particular classes of people – students, merchants, women, and so forth – while confessors' manuals and handbooks of moral theology analyzed the distinctive vices attendant on particular ranks or professions. Medical writing followed suit, with customized regimens directed not only at kings, but also at armies in the field, or students away at college (docs. 101–102).*

Did people really follow this advice? Living as we do amid a surfeit of medical admonition, we can be forgiven for being skeptical. But perhaps the degree to which people complied with regimen is less important than their evident appetite for it. Regimen literature was the channel through which the Galenic-Arabic model of the body, health, and disease came to define a European vernacular view of the human condition. Its doctrines quietly assumed a certain authority in regulating individual and community life, and even in resolving moral questions. Being a person of "regular habits" with regard to eating, sleeping, exercise, and so forth came to denote probity and respectability as well as health. Regimen was a secular ethics, based on an ideal of moderation; at the same time it flattered individuality by adjusting for physiological ˙complexion and social circumstance. Regimen was also a marker of freedom and social status, for only people who had the power and means to make choices in their lives could follow its prescriptions. Even if their advice was ignored in practice, these texts, so ubiquitous in the late Middle Ages, speak to a significant medicalization of everyday life. They also helped to shape the European concept of the self.

99. LIFESTYLE ADVICE FOR ALL (1): THE *SALERNO REGIMEN OF HEALTH*

The poem called Salerno Regimen of Health *(*Regimen sanitatis Salernitanum*) was one of the most popular medical texts of the Middle Ages; in consequence, it survives in many different versions. The basic framework is constant: the dedication to a king of England (sometimes a king of France) prefaces a catalogue of maxims for healthy living, often structured as numbered points with mnemonic clues (for example, five tests for good wine). In practice, however, the* Salerno Regimen *was highly elastic. Verses could be added or taken out without any perceptible break in continuity, so different copies might vary in length by several hundred lines. The earliest manuscript dates from the thirteenth century; its date and place of composition are not known with certainty.*

The version translated here was accompanied by a commentary and circulated in the late Middle Ages together with Arnau of Vilanova's Regimen for the King of Aragon. *The commentary came to be ascribed to Arnau, though it was not by him, and this borrowed authority boosted its popularity. An English version by Thomas Paynell was printed in 1528. The translation below is based on a new edition in 1617 of Paynell's translation of the commentary, with a fresh translation of the poem by the industrious Elizabethan physician and "translator-general," Philemon Holland (1552–1637). As usual, this revised version of the* Regimen *was designed for a popular market, but the formal occasion of its publication was the visit of King James I to Holland's home city of Coventry. The career of the* Salerno Regimen *illustrates the ironic truth that health advice for the masses always sells best when packaged as health advice for the elite.*

Source: trans. Philemon Holland, spelling modernized and text edited by Faith Wallis, from *Regimen sanitatis Salerni. The schoole of Salernes most learned and iuditious directorie, or methodicall instructions, for the guide and gouerning the health of man* ... (London: Imprinted by Barnard Alsop, and are to be sold by Iohn Barnes, at his shop in Hosier Lane, 1617), pp. 1–98, 109. Latin.

All Salerno School thus writes to England's king,
And for man's health these fit advices bring.
Shun busy cares, rash angers, which displease;
Light supping, little drink do cause great ease.
Rise after meat, sleep not at afternoon.
Long shalt thou live, if all these well be done.

When *Physic needs, let these thy doctors be:
Good diet; quiet thoughts; heart mirthful, free.

Sleep not too long in mornings, early rise,
And with cool water wash both hands and eyes.
Walk gently forth, and stretch out every limb:
Comb head, rub teeth, and make them clean and trim.
The brain and every member else these do relieve,
And to all parts continual comfort give.
Bathing, keep warm; walk after food, or stand:
Complexions [that are] cold do gentle warmth command [*require*].

Let little sleep or none at all suffice
At afternoon, but waking keep thine eyes.
Such sleep engenders *fevers, headaches, *rheums,
Dullness of soul, and belcheth up ill fumes
From forth thy stomach. All these harms ensue
By sleep in afternoons: believe it true!

Rheums from the breast, ascending through the nose
Some call *catarrhs, some *phthisis, some the *pose.

When wind within the belly is restrained
The body is by four diseases pained:
Cramps, *dropsy, colic, giddiness of brain
Wheeling it round. Break wind, and don't refrain!

Great suppers put the stomach to great pain:
Sup lightly, if good rest you mean to gain.

Thou shouldst not eat until thy stomach say
The food's digested which did pass that way.
For the true use of appetite to feed
Is Nature's diet: no more then shall [you] need.

Pears, apples, peaches, cheese and powdered [*preserved or cured*] meat,
Venison, hare, goat's flesh and beef to eat:
All these are *melancholy, corrupt the blood.
Therefore not feeding on them I hold good.

Your new-laid eggs, brisk cheerful-colored wine
And good fat broth, in Physic we define
To be so wholesome, that their purity
Doth nourish Nature very sovereignly.

The priest's fair daughter held it a law most true
That eggs be best when they are long, white, new.

Bread of red wheat, milk and new-made cheese,
Beast's testicles, port, marrow, brain of these,
Sweet wines, delicious meats, eggs that are rear [*slightly underdone*],
Over-ripe figs and raisins: these appear
To make the body fat, and nourish Nature,
Procuring corpulence and growth of stature.

Smell, savor, color, cheerful, fine:
These are the best tests of a cup of wine.
In choice of good wine, these are ever speaking:
Strength, beauty, fragrance, coolness, sprightly leaping.

The sweetest wines do most of all revive
And cheer the *spirits, being nutritive.

When too much red wine carelessly we drink
It binds [*constipates*] the belly, makes the voice to shrink.

I read [that] from garlic, nuts, herb-grace or rue,
Pears, radish-roots and *treacle do ensue
Such virtuous qualities that they all serve
As antidotes against poison to preserve.

He that takes garlic early in the morn
Needs let no drink by him to be forborne.
Diversity of countries he may see
And well enabled, if his mind so be.

Dwell where the air is clear, sweet, wholesome, bright,
*Infected with no fumes that hurt the spirit,
For sweetest airs do Nature most delight.

If overmuch wine hath thy brain offended
Drink early the next morning, and it's mended....

The springtime doth command our dinners be
But light and little, sparing in degree.
The summer season, being sultry hot,

Immoderate feeding should be then forgot.
The fall of leaf, or autumn, doth deny
Eating much fruit: great harm ensues thereby.
But in the winter, cold doth then require
Such a full meal as Nature can desire.

If in your drink washed sage is mixed with rue,
It is most wholesome poison to subdue.
Add thereto rose-flowers, if you feel the heat
Of Venus to wax wanton, or grow great.

Sea-water drunk with wine doth well defend thee
If on the sea, [sea-sickness do] offend thee.

Sage, salt and wine, pepper therewith applied,
Garlic and parsley: these have been well tried
To make good sauce for any kind of meat,
Procuring appetite when men would eat.

If thou wilt walk in health, let me advise,
Oft wash thine hands, chiefly when thou dost rise
From feeding at the table, for thereby
Thou gainest two benefits: it clears the eye,
Gives comfort to the palms, both which, well-tended,
Our health thereby the better is befriended.

Not over-old nor hot let be thy bread;
Hollow and light, but easily leavened,
Sparingly salted, of the purest wheat
And see that crusts thou do forbear to eat
Because that angry *choler they beget.
Thy bread well baked, light salted, sound of grain:
All these observe, [and] thou doest not eat in vain.

To feed on pork, whether we sup or dine,
Is worse than mutton if we have no wine;
But drinking wine therewith, it is sound food,
And *physic for the body very good.

The tripes or innards of the hog is best,
And better than of any other beast.

Sweet wine to urine is a stop or stay;
To looseness in the belly it makes way.
It harmeth both the liver and the spleen,
Causing the stone, as hath by proof been seen.

He that drinks water when he feeds on meat
Doth diverse harms unto himself beget:
It cools the stomach with a crude infesting,
And voids the meat again without digesting.

Flesh of young calves or veal is very good,
Quick in *digestions, nourishing the blood.

The hen, the capon, turtle-dove, and the starling,
The ring-dove, quail, lark, ousel fat and fair,
The partridge, robin redbreast, cock of the wood,
The pheasant, heath-cock, moorhen: all are good.
So the wild mallard and green plover too,
Eaten with wisdom as we ought to do....

Peas may be praised, and discommended too
According as their nature is to do.
The husks avoid, then the pulse [*the inner pea*] is good,
Well nourishing, not hurtful to the blood.
But in the husks they are a gnawing meat,
And in the stomach cause inflations great.

Goat's milk not camel's milk to drink is good
When *agues or *consumptions touch the blood
They nourish well. But beyond all, some say,
Milk of an ass doth nourish more than they.
But when a headache or hot fevers fall
The milk of cow and sheep are best of all.

Butter doth soften, moisten, and make loose besides
Those bodies where no fever doth abide.

Whey is incisive, washing, piercing too,
Cleansing and *purging where it's fit to do.

Cheese is by nature cold, stuffing, gross and hard,
Yet good with bread, where sickness is disbarred;
When being found in health, for them it's good,
But if not joined with bread, unwholesome food.

Cheese doth apologize in his own defense
When those unskilled in physic urge pretence
That it is hurtful, yet through ignorance
Know not whereby his hurtfulness doth chance:
The stomach's languishing cheese doth relieve,
And after stuffing food great ease doth [it] give.
A modicum thereof after all other food
By best physicians is allowed for good.

Often, yet little, drink at dinner-time;
But between meals you must from drink decline
That sickness may in power less prevail,
Which otherwise through drinking sharply doth assail....

By drinking ale or beer gross *humors grow,
Strength is augmented, blood and flesh also
Increaseth daily; urine they do procure,
Inflate the belly, as the learned assure.
And furthermore, of vinegar (they say)
Although it drieth, yet it cools its way
In passage, and it makes one lean
Being received fasting, so I mean.

It causeth melancholy, harms the seed
Of generation, and doth shakings breed.
Lean folk it hurteth, drying up their blood,
And unto fat folks greatly doth no good.

100. LIFESTYLE ADVICE FOR ALL (2): ALDOBRANDINO OF SIENA ON HEALTH THROUGHOUT THE LIFE CYCLE

Aldobrandino left his native Siena in Tuscany to become the personal physician of the countess Beatrix of Provence, mother-in-law of King Louis IX of France. To her he dedicated his Regimen for the Body *(*Régime du corps*), composed in 1256. This is probably the oldest medical text in French, and it survives in at least 35 manuscripts. There are also two Italian versions of the book. The fact that Aldobrandino wrote in the vernacular reflects both the courtly milieu in which he worked and the appetite of the literate laity of the thirteenth century for didactic literature.*

Aldobrandino's text is divided into four parts: the care of the body in general, broadly based on the six *non-naturals; a head-to-toe guide to the care of the individual parts of the body; advice on the properties of various foodstuffs; and, finally, a tract on physiognomy, the technique of reading character through physical traits. The extracts below are from the end of the first part, which deals with health in relation to the life cycle.

Aldobrandino's principal sources were Arabic works, notably Isaac Judaeus's Universal Diets *(for part 3), the works of Constantine the African (the chapter on the stomach), and particularly the* Canon *of Avicenna. The chapter on regimen for pregnant women and the care of infants reflects the Arab encyclopedists' concern with tailoring medicine to the particular circumstances of human life. This positions Aldobrandino's book somewhere between the generic advice of the* Salerno Regimen of Health *and more customized regimens.*

Source: trans. Faith Wallis from *Le régime du corps de Maître Aldebrandin de Sienne*, ed. Louis Landouzy and Roger Pépin (Paris: Campion, 1911), pp. 71–82. Middle French.

How a Woman Should Take Care of Herself When She Is Pregnant

In order to understand what we are saying to you, you must know that the child that is within the body of a woman is like the fruit upon a tree. For you see that in the beginning the flower from which the fruit comes is weakly attached to the tree and falls off with a little wind or rain and afterwards, when the fruit grows large, it holds on tightly and does not readily fall, and when it is ripe, it falls off lightly, like the flower.

You should also understand that a woman can lose her pregnancy in the first, second, or third month if she does not know how to care for herself. In the fourth or fifth month the danger is not so great, and one can bleed and *purge at this time, and perform medical interventions upon her if necessary, as Hippocrates says, because the child will hold on tight, just like a fruit which is not yet ripe. But the time when she is ready to deliver is dangerous, just as before, and to avoid the danger, we will teach how a pregnant woman should take care of herself.

First, she should avoid everything that is too salty, for as the philosophers say, because one eats such things the child can be born without nails and hair. [She should avoid] everything that provokes urination and menstruation, such as chick-peas, haricot beans, rue, parsley, lupins; and it is not good for her to eat too much at one time, nor a diversity of foods, but rather small amounts and often, and these should be good foods, such as chicken, partridge, blackbirds, kid, mutton, and all foods that concoct readily, and she should drink wine tempered with a bit of water. And she should avoid anger, labor, cogitation, fear, and trauma, and avail herself of things that give joy and solace, and this particularly in the first and last [trimester].

And it is not suitable for her to bathe, as we shall explain; nor to remain for long out in the sun, and she should inhale things that have a good perfume, and wear clothes that are fresh and clean. And to strengthen the appetite, one should get them to eat pears and pomegranates and sour apples; and let those who can have *electuaries made to strengthen the stomach and the whole body from one dram each of pearls that have never been pierced and of pyrethrum [*root of Spanish pellitory*], four drams each of ginger and mastic, and two drams each of zedoary root, cassia bark, cardamom, nutmeg, and cinnamon, and three drams each of root of sea lavender and long pepper: make a powder of all of these and then make electuaries with sugar.

And for those who cannot carry their infant to term: they can take an herb which the natural philosophers call "bistort" every day in a little wine mixed with water or they can make electuaries with it.

And when the time comes to deliver, fifteen days or three weeks in advance, she should bathe every day in water in which are steeped mallows, violets, linseed, fenugreek, barley, and camomile, and she should anoint her legs, thighs, and around her private parts with oil of camomile, chicken fat, foam from the top of butter, and *dialthea* [*a compound remedy made with the mucilaginous part of the marsh mallow*]. On emerging from her bath, if she is rich, let her drink two pennyweight of balsam in warm wine and if she is poor, let roots of costus and artemisia be cooked in wine and then in the wine drink two pennyweight of bull's bile. Let her make herself sneeze and hold her breath by the mouth and nose, and then force herself to walk, and to go up and down stairs, and then rest thereafter, and have her feet and hands rubbed, and inhale things that have a good perfume and perfume herself below with roots of costus and spikenard.

And if her appetite is weak, let her eat strained foods and eggs, but a little at a time and often, and drink wine tempered in a little water. And should it happen to be cold, let the air be warmed with lit coals and in summer let it be cooled and [the woman] can sit in lukewarm water up to her navel.

These things are beneficial in general for women who wish to deliver, but should it happen that the delivery is difficult and perilous, as when the child does not come out in the right position as it should, but with the feet or arms first – for you should know that it should come out naturally with the head first, the arms extended along the thighs – and if it happens as we said above, the only advice is that a midwife turn [the infant] around so that it can come out as it should.

And should it happen that the child is dead, it is incumbent on one to hasten the woman's delivery, because this is very dangerous.

Let her be given to drink water with fenugreek in which dates have been cooked, and let her be given this three or four times if necessary, or two drams of juice of rue in warm wine, or juice of juniper, or let her drink cinnamon and root of madder in wine.

And if she is fat, let her lie on her stomach and draw up her knees towards her head, and place a cushion under her belly, for if this is done it helps such women to deliver with greater ease.

And after she is delivered, she should bathe and be refreshed with good food and if pains and other ailments should occur, let medicines be made which are appropriate to the ailments.

How to Care for the Child When He Is Born

After the woman has delivered the child, you should know how to take care of the child.

Know that as soon as the child is born, it should be wrapped in crushed roses mixed with fine salt, and the umbilical cord should be cut to the length of four fingers, and put upon it powdered "dragon's blood" [*gum of East Indian climbing palm*], sarcocolla [*another exotic gum resin*], cumin, myrrh, and a linen bandage soaked in olive oil, and this is what many philosophers teach.

But it is safer to take a thread of twisted wool and to tie it onto the navel, and then lay on bandages soaked in oil, and leave them for four days; and [the cord] will fall off, and when it has fallen off, you should make haste to place upon it fine salt mixed with fine powder of costus, or of sumac, or of fenugreek, or oregano, and with this you can salt the whole body, particularly the nose and the mouth, in order to warm and solidify the navel and the whole body. For at the time the child is born, the whole body will be tender and soft, and it easily feels hot things and cold ones thereafter, which all too readily cause it grief and which can extinguish and change its natural form. And one can salt them more than once, if necessary, especially those who have a quantity of superfluities.

Afterwards, one should wash [the baby] and the nurse should clean out his ears and nostrils, and [the mother or nurse] should take care that her nails are trimmed so that she does not harm the baby, and she should place a little olive oil in the eyes. And the baby ought to fill its bottom nicely and be diligent to purge the superfluities, and press down nicely on the bladder, the better to urinate; and one should keep it from the cold as much as possible.

And when one wishes to swaddle [the baby], the members should be gently couched and arranged so as to give them a good shape, and this is easy for a wise nurse; for just as wax when it is soft takes whatever form one wishes to give to it, so also the child takes the form which its nurse gives to it. And for this reason, you should know that beauty and ugliness are due in large measure to nurses.

And when its arms are swaddled, and the hands over the knees, and the head lightly swaddled and covered, let it sleep in the cradle. The cradle should not be full of things which are hard and rough, but of soft things which will keep [the baby] from the cold, but not make too much heat. And take care that [the baby's] head is higher than the rest of the body, and that he sleeps straight, so that the body does not lean to one side and the head or any of the other members to the other. And the rooms where he sleeps should be dark, but not too much so, because great brightness can do considerable harm to his sight.

When he has slept enough, he should be washed if necessary, for it is the right time [for this], and it can be done two or three times a day, and if it is summer and the weather is hot, do it with water that is somewhat lukewarm, and if it is winter, let it be warmer. And in the bath, take care that water does not get into the ears, and one should take [the baby] by the right hand and the left foot, and stretch him, and then by the left toward the right, and gently bend the feet and legs to the back of the head to make the knee joints more free, and move them, and one should do thus with the other joints and move them, so that they can be more free. And when [the baby] has been bathed, he should be dried off with soft, dry towels, and put back to sleep, and make him lie first on his stomach and then on his back. And one should care for the infant in this manner, when the woman has delivered.

Now I shall tell you how he should be nursed. You should know that the milk that one should give him and the one that is best for him is his mother's milk, because this was what he was nourished on when he was in his mother's womb and after he is out of the womb the milk reverts naturally to the breasts.

And there should be enough [milk] to nurse [the baby] two or three times a day, for this is enough, and one should begin with a little bit, and it would be better before the baby suckles to put a small amount of honey into its mouth, and then it behooves one to press on the breast and bring a little [milk] out, and then after this he can nurse. And it is not good to nurse [the baby] to the point where he is bloated, but he should rest nicely after nursing, until the milk is swallowed and then gently be placed in the cradle.

But because mothers cannot always nurse their infants, we will teach you here what kind of nurse they ought to have. These things should be considered. One should consider her age, her form, her habits, her breasts, whether she has good milk, and whether the time since she had a child has been long or short, and if you find these things that we describe to be good, then you will do well to engage her.

First we shall speak to you about age. A woman who nurses a child should be twenty-five years old, for this is the age at which the natural heat for engendering good *humors is strongest. You should see that the woman resemble the mother as much as possible, that she has a good color (mingling red and white), and that she has a large, strong neck, a broad bosom, and firm flesh. And she should be neither too fat nor too thin, and should be healthy as far as one can tell, for sickly nurses kill children straight away.

About her habits: one should observe if she is of sound moral character; and it will not do if she is hot-tempered, or sad, or timid, or foolish, for these things upset the *complexions of children and make them become foolish and given to evil ways. For this reason philosophy taught of old that lords should have their children nurtured by nurses who were wise and of good life, because the malignity of their nurses can alter their noble form.

One should observe the form of the breasts; they should be firm and not too soft, nor should they be too large or too small, because breasts that are too large make children snub-nosed when they are put under their noses.

One should observe the quantity and nature of the milk, for the milk must be white, neither too clear nor too thick, not green or red or black; and the odor should not be too strong, or the taste too gross or too bitter or salty, but rather, sweet. And to know if it is too gross or too thin, take a drop and put it on your fingernail and if it drops off without your moving the nail, it is too clear and if it will not drop off until you turn the nail, it is too thick. So take [a nurse whose milk] is neither too thick nor too clear.

One should observe the time that has passed since the nurse had a child, for it should be at least one or two months since she had a child, and if it is the case that there has been one or two years, this is worthless. One who has had a son is preferable to one who has had a daughter. Make sure she went full term and that she did not lose her child before, or by trauma, or for some other reason.

These are the things which one must look out for in order to have a good nurse, and when you have her, it behooves the nurse to feed on good foods such as hot eggnog, lamb, kid, chicken, scaled fish, and purées of lettuce and borage; and she should avoid onions, rocket, wild mustard, parsley, mint, basil, and garlic, and all other things that cause bad blood. And she should work with moderation and not rest all day, and should take care not to sleep with a man, because this is what corrupts the milk, and she should not become pregnant, for a pregnant woman when she nurses kills and destroys children.

And when the nurse breast-feeds, she must shortly beforehand press on the breast, and then breast-feed, and she should give a little bit, but often, because to give too much at one time makes the belly grind and swell and [the baby to] throw up through the mouth. And when she has breast-fed, she should put [the baby] to sleep, but when he has rested a bit, and when the milk has been swallowed, she should move the cradle gently, and she should sing soft and lovely songs to put the baby to sleep.

The natural [age] for breast-feeding is up to the age of two, and afterwards the child should be systematically weaned, especially when his front teeth come in. And one must prevent him from chewing on hard things and so the nurse must give him bread that she has chewed in her mouth, and make porridge with bread-crumbs and honey and milk, and give him a small amount of wine. And if [the child] vomits or spits it out of the mouth, she should leave off and breast-feed him until the evil desires have passed. And one can give him puréed meat. And when he begins to chew, make for him pastries of bread and sugar in the form of dates.

And when [the child] begins to walk, one should not let his feet rest on anything hard, but on a soft and smooth place. And one leg should not be higher and the other lower, because this makes children lame. And one should not make children walk too much or stand on their legs too long before they are seven years old, because of the tenderness of the members, which can easily break and bend.

And when the teeth begin to come in, it is good to rub the mouth and gums with honey and salt and make [the child] to hold in his hand a peeled liquorice root which is not too dry, and a piece of gladiolus root, for these things strengthen the gums and dry out the humors that children have in their mouths.

And when he begins to speak, the nurse should rub his mouth with rock salt and honey, and then wash his mouth with barley water, especially if the child is slow to start speaking. And begin to say words such as "Mama" and "Papa" that do not contain letters that make the tongue move too much. And to make the teeth come in easily, one can anoint the gums with butter or chicken fat.

These teachings, which we have set out here, ought to be known to those who send their children out to be nursed. And if the children fall ill at the time of teething or at any other time, let them seek out good advice, for to give such here is not our intention.

How One Should Care for the Body at Each Age of Life

You have heard how to nourish your child in the first or second age [of life]. Now I will tell you how each individual can care for himself in the other ages [of life].

First, you should know that the natural philosophers say that there are four ages, namely: *adolescentia* [*adolescence, including infancy and childhood*], *juventus* [*youth, prime of life*], *senectus* [*old age*] and *senium* [*advanced old age*]. They say of the first that it is warm and moist, and in this time of life the body grows, and it lasts until twenty-five or thirty years of age. The second is hot and dry, and the body retains its vigor and power until age forty or forty-five. The third is cold and dry, and lasts until sixty years of age. The fourth is cold and moist, because of the abundance of cold humors which abound for lack of heat, and it lasts until death; and in this age, the body invariably goes into decline.

But if we wish to speak somewhat more subtly, it can be said that there are seven ages, namely: the first, when children are born and which lasts until teething, and this is *infantia* [*infancy*]. The next is *dentium plantatura* [*the embedding of the teeth*] and this is when the teeth have come, and it lasts until seven years of age. The third is *pueritia* [*childhood*] and lasts until age fourteen. And you should know that these three comprise the first [age] of which we spoke to you above, which is called *adolescentia*, and of these seven ages we have told you about two, namely *infantium* and *dentium plantatura* [in the preceding chapter]. Now we shall tell you what one ought to do in the others.

You should know that as soon as the child is seven years of age, he should be disciplined until he is well behaved and nothing should happen to anger him too much or make him to lie awake too much. And let him be given what he asks for and let there not remain in front of him anything that dries him out; and one should do this so that his nature may be well complexioned and filled with good habits, for this is the age when a child retains most and learns good habits and bad ones. And know that good habits are the guardians of the health of body and soul.

After this, one should give [the child] a bath two or three times a week, especially when he wakes from sleep; and when he has bathed, let him have something to eat, and then go out to play and frisk about. And when he comes back, give him something more to eat, and you may do this three times a day. And give him wine tempered with water to drink and ensure that he does not drink cold water on top of his food, for it can cause him trouble. And keep him away from milk, fruit and cheese as much as you can, for they can engender the [bladder] stone. And at this age, if you wish, send him to school and give him a teacher who knows how to teach properly without beatings and let him not be forced to remain at school, learning and being punished, any longer than he wishes.

After this, when he has passed fourteen years of age, it behooves one to take care that the humors do not abound too much, due to his excessive eating and drinking. And if they abound too much, they should be purged by bloodletting and light medicines. And he should avoid keeping too close company with women, because at this time nature and the complexions are too weak and for this reason it is better if he not frequent women before age twenty or twenty-five.

Those who have passed twenty-five years of age should undertake more vigorous activity, as we have told you, and avoid foods that engender red *bile, such as onions, leeks, and all other dry things; and they should consume things which are cold and moist, such as fish and the flesh of kids, and drink wine mixed with water, and avoid wine that is old and strong. And they should be bled and purged as the season and their natures demand, for this is the age when one can do this with the greatest safety.

When the thirty-fifth year is passed, one should avoid bloodletting as much as one can, save in cases of great necessity; and one should use medicine to purge evil humors, for at this age, [medicine] is more appropriate than bloodletting. And one should avoid frequenting women, for at this age, this is what accelerates aging. And to keep young and slow down aging, one should avoid sleeplessness, anger, and cogitation, and one should remain in joy and solace, and consume things that are very nourishing and that make the blood clear, and drink wine, and bathe once or twice a month to purge and cleanse the superfluities of the body....

But should one happen to pass sixty-five years of age, one should avoid purging and bloodletting unless the need is very great; and take good food that is lightly cooked, and drink old red wine, and stay away from wine that is white or new, and let it not be sweet, because anything sweet will cause [old people] trouble. And they should avoid working too hard; and should take baths and after the bath let themselves be rubbed down with the hands or with a towel that is not too coarse. And they should avoid the cold and perfume their beds and the chambers where they live with aloe wood, myrrh, amber, and storax. And they should take these electuaries, namely of *diacinamomi* [*compound medicine based on cinnamon*], *dyatrion piperon* [*"three-peppers"* *electuary*], *diagingibreos* [*electuary based on ginger*], *dyaireos* [*electuary based on iris*], *dianisi* [*electuary based on anise*], *diantos* [*confection based on rosemary flowers*], and other hot electuaries.

101. LIFESTYLE ADVICE, CUSTOMIZED (1): THE ARMY ON CAMPAIGN

The Regimen for Almería *(Regimen Almarie) was composed by Arnau of Vilanova for his patron, King James II of Aragon. The occasion was the campaign waged against the Muslim kingdom of Granada in 1309–10, when the Aragonese armies unsuccessfully besieged the city of Almería. Arnau himself was indirectly responsible for this campaign. While in service as a royal physician and ambassador, Arnau actively promoted his visionary project for the reform of Christian society. He persuaded both James and his brother, Frederick III of Sicily, that they had received a divine summons to lead this reformation. James was convinced that this included a campaign against Granada. As he prepared for war in the summer of 1309, he sent Arnau to the papal court at Avignon to solicit support. In Avignon, Arnau stunned his audience by proclaiming himself Christ's messenger, announcing the kings' divine mission, and attacking the whole structure of the Church. When word of this performance reached James, he ordered Arnau to return immediately and explain himself. During the sea voyage to join the king at Almería, Arnau, not knowing that the campaign was over, composed his regimen for the army in the field. It was probably intended to mollify his lord, but James nonetheless dismissed Arnau from his service.*

The Regimen for Almería *is short, and uncharacteristically disorganized. A regimen normally proceeds in the order of the six *non-naturals. Arnau begins by addressing "air" (where the camp should be sited), but then gets distracted by special instructions for the king and advice about clearing the road for the troops. He gets back on track with "water" but then drifts off into the prevention and treatment of diseases. There are no references to medical literature; indeed, there were almost no models for a work such as this. The* Regimen for Almería *is thus both original and revealing. Military medicine automatically evokes the image of the surgeon caring for the wounded, but Arnau focuses more realistically on sanitation and the prevention and treatment of disease.*

Source: trans. Michael R. McVaugh, "Arnald of Villanova's *Regimen almarie (Regimen castra sequentium)* and Medieval Military Medicine," *Viator* 23 (1992): 211–13. Latin.

The regimen that [Arnau of Vilanova] prepared for the king of Aragon during the crossing to Almería.

An army should not pitch camp in marshy regions for a long period of time. Wherever the camp may be located, the king should reside away from the side from which the land wind is blowing in off the mountains, called the zephyr or west wind; and every evening taking a chick-pea or lupine-seed's worth of pomander soaked in wine, place it on coals in the tent where he lies.

He will keep the crown that you know upon his head and, by day, will wear the necklace of stones around his neck hanging down to his breast.

When the army must move from one place to another, infantry shod with heavy-soled shoes should precede it by a mile or two, who will search in and around the route to see whether iron caltrops have been sown or scattered there, and [if so] pick them up. Likewise they will look in springs to see whether they find a moveable, hollow stone, or a fixed stake, and remove them before the water is drunk; similarly if there are dead plants floating there. In streams they should take note whether there is a long beam set across the stream; if it cannot be removed, then [water] should be drawn above it, or if below, then at least a mile downstream. Make the same examination in cisterns as well as in springs, and always be careful to see whether there is a gummy or greasy mass at the bottom, and [if there is] take it out; if it is a cistern, do not use the water, but if it is a well, [you may if you] drain it first. If you cannot make such an examination, then thoroughly moisten a fine white linen cloth in the water and fold it loosely; thus folded and tied with a cord, suspend it in the sun or the air and when it has dried, unfold it. If stains appear in it, of whatever color, the water is sure to be diseased, but if it is not stained, it is healthy.

And so that the army may be preserved from epidemic, let pits be dug everywhere outside its lines, like trenches, where animal wastes and bodies can be thrown; and when they are half full, cover them with earth. Everyone should take powdered coriander with their food, boiled in vinegar and then dried. To be protected more effectively, they should take the following powder on an empty stomach every fourth day: [take] one part of camomile flower, two parts of *kermes, three parts of usnea [*a type of lichen*], juice of rusty-black fern equal to the weight of all, and take one spoonful [of this] with plain sugar or rose sugar, followed by a little good wine; the poor can drink a cup of thrice-cooked *tisane prepared with a double measure of grass stalks. Let everyone wear a cap of *alcanna* covering the neck as well. The aforesaid tisane is made as follows: put a bowlful of barley in a clean glass vessel or a tin kettle with enough water to cover it, and let it come to a boil over a slow fire. Then strain it, and again boil it and strain it. Finally, the third time put it in ten bowls' worth of water with two handfuls of grass stalks, rinsed, and boil the whole over a bright slow fire until about half the water is gone; then take it off the fire and set it aside for future use, either strained or unstrained. Anyone suffering from *fever, of whatever age or sex or complexion, can take, fasting, one spoonful of powdered wood-sorrel added to the aforesaid tisane, drunk cold in summer and warm in winter. They should always use this tisane as drink when they have no wine.

All the wounded should use powder of lesser poligony daily as follows, taking a spoonful of it with wine, fasting – or, if they are poor, with the aforesaid water; and when the wound has been cleansed let [the powder] be sprinkled on externally too. If someone is poisoned, by an arrow or something else, he should take, fasting, one spoonful of the following powder with aromatic wine or the abovementioned tisane: [take] one part of citron seed, three parts of hart's tongue fern, and make a powder. Such patients can also be given cabbages with oil as food.

102. LIFESTYLE ADVICE CUSTOMIZED (2): A PHYSICIAN OF VALENCIA ADVISES HIS SONS, WHO ARE STUDYING IN TOULOUSE

*This letter by Dr Peter Fagarola of Valencia to his two sons, students at Toulouse in 1315, is found in a manuscript comprising mainly medical works written at Montpellier in the fifteenth century (London, British Library Sloan 3124, fols. 74r–77r). It is, in fact, a personal "regimen" organized according to Joannitius's six *non-naturals. It can be compared as well to a* consilium, *and as such it may have been copied and adapted for teaching medical students. One clue is the fact that the recipient of the advice is always addressed with the singular pronoun, even though there were two sons. In sum, this letter is at once a personal letter of advice and a generic* regimen sanitatis *for young men living away from home for the first time.*

Source: trans. Lynn Thorndike, "Translation of a Letter from a Physician of Valencia to His Two Sons Studying at Toulouse." *Annals of Medical History* n.s. 3 (1931): 17–20. Latin.

There follows a Regimen composed by Peter Fagarola, master of arts and medicine, which was sent by him from the city of Valencia to the city of Toulouse to his two sons, students residing in that city of Toulouse, in the year of our Lord one thousand, three hundred, and fifteen.

Of Foods, or How to Eat

Beware of eating too much and too often especially during the night. Avoid eating raw onions in the evening except rarely, because they dull the intellect and senses generally.

Avoid all very lacteal foods such as milk and fresh cheese, except very rarely. Beware of eating milk and fish, or milk and wine, at the same meal, for milk and fish or milk and wine produce leprosy.

Don't have fresh pork too often. Salt pork is all right.

Don't eat many nuts except rarely and following fish. I say the same of meat and fruit, for they are bad and difficult to *digest.

[Drink] twice or thrice or four times during a meal. Between meals drink little, for it would be better once in a while to drink too much at table than to drink away from table. Don't take wine without water and, if it is too cold, warm it in winter. For it is bad to grow used to strong wine without admixture of water.

Remember about the well water of Toulouse. Wherefore, boil it, and the same with the water of the Garonne [River], because such waters are bad.

Also, after you have risen from table wash out your mouth with wine. This done, take one spoonful of this powdered confection: of meat prepared with vinegar and dried coriander similarly prepared, a modicum each; of roast meat, fennel seed, flowers of white eyebright, two ounces each; of candied coriander, candied anise, scraped licorice, each one ounce and a half; of [cloves], mast, cubebs, each three drams; of galingale and cardamom, each two drams; of white ginger, six drams; of white loaf sugar, three drams; made into a powder and put in a paste. And keep this in your room in a [dry] place, for it will comfort your digestion, head, vision, intellect and memory, and protect from *rheum.

As to Sleep

Sufficient and natural sleep is to sleep for a fourth part of a *natural day or a trifle more or less. To do otherwise is to pervert nature. Too much is a sin, wherefore shun it, unless the case is urgent and necessary.

Avoid sleeping on your back except rarely, for it has many disadvantages, but sleep on your side or stomach, and first on the right side, then on the left.

Don't sleep in winter with cold feet, but first warm them at the fire or by walking about or some other method. And in summer don't sleep with bed slippers on your feet, because they generate vapors which are very bad for the brain and memory.

Don't go straight to bed on a full stomach, but an hour after the meal. Also, unless some urgent necessity prevents, walk about for a bit after a meal, at least around the square, so that the food may settle in the stomach and not evaporate in the mouth of the stomach, since the vapors will rise to the head and fill it with rheum and steal away and cut short memory.

Also, avoid lying down in a rheumatic place, such as a basement or room underground.

Of Air or One's Surroundings

Choose lodgings removed from all foul smells as of ditches or latrines and the like, since in breathing we are continually drawing in air, which, if it is *infected, infects us more and more forcibly than tainted food and drink do.

Likewise in winter keep your room closed from all noxious wind and have straw on the pavement lest you suffer from cold.

Furthermore, if you can have coals or chopped wood in a clay receptacle of good clay or if you have a chimneyplace and fire in your room, it is well.

Also, be well clad and well shod, and outdoors wear pattens [*wooden sandal-like overshoes with raised soles*] to keep your feet warm.

Also, don't make yourself a ["sausage"] cap [*with a long trailing point?*], as some do, for they are harmful.

And when you see other students wearing their caps, do [so] likewise and, if need be, put on one of fur.

And at night, when you study, you should wear a nightcap over the cap and about your cheeks.

And when you go to bed at night, have a white nightcap on your head and beneath your cheeks and another colored one over it, for at night the head should be kept warmer than during the day.

Moreover, at the time of the great rains it is well to wear outdoors over your cap a bonnet or helmet of undressed skin, that is, a covering to keep the head from getting wet. Indeed, some persons wear a bonnet over the cap in fair weather, more especially when it is cold, so that in the presence of the great they may remove the bonnet and be excused from doffing the cap.

Also, look after your stockings and don't permit your feet to become dirty.

Also, wash the head, if you are accustomed to wash it, at least once a fort-night with hot lye and in a place sheltered from draughts on the eve of a feast day towards nightfall. Then dry your hair with a brisk massage; afterwards do it up; then put on a bonnet or cap.

Also comb your hair daily, if you will, morning and evening before eating or at least afterwards, if you cannot do otherwise.

Also look out that a draft does not strike you from window or crack while you study or sleep or indeed at any time, for it strikes men without their noticing.

Also, in summer, in order not to have fleas or to have no more of them, sweep your room daily with a broom and [do not] sprinkle it with water, for they are generated from damp dust. But you may spray it occasionally with strong vinegar, which comforts heart and brain.

Exercise and Rest

If you will, walk daily somewhere morning and evening. And if the weather is cold, if you can, run on [an] empty stomach or at least walk rapidly, that the natural heat may be revived. For a fire is soon extinguished unless the sticks are moved about or the bellows used. However, it is not advisable to run on a full stomach but to saunter slowly in order to settle the food in the stomach.

If you cannot go outside your lodgings, either because the weather does not permit or it is raining, climb the stairs rapidly three or four times, and have in your room a big heavy stick like a sword and wield it now with one hand, now with the other, as if in a scrimmage, until you are almost winded. This is a splendid exercise to warm one up and expel noxious vapors through the pores and consume other superfluities. Jumping is a similar exercise. Singing, too, exercises the chest. And if you will do this, you will have healthy limbs, a sound intellect and memory, and you will avoid rheum. The same way with playing ball. All these were invented not for sport, but for exercise. Moreover, too much labor is to be avoided as a continual practice.

On Accidents of the Soul

Accidents of the soul have the greatest influence, such as anger, sadness, and love of women, fear, excessive anxiety: concerning all which I say nothing more than that you [should] avoid all passions of the soul harmful to you and enjoy yourself happily with friends and good companions, and cultivate honesty and patience, which bring more delights to the soul, and especially if you love God with your whole heart....

103. MEDICALIZING THE TABLE AND THE HOME: THE *TACUINUM SANITATIS*

Ibn Butlan (d. 1066), a Christian Arab physician trained in Baghdad, distilled the precepts of Galenic preventive medicine into forty takwim *or tables. These charts listed 280 separate entities, grouped roughly according to the same scheme of the six *non-naturals found in the regimens of health: food and drink, states of mind, etc. Reading across the fifteen columns of the chart, the doctor could learn what the primal qualities of the entity were and in what *degree; how to recognize the best variety; what its benefits and potential adverse effects were; and how adverse effects could be mitigated. More complex and sophisticated choices were thus introduced into the basic medieval formula for staying healthy.*

These Takwim al-sihha *or* Tables of Health *were translated into Latin in southern Italy in the mid-thirteenth century under the title* Tacuinum sanitatis *— the first word being a simple transcription of the Arabic* takwim. *In the late fourteenth and early fifteenth centuries, a group of manuscripts was produced for noble patrons in northern Italy that did away with the tabular format of the* Tacuinum *and recast the text in condensed prose. But the principal interest of these books lies in their illustrations — lavish and lively scenes of people growing and preparing food, enjoying exercise and entertainment, taking baths, expressing their emotions, and facing the wind and weather. The text and images reproduced here come from a manuscript made around 1400 for George of Lichtenstein, bishop of Trent. They illustrate three aspects of the* Tacuinum *that set it apart from the general run of regimens of health, namely the attention given to foods that have been processed by cooking and preservation (soups, breads, and even pasta), to textiles for clothing, and to the arrangement of houses. The quest for health was colonizing every corner of medieval daily life.*

Source: trans. Oscar Ratti and Adele Westbrooke, in Luisa Cogliati Arano, *The Medieval Health Handbook* (New York: Braziller, 1976): extracts from the Vienna manuscript of the *Tacuinum sanitatis* (Vienna, Österreichische Nationalbibliothek MS ser. nov. 2644), color plates XLII and XLVII; black and white plate and caption no. 116. Latin.

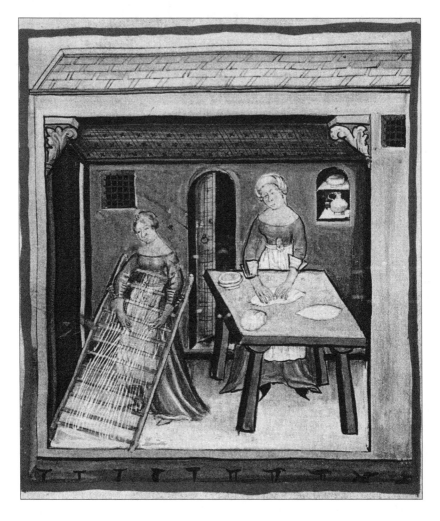

Pasta (fol. 45v)

Nature. Warm and moist in the second *degree. **Optimal**. That which is prepared with great care. **Usefulness**. It is good for the chest and for the throat. **Dangers**. It is harmful to weak intestines and to the stomach. **Neutralization of the Dangers**. With sweet barley. **Effects**. Very nourishing. It is good for a hot stomach, for the young, in winter, and in all regions.

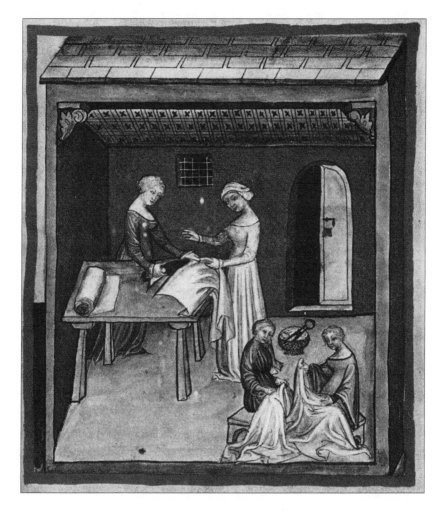

Linen Clothing (fol. 105v)

Nature. Cold and dry in the second degree. **Optimal**. The light, bright, beautiful kind. **Usefulness**. It moderates the heat of the body. **Dangers**. It presses down on the skin and blocks transpirations. **Neutralization of the Dangers**. By mixing it with silk. **Effects**. It dries up ulcerations. It is primarily good for hot *temperaments, for the young, in summer, and in southern regions.

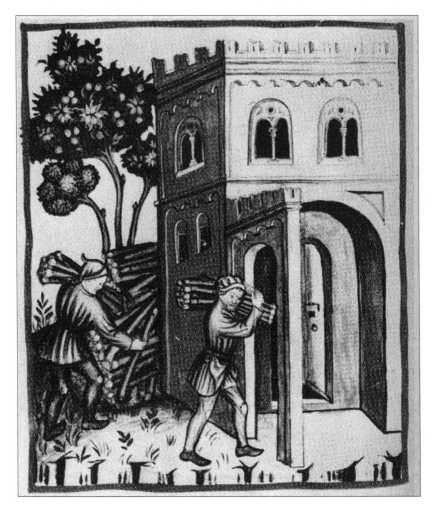

Winter Rooms (fol. 97v)

Nature. They must be of moderate warmth. **Optimal**. Those with a temperature similar to that at the end of spring. **Usefulness**. They reawaken the faculties made drowsy by the cold air. **Dangers**. They cause thirst and allow food not properly *digested to pass through [the body]. **Neutralization of the Dangers**. By placing them towards the northerly side. They are suitable above all to cold temperaments, to very old people, in extremely frigid temperatures, and in mountainous regions.

104. MEDICALIZING SEX: CONSTANTINE THE AFRICAN

It is virtually certain that Constantine the African (see doc. 32) translated or adapted On Sexual Intercourse *(De* coitu*) from one or more Arabic works, but no source has been identified. The treatise was widely read in the Middle Ages and played an important role in transforming sex into a medical issue, one that was explicable in physiological terms and susceptible to being discussed from a purely hygienic point of view. Joannitius, it will be recalled, listed sexual intercourse as one of the **non-naturals*. As such, sex was in principle essentially neutral; it could be beneficial or harmful only insofar as it affected the body's **humoral balance. Constantine's treatise begins with theory (c. 1–12) and then moves into therapies for sexual problems (c. 13–17). The point of view is exclusively masculine and the author does not blush to furnish recipes for aphrodisiacs. In* The Merchant's Tale *Chaucer professed shock that this "cursed monk" should write such things. Indeed, the treatise hovers uneasily on the frontier between medicine and eroticism.*

Source: trans. Faith Wallis from *Constantini Liber de coitu. El tratado de andrología de Constantino el Africano*, ed. Enrique Montero Cartelle (Santiago de Compostela: Universidad de Santiago de Compostela, 1983), pp. 76–184. Latin.

Prologue

The Creator, desiring the race of animals to persist in a steadfast and consistent way, and not perish, arranged that it should be renewed by intercourse and by generation, so that being thus renewed, it should not utterly be destroyed. Therefore, he fashioned natural members for animals that would be fit and proper for this task, and he implanted within them such marvelous power and such lovely delight that there is no animal that does not take enormous pleasure in sexual intercourse. For if animals disliked sexual intercourse, the race of animals would surely perish. Sexual intercourse is so innate in animals that if they are hindered [from it] for a long time, they will do it the moment the opportunity presents itself, disregarding almost everything else. Sexual intercourse takes place between two animals; semen is emitted by one, and the other, joining with [the first], receives [the semen] in its deep cavity, which is closed on all sides lest it be spilled and scattered abroad.

1. How Many Things Are Involved in Sexual Intercourse and Where They Come From

There are, in fact, three things involved in sexual intercourse; appetite, which arises from fantasizing thoughts; *spirit; and humor. Appetite comes from the liver, spirit from the heart, and humor from the brain; for since there is a delightful motion in sexual intercourse, all the parts of the body are warmed through this motion, and the humor in the brain is liquefied by this warmth and when it is liquefied, it is drawn through the veins which are behind the ears and which lead down to the testicles and thence it is ejected by the penis into the vulva. For as Hippocrates says, conception is impossible for people who have had the veins which pass behind the ears cut, for the semen does not flow. And if they emit anything at all, it is not semen, but a watery moisture, and so no conception can take place.

2. Different Types of People Who Engage in Sexual Intercourse

Because some men have an erection and perform intercourse frequently but are unable to emit semen, while others emit semen even if they do not wish to and do not have an erection, and still others have no desire for sex, do not have an erection, and do not emit semen, it is incumbent upon us to explain all these things. When appetite arises in the liver, as we said, spirit is displaced from the heart and descends through the arteries to the penis; it fills the hollow of the penis and by filling up like a uterus, [the penis] grows erect, hard, and rigid. And yet it cannot emit semen if there is an insufficiency or lack of seminal humor in the brain. When there is an excess of this humor in the brain and an insufficiency and defect of "wind" in the heart, semen is emitted involuntarily, but the penis is not erect. But if there is insufficiency or lack of both, the penis will not be able to become erect and neither will semen be emitted. But those who have sex with all of these three in sound condition will be successful in generating: semen will be drawn from the brain through the veins which descend behind the ears, and be emitted through these [veins] into the spinal cord, and then from the spinal cord into the kidneys, and from the kidneys to the testicles, and from the testicles it will be emitted via the penis – not indeed by the urinary duct, but by another which is especially for the semen.

3. What Semen Is

Now that we have discussed these things, we should say what semen is, and how Galen defines it. For he says: semen is a pure, warm, humid substance from which a human being is made. And again: semen is a warm and mobile spirit and its motion impels the moisture of the body, producing in it an effect that is similar to the one from whom it proceeds. Again, Galen says in his book on the treatment of the members [*Usefulness of Parts* 14.9]: semen is spirit and frothy moisture. The moisture is made frothy by motion, as we see during a storm at sea. It is described this way because when semen is ejaculated it appears abundant and then after a little while it diminishes considerably; it does not remain homogenous like sputum or mucus, because these are liquid and raw, while semen is *concocted and dense. When it falls into an appropriate place, being full of *vital spirit, it is formed into a human being. But if it falls into a place which is not appropriate, the spirit within it evaporates, and the liquid diminishes and disperses.

4. What Semen Is Made From

Now we should say what the causes are from which semen is made. For it is a superfluity, and a highly moderate one: "moderate" means *tempered between warm and moist. And because the testicles are among the principal and fundamental members, and because they both collect and transform semen and (because they are close to the penis) transmit it, it behooves us to discuss their nature.

The vital power of semen is either tempered or distempered. If the nature of the testicles is warm and humid — that is, tempered — the semen will be tempered. If it is distempered, it is not good for anything. The quality [of the testicles] is distinguished under two headings: *simple and compound, like the quality of the whole body. The simple [quality is the one that] predominates and is superior, such as warm, moist, cold and dry; the compound [qualities] are warm and moist, cold and moist, warm and dry, and cold and dry: and as the ancients say, semen changes in relation to these four qualities. Heat makes semen subtle and watery by dissolving and diffusing it; cold makes semen thick and gross by coagulating and condensing it; dryness reduces semen, while moisture increases it and makes it copious. If they combine, these qualities produce six others, just as in other bodies: four arise from these in a fitting manner, but two in a faulty way. The four are: warm and moist; warm and dry; cold and moist; cold and dry, and these are useful. The two useless ones are: warm and cold, moist and dry, which repulse one another. And because thin semen is made from warmth and thick [semen] from cold, scanty semen from dryness and abundant semen from moisture, as we said, these four produce four other useful [compounds]: thin and abundant, thick and abundant, thin and scanty; thick and scanty. Two are useless: thin and thick, scanty and abundant. They repel one another at every turn. An explanation of this is to be found in the book which we wrote about leprosy.

5. Who Is Capable of Emitting Semen?

Now that we have covered these topics, let us speak first about those men who are potent and who are superior at emitting semen. In these men, the testicles are indubitably tempered, warm, and moist. For example, if they are men who drink much wine, they abound in appetite and [thus] in semen, and the same is true if it is spring-time, [a season] which is tempered, warm and moist. Heat increases appetite and manliness; but cold diminishes appetite and makes for womanliness. So if the nature of the testicles is warm, appetite for lechery will be great and more male children will be conceived, and the hair in the pubic area and on the rest of the body will appear at the right time. But if it is cold, the men will be effeminate, and appetite will be wanting, and the hair will grow in late, and it will be scanty in the pubic area and the groin. If it is dry, the appetite will be low and the semen scanty. If it is moist, the semen will be plentiful and the hair grow in straight and soft. So much for the simple nature of the testicles.

If their composite [nature] is warm and moist, the heat will produce a strong appetite and much hair; from moisture will come abundance of semen and frequent copulation without adverse effects, nor will the man be able to bear abstinence, as Galen says. If it is warm and dry, the semen will be scanty due to the dryness, and the pleasure upon ejaculation will be great, and the children will be males and numerous, and the appetite will be great and urgent at the outset of puberty, and hair will spread over the pubic area up to the navel and to the middle of the thighs. These people greatly desire sexual intercourse and they finish quickly, for if they persist at it, they suffer for it. If it is cold and dry, there will be no appetite because of the cold and the semen will be scanty because of the dryness. If it is cold and humid, the appetite will be low because of the cold, and hair will grow only on the pubic area, and daughters will be born for the most part. The semen will be abundant because of the moisture, and there will be frequent nocturnal emissions during sleep, because a large amount of moisture makes haste to exit and an effusion of semen is produced without great pleasure. These people experience emissions when the sight of women gives them pleasure and when they recall them in their sleep, they provoke nocturnal emissions. Unlike the others, these emissions are not due to an abundance of humidity. The signs of the nature of the testicles that we have mentioned are to be observed on the whole body.

6. Why the Testicles Are Considered Principal Members

The ancients said that the testicles are among the principal members. Both Hippocrates and Galen say that power is discharged from the testicles to the whole body, just as the brain discharges the power of motion and sensation to the penis and the heart, through the arteries, discharges the power of erection, and desire. The power that is in the testicles is discharged to the whole body, because it makes male and female, and therefore the testicles are the foundation and root of the power that bestows great warmth to the whole body. In consequence, those who are castrated do not grow beards, nor are they hairy, and their veins are like the veins of women, nor do they have sexual appetite. For these reasons the testicles are said to be among the principal members.

7. The Nature of the Right and Left Testicles

Now it is said that warmth is the cause of masculinity and cold of femininity, and because this is the case, the members on the right generate males and those on the left, females. Hippocrates says that these members assist one another. Galen also states that it is no wonder that the warmth of the right testicle and the right part of the uterus is greater than the warmth of the left testicle and the left part of the uterus, because [organs on the right] are closer to the liver and are nourished with pure, clear blood. Therefore, males come from the right and females from the left. Hippocrates also says: if a boy at the time of puberty sees that his right testicle is larger and more prominent, he will engender boys, and if his left one [is larger], girls. Hippocrates tells us to notice that during puberty a boy will become more robust and his voice will change and become rough. This comes about from two causes: one from the female, one from the male. For if warm semen falls upon the mouth of the womb and reaches the left part, it will generate a female, and if it reaches the right part, it will produce a male. It sometimes happens that the power of this warmth is overcome. For some doctors have said that if semen that proceeds from the right side [of the man] falls into the left side of the uterus, it will produce an effeminate man; and if what is emitted from the left [testicle] falls into the right [side of the womb] it will make a masculine woman. Beyond this, however, God is able to grant male children to those who wish them and female children to those who wish them, as he himself designs. We have spoken with reference to warmth and cold. After this, we shall speak of the things that foster semen, and of the things that harm it.

8. Why Sexual Intercourse Is Beneficial and Why It Is Harmful

In their books, the ancients said that the things that preserve health are exercise, baths, food, drink, sleep, and sexual intercourse. We should say how sexual intercourse is beneficial, how and when it ought to be carried out, and how it benefits or harms, and what happens to those who do it frequently. For Galen says in his book on *The Art [of Medicine]*, where he replies to what Epicurus said (namely, that no one who has sex is healthy), that in fact intercourse promotes health and he shows how it ought to be done. For he declares when it is appropriate to do it and at what intervals, so that the person performing the act feels no injury. For if someone who is sluggish and weak has intercourse, his body will afterwards feel more buoyant than before and his mind more cheerful.

But there is a suitable time for intercourse: when the body is in a tempered state with respect to all external influences, that is, it is neither full of food nor totally empty, nor cold nor warm nor dry nor moist, but tempered. If the person departs from this norm, and then has sex, it is preferable that he be warm rather than cold, replete rather than fasting, moist rather than dry. And it is preferable [that he do it] before rather than after sleep, because if he falls asleep afterwards, he will rest from his exertion and therefore it will be more beneficial for his vital *powers. Rufus [*of Ephesus, Greek physician and author, fl. 100 CE*] proclaims this when he says: if intercourse takes place in the manner we have described, it will be better for conception and for the embryo, and it will be better for the man if it is done thus, and even for the woman, because if she falls asleep afterwards, the woman retains the semen better. And this happens naturally, even without benefit of [medical] instruction. So overall it is better to have sex in the manner we have described. And if someone has intercourse in the middle of the night, he makes a mistake, because his food is [only] half *concocted. Likewise, if he does it in the morning before eating, he makes a mistake, and the emission will be thin, because everything is *digested. Some observant doctors have declared that if someone full of food has intercourse before it is completely digested, the fetus that results from such coitus, while fully formed, will nonetheless have an abnormally large head and will be mentally defective. And that is why we said that anyone who has intercourse before his meal is digested is making a mistake. The morning is also not appropriate, for the reason we stated above, and because weakness inevitably follows sexual intercourse, it is not appropriate to exert oneself in any way afterwards. Therefore, it is evident from this that intercourse is better before sleep than after sleep, because when one falls asleep, one rests from exertion; if one wishes to have sex in the morning, one should restrain one's body so that it will be capable of tolerating exertion.

9. The Benefits and Drawbacks of Sexual Intercourse

Now it is time to discuss who benefits from intercourse and who is harmed by it. We say that it is beneficial in two ways, according to what Galen says in his commentary on [Hippocrates's] *Epidemics*: on the one hand, [it benefits] a person who has an excess of *phlegm that is not viscous and who is vigorous; and on the other hand, a person in whom a sharp, volatile smoky vapor (*fumus*) abounds, which by its very nature *infects the body's *temperament. It is, indeed, beneficial for these two.

It is beneficial for someone with an excess of non-viscous phlegm, if he is robust, because the humor is *evacuated by intercourse; and [intercourse] should not be infrequent, because the warmth that is generated from the rapid motion of coitus condenses and dries. If there is debility of vital powers with the abovementioned phlegm, frequent intercourse is very harmful because the body is rendered extremely cold and weak. Were someone to ask us why we drew this distinction between strong vital power and weak, we would say that [intercourse] benefits one whose vital power is strong and harms one whose vital power is weak because it alters his body in the direction of extreme cold and weakness. For Galen declares that frequent intercourse dries the body, just as it happens to a fat man when his body threatens to dissolve. Some people think that intercourse does not warm the body, but always cools it. But when the vital power and natural heat are strong, it warms the body. When vital power and natural heat are weak, [intercourse] warms while it is going on, but afterwards, when it is over, there is a profound chilling. And so we distinguish between strong and weak vital power, and we say that [intercourse] benefits one whose vital power is strong and harms one whose vital power is weak because it chills, as Galen says.

10. The Usefulness of Intercourse

Intercourse is useful in another way, namely to the person in whom sharp smoky *vapor abounds, which infects his temperament. For if this smoky vapor is enclosed in his body and not dissolved, it causes great injury, but if he has sex, the superfluities are dissolved and the body rests and cools down and is assisted. But it should not happen frequently, unless necessary, and then it should be done in the proper fashion.

We said that intercourse benefits people in two ways. Rufus [of Ephesus] says that intercourse eliminates a harmful condition in the body and reduces rage; it benefits *melancholics, brings the insane to their senses, and relieves a lover from his passion, provided he can lie with the woman he desires. And so Galen says: a wild animal is ferocious before intercourse and after intercourse it is more tame. Hippocrates says: intercourse is very harmful for someone whose illness is getting worse.

11. The Weakness Which Those Having Intercourse Experience, and Other Incidents

Since the subject has come up, it is incumbent upon us to show why and whence comes this weakness in the animal [spirits], and under what circumstances some men experience paralysis and sadness during intercourse, some a tremor, some a bad smell, while in others the stomach swells during sex, others are overcome by a shrill sound, while others have a headache or similar problem after sex.

We say that the fluid that is emitted from the body when semen is ejaculated is substantial, and it has its essence from the members; it is not like the fluid lost during evacuation, because this [fluid], being a superfluity in the members, is accidental. Likewise, Hippocrates says in his book on the fetus: when our semen is emitted voluntarily, weakness often supervenes. In this statement, Hippocrates wishes to teach us that semen takes its origin from the essence of the healthy members and that the members are composed of this fluid. It should be known that what is healthy comes from healthy members and what is diseased, from diseased [members]. In the same vein, Galen says in his book *On Semen* on the subject of those who have intercourse too often: not only does fluid proceed from the members, but vital spirit exits as well through the arteries along with semen, and for this reason it is no wonder that those who couple frequently are weakened. For when the body is drained of these two [namely, fluid and spirit] and only appetite and pleasure remain, the vital spirit is dissipated, and many have died because of this. And because this is the case, what Galen says is not to be wondered at. It is evident, then, that the animal that has intercourse to excess will rapidly expire and the one that has intercourse infrequently will live longer. For this reason, eunuchs are longer-lived, because they cannot have sex, since in their case the sinew that governs erection has been cut and semen does not descend in the accustomed way. Galen says this is the reason for the [long] life of eunuchs and explains why they seem to be insane to all who converse with them, because every perturbation of the mind is calmed by an emission of semen, according to what Rufus said. From the nature of their perturbation, their faces become turbulent, like their [bodily] condition. And therefore we find that animals are fierce before intercourse and tame after intercourse. For this reason animals which have sex frequently live for a short time, because [sex] is carried out by the soul and by nature: by the soul, because it desires and takes pleasure, and by nature, because it is on fire during the act. And because we move around a good deal during intercourse, some *animal spirit is released, and some *natural spirit. We have conveyed what Galen says on this subject and explained it. We have also conveyed what the ancients said about this.

12. Why Shivering Occurs in Sexual Intercourse

The reason why shivering and sadness occur during intercourse is bad mixing of the humors and because of the warmth which supervenes during intercourse, for any body which has bad humors will shiver if it is suddenly warmed; and when this shivering comes upon it, sadness comes upon it. In those who experience trembling, it happens because of a bad quality in a superfluity. In those who experience a noxious smell, it happens because of a *putrid mixture that is released during intercourse by warmth. In those whose stomach bloats during intercourse, this presents itself because natural warmth is weak in these people, and this cause and infirmity come from melancholy. In their case, they always crave intercourse because of the great quantity of *windiness that is contained at the time of intercourse; and because it is contained within, they also experience rumbling and noise [in the bowels]. In fact, some people hear this externally, like a shrill sound. Some have a headache after intercourse; the cause is smoky vapor from the moisture of the blood and the superfluities of the body and from an evil mixture [of the humors] that ascends into the head because of the agitation. This is the opinion of Galen, expressed in his commentary on the *Epidemics*. But we, briefly expounding the essentials on this subject, will turn to the things that stimulate intercourse, according to what we said. For there are some people who are incapable of intercourse, but crave it, and we have explained why they cannot satisfy their desire.

13. Foods That Generate Semen and Foods That Extinguish It

It is important for us to know what foods generate semen and stimulate desire for intercourse and on the other hand, what [foods] dry out and diminish semen, so that men may abstain from what is contrary and make use of what is suitable. We shall set forth these things concisely.

The ancients indicated the foods that generate semen and those that extinguish it, those that stimulate the appetite, and those that suppress it, those that generate and attract what was not, and those that suppress and extinguish what was, and what fires the appetite for intercourse. The things that repel it are contrary to these.

That which nourishes and fills and is assimilated to the essence of semen, produces semen. Foods that bring these things about generate semen, and if they cannot have all three of these [qualities], they should at least have one or two. So foods that are very nourishing generate semen; those that are not very nourishing do not generate semen. For we said that the nature of semen consists of liquid and spirit and it comes from moisture in the food; therefore, it is necessary that foods that generate semen be very nutritious and produce windiness and these things are suited to the essence of semen. And things that do not have both these [qualities] will nevertheless be of use if they have one of them; either they will through heat attract it, and extract it and carry it off in hidden channels, or they will be mixed with the nutriment, and the three [qualities] will be produced from this.

Likewise, when we wish to prepare food which is suitable, we should combine these three [qualities] together or at least one or two of them. We declare that the chick-pea possesses [all] three: it is very nutritious, it generates windiness, and it is warm and humid. It generates semen naturally by itself. Approximating it is what is called in Arabic *erice* [*possibly colophony, or pine resin*], especially if it is combined with bone marrow. The same is true of turnips. And if you wish to mix two foods, you should do it this way: because broad beans nourish and make windiness, but nonetheless as food they border on coldness, they lack one [quality] and possess two. Long pepper, ginger, black pepper, and the like are merely hot, and none of them provide what will generate semen. If you mix one of these things with broad beans, the result will be a food that generates semen and augments intercourse, because it possesses [all] these three [qualities]. And in this way one should compound one food from two by taking into account the action of each, as we have said.

14. Drinks

Now we should speak about drinks and the things that generate and draw out semen. There are the foods like the ones we spoke about – pepper and octopus, pine-nuts, figs, fresh meat, brains, and eggs yolks. Suitable for ˙potions as well are skink, and "wolf-testicles" – that is, rag-wort – because it rouses lust like the skink. Dioscorides also says that if this root is held in the hand, it stimulates erotic desire and if drunk with wine, it inflames it even more. Ginger also provokes and inflames erotic desire. Red and white behen-nuts, sweet costus, oriental crocus, and flax seeds eaten in quantity – if they are cooked in honey, with pepper added – inflame erotic desire; so do cardamom, nettle seed, anise, and similar things. Some of these are foods and some are medicines, and you will cure contraries with these, because contraries are cured by contraries.

15. Things That Dry Out Semen

These are the things that do not generate semen, but dry out and dissolve windiness, namely: anything that is warm and dry such as dill, rue, and the like. And therefore Rufus says that rue is contrary to semen if it is eaten in quantity, but it is useful because it rouses appetite in the stomach and provokes urination. The things that constrain, suppress, and thicken semen, and which extinguish lust, are cold foods such as lettuce, purslane, gourds, white chard and red chard, mulberries, pumpkins, cucumbers, melons, and anything that is cold and humid, such as tuna and other fish, and things of this kind. Whatever is cold and dry constrains erotic desire, such as sumac, vinegar, and sour grapes; and should anyone wish, combine two or three of these in order to extinguish semen and constrain lust. More effective than these for constraining the appetite for intercourse is to cook lentils with lettuce seed, and drink the liquid: the appetite of lust is extinguished. Other things that extinguish the appetite of lust and dry out semen are hemp seed and the seed of wild purslane. Mix these two with the juice of field purslane and give it to be eaten as necessary. In the same way, if necessary, the *simples and the compounds which we mentioned should be taken.

16. Medicines That Promote Intercourse

Now we should speak about the medicines that benefit those incapable of intercourse, and because compound potions are found to promote intercourse and are found commonly among rich and poor, such as nutmeg *electuary and the great *trifera* [*a compound medicine, for which there are various recipes*], nuts in honey, rag-wort in honey, preserved ginger, nut syrup, honey syrup, syrup of raisins, and the like, we will leave these aside, because they are found in the hands of many; and we will speak of those that we have tested ourselves and that our authorities employ, that work quickly and produce their effects gently. For we know other things that, if added into the above-mentioned *potion, augment lust – for example, a light heart and daily happiness, as Philumenus says [*Greek physician: see doc. 5*]. For he says that lust is produced in different ways, because whatever touches it sets it on fire, such as signs of love, the recollection of love, kisses on the cheek, squeezing the hand, sucking the tongue, gazing on the face of the beloved, sighs, and whispers. These and others of the kind increase lust....

Another electuary – none better can be found – for increasing lust. Take roots of garden carrots, discard the inner part and pound up the peels for a long time, [add] one pound of gum arabic, put it in a pan with one ounce of sesame oil and fry it. Afterwards add 3 pounds of honey and let it cook until it is thickened. Add five egg yolks and after a short time remove from the heat and add 2 drams of galingale, 2 drams each of cole-wort seed, long pepper, cinnamon, cloves, ochre, sweet cicely seed, turnip seed, onion seed, and carrot seed. Mix well together and if you wish to alter the color, add 2 drams of saffron. Store in a glass container and use as needed....

I made this [recipe] for men who are impotent. Take one dram of cloves; drink it in milk in the morning. Cow's milk taken every day in the morning also increases lust....

Pills for the impotent. Take equal quantities of seed of white onions, rag-wort, the brains of sparrows, flowers of male palm, and white incense. Temper with warm water and shape into pills the size of chick-peas. Give seven in the morning, with wine – and no more, because if you give more, the woman will faint beneath him. But if he wishes to extinguish desire, let him drink a bunch of rue [steeped] in warm water.

Another medication to be taken before intercourse, because it stimulates marvelously. Take the brains of thirty male sparrows and dissolve them for a long time in a glass container. And immediately after it is killed, take an equal quantity of the fat that is around the kidneys of a billy-goat and melt it over a fire. Add the brains and add as well a sufficient quantity of honey. Mix it up in a pan and cook it until it hardens. Afterwards, make it into pills the size of hazelnuts and give one before intercourse.

17. Ointments Which Rouse One to Intercourse

Lo, we have spoken of things one can take to strengthen and augment sexual desire. Now we must speak briefly about things that are applied on the surface [of the body], and so the book will end.

Anoint the penis and testicles and the area around and below them with the following ointment. Take oil of iris, oil of wild onions prepared with sesame, pellitory, stavesacre, and nettle seed. Grind them up together and cook them in their oils and apply as ointment....

An ointment made from ants. Take large black ants, put them alive into a glass bottle and add good oil of elder on top. Hang it in the sun for several days, and strain it afterwards. Anoint the testicles and the soles of the feet: this is very good.

A lotion that stimulates coitus. Take 6 drams of *scammony and 1 ½ drams of euphorbia. Pound them up separately. Strain 9 drams of white wax, and when it is melted gradually add in the aforementioned [herbs]. Stir vigorously and set it aside. When it is needed, pour it onto a cloth and place it over the testicles and penis. When they are warm, take [the cloth] off and perform coitus. And if you wish to extinguish [desire], anoint the aforementioned members with water in which opium has been dissolved.

CHAPTER FIFTEEN

SATIRES AND CRITIQUES OF MEDICINE

In the comic Middle English poem entitled "The Fox and the Wolf in the Well," a hungry fox breaks into a hen-house and devours three hens. The survivors fly to the rafters, from where the rooster angrily chides the fox. The sardonic fox replies that he was doing the hens a favor: they were ailing and if he had not opened their veins out of charity, they would surely have died. Since the rooster is plainly suffering from an over-heated spleen, perhaps he should come down from his perch and submit to the same therapy before it is too late!

Getting the joke in "The Fox and the Wolf" depends on some rather detailed knowledge of Galenic physiology and pathology, as well as an understanding of the purpose of bloodletting. It also assumes that listeners were sufficiently familiar with medical practice to appreciate the humor in comparing it to legalized murder. Whether it takes the form of comic burlesque (like these beast-tales, or like Nigel of Longchamps's fable of Burnel the Ass in doc. 105) or of sarcastic invective (as dispensed by Petrarch in doc. 106), a satire is only successful if the audience accepts an ideal that the satire will expose as wanting. In a sense, teasing doctors for using obscure words is a backhanded way of acknowledging the scientific prestige of scholastic medicine. To excoriate doctors for charging exorbitant fees tacitly admits that health care can be sold, because criticizing unfair market practices assumes a knowledge of what fair practices are. Of course, there were serious critiques of medicine's failings, but from the historian's perspective, satire and scolding are important gauges of how deeply embedded in medieval society medicine had become.

105. DR GALEN AND BURNEL THE ASS

The author of this rollicking comic poem about an ambitious ass was a Norman whose family settled in England in the early twelfth century. By 1170, Nigel of Longchamps, erstwhile student of the schools of Paris, was a monk at Canterbury Cathedral, where he spent the remainder of his life. His learning was humanist in character – he was well versed in the ancient poets, notably Ovid, Virgil, and Juvenal – but he was also steeped in the Bible, the Fathers, and the moralistic and hagiographic literature of the Middle Ages. He found much to criticize in the students of his day, particularly their mania for dialectic and their vaulting careerism.

A Mirror for Fools is cast in the popular satirical mode of the beast-fable. The protagonist is Burnel the Ass, who longs for a tail equal in length to his ears and who symbolizes the monk or cleric greedy for advancement. Burnel tries both Salernitan medicine and academic studies in Paris, but he fails to gain promotion by either route. In the end, his old master catches up with him and **"cauterizes" his ears so that they finally match his tail.*

The satire against medicine targets the profession's duplicity and hypocrisy. Dr Galen first invokes Nature (and quotes Hippocrates) to tell Burnel that it is futile to want a longer tail and then proceeds to compose a burlesque prescription for a remedy. The message here is that doctors vaunt the difficulty of a cure in order to enhance the mystique of the treatment and justify its cost, all the while absolving themselves of responsibility for the results (see doc. 93). Dr Galen's counterpart is Trickman the English merchant, who has been sent to Salerno to find a cure for his bishop's mis-shapen nose – a sly reflection of Burnel's quest for a longer tail. The numerous casual references to doctors and cures scattered throughout the text indicate how widespread and commonplace interest in learned medicine had become in the twelfth century.

Source: trans. J.H. Mozley, *A Mirror for Fools, or, The Book of Burnel the Ass* (Notre Dame, IN: University of Notre Dame Press, 1963), pp. 3–4, 20–22, 24–26, from the critical edition of Nigel of Longchamps, *Speculum stultorum*, ed. John H. Mozley and Robert R. Raymo (Berkeley: University of California Press, 1960). Latin.

Burnel the Ass leaves his master and consults Dr Galen about medical intervention to lengthen his tail. Dr Galen's address to Burnel parodies Hippocrates's first Aphorism: "Life is short, the Art is long; opportunity is elusive, experiment is dangerous, judgment is difficult...."

> There was an Ass with ears of monstrous size,
> Who wished with them his tail to equalize.
> It was too short – though not for use, he said;
> He grieved because it did not match his head.

So, lest it suffer more abbreviation,
He called the doctors in for consultation;
For they, he thought, might all their art apply,
And so make good Nature's deficiency.
But Galen said: "Two feet of tail suffice
For any donkey; just take my advice,
Don't try for more; the more you lengthen it,
Letting it trail along the muddy street,
The filthier it will be. So be content,
Or else you may well find, whereas you meant
To make it long you'll only make it short.
Value what Nature sends, nor hold as nought
What she has given. Believe me, that old tail
Stuck on your rump is of far more avail
Than one that's new. But no, it doesn't please,
You want a better. All our surgeries
Will only make a worse one. Any moke
Can have his tail cut off; but it's no joke
To make a new one grow. Life's short, Art's long,
No time to lose when things are going wrong.
Treatment oft fails and cures are hard to work;
Dangers remain for sure, and causes lurk
Concealed; the laws of medicine differ far
From what both you and others think they are.
Not even high skill can always sickness heal,
Medicine is set in balance, tips the scale
In equal measure both to good and ill,
Heals one, but not another. Though the will
Be there, the power oft lacks, the doctor fails
To give the longed-for help to him who ails.
God's Grace performs, he doth but minister.
The precepts of our art, then, we who hear
Must practice faithfully; yet even so
We cannot what you wish on you bestow.
'Tis God alone that heals; the will is ours,
But his the power; they whom his aid empowers
Can heal, our aid he needs not; we make use
Of varied kinds of pigment, herb and juice;
His word alone makes whole; healers are we
In name, but God in true reality.
Remember then, that tail he gave retain,

You foolish ass, nor further things in vain
Seek after, and to what you have hold on,
Lest what you have you haply find is gone.
Stay as your doctor left you, I entreat,
Till [God] return himself and change your state.

Dr Galen tells a fable about a cow who rashly cut off her tail to escape a frozen pond in the winter, only to be tormented to death by flies in the summer.

All this I saw myself and now have told,
Burnel, for your instruction. What you hold
Let that suffice, for if the truth be said,
Saving your honor, you're a muttonhead,
And your scheme's folly. Best go home. You can't
Find any drugs to do the thing you want.
Though every leech you in the world could find
Swore he could graft a tail on your behind,
'Twould be but words – though I will not deny
A tail might grow if treated properly.
Broken or bruised – can be made whole again;
But severed – so for ever must remain.
What's cut but not cut off can treatment bear,
But dead with living never can cohere.
Let tail with body in due compact be,
Tail then might grow in length considerably.
But mind – the cost we have to calculate;
The drugs are numerous and the outlay great.
Difficult cures must swollen purses bleed,
And deep-set wounds of deep-laid wealth have need.
Would it not be enough to made addition
Of a whole ell, to meet your high ambition?"
He murmured his assent with smiling face;
The noise re-echoed through the market-place.
Galen went on: "Off to Salerno then,
And with all speed be out and back again.
Buy there whate'er you need; see you don't waste
Time on the road; with all four feet make haste,
Add a fifth if you can! Just pay the cost:
I'll see you find none of my labor's lost.
You pay the money, I'll supply the skill,
If their old power my hands remember still.

Quick then and get your passport, that will lend
Speed to your journey. You have many a friend,
Some dear ones, who will money gifts supply.
Easy perhaps to find the cures; yet I
Fear they may not be found so easily.
But take for them, to bring them home again,
Vessels in plenty. Spare no toil or pain
In packing, lest they perish on the way,
And seal them too, lest aught should go astray.
And now (you've skill to write) on parchment clear
Write down the cures which you'll have need of here.
Some marble-fat, fresh milk of kite or goose,
Some fear of wolf, some speed of running luce [*a pike (fish)*],
Cool shade of furnace heated seven times hot,
A foal that on a she-mule has been got,
A seven years' treaty between hare and hound;
Of peacock's scream (tail not yet grown) – a pound;
Some warpless cloth unwoven, red of hue,
Some ass's laughter (found of course by you),
Some saffron milt of herring or of bee,
Some kisses which the lark has lovingly
Sent to her falcon, liver of cheese-mite
Or foot or blood; of blessed Christmas night,
Which for your use full long enough should prove,
A little portion; from the Mount of Jove
Three pounds and fifteen ounces should you bring;
And while among the Alps you're traveling
During the night of John the Baptist [*24 June*] take
A little snow that's fallen; tail of snake
And scarlet viper – very useful they,
But not a penny for them should you pay.
Collect all these (they must be new), then pack
Them carefully and hoist them on your back."
So Galen spoke; and the ass stooping low
His suppliant head down to the ground did bow....

Burnel takes his leave of Galen and journeys to Salerno, where he puts up at an inn.

Rising next morn he seeks the goods to buy,
But baffled goes in sad perplexity.
Four days about the city streets he fares,

In fruitless search for non-existent wares.
A London merchant spied him as he strayed,
Took note of him and thus accosting said:
"You are a deputy of note, I see;
Important are those wares in high degree
For which you seek. Whoever sent you here
Was wise and wealthy also, that is clear.
Your face and figure plainly indicate
Both who you are and whence you've come – a great
Person indeed; though foreign garb you wear,
In your own land you'll be no foreigner.
All your great house, how they must feel concern,
What vows and prayers uplift for your return!
England's my birthplace, London is my home;
On bishop's business lately did I come.
Nature had set his nose a-tilt, and he
Required that Art [of medicine] should find a remedy.
So on account of this unhappy – bent,
Four of us to these foreign parts were sent.
One year passed, then another: now bereft
Of my three friends by one fell stroke I'm left.
Look, I have wares, which would effect, I'm sure
Could you but take them home, a wondrous cure.
All that you came to look for here abroad
I've got it in my house all sealed and stored.
I can't get home; I've fallen into debt;
The expenses were too great, and here I'm set!
But how I miss the land I hold so dear
All the more keenly that I'm stranded here.
News has just come, my father's passed away;
And so has my old master, so they say.
Now look, I've ten glass jars, filled to the top
With all your paper mentions, in my shop.
Just give me what I paid myself, and then
Tomorrow, well-equipped, start home again.
Beyond that sum I would not ask a bean –
We're strangers here together – I'm not so mean.
Yet this I ask: you have a saintly air,
So don't forget me when you say a prayer."
Then straightway Burnel counted out the cash,
And took for it ten vessels full of trash;

And then the contract thus to stabilize
He asked the merchant's name: he thus replies:
"Trickman I'm called, my father just the same;
I'm London born; Jill is my mother's name;
Julie's my sister, known in many lands,
Trickie's my wife, joined in true wedlock's bands.
Now you tell me what noble name you own,
That I may not forget you when you're gone."

Burnel sets off for Lyons but loses his pharmaceutical "ingredients" – and part of his tail – when he is attacked by dogs. Then he repairs to Paris, where he fails to learn anything in the schools. Ambitious to become a bishop, he takes the road to Rome, but he then repents and decides to enter a religious order. After considering each of the orders in turn, he finally decides to found his own, with a rule that includes all the indulgences and concessions of the other orders. He meets up with Dr Galen once more and vents his disillusionment with the corruption of church and state. Finally, Burnel's old master shows up and takes the errant donkey home.

106. PETRARCH LASHES OUT AGAINST THE DOCTORS

*When Pope Clement VI was ill from December 1351–February 1352, Petrarch sent him two letters (*Letters of Old Age *16.3 and* Familiar Letters *5.19) advising him to rely on a single trustworthy physician and avoid a crowd of consultants. One of the pope's doctors attacked Petrarch for interfering, and this provoked the first of the poet's* Invectives. *The sniping continued until Petrarch left the papal court in May 1353. Petrarch would later augment his invective against the doctor with further diatribes against ecclesiastical pomp, scholastic philosophy, and French culture. All four* Invectives *were revised and published in 1355.*

Petrarch consistently protests that his hostility is directed at bad doctors, not at doctors in general. Nonetheless, he has a very low opinion of the whole enterprise of medicine. It is a "mechanical" craft unworthy to be compared to the liberal arts or poetry. Yet doctors shamelessly appropriate the title of "philosopher" and dare to open their mouths in the presence of a true man of letters. These are vulgar people, who take fees, poke their noses into urine and excrement, lie and quarrel, and whose vaunted authorities are pagans like Galen, or free-thinking Muslims like Averroes. Doctors are intellectually beneath contempt; to top it all, they are not much good at healing.

Source: trans. David Marsh from Petrarch, *Invectives*, I Tatti Renaissance Library 11 (Cambridge, MA: Harvard University Press, 2003), pp. 5–13, 17–19, 25–27, 29–31, 33, 41–42, 71–73, 79–81. Latin.

For my part, I remember clearly that I did not criticize the medical profession, but merely its professionals – and not all of them, but only the insolent and factious ones. Yet in your guilt, you and many others were inwardly distressed and enraged to an amazing degree. I don't know what's the matter. Attack slow-witted philosophers, goad unskillful poets, and disparage inelegant orators: Plato and Aristotle, Homer and Virgil, Cicero and Demosthenes will never be angry. But reproach ineffective and ignorant physicians, and nearly all of them rant and rave....

If I weren't familiar with your ignorance and lack of confidence, I would be surprised that my advice had fanned your anger against me. As I later discovered, even the most learned of your colleagues say that a patient should be entrusted to one trustworthy physician who seldom errs. Otherwise, by consulting many physicians, he may be exposed to the errors of many. You are clearly not that doctor. If you were, you would never have written such a windy letter to answer my criticisms of factious and ignorant physicians. You must have been cut to the quick to have cried out so loudly.

In your confused babbling, you did not scruple to insinuate that I fawn on the pope. But how could I, of all people, fawn on anyone? As is commonly known, it is my policy to despise everything but virtue and my good name. What could persuade me to change what I have been since my early years? Ask the very man we are discussing. He will tell you that he often volunteered to give me more favors than you could dare to wish for, as importunate as you are. And he will tell you that I refused them all out of my love of freedom, a virtue of which you have no experience or knowledge. Cease, then, to 'infect people in good health with your leprosy and with the maladies of your ambition and avarice. You are a manipulator of your patients, an insincere and disgusting adulator, if I correctly judge your nature. In the hope of a vile little gain, you frequent the latrines of both popes and paupers. By contrast, it is my custom to frequent verdant woods and solitary hills, desiring only knowledge or glory....

What could be more intolerable than an insolent fellow, who has renounced all shame and will deny anything you say to him? What great impudence! What meretricious effrontery! You deny that physicians disagree, when the whole human race openly complains of the fact. If only this were the case! I wish I were lying, although I could not lie about this. Indeed, I wish I were mistaken and that everyone were healthy. Indeed, I speak the truth and thousands of people are in danger because they are governed by the factious, divergent, and uncertain authority of physicians. You say that you physicians agreed about the pope's recent care. Beware, but not that you lie: for you physicians are all notorious for lying every day. Beware lest the truth itself refute you with mighty proofs. Perhaps you all agreed once the pope's health had improved. But no one, including the pope, doubts that he would have recovered much sooner, if *you* at least had spent the entire period of his illness living on the distant shores of India.

But suppose – I shudder to think of it! – that the pope had paid his debt to nature. Even the vicar of immortal God is mortal. What great and unresolved discord there would have been among you concerning his pulse, his *humors, his *critical day, and his medications! Ignorant of the real cause of his illness, you would have filled heaven and earth with dissonant cries. Wretched are the sick who trust in your aid! But Christ, who holds all human salvation in his hands, saved him despite your ignorance. I pray that Christ may do all that is necessary for him and the Church he governs. You physicians appropriate the results of God's beneficence and the excellence of the pope's own physical constitution, and claim to have revived him from the dead. Now that the danger is past, you all agree with subtle cunning. In this way, our learned father will not sense your discord, even though by his insight and experience he understands and foresees many things. (I don't say he understands *all* things, as you do, flatterer.) Otherwise, he would dismiss, spurn, and detest you as reckless guides on a dangerous path....

But I am surprised by your furious rage. I had never written to you before, and even now I am loath to speak to someone who won't understand me. I did write a brief letter to the Roman pontiff, dictated by my fear and devotion when he was seriously ill. Unless I am mistaken, this letter was useful to him, if perhaps not to you. I warned him to avoid carefully the crowd of quarreling physicians, as well as any doctor who pays more attention to empty eloquence than to his science: for our age offers a vast multitude of such men. Even if you rage with indignation, I don't regret my advice. Nor did I think I should be stoned to death because I offered loyal advice to this man, even if he didn't need it. All of us who glory in being called Christians owe him not only our advice, but our allegiance and obedience as well.

If you were sane, you would have replied to the pope, not to me, since I didn't write to you. Perhaps, with your herbal and medicinal eloquence, you might have persuaded him to entrust his life and his affairs to you and to place his hopes for life and health in your hands alone. In turn, he might have shunned me and my fellow scholars as a harmful and useless breed, whether you chose to call me a poet or something else. I think you will go to any lengths, ignoramus. In your hatred of me or rather your hatred of the truth, you unjustly inveighed against poets. In fact, I wrote nothing poetical on this subject; and if you weren't so completely stupid, my very style would prove this to be the case. Perhaps your impudence should compel me to write about you in my poetry, exposing you to be torn apart by future generations. But you seemed unworthy of a place in my little works that would make you known to posterity.

But why do I force colors on a blind man, or noises on a deaf one? Ply your trade like a mechanic, I pray you. Cure your patients, if you can. If not, kill them, and demand payment when they are dead. Thanks to the blindness of the human race, you alone are the lord of life and death, as you boast, and are granted immunity that no emperor or king enjoys. Enjoy your deadly privilege. You have devoted your brain to an excellent art that offers you the greatest security. When someone survives, he owes you his life. When someone dies, you owe him nothing but the lessons of the experience. Death can be blamed on nature or the patient. Only you bestow life. When Socrates had learned of a painter who had become a physician, he justly observed: "What prudence! He abandoned an art in which faults are exposed, and embraced one whose mistakes are buried in the earth." ...

I know that your art is useful; and although it gained acceptance late among our people, it was afterwards held in honor. Indeed, this art was attributed to the invention of the immortal gods, for it seemed too great to be a human discovery. A more reliable authority confirms this opinion in Ecclesiasticus [38:4]: "The Most High has created medicine out of the earth." In fact, this is true in common of everything. What are all our experience, all our knowledge, and our wisdom but a divine creation and a gift from God? It is written at the beginning of the same book: "All wisdom is from the Lord God [Ecclus. 1:1]." Lest you become complacent in the special merit of your mechanical art, hear what is written in the same book concerning the mechanical art of agriculture: "Hate not laborious works, nor the husbandry created by the Most High [Ecclus. 7:17]."

What do you possess that you can exalt above any farmer? Both arts derive from the same source, for both were created by the Most High. Indeed, what reason do you have for comparing yourself to a farmer? He benefits human life, while you undermine it, though you profess to do the opposite. He aids humankind by his labors; you harm it by your idleness. Naked out in the fields, he keeps the people well-fed by his hunger; lavishly dressed in their bedrooms, you destroy people's health by your words....

You [physicians] wish to speak about any subject whatsoever, and forget your own profession which, in case you don't know, means inspecting urine and other things that shame forbids me to mention. But you are not ashamed to insult people who are concerned with virtue and the soul....

I leave lying to you physicians, including the worst kind of lie, one that causes great peril and harm to those who believe it. If you don't believe me, ask the common people, who have made such behavior proverbial. They tell a patent liar: "You lie like a physician." As for the poets – and I hardly dare dignify myself with this name, which you in your madness cast at me as a reproach – the poets, I say, strive to adorn the truths of the world with beautiful veils. In this way, the truth eludes the ignorant masses, of which you are "the very dregs." But for perceptive and intelligent readers, it is just as delightful to discover as it is difficult to find....

If you had spoken kind words, you would have heard kind words. Instead, you heard what you deserved to hear, not what I usually write. Remain silent for a while and reflect. Forgive yourself for starting this quarrel. I have said enough. I would be mad to speak longer with you. At the end of your letter, you transcend the ridiculous by serving notice of my death in the name of Medicine. Medicine might do something to postpone my death; you can do nothing. Indeed, you can do much to hasten it. You have been blessed with a famous trade: you know how to deliver a body from the diseases of old age. If Medicine could speak, I am sure she would thank me warmly for exposing the infamy of today's physicians, whose modern errors have extinguished her ancient glory....

Let us hear what you say and how you present yourself: "I am a physician." Do you hear this, Apollo, who discovered medicine or you, Asclepius, who enlarged it? "Consequently, I am a philosopher." Do you hear this, Pythagoras, who first invented this name? Weep, discoverers of the arts! Graced with a priestly fillet, an ass tramples your territory, boasting that he is a philosopher and claiming philosophy for his own. "Our philosophy," he says. Alas, what is this? We shall hear worse if we live longer. By now, I suspect, we are approaching the end of the world. "There shall be signs in the sun, and in the moon, and in the stars [Luke 21:25]." But this sign is not found in the Gospel: when an ass can philosophize, the heavens will fall. What can I tell you? I feel sorry for philosophy, if it belongs to you. But at my peril I would go so far as to swear that you don't know what a philosopher is. Let me not pile up all my arguments on this single point. I have many things to discuss with you on this subject. But I have prefaced my remarks in this way so that you know that I don't consider you a philosopher.

And then, what is the next thing adduced by this presumptuous fool? Armed with these arts, he claims that he can cure not only bodily maladies, but those of the soul as well! Health and salvation do not always come from the Jews. Here is a half-barbarian savior. And you call me proud! Read my letter again. It made you rage and now it will make you die. When did I claim philosophy or poetry as mine? When did I call myself a philosopher or poet? When was I anything but a scorner of your character and intellect – a role I deemed not merely legitimate, but my obligation? In his modesty, Augustine merely calls himself a master [*that is, a teacher*] of rhetoric [*Confessions*

5.13.23]. You call yourself a philosopher and a physician; and then you add a third title: lord of rhetoric. Since you delight in titles, we may add a fourth: you are a large and deep sewer, as Seneca says [*Controversies* 3.pr.16]....

Philosophers spurn money, in case you don't know. You cannot put philosophy up for sale. Who can sell what he does not possess? Even if you did possess philosophy, you could not put it up for sale; rather, philosophy would prohibit you from selling yourself. As it is, philosophy does not bring you honor, nor do you bring honor to philosophy. Instead, by your base greed you dishonor her name. Listen to me, you windy sophist. (Pardon me if I call you a sophist, O noble logician, but I am compelled by reality. When I see the facts, I cannot use words at odds with them.) Spin out a sophistical argument. Place me on the rack. You may force me to confess, but never to agree.

How can I believe that you are a philosopher, when I know you are a mercenary mechanic? I gladly repeat this term, since I know that no other reproach stings you more. I often called you a mechanic, not by chance but by choice; and I call you a second-rate one, to cause you more pain. Ask the authors who have discussed the mechanical trades. They will point you to your rightful place there. But you spurn them, and wish to appear a philosopher. To achieve this – a farce that calls out for comic laughter – you repeatedly use the word "method." What a crafty intellect! You arrive at your goal by a shortcut. By now, others may be calling you a philosopher. But I shall not consider you a philosopher, no matter how many "methods" you can cram into every line you write. Often, I grant you, even the minds of fools can conceive a reckless and precipitous desire for glory. I can't remove this desire from you. For the human will is indomitable, especially in madmen....

But since at present you lack everything that makes a philosopher, how can you brazenly usurp the name of philosopher? Or, to stay with my topic, how can you claim the venerable pallor of a philosopher's face, which comes from nocturnal studies?

Your own wasted pallor comes from the chamber-pots you study every day. If it were inspired by the sympathy of friendship, by compassion for the poor, or by the love you feign for the commonwealth, such pallor would not be disgraceful, but glorious. But now it is your greed for a handful of gold that drags you miserably through the sewers, and changes you into such a creature that, if you saw yourself, you would flee in terror, and rightly so. Don't blame your public service for what you are, but your desires. Don't denigrate your studies, but your way of life. O perceptive philosopher, you haven't seen the true cause of your pallor, although it lies open to view. And you seek to see what is hidden in organs and tissues? You don't see what lies in plain sight!

Even though I am no physician and lack dialectic, I shall show you the cause of your pallor. Even against your will, you shall realize that this is true. You move in dark, livid, fetid, and pallid places. You rummage around in sloshing chamber-pots. You examine the urine of the sick. You think about gold. Is it any wonder, if in the midst of pallid, dark and sallow places you yourself become pallid, dark, and sallow? If the wisest patriarch's flock changed color when it was exposed to mottled branches [Gen. 30:32–42], it is strange that the same thing happens to you? You're waiting for me to say that your color comes from gold. No, it comes from what you are exposed to.

I have spoken at great length, and would rather have been silent. But the subject demands its true name which may be tolerated here a single time – a name which is often found in the Holy Scriptures. I say that your color, smell and taste come from the stuff to which you are exposed – shit.

107. THE DOCTOR AS COMIC RELIEF IN THE *CROXTON PLAY OF THE SACRAMENT*

The subject matter of the late-fifteenth-century English miracle play known as the Croxton Play of the Sacrament *is no laughing matter, whether read through medieval or modern eyes. It concerns a miracle that allegedly occurred in Spain in 1461. A group of Jews got possession of a consecrated Mass wafer – which, according to the doctrine of transubstantiation, was now the actual body of Christ – and proceeded to re-enact the Passion by "torturing" and "crucifying" it. Their purpose was to disprove the miracle of the Mass, and this motive has led some scholars to argue that the target of the play was Christian heretical and anticlerical skepticism, not Jews as such (the Jews had officially been expelled from England in 1291). Be that as it may, the play certainly exploits ugly legends of Jewish acts of desecration, and even ritual murder. In the Croxton play, the Host not only bleeds in response to its torments, but takes revenge on the chief Jewish conspirator by sticking to his hand and pulling it off from his arm. Medical help is clearly in order, and on cue a drunken doctor and his boisterous servant appear on the scene. The doctor is a stock figure of fun in folk entertainments such as mummers' plays, where he pops in to resurrect the slain hero (or sometimes his adversary). In the case of the* Play of the Sacrament, *the joke is even more pointed in that Christ himself, re-crucified by the Jews in their desecration of the Host, will burst out of the pot in which he has been "buried" at the climax of the play in a true resurrection. The episode of Colle and Master Brownditch given below is pure comic relief, but it plays to audience prejudices that were as stereotyped as the image of the Jew. The name "Brownditch" is undoubtedly an allusion to the excrement that Petrarch identified with the doctor's calling.*

Source: trans. Faith Wallis from *Croxton Play of the Sacrament*, in *Medieval Drama: an Anthology*, ed. Greg Walker (Oxford: Blackwell, 2000), lines 445–572; pp. 224–27. Middle English.

Here shall a doctor's servant come onto the stage, saying:

COLLE

  Aha, here is fair fellowship!
  Although I am not prepared to do so, I long to slip away.
  I have a master – I wish he had the pip [*were sick*],
  I tell you in confidence!
  He is a man whose knowledge is complete –
  Except for thrift. I can with you dispense [with niceties].
  He sits with some tapster in the bar;
  His hood he will sell [for drink] there.

  Master Brownditch of Brabant,
  (I tell you: he is that same man)
  Called the most famous physician
  That ever saw urine.
  He sees as well at noon as at night
  And sometimes by a candle-light
  Can give a judgment just as well
  As one that has no eyes at all.

  He is also a bone-setter:
  I know no man who is better!
  In every tavern he is debtor,
  That is a good symptom!
  But I wonder why he is taking so long,
  I fear that something is going wrong,
  For he has deserved to be hung;
  May God never send worse news!

  He had a lady lately to cure;
  I know by now she is taken care of!
  She is where no Christian creature
  Will hear her tell her tale!
  If I stood here till midnight
  I could not declare aright
  My master's cunning insight –
  That he has in new ale!

  But what the devil ails him that he tarries so long?
  A sick man might soon come to harm.

Now all the devils of Hell curse him!
God grant me my boon!
I think it best we make a proclamation:
If any man can him spy,
Lead him to the pillory!
In faith, it shall be done.

Here he shall stand up and make a proclamation, thus:

COLLE

If there be either man or woman
That saw Master Brownditch of Brabant,
Or ought of him can tell,
They shall be well rewarded.
He has a trimmed beard and a flat nose,
A threadbare gown and torn hose;
He never speaks good sense or to the purpose.
To the pillory lead him!

MASTER BROWNDITCH

What, boy? What are you prattling about?

COLLE

Ah, master, master! Only about the reverence you are due!
I thought never to see your goodly face again,
You have tarried so long from here.

MASTER BROWNDITCH

What have you said in my absence?

COLLE

Nothing, master, save to your reverence
Have I told this audience;
[*Aside*] And some lies mixed in!
But master, I pray you, how goes your patient
That you had lately under your treatment?

MASTER BROWNDITCH

I warrant she feels no pain.

COLLE

> Why, is she in her grave?

MASTER BROWNDITCH

> I have given her a drink made full well
> With *scammony and with *oxymel,
> Lettuce, sage, and pimpernel.

COLLE

> Nay, then is she full safe!
> For now you are come, I dare well say
> That in my judgment there is no one
> From Dover and Calais
> So cunning, by my faith.

MASTER BROWNDITCH

> Cunning? Yea, yea, and with practice
> I have saved many a man's life.

COLLE

> On widows, maids and wives
> Your cunning you have just about all spent.

MASTER BROWNDITCH

> Where is my bag with the drink I so enjoy?

COLLE

> Here, master – master, be careful how you chug!
> The Devil, I think, moves within,
> For it goes "glug, glug."

MASTER BROWNDITCH

> Here is a great congregation [*that is, the audience*],
> And all are not healthy, without negation.
> I would have a declaration:
> Stand up and make a proclamation.
> Do it fast, make no delay,
> But boldly make a declaration
> To all people who wish to get help.

Here for a time [Colle] *will make a declaration.*

COLLE

> All manner of men that have any sickness,
> Direct yourselves to Master Brownditch!
> No matter what disease or sickness you have,
> He will never leave you until you're in your grave.
> Who has a cancer, colic, or the *flux,
> The *tertian, the *quartan, or the burning aches;
> For worms, for gnawing, grinding in the stomach or in the *boldyro*
> > [*penis or testicles?*]
> All kinds of red eyes, bleary eyes, and migraine too;
> For headache, boneache, and toothache as well;
> He will take on men with the colt-evil [*swollen penis*] or a hernia,
> All that have the head-cold or *consumption.
> Though a man were right healthy, he would soon make him sick!
> Inquire at the coal-shed, for there is his lodging,
> Just beside Babwell Mill, if you take my meaning.

MASTER BROWNDITCH

> Now, if there be either man or woman
> That needs the help of a physician ...

COLLE

> Indeed, master, I can tell you [of one]
> As you will understand.

MASTER BROWNDITCH

> Know you any about this place?

COLLE

> Yea, that I do, master, may I have grace!
> Here is a Jew named Jonathas,
> Who has lost his right hand.

MASTER BROWNDITCH

> Fast to him I would inquire.

COLLE

> Before God, master, his gate is here.

MASTER BROWNDITCH

> Then to him I will go near.

My master, well met!

JONATHAS

What are you doing here, fellow? What do you want?

MASTER BROWNDITCH

Sir, if you now need any surgeon or physician
I can well help you with your disease,
Whatever hurt or harm it is.

JONATHAS

Sir, you are ignorant if you come so casually
And appear in my presence so impertinently.
Get out of my sight, and quickly,
For you are ill-advised.

COLLE

Sir, the harm to your hand is known far and wide,
And my master has saved many a man's life.

JONATHAS

I think you have come to make some trouble.
Be off quickly, or you'll be punished.

COLLE

Sir, you know well it can't go wrong;
Men that are masters of science are useful.
If you piss into a pot right now
He can tell you if it's curable.

JONATHAS

Go away, fellows. I don't like your babbling!
Sweep them away both, and that right soon!
Give them their reward, that they be gone!

GLOSSARY

adust: burnt or scorched. A °humor can be adust when subjected to excessive heat and dryness. Adust humors are morbific and need to be °evacuated.

ague: an acute fever, particularly the type of fever typical of malaria, with cycling hot, cold, and sweating stages.

alter, alterative: to change a quality or bring about a mutation of the °complexion, for better or worse. An alterative is a remedy that cures by changing and thus correcting an imbalance in the °humors or their qualities.

analepsy: in pre-modern medicine, a type of epileptic attack thought to arise from the gastric region (*ana-* is the Greek prefix meaning "upwards").

animal (spirits): see °spirits.

antidotarium: a compilation of recipes for compound medications, i.e., those made from more than one substance.

aperient: a drug that has the quality of opening the pores or channels in the body (hence the "aperitif" drunk before dinner to "open" the stomach).

apoplexy: cerebral hemorrhage or stroke.

aposteme: a morbid localized swelling (e.g., a boil, tumor, etc.).

apostolicon: an ointment containing waxes, pitch, and vinegar.

asafoetida: gum resin from the root of the plant *Ferula asafoetida*.

Armenian bole: earth containing iron oxide (from the Latin *bolus*, "clod of earth"). It was frequently employed in ancient and medieval pharmacy.

biduan: term designating a °fever which reaches paroxysm every other day.

bile, black: see °melancholy.

bile, red: see °choler.

blessed oil: a liquid obtained by heating powder made from bricks soaked in oil, used for medical purposes.

carbuncle: boil.

carminative: a medicine with the property of expelling flatulence.

castoreum: reddish glands found in the groin of the beaver and widely used in medieval medicine, notably as an °emetic.

cataract: clouding of the crystalline lens of the eye resulting in loss of sight. The name derives from the theory that the eye was filling up with excess °humor from the brain.

catarrh: dripping from the nose; by extension, a head cold.

causus: a kind of continuous °fever.

cautery: the application of a heated metal instrument to the body to sear the tissue (e.g., in order to close off a ruptured blood vessel). In ancient and medieval medicine, cautery was also used to divert the flow of °humors through the body. A "potential cautery" is a topical application used for a similar purpose.

cerote (or cerate): a thick, wax-based topical application.

choler: one of the four °humors of the body, also known as red or yellow bile. Its °temperament is hot and dry.

cholera: in pre-modern medicine, an acute gastrointestinal ailment marked by vomiting, severe but blood-free diarrhea, and colic.

chyle: the initial product of the "first digestion" of food in the stomach: coarsely mashed and mixed food. The next phase is °chyme.

chyme: the pulpy, more liquefied stage of °chyle as it is further digested.

clyster: enema used to administer a °purgative.

coction/concoction: the action of the innate heat of the body in "cooking" food or morbific matter, permitting its °digestion.

collyrium: medicated drops or ointment for the eyes.

complexion: the blending of qualities or °humors which is natural to an individual person, an organ of the human body, or a humoral type; °temperament. The term survives today to denote the quality of the skin of the face, because pre-modern physicians made an initial determination of the patient's complexion from examining the face.

consimilar members: see °similar.

consumption: wasting away or progressive emaciation; in particular, the wasting that is a symptom of pulmonary tuberculosis, and hence the common pre-modern name for this disease.

contra-naturals: in the Galenic system expounded, for example, by Joannitius (doc. 33), a generic category encompassing diseases and trauma that threaten the constitution of the body (see °naturals).

corrupt, corruption: the state of a substance (e.g., air, food) or a °humor that has been transformed into a morbid state through qualitative excess (e.g., too much heat), or through °infection. The core metaphor is one of putrefaction: an internal disease is visualized as a collection of rotting organic matter that needs to be diverted away from important organs and then °evacuated, or as an internal wound that is suppurating with diseased matter.

crisis: a sudden change in the course of an illness which either restores the patient to health or leads to death.

critical (day): a day on which a crisis is likely to occur.

cupping: the operation of evacuating blood through the skin by applying

a heated glass cup to the surface of the skin (which may be °scarified in
advance).

decoction: the fluid resulting from boiling a herb or other substance: e.g.,
°ptisane is the decoction of barley.

degree: Galen assumes that each foodstuff or each basic ingredient of a
compound medicine not only exhibits the primal qualities of heat, cold,
moisture, and dryness, but does so to a greater or lesser extent. Arabic
Galenists systematized this by positing four degrees for each quality,
from barely perceptible (the first degree) to extremely intense (the fourth
degree). Ingredients were held to possess two qualities, one from the
hot-cold and one from the moist-dry binary.

determine: in the jargon of the medieval university, to make an
authoritative declaration on a topic, notably by resolving a disputed
question or constructing a logical argument.

diacastoreum: an °electuary made with °castoreum.

diaciminum: a compound medicine whose principal ingredient was
cumin.

diaphoretic: a treatment to induce sweating.

diaprunum: a compound medicine whose principal ingredient was
the common plum. It was generally administered as a cathartic and
emollient.

digest, digestion: a term with both a primary and an extended meaning,
digestion can refer to the physiological process of refining and
transforming food, or even air, into a form the body could absorb. It
is understood to proceed in stages: the first digestion in the stomach
produces °chyle, the second digestion in the liver produces blood, and
the third digestion is when the blood is taken up into the members.
All three produce waste products, which must be expelled by the body.
Digestion also had an extended meaning when applied to pathology. A
wound or internal disease required that the °corrupt or °peccant disease
matter be "digested" and the body's normal continuity or °temperament
restored. Drug therapy and wound dressing in particular aimed to
promote this digestion.

dropsy: accumulation of fluid in the abdomen.

dyscrasia: disruption of an individual's °complexional or °humoral balance.

dyspnoea: difficulty in breathing.

electuary: a drug administered in the form of a paste that was licked from
a spoon.

emetic: a drug that provokes vomiting. Some compounds had distinctive
names, such as "Patriarchal Emetic Filtrate" (doc. 49).

emunctory: channel by which morbific matter is drawn off from the internal organs to the surface of the body.

ephemeral: term designating a °fever that attacks the °spirits.

erysipelas: a streptococcal skin infection characterized by sudden high fever, malaise, and a painful, swollen rash with blistering and discoloration of the skin.

etiology: the branch of medical theory concerned with disease causation.

evacuate, evacuative: any procedure designed to expel disease matter (e.g., °corrupt or °peccant humor) from the body. The body will do this naturally through vomiting, bowel movements, etc., but the physician may assist the weakened body at the suitable moment by administering a °purge, or by opening a vein (bloodletting or °phlebotomy).

experiment: when applied to medicine, the word denotes a tried-and-true remedy, one that has been proven effective by experience (*experimentum*), but whose action cannot necessarily be explained by pharmacological theory.

fantasy: according to ancient notions of cerebral localization of mental faculties, fantasy or imagination is connected with the anterior part of the brain, reason with the mid-section, and memory with the posterior part.

fever: unnatural heat of the body. Fevers were classified by the periodicity of their paroxysms: "continuous" fevers never broke, "quotidian" fevers peaked every day, "biduan" every other day, "tertian" fevers peaked every third day (counting inclusively), "quartan" fevers every fourth day, and so forth. Fevers were also classified according to the matter affected: "ephemeral" fevers attacked the °spirits, "putrid" fevers the °humors, and "hectic" fevers the solid parts of the body.

fistula: an ulcer that takes the form of a channel or pipe.

flux: literally, "flow"; usually applied to morbid discharge from the bowels (diarrhea). A "bloody flux" is diarrhea where blood is present in the excrement.

foment/fomentation: a warm topical application, usually of a cloth steeped in water or a medicated °decoction.

fumigation: burning a medicinal substance to produce smoke, which is channeled into a body orifice. Fumigation was typically used to introduce medicine into the female reproductive organs. The patient would crouch on a stool over a small brazier.

hectic (fever): see °fever.

hemitreus: a particularly severe form of °tertian fever.

hiera: literally, "something holy." *Hiera* or *gera* was a generic and honorific title for certain noteworthy compound medicines. The most widely known was *hiera* (or *gera*) *pigra*, "holy bitters," a cathartic of which the principal ingredient was tincture of aloes. *Hieralogodion* was used to treat melancholy.

homeomerous: having or consisting of ˚similar parts.

humor: depending on context, either (a) moisture or fluid of some kind, or (b) one of the four bodily fluids deemed to constitute the physiological basis of human life. The classic humors are blood, red bile (also called yellow bile or ˚choler), ˚phlegm and black bile (or ˚melancholy).

hydromel: a drink of honey mixed with water.

infect, infection: in pre-modern medicine, a term that denotes tainting with a poison or morbid substance, such as ˚corrupt air. The underlying idea is not so much invasion (as it is for modern people who are accustomed to the concept of germs), but rather staining, pollution, or contamination. Water and earth can be "infected" by corrupt air; corrupt humors within the body "infect" the spirits, etc.

intention/remission (of forms): a scholastic philosophical term, which in a medical context denotes a theoretical model for expressing the relationship between variations in human health (on a scale from perfectly healthy at one end, to dead at the other) and variations in the mixture of the four ˚humors. There was considerable debate, for instance, on exactly how far one could depart from a perfectly temperate condition, with all four humors in balance, before one actually was sick. This had implications for pharmacy: what ˚degree of a quality in a drug would actually restore the patient to a more or less temperate condition? How much of that drug would have to be administered?

kermes: the pregnant female insect *Coccus ilici*. In the Middle Ages, it was thought to be a berry and was collected from a species of evergreen oak.

lientery: diarrhea in which particles of undigested food can be observed.

melancholy: black bile. One of the four ˚humors of the human body, its qualities are cold and dry. It also refers to a disease state caused by excess of this humor, or by ˚adust blood or black bile, and characterized by mental gloom, obsession, and other psychic disturbances.

mithradatum: a weak opium preparation.

morbific: causing disease.

mortify, mortification: depending on context, "mortify" can mean either (a) to subdue or bring under control (a disease or a poison) or (b) to rot or corrupt (e.g., in cases of gangrene the flesh is "mortified").

myrobolans: dried fruit of a plum, *Prunus cerasifera*, imported from the East.

natron: hydrous sodium carbonate, a mineral salt found in dried lake beds, e.g., in Egypt.

natural (spirits): see ˚spirit.

natural day: an "artificial" day is 24 hours; a "natural" day is the period from sunrise to sunset, which varies in length throughout the year.

naturals: in Arab-Galenic physiology, the term "naturals" or "things natural" refers to the unalterable "givens" of the physical world and the human body: the elements, complexions, °humors, organs, etc. See also °non-naturals and °contra-naturals.

nerve: the Latin word *nervus* means both "nerve" and "sinew"; the two meanings were technically distinct, though in practice they can be difficult to disentangle.

nitre: a term applied to various alkaline substances, e.g., soda, potash.

noli me tangere: "touch me not": a name applied by pre-modern physicians to ulcerative conditions of soft tissue and bone, notably lupus. Its name allegedly derived from the fact that it seemed to worsen if handled. It was classed as a cancer by medieval writers.

non-naturals: in the Galenic system, the term "non-naturals" or "things non-natural" refers to environmental and behavioral factors which are variable, and which exert an influence on the °naturals. These include air, food and drink, sleep and wakefulness, rest and motion, retention and elimination, and emotional states.

occlusion: a blockage.

official: in anatomy, an organ or body part, such as the heart or hand, that performs a specific "office" or function; in pathology, a disease that affects an official part, such as gout, which attacks the foot. See also °similar.

ophthalmia: an inflammation of the eye.

oppilation: a blockage.

oximel, oxymel: a medicinal drink made of wine and honey.

oxysaccharum: a medicinal preparation of vinegar and cane sugar.

palsy: the condition of paralysis or weakness, sometimes accompanied by tremor.

peccant (humor): a bodily °humor that has become excessive or °corrupt (e.g., by being °adust), and hence transformed into °morbific matter, which leads to (literally, is "guilty of") disease. The doctor aims to °evacuate peccant humors.

pessary: a vaginal tampon, soaked in medicine and used to administer medication to the vagina or womb.

petroleum: a generic term for various kinds of mineral oil, including pitch.

phantasy: see °fantasy.

phlebotomy: bloodletting.

phlegm: One of the four °humors of the human body. It is cold and wet.

phlegmon: an inflamed, red swelling, boil or tumor. The old-fashioned English equivalent was carbuncle, a word that also means "ruby."

phthisis: synonym for °consumption (from the Greek word meaning "wasting away").

physic: the branch of natural philosophy that considers questions about the natural world. After the twelfth century, *physica* becomes a synonym for learned medicine. It can also denote a medicament, e.g., "to take physic."

plethora: a state of being dangerously replete with °humors, particularly blood. Since the liver was held to manufacture blood continuously from food, overindulging could result in plethora. The solution was °evacuation by bloodletting.

pose: synonym for °catarrh.

potion: internally administered medicine in liquid form; often generalized to cover any internally administered medicine.

power(s) (Latin *virtus, virtutes*): in Galenic medicine, as adumbrated by Joannitius, for example (see doc. 33), the natural principles within the body that organize and execute the three major functions of life: nutrition, growth, and reproduction (natural power); respiration, heat, and emotion (spiritual or vital power); sensation, voluntary motion, and cognition (animal power). The powers are the manifestations of the °spirits.

procatarctic: pertaining to an external or immediate cause of a disease.

proegumenal: pertaining to an internal or predisposing cause of a disease.

ptisane: see °tisane.

purge, purgative: to "clean" or °evacuate the body of disease matter or °peccant humor by provoking vomiting (using an °emetic or cathartic) or a bowel movement (using an enema). A purgative is a medicine administered to effect purging, or which has the property of purging.

putrid (fever): see °fever.

quartan (fever, ague): a °fever or °ague where the paroxysms occur on every fourth day, counted inclusively. This pattern is characteristic of malaria.

quinsy: inflammation or swelling in the throat causing choking or suffocation.

quintal: a hundredweight.

quotidian: see °fever.

remission: see °intention.

repellent: a treatment that contains morbid matter, and forces it away from vital organs and toward the exterior of the body.

resolution: dissolving or dispersing of °corrupt humors.

resolve, resolvent: a treatment that dissolves and disperses °corrupt humors.

rheum, rheumatic: a morbid discharge of °phlegm in the head (e.g., a runny nose), eyes, joints, etc.

ripe, ripen: the process whereby an °aposteme reaches a mature state in which the °morbific matter can be °digested.

sanguine: referring to blood as a °humor, or to a °complexion dominated by blood.

sanies (*adj.* sanious): the thin, clear fluid that oozes from a wound, composed of pus and blood serum.

scammony: a strong °purgative made from the roots of *Convolvulus scammonia*.

scarify: to make shallow cuts in the skin, or to raise a blister by the application of a hot iron, acid, or boiling pitch. The formation of liquid in the blisters was seen as a sign that the body was acting to drain away dangerous °humors.

semiotics: in medicine, the study of the nature and interpretation of diagnostic and clinical signs.

similar: with reference to anatomy, a term referring to the homogenous parts, such as bone or muscle, that are found in various different organs or members. With reference to pathology, it refers to diseases which affect °humors or similar parts, such as °fevers. See also °official.

simple: a drug composed of a single, usually herbal, substance; a herb used for medicinal purposes.

solution of continuity: a rupture or dissolution of the continuity of bone or flesh, i.e., physical trauma in the form of breakage, tearing, or wounding.

solutive, solvent: see °resolvent.

specific form: a power that inheres in a substance by its very nature, and that is not reducible to the sum of the qualities of which it is composed. Also called "total species," this concept was used to explain, among other things, the specific action of drugs like °theriac.

spirit(s): in Galenic medicine, the subtle life-forces that organize the principal functions of the body. The natural spirit, whose seat is the liver, controls nutrition, growth, and reproduction; the vital (or spiritual) spirit in the heart controls respiration, vital heat, and to some degree, motion and emotion; the animal spirit in the brain governs sensation, voluntary motion, and in humans, reason. The "spiritual members" are the heart and lungs. See also °power.

spodium: a fine ash obtained from wood, metal, ivory, etc. by calcination.

stasis: the high-water mark, so to speak, of a disease. Galenic theory staged acute diseases into "onset" (*principium*), "intensification" (*augmentatio*), and "decline" (*declinatio*). Stasis (*status*) preceded decline.

strangury: difficulty in urinating.

strychnos: one of the numerous members of a genus of flowering plants of the family Loganiacae. The most likely candidate in a medieval text is *Strychnos nux-vomica*, a tropical Asian plant, from which the poison strychnine is extracted. It is a powerful °emetic.

stupe: a piece of towel or flannel with which a °fomentation is applied.

styptic: property of a substance that acts as an astringent, contracting tissue; also applies to something that binds the stomach and bowels, restraining °evacuation.

subtiliative: having the property of rendering smooth, thin, or fine in texture.

suffumigate: see °fumigate.

syncope: fainting.

synectic: producing an effect without an intermediary.

synocha(l): a kind of continuous °fever, ascribed to putrefaction of the blood.

syrup: in the medical sense, a drug administered in sugar syrup. The sugar syrup medium acted as a preservative agent, and thus the syrup itself was held to have medicinal, preservative effect.

temper, temperament: the proper or balanced mixture of the four elements, qualities (hot, cold, wet, dry), or °humors. In pharmacy, the qualities of one ingredient will be tempered (mitigated, balanced out) by the addition of an ingredient of contrary qualities. With reference to human physiology and psychology, temperament can refer to generic type ("the melancholy temperament") or individual °complexion.

tenesmus: strong sensation of discomfort in the lower bowel and desire to defecate; straining results in the passage of mucus and often blood.

terra sigillata: red clay, originally from the Aegean island of Lemnos, formed into tablets and impressed with a seal: a popular remedy in ancient Rome, and used in medieval medicine as an antidote and astringent.

tertian: see °fever.

theriac: an elaborate compound drug, used as a panacea or universal antidote to poison.

tisane: water in which barley has been boiled.

treacle: common English word for °theriac.

troche, trochee: a powdered medication mixed with a binder such as gum arabic and formed into small tablets that are then dried.

vapors: internal fumes produced by °digestion. These could be benign or morbid, depending on the state of digestion or the predominance of certain °humors.

venter: body cavity. There are three venters in Galenic medicine: the abdomen, the chest, and the skull.

ventose/ventosity: internal "windiness," a condition in which the body's humors, °vapors or °spirits are chaotically mobile. Windiness is sometimes used to denote flatulence.

ventricle: a small cavity or hollow space within an organ. Medieval doctors recognized not only the ventricles of the heart, but also ventricles in the brain. To the three main ventricles, they assigned different cognitive functions (imagination, reason, memory).

virtue: synonym for °power.

visible/visual spirit: according to one ancient/medieval theory of the physiology of vision, the eye emits a subtle ray – a visible spirit – which contacts the object of sight and connects the mind to it.

vital (spirits): see °spirits.

wind(iness): see °ventose.

INDEX OF TOPICS

The references in this index are to the document numbers.

SOURCES

1. "Isidore of Seville: The Canon of Medicine," from Isidore, *Etymologiae,* book 4, trans. by William D. Sharpe, *Isidore of Seville: The Medical Writings.* Philadelphia: American Philosophical Society, 1964. Reprinted by permission of the American Philosophical Society.

3. "Teaching the Alexandrian Curriculum in Sixth-Century Italy: Agnellus of Ravenna's Commentary on Galen's *On Sects,*" from Agnellus of Ravenna, *Lectures on Galen's 'De sectis,'* ed. and trans. David O. Davies and L.G. Westerink *et al.* Buffalo: Dept. of Classics, SUNY Buffalo, 1981. Copyright © 1981, State University of New York, all rights reserved. Reprinted by permission of SUNY Press.

12. "A Sixth-Century Byzantine Saint Dispenses Medical Advice: Theodore of Sykeon," from Elizabeth Dawes and Norman H. Baynes, *Three Byzantine Saints: Contemporary Biographies Translated from the Greek.* Oxford: Blackwell, 1948. Reprinted by permission of Blackwell Publishing Ltd.

13. "The Medical World of Gregory of Tours: Plagues, Doctors, and Saints," from Gregory of Tours, *Historiae* 9.21–22, trans. O.M. Dalton, *Gregory of Tours: The History of the Franks.* Oxford: Clarendon Press, 1927; excerpts from *Liber de virtutibus sancti Martini episcopi,* trans. Raymond Van Dam, *Saints and their Miracles in Late Antique Gaul.* Princeton: Princeton University Press, 1993. Copyright © 1993 Princeton University Press. Reprinted by permission of Princeton University Press.

14. "A Reluctant Bishop-Healer: John of Beverley," Bede, *Ecclesiastical History of the English People,* ed. and trans. Bertram Colgrave and R.A.B. Mynors. Oxford: Clarendon Press, 1969. Reprinted by permission of Oxford University Press.

19. "Dietary Advice for a Merovingian King," from Anthimus, *On the Observance of Foods,* ed. and trans. Mark Grant. Totnes: Prospect Books, 1996. Copyright © 1996 by Mark Grant. Reprinted by permission of Prospect Books.

21. "The Care of the Sick at the Monastery of Vivarium," from Cassiodorus, *Institutes of Divine and Human Learning* 1.31, trans. Leslie Webber Jones, *An Introduction to Divine and Human Readings.* New York: Columbia University Press, 1946. Copyright © 1946 Columbia University Press. Reprinted by permission of Columbia University Press.

22. "Medical Injunctions in the *Rule of St Benedict,*" from *St Benedict's Rule for Monasteries,* trans. Leonard J. Doyle. Collegeville, MN: Liturgical Press, 1948. Copyright © 1948, 2001 by The Order of Saint Benedict, Inc. Published by Liturgical Press, Collegeville, Minnesota. Reprinted by permission of Liturgical Press.

24. "*The Plan of St Gall*: Medical Facilities within an Ideal Monastery," from Laura Price, Walter Horn and Ernest Born, *The Plan of St. Gall in Brief.* Berkeley and Los Angeles: University of California Press, 1982. Copyright © 1982 by the Regents of the University of California. Reprinted by permission of University of California Press.

25. "Medicine, Morality, and Meditation in a Monastic Herb-Garden: Walahfrid Strabo's *The Little Garden,*" from Walahfrid Strabo, *Hortulus. De cultura hortulorum,* trans. R. Payne. Pittsburgh: Hunt Botanical Library, 1966. Reprinted by permission of Hunt Botanical Library.

26. "Medical Networks of Eighth-Century Anglo-Saxon Missionaries," extract from the *Hodeporicon* of Willibald, trans. C.H. Talbot, *The Anglo-Saxon Missionaries in Germany.* London: Sheed and Ward, 1954.

29. "Letters of Medical Advice from Bishop Fulbert of Chartres and his Circle," from

The Letters and Poems of Fulbert of Chartres, ed. and trans. Frederick Behrends. Oxford: Clarendon Press, 1976. Reprinted by permission of Oxford University Press.

30. "*Bald's Leechbook* and *Leechbook III*," excerpts from *Bald's Leechbook* and *Leechbook III*, trans. M.L. Cameron, *Anglo-Saxon Medicine*. Cambridge: Cambridge University Press, 1993. Reprinted by permission of Cambridge University Press.

35. "Salernitan Anatomy: The *Second Salernitan Demonstration*," from *The Second Salernitan Demonstration* (ascribed to Bartholomaeus of Salerno), trans. George W. Corner, *Anatomical Texts of the Earlier Middle Ages*. Washington, DC: Carnegie Institute, 1929.

36. "The Practice of Pharmacy Rationalized: *Circa instans*, the *Antidotarium Nicolai* and Its Commentary," from Nicholas of Salerno, *Antidotarium Nicolai*, trans. Michael R. McVaugh in *Sourcebook in Medieval Science*, ed. Edward Grant. Cambridge, MA: Harvard University Press, 1974; Matthaeus Platearius, extracts from the introduction to his commentary on the *Antidotarium Nicolai*, trans. Michael R. McVaugh in *Sourcebook in Medieval Science*, ed. Edward Grant. Cambridge, MA: Harvard University Press, 1974. Copyright © 1974 by the President and Fellows of Harvard College. Reprinted by permission of Harvard University Press. All rights reserved.

38. "The Practice of Surgery Rationalized: The *Surgery* of Roger Frugard," from Roger Frugard, *Chirurgia*, trans. Michael R. McVaugh in *Sourcebook in Medieval Science*, ed. Edward Grant. Cambridge, MA: Harvard University Press, 1974. Copyright © 1974 by the President and Fellows of Harvard College. Reprinted by permission of Harvard University Press. All rights reserved.

39. "The Salernitan Tradition of Gynecology: *The Trotula*," from *The Trotula: A Medieval Compendium of Women's Medicine*, ed. and trans. Monica Green. Philadelphia: University of Pennsylvania Press, 2001. Reprinted by permission of University of Pennsylvania Press.

44. "Is Medicine a Science? (2): Arnau of Vilanova Argues That Medicine Transcends Theory," from Arnau de Vilanova, *Lecture on the Text "Life is Short"* (*Repetitio super canonem "Vita brevis"*), trans. Michael R. McVaugh and Luís García Ballester, "Therapeutic Method in the Later Middle Ages: Arnau de Vilanova on Medical Contingency," *Caduceus* 11 (1995): 75–86. Reprinted by permission of Southern Illinois University.

48. "Academic Dissection as 'Material Commentary' (2): Anatomical Illustration," the "Five Picture Series": MS Munich, Bayerische Staatsbibliothek CLM 13002 fols. 2v–3r, reproduced in Nancy Siraisi, *Medieval and Early Renaissance Medicine*. Chicago: University of Chicago Press, 1990. Reprinted by permission of Bayerische Staatsbibliothek, Munich.

50. "Signs and Diagnosis (1): Gilles of Corbeil on Urines," trans. Michael R. McVaugh in *Sourcebook in Medieval Science*, ed. Edward Grant. Cambridge, MA: Harvard University Press, 1974. Copyright © 1974 by the President and Fellows of Harvard College. Reprinted by permission of Harvard University Press. All rights reserved.

51. "Signs and Diagnosis (2): *Epitome on Pulses*," from *Summa pulsuum*, trans. Michael R. McVaugh in *Sourcebook in Medieval Science*, ed. Edward Grant. Cambridge, MA: Harvard University Press, 1974. Copyright © 1974 by the President and Fellows of Harvard College. Reprinted by permission of Harvard University Press. All rights reserved.

55. "Scholastic Pharmacology: Bernard of Gordon," extracts from Bernard of Gordon, *On the Preservation of Human Life*, trans. Michael R. McVaugh, "Quantified Medical Theory and Practice at Fourteenth Century Montpellier." *Bulletin of the History of Medicine* 43 (1969): 409–13. Copyright © 1969 by Bulletin of the History of Medicine. Reprinted by permission of the Johns Hopkins University Press.

56. "A Primer on Bloodletting (1): Lanfranc of Milan's Scholastic Phlebotomy," from Lanfranc of Milan, *Magna chirurgia*, tract 3, doctrine 3, chapter 16, trans. Michael R. McVaugh in *Sourcebook in Medieval Science*, ed. Edward Grant. Cambridge, MA: Harvard University Press, 1974. Copyright © 1974 by the President and Fellows of Harvard College. Reprinted by permission of Harvard University Press. All rights reserved.

59. "Is Surgery a Science? (2): Henri of Mondeville Defends the Scientific Credentials of Surgery," from the French version of the *Chirurgia* edited by E. Nicaise, *Chirurgie de Maitre Henri de Mondeville* (Paris, 1893), trans. Michael R. McVaugh in *Sourcebook in Medieval Science*, ed. Edward Grant. Cambridge, MA: Harvard University Press, 1974. Copyright © 1974 by the President and Fellows of Harvard College. Reprinted by permission of Harvard University Press. All rights reserved.

60. "Is Surgery a Science? (3): Guy of Chauliac's History of Surgery," from Guy de Chauliac, *Inventiarium*, trans. James Bruce Ross in *The Portable Medieval Reader*, ed. Mary Martin McLaughlin. New York: Viking, 1949. Copyright © 1949 by James Bruce Ross. Reprinted by permission of Viking Penguin, a division of Penguin Group (USA) Inc.

62. "A Surgical Sampler (2): Teodorico Borgognoni and the New Surgical Diseases," from Teodorico Borgognoni, *The Surgery of Theodoric ca. AD 1267*, trans. Eldridge Campbell and James Colton. New York: Appleton-Century-Crofts, 1960. Reprinted by permission of Prentice-Hall, Inc., Upper Saddle River, NJ. An imprint of Pearson.

63. "A Surgical Sampler (3): Ophthalmic Surgery," from Benvenutus Grassus, *De oculis eorumque egritudinibus et curis*, trans. Casey A. Wood. Stanford, CA: Stanford University Press, 1929.

64. "A Surgical Sampler (4): Surgical Anesthesia?," from Teodorico Borgognoni, *The Surgery of Theodoric ca. AD 1267*, trans. Eldridge Campbell and James Colton. New York: Appleton-Century-Crofts, 1960. Reprinted by permission of Prentice-Hall, Inc., Upper Saddle River, NJ. An imprint of Pearson.

67. "Roger Bacon: Alchemy and the Medical Payoff of 'Experimental Science'," extracts from Roger Bacon, *Opus maius*, trans. Robert Belle Burke. Philadelphia: University of Pennsylvania Press, 1928. Reprinted by permission of University of Pennsylvania Press.

68. "Bisticius: A Florentine Goldsmith and Medical Alchemist," trans. Lynn Thorndike, *Science and Thought in the Fifteenth Century*. New York and London: Haffner, 1967; reprinted from Columbia University Press, 1929. Copyright © 1929 Columbia University Press. Reprinted by permission of Columbia University Press.

69. "Interpreting Symptoms: The Difficult Case of Leprosy," from Gilbert the Englishman and Jordanus de Turre, trans. Michael McVaugh in *Sourcebook in Medieval Science*, ed. Edward Grant. Cambridge, MA: Harvard University Press, 1974. Copyright © 1974 by the President and Fellows of Harvard College. Reprinted by permission of Harvard University Press. All rights reserved.

73. "Prophecy and Healing: The Meaning of Illness According to Hildegard of Bingen," excerpts from *The Letters of Hildegard of Bingen*, trans. Joseph Baird and Radd K. Ehrmann. Oxford: Oxford University Press, 1998. Copyright © 1988 Joseph Baird and Radd K. Ehrmann. Reprinted by permission of Oxford University Press.

74. "Should Clergy and Monks Practice Medicine?," from Canon 8 of Pope Alexander III Enacted at the Council of Tours, 1163, trans. Darrel W. Amundsen, "Medieval Canon Law on Medical and Surgical Practice by the Clergy," *Medicine, Society, and Faith in the Ancient and Medieval Worlds*. Baltimore: The Johns Hopkins University Press, 1996. Originally published in *Bulletin of the History of Medicine* 52 (1978): 22–44. Copyright © 1996 by Bulletin of the History of Medicine. Reprinted by permission of the Johns Hopkins University Press.

75. "The Faculty of Medicine of Paris *vs.* Jacoba Felicie," trans. James Bruce Ross in *The Portable Medieval Reader*, ed. Mary Martin McLaughlin. New York: Viking, 1949. Copyright © 1949 by James Bruce Ross. Reprinted by permission of Viking Penguin, a division of Penguin Group (USA) Inc.

76. "The Faculty of Medicine of Paris *vs.* Jean Domrémi," trans. Faith Wallis, in Geneviève Dumas and Faith Wallis, "Theory and Practice in the Trial of Jean Domrémi," *Journal of the History of Medicine and Allied Sciences* 54 (1999): 55–87. Copyright © 1999 Journal of the History of Medicine and Allied Sciences. Reprinted by permission of Oxford University Press.

78. "The Doctor at the Bedside (1): Precept According to Archimatthaeus," trans. Henry E. Sigerist, "Bedside Manners in the Middle Ages: The Treatise *De cautelis medicorum* Attributed to Arnold of Villanova," in *Henry E. Sigerist on the History of Medicine*, ed. Félix Marti-Albañez. New York: MD Publications, 1960. Originally published in *Quarterly Bulletin, Northwestern University Medical School* 20 (1946): 135–43.

79. "The Doctor at the Bedside (2): Precept According to Arnau of Vilanova" trans. Henry E. Sigerist, "Bedside Manners in the Middle Ages: The Treatise *De cautelis medicorum* Attributed to Arnold of Villanova," in *Henry E. Sigerist on the History of Medicine*, ed. Félix Marti-Albañez. New York: MD Publications, 1960. Originally published in *Quarterly Bulletin, Northwestern University Medical School* 20 (1946): 134–37.

84. "The Special Challenges of Plague (1): The Report of the Paris Medical Faculty, October 1348," trans. Rosemary Horrox, *The Black Death*, Manchester Medieval Sources Series. Manchester and New York: Manchester University Press, 1994. Reprinted by permission of Manchester University Press, Manchester, UK.

85. "The Special Challenges of Plague (2): Guy of Chauliac on the Black Death," from Guy de Chauliac, *Ars chirurgicalis Guidonis Cauliaci medici*, trans. Michael R. McVaugh in *Sourcebook in Medieval Science*, ed. Edward Grant. Cambridge, MA: Harvard University Press, 1974. Copyright © 1974 by the President and Fellows of Harvard College. Reprinted by permission of Harvard University Press. All rights reserved.

86. "The Special Challenges of Plague (3): John of Burgundy's *Treatise on the Epidemic*," trans. Rosemary Horrox, *The Black Death*, Manchester Medieval Sources Series. Manchester: Manchester University Press, 1994. Reprinted by permission of Manchester University Press, Manchester, UK.

87. "Professional Character in the Early Middle Ages: Variations on Hippocratic Themes," from *Letter of Arsenius to Nepotian*, trans. Loren MacKinney, "Medical Ethics and Etiquette in the Early Middle Ages: The Persistence of Hippocratic Ideals," *Bulletin of the History of Medicine* 26 (1952): 11–12. Copyright © 1952 by Bulletin of the History of Medicine. Reprinted by permission of the Johns Hopkins University Press.

90. "Licensing and Accountability (1): Malpractice in Crusader Palestine," extracts from the *Livre des Assises de la Cour des Bourgeois*, trans. Vivian Nutton, in Piers D. Mitchell, *Medicine in the Crusades: Warfare, Wounds and the Medieval Surgeon*. Cambridge: Cambridge University Press, 2004. Reprinted by permission of Cambridge University Press.

91. "Licensing and Accountability (2): Legislation Governing Doctors in the Thirteenth-Century Kingdom of Sicily," excerpts from the *Constitutions of Melfi*, trans. Edward F. Hartung, "Medical Regulations of Frederick the Second of Hohenstaufen," *Medical Life* 41 (1934): 592–94.

92. "Licensing and Accountability (3): Examining and Supervising Practitioners in Fourteenth-Century Valencia," extracts from *Medical Licensing and Learning in Fourteenth-Century Valencia,* ed. and trans. Luis García-Ballester, Michael R. McVaugh and Agustín Rubio-Vela, Transactions of the American Philosophical Society 79, part 6. Philadelphia: American Philosophical Society, 1989. Reprinted by permission of the American Philosophical Society.

94. "The Organization and Ethos of a Medieval Hospital (1): The Jerusalem Hospital," trans. E.J. King, *The Rule, Statutes and Customs of the Hospitallers, 1099–1310.* London: Methuen, 1934. Reprinted by permission of Associated Book Publishers (U.K.) Ltd.

96. "The Organization and Ethos of a Medieval Hospital (3): A Twelfth-Century English Leper Hospital," trans. Edward J. Kealy, *Medieval Medicus: A Social History of Anglo-Norman Medicine.* Baltimore: The Johns Hopkins University Press, 1981. Copyright © 1981 The Johns Hopkins University Press. Reprinted by permission of the Johns Hopkins University Press.

98. "Medical Care in a Medieval Hospital (2): John of Mirfield at St Bartholomew's Hospital, London," extracts from John of Mirfield, *Breviarium Bartholomei,* trans. Percival Horton-Smith Hartley and Harold Richard Aldridge, *Johannes de Mirfeld of St Bartholomew's, Smithfield; His Life and Works.* Cambridge: Cambridge University Press, 1936. Reprinted by permission of Cambridge University Press.

101. "Lifestyle Advice, Customized (1): The Army on Campaign," from Arnau of Vilanova, *Regimen for Almería, Arnaldi de Vilanova Opera Medica Omnia,* vol. 10, pt. 1, ed. Michael R. McVaugh; trans. Michael R. McVaugh in "Arnald of Villanova's *Regimen almarie (Regimen castra sequentium)* and Medieval Military Medicine," *Viator* 23 (1992): 201–13. Copyright © 1992 by the Regents of the University of California. Reprinted by permission of University of California Press.

102. "Lifestyle Advice, Customized (2): A Physician of Valencia Advises His Sons, Who Are Studying in Toulouse," from Peter of Fagarola, trans. Lynn Thorndike, "Translation of a Letter from a Physician of Valencia to his Two Sons Studying at Toulouse." *Annals of Medical History* 3 (1931): 17–20.

105. "Dr Galen and Burnel the Ass," from Nigel of Longchamps, *Speculum stultorum,* trans. J.H. Mozley, *A Mirror for Fools, or, The Book of Burnel the Ass.* Notre Dame, IN: University of Notre Dame Press, 1963, from the critical edition of Nigel of Longchamps, *Speculum stultorum,* ed. John H. Mozley and Robert R. Raymo. Berkeley: University of California Press, 1960. Copyright © 1960 by the Regents of the University of California. Reprinted by permission of University of California Press.

106. "Petrarch Lashes Out against the Doctors," from Petrarch, *Invectives,* trans. David Marsh. Cambridge, MA: Harvard University Press, 2003. Copyright © 2003 by the President and Fellows of Harvard College. Reprinted by permission of Harvard University Press. All rights reserved.

READINGS IN MEDIEVAL CIVILIZATIONS AND CULTURES
Series Editor: Paul Edward Dutton

"Readings in Medieval Civilizations and Cultures is in my opinion the most useful series being published today."
— William C. Jordan, Princeton University